Health

The Basics

SIXTH EDITION

REBECCA J. DONATELLE
Oregon State University

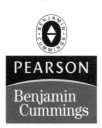

PEARSON

Benjamin
Cummings

San Francisco   Boston   New York
Cape Town   Hong Kong   London   Madrid   Mexico City
Montreal   Munich   Paris   Singapore   Sydney   Tokyo   Toronto

Publisher: Daryl Fox
Senior Acquisitions Editor: Deirdre Espinoza
Development Manager: Claire Alexander
Project Editor: Susan Malloy
Assistant Editor: Christina Pierson
Production Supervisor: Steven Anderson
Manufacturing Buyer: Stacey Weinberger
Cover Designer: Yvo Riezebos Design
Text Designer: Kathleen Cunningham Design
Production and Composition: The Left Coast Group
Photo Research: Brian Donnelly, Cypress Integrated Systems, Inc.
Copy Editor: Deborah Kopka
Proofreader: Martha Ghent
Cover Printer: Coral Graphics
Text Printer: Courier Kendalville

Cover Photo: Jud Guitteau / Illustration Works

Credits can be found on page C-1.

ISBN 0-8053-2852-1
ISBN 0-8053-6028-X (p-copy)

Library of Congress Cataloging-in-Publication Data
Donatelle, Rebecca J., 1950–
  Health the basics / Rebecca J. Donatelle.—6th ed.
    p. cm.
  Includes bibliographical references and index.
  ISBN 0-8053-2852-1 (pbk.)
  1. Health. I. Title.
  RA776.D663 2005
  613—dc22
                          2004001934

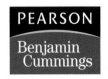

PEARSON
Benjamin
Cummings
www.aw-bc.com

1 2 3 4 5—CRK—07 06 05 04

Preface

Has there ever been an era in which more people have been concerned with health? Whether trying to improve appearance, lose weight, exercise more, feel better, enhance interpersonal relationships, or avoid disease-causing pathogens, more and more people are tuned in to health issues and topics.

Not too long ago, disease and illness were seen as phenomena people had little power over. People who became sick from an infectious disease either weathered the illness and recovered or, in all too many cases, died. Few choices were available in foods, medicines, and services; consequently, health care decisions usually focused on cleanliness, avoiding known hazards, and staying away from others who were sick.

In sharp contrast, today's health-conscious individuals have choices surrounding health that their parents and grandparents could not have imagined: pharmacies loaded with prescription and over-the-counter drugs, health food stores with thousands of products that claim to promote wellness and prevent illness, Yellow Pages filled with doctors and alternative practitioners to choose from, grocery stores and fast-food restaurants packed with every imaginable food, and transportation moving people to and from far-flung continents in a matter of hours. Books, television, the Internet, and other media-driven sources are constantly luring consumers into buying miracle products. Talk show hosts offer formulas for relationship success, sexual prowess, and a slew of other behaviors and products that promise happier and healthier living.

While being bombarded with marketing choices, individuals have to deal with the threat of both real and imagined adversaries. Violent acts are reported on the nightly news and in newspaper headlines. Divorce statistics seem to spell doom and gloom for the American family. Obesity, soaring drug use and abuse, epidemic depression and mental illness, increasing rates of infectious and noninfectious diseases, threats from emerging and resurging diseases, tales of environmental destruction, and a host of other bad news topics seem to permeate the culture.

Juxtaposed against the threats to health are advances in medical research, new opportunities for personal choice, increased attention to policies designed to preserve health and protect against harm, and improved strategies for promoting health and preventing premature disease and disability. Technologies continue to be developed, with concomitant improvements in diagnosis of disease and treatment occurring daily. At no time in history has it been more evident that by taking action, an individual can prevent illness and prolong a productive, fully functional life. Regardless of whether changes in public policy and community and corporate behavior are necessary to help improve health status, this much is true: The better individuals prepare themselves to make wise decisions, and the more community leaders and representatives of the health care system work together to help achieve and maintain excellent health status, the more likely that everyone's quality of life will improve.

Each new class of college students represents a more savvy group of health consumers, complete with its own unique perspectives on health. An astounding, often contradictory and confusing, array of health information is available through the simple click of a mouse, the routine turn on of the television, or the casual perusal of a magazine. Because there is no one recipe for achieving health, it is important to consider the various opinions and options available to determine what information is the most scientifically defensible and which poses the least amount of risk to wellness.

After more than 30 years of teaching public health students from a wide range of health and other disciplines and after working on several editions of this book, I continue to be excited about the tremendous opportunities that students today have to *make a difference* to their health, the health of their loved ones, and the health of others. Part of my goal in writing this book is to help students be better "change agents" as they view the health controversies of today and those that will shape their future—not just in the arena of personal health behaviors, but also in the larger realm of policy changes and community behaviors, which ultimately can assist the global population in living smarter, longer, and better. In short, this book is designed not just to teach health facts but to present health as a much broader concept, something that everyone desires and deserves. By understanding the factors that contribute to health risk, exploring concepts provided in this text, contemplating action plans that might serve to reduce risk, and using the technological tools provided, students can take the first steps in accessing better health.

New to the Sixth Edition

Every year as I face a new class of students, I am struck by the fact that these students will face a new set of health challenges surpassing anything that their parents or I could imagine at their age. These students must be able to find and assess accurate information about health, understand basic foundational material, and choose from a myriad of alternatives as they seek to maintain or improve their health. Each page of this text is designed to provide the latest information, engage students in active thinking and learning, and guide students to make health decisions based on the best science, rather than pop mythology.

As with previous editions of this text, I have been committed to ensuring that this new edition provides students with the latest in cutting-edge research as well as describing the latest discoveries, controversies, and realities that today's students face on a daily basis. Page by page, *Health: The Basics* is designed to pack maximum information into a smaller and relatively moderately priced text. It is designed to be engaging, and to move students from just thinking about health improvements to being actively involved in their own health behavior changes. In keeping with my philosophy of leading the market in covering the "hottest" health topics for each new group of students, this edition of *Health: The Basics* includes the following major enhancements and additions.

- **New Make It Happen! sections** at the end of each chapter reinforce the results of each chapter's self-assessment, give students the steps to follow for making a behavior change, and describe one student's behavior change in the area covered in the chapter. We hope to give students the tools that they need to make real and lasting behavior changes, and to see these changes as something that can continue long after they have completed their health class.
- **New In the News selections** at the beginning of each chapter give a preview of a *New York Times* article describing the latest research or developments in that chapter's subject. This encourages students to make connections between the content they are learning in school and "real world" issues. Students can access the complete, unabridged text of the article on this book's free website.
- **New Behavior Change Contracts** found at the end of the book give students contracts to fill out as part of their Make It Happen! behavior change plan. Examples of completed contracts are included.
- **Expanded coverage of bioterrorism and microbial threats** in the post 9/11 era. This material provides a realistic perspective on risks and threats, as well as helping students understand the numerous efforts being made to protect the public's health.
- **New information on the phenomenon of self-mutilation and cutting behavior** engaged in by many students. Distinctions between self-inflicted violence and suicide, the

lure of extreme sports, and related behaviors will help students better understand who is at risk, options for assistance, and ways to reduce risk.
- **Greatly expanded information on the global epidemic of obesity and unique problems facing Americans who are overweight or obese.** In addition, information on portion distortion and changes in portion size over recent decades are discussed and illustrated.
- **New information on popular diets, including the newest research on low carbohydrate diets.** Other nutritional updates include changes to the Food Guide Pyramid, and guidelines on trans-fats in the diet.
- **Expanded coverage of relaxation techniques to cope with stress** and the importance of stress management in healthy immune functioning and the prevention of chronic disease
- **Discussion of new research on Syndrome X** and its role in the development of hypertension and cardiovascular disease
- **New coverage on the Female Athlete Triad** and the unique challenges faced by athletes as they face the pressures to be successful in competitive sports
- **New coverage of OxyContin, Ecstasy, ephedra, and other substances** young adults widely discuss but whose risks are often misunderstood
- **Expanded coverage of the role of technology in increasing health risks;** "technostress" and other pressures are highlighted.
- **New research on the safety of cell phones,** as well as important considerations in using them for prolonged periods
- **Updated information on the newest contraceptive methods** available to students today, including their relative effectiveness, issues with use, and other key aspects of effective use. Plan B, NuvaRing, Ortho Evra, and Mirena are among the products described and assessed.
- **Updated and expanded coverage on the dual epidemic of diabetes and obesity,** including the relationship between the two and the importance of diet and exercise in risk reduction
- **New information on exercise programs that are attracting interest on college campuses,** including Pilates, newer forms of yoga, and tai chi

Maintaining a Standard of Excellence

With every edition of *Health: The Basics,* the challenge has been to make the book better than before and to provide information and material that will surpass the competition at every level. The fact that there are many fine health texts on the market today makes the task even more difficult. As such, I have painstakingly considered our reviewer feedback, student comments, focus group discussions, and the broader health marketplace in designing a book that reflects the **three Rs** for a successful book: **relevance**—reflects real-world issues and problems that students can identify with and have special meaning/importance to them; **reliability**—reflects cutting-edge consensus research from reliable and valid research studies; **readability**—captures the attention of today's techno-influenced students with non-judgmental writing that engages them and inspires them to read on.

Of equal importance to the above are the pedagogical standards that have been built upon with each successive edition of *Health: The Basics*.

- Chapter 1, "Promoting Healthy Behavior Change," establishes a dual approach used throughout the text: the individual and social context of health and disease and the importance of health to society as a whole.

- To assist students in their efforts to achieve health, the book provides a foundation of information and thought-provoking questions to help them think about specific, negative health behaviors and what strategies might promote behavior change. Additionally, students are challenged to think how their actions may impact others now and in the future. The text guides students through their own health evolution. Rather than just advising students on how to behave in a particular manner, the text emphasizes behavior choice by presenting students with various health options.

- Pedagogical aids such as the What Do You Think? questions throughout the chapter encourage students to apply information acquired from the chapter to their own lives.

- A broad approach to diversity, both within the United States and in the global community, is incorporated throughout the text, emphasizing the fact that health discussions can no longer be limited to populations that reside inside U.S. borders, but must encompass the potential impact of health policies and behaviors on other nations, cultures, ideologies, and perspectives.

- The roles of community, health policies, and health services in disease prevention and health promotion are integrated throughout the text. The public health approach is often ignored in health texts in favor of a pure individual focus. Optimum health changes will occur only in environments that are conducive to change, in which individuals are informed and can maximize resources to make long-term behavior changes.

- Within a strong pedagogical framework, the importance of building health behavior skills is emphasized and integrated consistently throughout the text. Readers will learn specific applications to their own lives in every chapter through the Assess Yourself, Reality Check, and Skills for Behavior Change boxes offered throughout the text.

Special Features

Each chapter of *Health: The Basics* includes several of the following special features in various combinations. These features are designed to help students think about healthy behavior skills and how to apply concepts found in the boxes to their everyday lives.

- **Assess Yourself** boxes provide quick, general indicators of personal health status in various areas, which students may consider when initiating behavior change.
- **Skills for Behavior Change** boxes focus on practical strategies that students can use to improve their personal health and reduce their risks from harmful health behaviors.
- **Reality Check** boxes focus attention on potential risks and safety issues, often as they relate to college-age students. Statistical information and trends help students recognize risks as they relate to particular behaviors and outcomes.
- **Health in a Diverse World** boxes increase awareness and appreciation for individual and cultural differences. They promote acceptance of diversity on college campuses and help students thrive in an increasingly diverse world. In particular, these boxes focus on health implications and issues for diverse populations.
- **Women's Health/Men's Health** boxes help students better understand some of the unique aspects of men's and women's health, as well as the challenges faced by each group as they attempt to achieve optimal health.
- **Consumer Health** boxes promote consumer skills by increasing awareness about the health market and focusing on particular consumer issues.
- **New Horizons in Health** boxes report on late-breaking health news and topics of recent concern. They show students that health is a dynamic and constantly changing field.

Learning Aids

- Each chapter is introduced with **Chapter Objectives** to alert students to the key concepts to be covered in upcoming material.
- Designed to spark student interest and demonstrate the relevance of health to everyday life, **In the News selections** complete the introduction to each chapter.
- Groups of **What Do You Think? questions** that encourage students to think critically are highlighted and strategically placed throughout each chapter.
- To emphasize and support understanding of material, pertinent health terms are boldfaced in the text and defined in the **running glossary** appearing at the bottom of text pages.
- At the end of each chapter, the **Taking Charge** section wraps up the chapter content with a focus on application

by the student. The **Make It Happen!** section integrates the self-assessment results with the steps of behavior change and encourages student participation. In addition, the Summary, Questions for Discussion and Reflection, Accessing Your Health on the Internet, and Further Reading sections offer more opportunities to explore areas of interest.

Student Supplements

Available with *Health: The Basics,* sixth edition, is a comprehensive set of ancillary materials designed to enhance learning:

- **MyHealthClass (www.myhealthclass.com).** This online resource lets students access a wide range of print and media supplements that make studying convenient and fun. Content includes the Take Charge of Your Health! Worksheets; Behavior Change Log Book and Wellness Journal; Study Guide for StudentBody101.com; and links to Research Navigator™, StudentBody101.com, and the text's Companion Website (all described further below). The instructor resources on the site are described later in this preface.
- **Companion Website (www.aw-bc.com/donatelle).** This easy-to-navigate site offers the complete articles highlighted in the text's In the News feature, interactive self-assessment activities, practice quizzes, open-ended critical-thinking questions, hypothetical case studies, Web links, and audio and video clips. The website also includes the Flashcard program, with the entire list of terms and their definitions from the textbook available for study, and eThemes of the Times, containing 30 *New York Times* articles reporting on the latest health news and research.
- **StudentBody101.com (www.studentbody101.com).** This dynamic website, accredited by Health on the Net, contains current health news articles, self-assessments, online discussions, and behavior-change tips.
- **Study Guide for StudentBody101.com (0-8053-4793-3).** This study guide supplements the website with new exercises, additional Web links, interviews with health experts, and more.
- **Take Charge! Self-Assessment Workbook with Review and Practice Tests (0-8053-6038-7).** This workbook includes quizzes, 90 assessment worksheets, behavior change projects, and review/practice tests for students.
- **Take Charge of Your Health! Worksheets (0-8053-6037-9).** This pad of 38 self-assessment activities (selected from the *Take Charge Workbook)* is available separately from the workbook.
- **Behavior Change Log Book and Wellness Journal (0-8053-5548-0).** This assessment tool helps students track daily exercise and nutritional intake and create a long-term nutrition and fitness prescription plan. It also includes a Behavior Change Contract and topics for journal-based activities.

Instructor Supplements

A full resource package accompanies *Health: The Basics* to assist the instructor with classroom preparation and presentation.

- **MyHealthClass.** This online resource provides everything instructors need to teach health in one convenient location. MyHealthClass' course management system is loaded with valuable free teaching resources that make giving assignments and tracking student progress easy. Powered by CourseCompass™, the preloaded content in MyHealthClass includes PowerPoint slides, Test Bank questions, Instructor's Manual material, and more.
- **Discovery Health Channel Health and Wellness Lecture Launcher Videos (Volume I, 0-8053-5369-0, Volume II, 0-8053-6001-8).** Created in partnership with Discovery Health Channel, this two-volume set of VHS tapes offers lecture-launcher clips on topics from nutrition to stress management to substance abuse. There are 24 segments in all, ranging in length from 5 to 12 minutes. This supplement is also available on CD for digital presentation.
- **Instructor's Resource Binder (0-8053-5567-7).** This three-ring binder accommodates all print supplements that accompany *Health: The Basics.*
- **Instructor's Resource Manual (0-8053-6032-8).** This teaching tool provides student and classroom activities, chapter objectives, lecture outlines, and Companion Website resources to reinforce chapter concepts and develop effective student learning. It also includes ideas for incorporating the Discovery Health Channel video clips into your course and discussion questions for the In the News articles.
- **Great Ideas: Active Ways to Teach Health and Wellness (0-8053-2857-2).** This new publication provides instructors with effective, proactive strategies contributed by health educators from around the country for teaching health topics in a variety of classroom settings.
- **Printed Test Bank (0-8053-6036-0) and Computerized Test Bank (0-8053-6035-2).** The questions in the comprehensively revised test bank were reviewed by a panel of instructors for relevance and accuracy. The Test Bank includes approximately 1,500 multiple-choice, short-answer, true/false, matching, and essay questions, all with answers and page references. The cross-platform TestGen CD-ROM enables you to create tests, edit questions, and add your own material to existing exams.
- **PowerPoint Presentation CD-ROM (0-8053-6033-6).** This cross-platform CD-ROM includes all of the figures and tables from the book, plus lecture outlines that may be customized for lecture presentation.
- **Transparency Acetates (0-8053-6034-4).** The figures and tables from the text are also available as full-color transparencies.
- **Course Management.** In addition to MyHealthClass, WebCT and Blackboard are also available. Contact your Benjamin Cummings sales representative for details.

- **EduCue Personal Response System.** This polling system can help you take attendance, pose questions, and assess your students' progress instantly. Each student uses a wireless transmitter ("clicker") to communicate their answers to your questions in class; a receiver immediately tabulates answers and displays them graphically. You can record the results for grading or simply use them as a discussion point.
- **Instructor's Guide for StudentBody101.com (0-205-35084-4).** Using journal articles and online resources from StudentBody101.com, this manual provides tips for conducting discussion sessions, assigning writing activities, spurring debates, and encouraging self-assessment.

Acknowledgments

After writing six editions of *Health: The Basics,* I can only marvel at the dedication and professionalism of the many fine publishing experts who have helped make such a text successful. With each subsequent edition of *Basics,* their skills in dealing with the complexities and considerations of the publication process have become more apparent. I have been extremely fortunate in having a steady stream of fine publishing teams to help me create the foundations of a text that was responsive to students, creative in approach, and reflective of the most important health trends of the times.

Since the acquisition of *Health: The Basics* by the Benjamin Cummings group, I have been extremely pleased by the professionalism, dedication, and attention to detail that this publication team has displayed as we've progressed through several editions of the text. They are truly outstanding and a pleasure to work with. From the highly skilled and enthusiastic Acquisitions Editor, Deirdre Espinoza, and Publisher Daryl Fox, to the outstanding editorial staff, I have been uniformly amazed at their consistent efforts to produce a great finished product. Although I wouldn't have thought it was possible to beat past publishing efforts, I must honestly say that my experiences with Benjamin Cummings have been the best of my publishing years, and remarkably, it just keeps getting better! They personify key aspects of what it takes to be successful in the publishing world, from this author's perspective: (1) drive and motivation for hard work and efficient process, (2) commitment to excellence, (3) a vibrant, youthful, and enthusiastic approach that is in tune with college student needs, and (4) personalities that motivate an author to continually strive to produce market-leading texts. From the wonderful guidance, thoughtful suggestions, and patient prodding demonstrated by Susan Teahan, my initial project editor with *Health: The Basics,* to the superb effort, expertise, level-headed perspective, and guidance shown by Susan Malloy in subsequent editions and related supplements, I have been extremely impressed by the high level of skill that the editorial staff exhibits. Susan Malloy is, quite simply, an outstanding employee and ambassador for the BC group, and I feel fortunate to have worked

with her over the last editions of my texts. Without her efforts, in particular, these texts would not have come to fruition or enjoyed the successes that they have achieved. Having worked with many people in comparable positions over the years, I can say without question that she is one of the finest project editors any author could work with. Thank you, Susan!

In addition, I would like to acknowledge the wonderful editorial assistance provided by Developmental Editor Alice E. Fugate, who did an outstanding job in a short time frame to merge some of the newest features of *Health: The Basics* with content from *Access to Health* and in suggesting revisions and modifications based on reviewer comments and market demands. This was a huge and complicated task, and Alice did a remarkable job.

Although these women were key contributors to the finished work, there were many other people who worked on this revision of *Health: The Basics.* In particular, I would like to thank The Left Coast Group for their invaluable assistance in final book development and refinement, and Christina Pierson, Assistant Editor, for overseeing the complete supplements package. I would also like to thank the Benjamin Cummings marketing and sales force, particularly Marketing Manager Sandra Lindelof, who spent countless hours making sure that *Health: The Basics* got into instructors' hands. Part of the success of any book depends on the efforts of those who work diligently to make sure that the strengths of the book are outlined and that instructors are able to make good decisions about what their students will be reading. In keeping with my overall experiences with Benjamin Cummings, the sales staff and editorial staff are among the best of the best. I am very lucky to have them working with me on this project and want to extend a special thanks to all of them!

Contributors to the Sixth Edition

Many colleagues, students, and staff members have provided the feedback, reviews, extra time and assistance, and encouragement that have helped me meet the demands of rigorous publishing deadlines over the years. With each edition of the book, your assistance has made the vision for *Health: The Basics* a reality. Rather than just creating an upscale version of a shorter format high school text, we have worked diligently to provide a text that is "alive" for readers. With each edition, we would not have developed a book like this one without the outstanding contributions of several key people. Whether acting as reviewers, generating new ideas, providing expert commentary, or writing chapters, each of these professionals has added his or her skills to our collective endeavor.

I would also like to extend a personal thank you to Dr. Patricia Ketcham, Director of Health Promotion Programs in Student Health Services (Oregon State University). Since the first edition of *Access to Health* more than 15 years ago, she has been a consistent and solid contributor to each new edition of my texts. Her insights into the problems faced by students on today's campuses and her background in public health have helped shape chapters focusing on reproductive choices, addictions, tobacco, and substance abuse; as always, these chapters represent the latest and most important issues facing students. Specific chapters contributed by Dr. Ketcham in this edition are Chapter 6, "Birth Control, Pregnancy, and Childbirth," Chapter 7, "Licit and Illicit Drugs," and Chapter 8, "Alcohol, Tobacco, and Caffeine." In addition, chapters focusing on death and dying and sexuality were contributed by Dr. Donna Champeau, Assistant Professor in the Department of Public Health (Oregon State University) to *Access to Health* and these were adapted and revised for use in *Health: The Basics*. Many thanks to Dr. Champeau for her contributions to these chapters.

Reviewers for the Sixth Edition

The expertise of many professionals is necessary to create a finished work that represents the best available health information source for college level students. Clearly, *Health: The Basics* continues to be an evolving work in progress incorporating the help of many fine minds in ensuring a quality product. Each new edition builds on the combined expertise of many colleagues throughout the country who are dedicated to the education and positive behavioral change of students and the health of the population as a whole. My thanks go to the following reviewers who have helped us with this admirable tradition: Judy Ary, North Dakota State University; Jeremy Barnes, Southeast Missouri State University; Joseph Bell, Abilene Christian University; Jeanne Boone, Palm Beach Community College; Cheryl Boron, Paradise Valley Community College; Kristine Brown, California State Polytechnic University; Duane Crider, Kutztown University; Sherri Dawson, Southwest Virginia Community College; Robert Dollinger, Florida International University; Brian Findley, Palm Beach Community College; Pamela Homiak, University of Maryland; John Kalinowski, College of New Jersey; Karen Lew, Southeast Louisiana University; Pamela Manning, University of Maryland; Kathleen Masket, College of San Mateo; Susan Masden Moore, Western Illinois University; Debbie Murray, University of North Carolina; Miguel Perez, California State University, Fresno; Linda Rankin, Idaho State University; Gina Sirach, Southeastern Illinois College; Margaret Snooks, University of Houston, Clear Lake; Jiri Stelzer, Valdosta State University; Eric Templet, Southeastern Louisiana University; B. McKinley Thomas, Augusta State University;

Jane Vatchev, College of DuPage; Becky Vidourek, University of Cincinnati; Kirk Westre, Whitworth College.

We also had a panel of reviewers who scrutinized the Test Bank and made innumerable helpful comments and critiques: Steve Hartman, Citrus College; Ping Johnson, Kennesaw State University; Raeann Koerner, Ventura College; Susan Masden Moore, Western Illinois University; Phil Sparling, Georgia Technical University; Michael Teague, University of Iowa.

The colleagues who attended our Health Summits contributed invaluable feedback as well: Lynda Armona, County College of Morris; Robert Axtell, Southern Connecticut State University; Michael Ballard, Eastern Kentucky University; Michael Basile, Borough of Manhattan Community College; Jeanne Boone, Palm Beach Community College South; Karen Camarata, Eastern Kentucky University; David Carey, Ventura College; Mary Ann Carr, Middle Tennessee State University; Charlie Chatterton, Eastern Connecticut State; Yosuke Chikamoto, California State University, Fullerton; Steve Contarsy, Santa Monica College; Olivia Cousins, Borough of Manhattan Community College; Kathryn L. Davis, Slippery Rock University; William Dunscombe, Union County Community College; William Elizuk, Broward Community College; Augie Eosso, Raritan Valley Community College; Jeremy Erdmann, Murray State University; Brian Findley, Palm Beach Community College South; Marisha Fortner, University of Notre Dame; Robert Grueninger, Morehead State University; David Harackiewicz, Central Connecticut State University; Janet Heller, Bronx Community College; Jennifer Howard, Morehead State University; William Huber, County College of Morris; Vincent Merill, California State University, Fullerton; Marilyn Miller, Bloomsburg University; Mary Miller, Morehead State University; Kevin Petti, Miramar College; Jeff Schlicht, Western Connecticut State University; Lydia Strong, Santa Monica College; Michele Sweeney, Salem State College; Lynn Spadine Taylor, Slippery Rock University; Nanette Tummers, Eastern Connecticut State; Malinda Tuttle, University of Louisville; Robert Walker, John Brown University; Molly Whaley, Middle Tennessee State University; Matt Wiggins, Murray State University.

Rebecca J. Donatelle
Health & Kinesiology
Benjamin Cummings
1301 Sansome Street
San Francisco, California 94111

Brief Contents

Contents

Part Six
Facing Life's Challenges

Chapter 15
Life's Transitions: The Aging Process 399

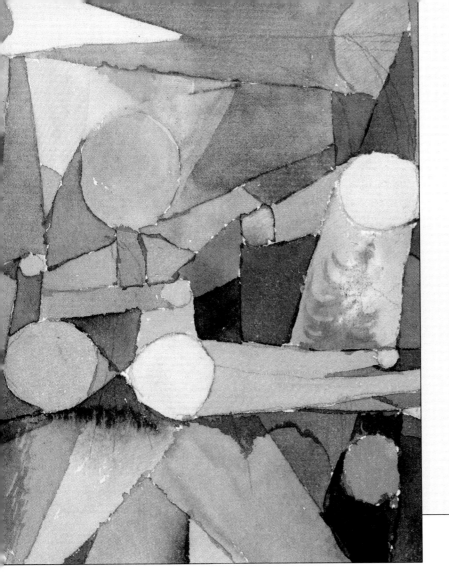

Promoting Healthy Behavior Change

Objectives

* Discuss health in terms of historical perspectives and its multidimensional elements.

* Explain the importance of a healthy lifestyle in preventing premature disease and disability.

* Discuss the health status of Americans and the importance of *Steps to a HealthierUS, Agency for Health Care Research and Quality Guidelines*, *Healthy People 2000, Healthy People 2010,* and other initiatives in establishing national goals for promoting health.

* Evaluate the role of gender in health status, health research, and health training.

* Provide a rationale for focusing on current risk behaviors as a means of influencing current and future health status.

* Examine how predisposing factors, beliefs, attitudes, and significant others affect a person's behavior changes.

* Assess behavior-change techniques and apply them to your own situation.

The New York Times
In the News

Hormone Studies: What Went Wrong?

By Gina Kolata

For nearly nine months, doctors and researchers have been struggling with an intractable problem: how could two large high-quality studies come to diametrically different conclusions about menopause, hormone therapy and heart disease?

The question arose in July, when scientists saw data from a large federal study called the Women's Health Initiative, which was ended early when it became clear that a widely used hormone-replacement drug, Prempro, had risks, including heart attacks, that exceeded its benefits.

That finding directly contradicted previous studies showing that the hormones reduced heart disease risk, in particular, the Nurses' Health Study, a large research effort that has been going on for years.

The question is why.

To answer it, researchers are reviewing the data, scrutinizing the design of each study and examining other research that may help reconcile the disparate findings. But so far, as they noted at a recent symposium at the Harvard School of Public Health, they have had no luck. As one explanation after another fails to hold up, the mystery deepens.

Read the complete article online in the eThemes section of this book's website: www.aw-bc.com/donatelle.

Concerned about your health? You are not alone. At no time in U.S. history have so many individuals, government agencies, educational systems, community groups, businesses, and health care organizations been so concerned about health or so vocal in their attempts to influence health habits. Billboards graphically display the dangers of drinking and driving and the impact of cigarette smoke, even on people who don't smoke. Television ads warn of the dangers of unsafe sexual activity and illegal drugs while touting the miraculous benefits of medicines that appear to "fix" everything. Even the President has warned U.S. citizens that over half of us are overweight and unfit, and the health of the country is in jeopardy due to epidemic rates of obesity, diabetes, and other lifestyle-related maladies. On a daily basis, you are challenged to "Just do it, but don't overdo it"; "Be all you can be, but be yourself"; "Eat cruciferous vegetables, but buy organic"; and exercise, but not to the point of being obsessed!

Conflicting health claims abound, and research that would clarify their authenticity is scarce or written in technical language that is hard to interpret. As a result, many people are confused about what they should and should not do when it comes to their health. We often assume that the government and the medical profession will protect us, only to find out that what we have been told is true may in fact be false. For example, for the past three decades doctors have advised women who have gone through menopause to take hormone replacement therapy (HRT) as protection against heart disease and stroke. Research appeared to support this recommendation. However, in 2002 and 2003, studies appeared that contradicted the safety of this treatment. The Women's Health Initiative found that HRT actually increases the risk of heart disease, stroke, and blood clots; Cancer Research UK found that combined HRT doubled a woman's normal risk of developing breast cancer.[1]

In these cases, health researchers and practitioners, and others on whom we rely for information, appear to have based long-standing prevention and treatment regimens on faulty premises. How many other health recommendations are false or misleading? Even the best scientists must struggle to determine which research is valid and which provides only a preliminary indicator of hazards or benefits. How can the average person figure out what is accurate and what is bogus?

Answering these questions is not an easy task. Thus, it is fairly easy to see why individuals struggle so hard to "get it right" when it comes to making the best health decisions for themselves or those they care about. And, in spite of all of the emphasis on health in society today and all of our resources aimed at prevention, intervention, and treatment, the health status of Americans continues to be plagued by old problems.

Why is being healthy so challenging for so many of us? What can we do to make better decisions and become wiser, more responsible health consumers? There are no easy answers, because health is influenced by a myriad of factors—some that we can control and some that we can't. But the good news is that many people have found the skills and motivation to look objectively at where they are, plan carefully, and make decisions that improve their life and health. They have learned how to use technological and community resources to enhance rather than diminish their health. Perhaps more importantly, they have found their own unique ways to make long-term behavior changes. Have you ever

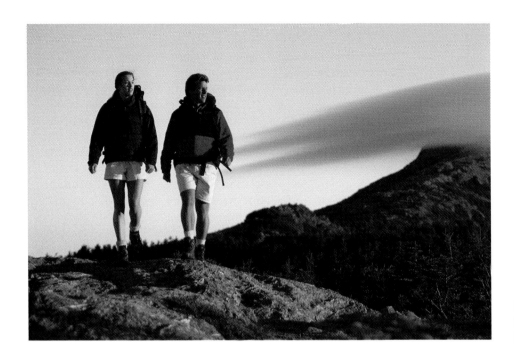

Today, health and wellness mean taking a positive, proactive attitude toward life, living it to the fullest.

wondered, for example, how one of your friends lost weight and is now running in triathlons, when you can't lose an ounce, and your latest trip up the stairs leaves you panting for breath? Or why another friend seems to thrive under pressure, while it makes you break down into a screaming fit? Why do so many good health intentions remain only intentions without progressing to the action phase?

This text is not designed to provide a foolproof recipe for achieving health or to answer all of your questions. It *is* designed to provide fundamental knowledge about health topics, to help you use personal and community resources to create your own health profile, and to challenge you to think more carefully before making decisions that affect your health or the health of others. It shows how policies, programs, media, culture, ethnicity, gender, and socioeconomic status directly and indirectly influence health in the United States and around the world. It is our hope that you will gain appreciation for the many achievements that we have made in health and the many challenges that lie ahead. In addition, we hope that you will begin to look at health not in an ethnocentric way, in which you are only able to appreciate those who look and talk like you and have habits and customs like you, but rather, that you begin to look at global health in a more inclusive way.

Health decisions should be based on the best available research and should be consistent with who you are, your values and beliefs, and who you want to become. Although health is not always totally within your control, certain behavior choices will affect you positively today and reduce future health risks. For those risk factors beyond your control, you must learn to react, adapt, respond appropriately, and use a reasoned rather than purely emotional rationale for your choices. By making informed, rational decisions, you will improve the quality and the length of your own life and have a positive influence on those around you.

Putting Your Health in Perspective

Although we use the term *health* almost unconsciously, few people understand the broad scope of the word. For some, *health* simply means the antithesis of sickness. To others, it means being in good physical shape and able to resist illness. Still others use terms such as *wellness,* or *well-being,* to include a wide array of factors that lead to positive health status. Why all of these variations? In part, the differences in perception are due to an increasingly enlightened way of viewing health that has taken shape over time. As our understanding of illness has improved, so has our ability to understand the many nuances of health. Although our current understanding about health has evolved over centuries, we have a long way to go in achieving a truly comprehensive view of this complex subject.

Health: Yesterday and Today

Prior to the 1800s, if you weren't sick, you were not only regarded as lucky, but also healthy. When deadly epidemics such as bubonic plague, influenza, and cholera killed millions of people, survivors were believed to be of hearty, healthy stock, and they congratulated themselves on their good fortune. Poor health was often associated with poor hygiene and unsanitary conditions, and a stigma was attached to households that harbored illnesses. Not until the late 1800s did researchers discover that victims of epidemics were not simply unhealthy or dirty. Rather, they were victims of environmental factors such as microorganisms found in contaminated water, air, and human waste over which they often had little control. Public health officials moved swiftly to address these problems. As a result, health became synonymous with good hygiene. Colleges offered courses in health and hygiene, the predecessors of the course you are taking today.

Investigation into the environment as the primary cause of disease continued into the twentieth century as outbreaks of tuberculosis, pneumonia, and influenza surged in many regions of the world. People who made it through the first few years of life without succumbing to an infectious disease usually were able to survive to old age. (Keep in mind, however, that the average life expectancy in 1900 was only 47 years.) Continued improvements in sanitation brought dramatic changes in life expectancy. The development of vaccines and antibiotics added even more years to the average life.

By the 1940s, progressive thinkers began to note that there was more to health than hygiene or disease. At an international conference in 1947, the World Health Organization took the landmark step of trying to clarify what health truly meant: "Health is the state of complete physical, mental, and social well-being, not just the absence of disease or infirmity."[2] For the first time, the concept of health came to mean more than not being ill.

Not until the 1960s and 1970s, however, did the definition of health begin to mirror the comprehensive model that public health professionals had advocated for decades. Scientists argued that **health** was much more than the absence of disease; it includes the physical, social, and mental elements of life, as well as environmental, spiritual, emotional, and intellectual dimensions of life. To be truly healthy, a person must be capable of functioning at an optimal level in each of these areas, as well as interacting with others and the greater environment. In addition, public health leaders argued that it wasn't just length of life or the number of disease-free years that mattered, but rather achieving your potential for a happy, healthy, and productive life. Today, quality of life is considered as important as years of life.

Since most childhood diseases are preventable or curable and since massive public health efforts are aimed at reducing the spread of infectious diseases, many people are living well into their 70s and 80s. According to **mortality** (death rate) statistics, people are now living longer than at any time in our history. **Morbidity** (illness) rates also indicate that people less frequently contract the common infectious diseases that devastated previous generations. However, longer life and less frequent disease are not proof that people are indeed healthier.

Health   Dynamic, ever-changing process of achieving individual potential in the physical, social, mental, environmental, spiritual, emotional, and intellectual dimensions of life.

Mortality   Death rate.

Morbidity   Illness rate.

Wellness   The achievement of the highest level of health possible in each of several dimensions.

Activities of daily living (ADLs)   Tasks of everyday living, such as bathing and walking up stairs.

The Evolution toward Wellness

René Dubos, biologist and philosopher, aptly summarized the thinking of his contemporaries by defining health as "a quality of life, involving social, emotional, mental, spiritual, and biological fitness on the part of the individual, which results from adaptations to the environment."[3] The concept of adaptability, or the ability to successfully cope with life's ups and downs, became a key element of the overall health definition. Eventually the term **wellness** became popular and not only included the previously mentioned elements, but also implied that there were levels of health in each category. To achieve high-level wellness, a person would move progressively higher on a continuum of positive health indicators. Those who fail to achieve these levels may move to the illness side of the continuum. Today, the terms *health* and *wellness* are often used interchangeably to mean the dynamic, ever-changing process of achieving one's potential in each of several interrelated dimensions. These dimensions typically include those presented in Figure 1.1 and described below.

The dimensions of health are:

- *Physical health.* This dimension includes characteristics such as body size and shape, sensory acuity and responsiveness, susceptibility to disease and disorders, body functioning, physical fitness, and recuperative abilities. Newer definitions of physical health also include our ability to perform normal **activities of daily living (ADLs),** or those tasks necessary to normal existence in today's society. Being able to get out of bed in the morning, bend over to tie your shoes, and other usual daily tasks are examples of ADLs.
- *Social health.* This dimension refers to the ability to have satisfying interpersonal relationships, including interactions with others, adaptation to social situations, and appropriate daily behaviors.
- *Intellectual health.* This dimension refers to the ability to think clearly, reason objectively, analyze critically, and use brain power effectively to meet life's challenges. It means learning from successes and mistakes and making responsible decisions that take into consideration all aspects of a situation.
- *Emotional health.* This dimension refers to the feeling component—expressing emotions when it is appropriate, controlling them when it is not, and avoiding expressing them inappropriately. Self-esteem, self-confidence, self-efficacy, trust, love, and many other emotional reactions and responses are all part of emotional health.
- *Environmental health.* This dimension refers to an appreciation of the external environment and the role individuals play in preserving, protecting, and improving environmental conditions.
- *Spiritual health.* This dimension may involve a belief in a supreme being or a way of life prescribed by a particular religion. Spiritual health also includes the feeling of unity with the environment—a feeling of oneness with others and with nature—and a guiding sense of meaning or

value in life. It also may include the ability to understand and express one's purpose in life; to feel a part of a greater spectrum of existence; to experience love, joy, pain, sorrow, peace, contentment, and wonder over life's experiences; and to respect all living things.

Although typically not considered a dimension in most wellness continuums, **mental health** is an important concept. Often confused with emotional, social, spiritual, or intellectual health, it is a broader concept that encompasses all of these dimensions. According to the U.S. Surgeon General, this umbrella term refers to the "successful performance of mental function, resulting in productive activities, fulfilling relationships with others, and the ability to adapt to change and cope with adversity. From early childhood until late life, mental health is the springboard of thinking and communication skills, learning, emotional growth, resilience, and self-esteem."[4] Mental health is a critical public and community health priority.

A well individual might display these characteristics.

- A realistic sense of self, including personal capabilities and limitations
- An appreciation of all living things, no matter how ugly or beautiful, how unique, or how great or small
- A willingness to understand imperfection, forgive others' mistakes, and grow from personal mistakes or shortcomings
- The ability to laugh, cry, and genuinely feel emotions without getting lost in emotional upsets
- The ability to function physiologically at a reasonable level
- The ability to maintain and support healthy relationships with family, friends, and intimate partners, and to interact appropriately with strangers
- An appreciation for one's role in preserving and protecting the environment
- A sense of satisfaction with life and an appreciation for the stages of the life experience
- A zest for living, coupled with a curiosity about what each new day will bring
- A respect for self and a respect for others
- A realistic perspective about life's challenges and stressors and the skills to cope with them
- A balance in all things

Many people believe that wellness can best be achieved by adopting a *holistic* approach, which emphasizes the integration of and balance among mind, body, and spirit. Achieving wellness also means attaining the optimum level of wellness for a person's unique limitations and strengths. A physically disabled person may function at his or her optimum level of performance; enjoy satisfying interpersonal relationships; maintain emotional, spiritual, and intellectual health; and have a strong interest in environmental concerns. In contrast, those who spend hours lifting weights to perfect the size and shape of each muscle but pay little attention to nutrition may *look* healthy but may not have a good balance in all areas of health. Although we often consider physical attractiveness and other external trappings in measuring overall

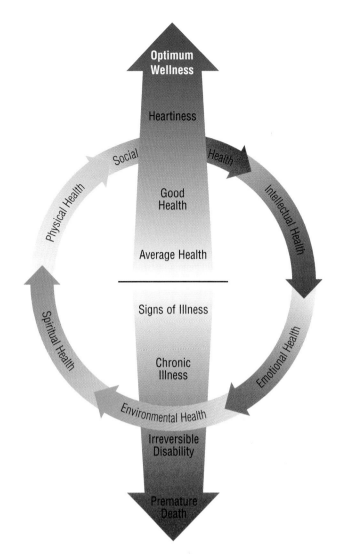

Figure 1.1
The Dimensions of Health and the Wellness Continuum

health, appearance is actually only one sign of wellness and indicates little about the other dimensions.

How healthy are you? Complete the Assess Yourself box on the next page to gain perspective on your own level of wellness in each dimension.

What do you think?
Based on the wellness dimensions discussed, what are your key strengths in each dimension?
✷ *What are your key deficiencies?* ✷ *What one or two things can you do to enhance your strong areas?* ✷ *To improve your weaknesses?*

Mental health An umbrella concept encompassing emotional, social, spiritual, and intellectual health.

How Healthy Are You?

Although we all recognize the importance of being healthy, it can be a challenge to sort out which behaviors are most likely to cause problems or pose the greatest risk. Even when we recognize our unique risks and know what to do, it isn't always easy to stay motivated enough to maintain a specific set of health behaviors. Before you decide where to start, it is important to take a careful look at your current health status. Think carefully about where you believe that you are today in each dimension of health. Rate your health status in each of the following dimensions by circling the number that comes closest to describing the way you are most of the time.

	Poor Health		Average Health		Excellent Health
Physical health	1	2	3	4	5
Social health	1	2	3	4	5
Intellectual health	1	2	3	4	5
Emotional health	1	2	3	4	5
Environmental health	1	2	3	4	5
Spiritual health	1	2	3	4	5

After completing the above section, how would you rate your **overall** health? 1 2 3 4 5

Which area(s), if any, do you think you should improve? _____

If we were to ask your closest friends how healthy they think you are, which area(s) do you think they would say you need to improve? _____

By completing the following assessment, you will have a clearer picture of health areas in which you excel and those that need improvement. Taking this assessment also will help you to reflect on various components of health that you may not have thought much about.

Use the results from this assessment as a guide to begin analyzing potential areas for improvement and/or maintenance. Answer each question. Then write your score for each section on the Personal Checklist at the end of this assessment for a general understanding of your health profile. Think about the behaviors that influenced your score in each category. Would you like to change any behaviors? Choose the area you would like to improve, then complete the Behavior Change Contract at the end of this book. Use the contract to implement a behavior change over the course of this class.

This assessment is not a substitute for the advice of a qualified health care provider. Consider scheduling a thorough physical examination with a licensed physician or setting up an appointment with a mental health counselor at your school if you think you need help making a behavior change.

For each of the following, indicate how often you think the statements describe you.

PHYSICAL HEALTH

	Never	Rarely	Some of the Time	Usually or Always
1. I am happy with my body size and weight.	1	2	3	4
2. I engage in vigorous exercises such as brisk walking, jogging, swimming, or running for at least 30 minutes per day, 3–4 times per week.	1	2	3	4
3. I do exercises designed to strengthen my muscles and increase endurance at least 2 times per week.	1	2	3	4
4. I do stretching, limbering up, and balance exercises such as yoga, pilates, or tai chi to increase my body awareness and control and increase my overall physical health.	1	2	3	4
5. I feel good about the condition of my body and would be able to respond to most demands placed upon it.	1	2	3	4
6. I get at least 7–8 hours of sleep each night.	1	2	3	4

	Never	Rarely	Some of the Time	Usually or Always
7. I try to do moderate activity each day, such as taking the stairs instead of the elevator and walking whenever I can instead of riding.	1	2	3	4
8. My immune system is strong, and my body heals quickly when I get sick or I am injured.	1	2	3	4
9. I have lots of energy and can get through the day without being overly tired.	1	2	3	4
10. I listen to my body; when there is something wrong, I make adjustments to heal it or seek professional advice.	1	2	3	4

SOCIAL HEALTH

	Never	Rarely	Some of the Time	Usually or Always
1. When I meet people, I feel good about the impression I make on them.	1	2	3	4
2. I am open, honest, and get along well with other people.	1	2	3	4
3. I participate in a wide variety of social activities and enjoy being with people who are different from me.	1	2	3	4
4. I try to be a "better person" and work on behaviors that have caused problems in my interactions with others.	1	2	3	4
5. I get along well with the members of my family.	1	2	3	4
6. I am a good listener.	1	2	3	4
7. I am open and accessible to a loving and responsible relationship.	1	2	3	4
8. I have someone I can talk to about my private feelings.	1	2	3	4
9. I consider the feelings of others and do not act in hurtful ways.	1	2	3	4
10. I try to see the good in my friends and do whatever I can to support them and help them feel good about themselves.	1	2	3	4

INTELLECTUAL HEALTH

	Never	Rarely	Some of the Time	Usually or Always
1. I carefully consider my options and possible consequences as I make choices in life.	1	2	3	4
2. I learn from my mistakes and try to act differently the next time.	1	2	3	4
3. I follow directions or recommended guidelines, avoid risks, and act in ways likely to keep myself and others safe.	1	2	3	4
4. I consider myself to be a wise health consumer and check reliable information sources before making decisions.	1	2	3	4
5. I am alert and ready to respond to life's challenges in ways that reflect thought and sound judgment.	1	2	3	4
6. I have at least one hobby, learning activity, or personal growth activity that I make time for each week.	1	2	3	4
7. I actively learn all I can about products and services before making decisions to buy them.	1	2	3	4
8. I manage my time well rather than let time manage me.	1	2	3	4
9. My friends and family trust my judgment.	1	2	3	4
10. I think about my self-talk (the things I tell myself) and then examine the evidence to see if my perceptions and feelings are sound.	1	2	3	4

(continued)

EMOTIONAL HEALTH

	Never	Rarely	Some of the Time	Usually or Always
1. I find it easy to laugh, cry, and show emotions like love, fear, and anger and try to express these in positive, constructive ways.	1	2	3	4
2. I avoid using alcohol or other drugs as a means of helping me forget my problems.	1	2	3	4
3. When confronted with a challenging situation, I tend to view the glass as "half full" rather than "half empty" by perceiving problems as opportunities for growth.	1	2	3	4
4. When I am angry, I try to resolve issues rather than stew about them.	1	2	3	4
5. I try not to worry unnecessarily and try to talk about my feelings, fears, and concerns rather than letting them become chronic unresolved issues.	1	2	3	4
6. I recognize when I am stressed and take steps to relax through exercise, quiet time, or other calming activities.	1	2	3	4
7. I feel good about myself and believe others like me for who I am.	1	2	3	4
8. I try not to be too critical and/or judgmental of others and to understand differences or quirks that I may note in others.	1	2	3	4
9. I am flexible and adapt or adjust to change in a positive way.	1	2	3	4
10. My friends regard me as a stable, emotionally well-adjusted person whom they trust and rely on for support.	1	2	3	4

ENVIRONMENTAL HEALTH

	Never	Rarely	Some of the Time	Usually or Always
1. I am concerned about environmental pollution and actively try to preserve and protect natural resources.	1	2	3	4
2. I buy recycled paper and purchase biodegradable detergents whenever possible.	1	2	3	4
3. I recycle my garbage, purchase refillable containers when possible, and try to minimize the amount of paper and plastics that I use.	1	2	3	4
4. I try to wear my clothes for longer periods between washing to reduce water consumption and the amount of detergents in our water sources.	1	2	3	4
5. I vote for pro-environment candidates.	1	2	3	4
6. I write my elected leaders about environmental concerns.	1	2	3	4
7. I turn down the heat and wear warmer clothes at home in winter and use the air conditioner only when necessary or at higher temperatures in the summer.	1	2	3	4
8. I am aware of lead pipes in my living area, chemicals in my carpet, and other potential environmental hazards and try to reduce my exposure whenever possible.	1	2	3	4
9. I use both sides of the paper when taking class notes or doing assignments.	1	2	3	4
10. I try not to leave the water running too long when I brush my teeth, shave, or shower.	1	2	3	4

SPIRITUAL HEALTH

		Never	Rarely	Some of the Time	Usually or Always
1.	I believe life is a precious gift that should be nurtured.	1	2	3	4
2.	I take time to enjoy nature and the beauty around me.	1	2	3	4
3.	I take time alone to think about what's important in life, such as who I am, what I value, where I fit in, and where I'm going.	1	2	3	4
4.	I have faith in a greater power.	1	2	3	4
5.	I engage in acts of goodwill without expecting something in return.	1	2	3	4
6.	I feel sorrow for those who are suffering and try to help them through difficult times.	1	2	3	4
7.	I look forward to each day as an opportunity for further growth.	1	2	3	4
8.	I work for peace in my interpersonal relationships, in my community, and in the world at large.	1	2	3	4
9.	I have a great love and respect for all living things, and regard animals, etc., as important links in a vital living chain.	1	2	3	4
10.	I experience life to the fullest.	1	2	3	4

Although each of these six dimensions of health is important, there are additional factors that don't readily fit one dimension. College students face some unique risks that others may not have. For this reason, we have added an additional section to this self-assessment that focuses on personal health promotion and disease prevention. Answer these questions and add your results to the Personal Checklist that follows.

PERSONAL HEALTH PROMOTION/DISEASE PREVENTION

		Never	Rarely	Some of the Time	Usually or Always
1.	I know the warning signs of common sexually transmitted infections, such as genital warts, chlamydia, and herpes, and read new information about these diseases as a way of protecting myself.	1	2	3	4
2.	If I were sexually active, I would use protection such as latex condoms, dental dams, and other means to reducing my risk of sexually transmitted infections.	1	2	3	4
3.	I find ways other than binge drinking when at parties or during happy hours to have a good time.	1	2	3	4
4.	When I have more than 1 drink, I ask someone who is not drinking to drive me home.	1	2	3	4
5.	I have eaten too much in the last month and have forced myself to vomit to avoid gaining weight.	4	3	2	1
6.	I have several piercings and enjoy the rush that comes with each piercing event.	4	3	2	1
7.	If I were to get a tattoo or piercing, I would go to a reputable person who follows strict standards of sterilization and precautions against blood-borne disease transmission.	1	2	3	4
8.	I engage in extreme sports and find that I enjoy the highs that come with risking bodily harm through physical performance.	4	3	2	1

(continued)

	Never	Rarely	Some of the Time	Usually or Always
9. I do not mix alcohol or other drugs with prescription and over-the-counter drugs.	1	2	3	4
10. I practice monthly breast/testicle self-examinations.	1	2	3	4

PERSONAL CHECKLIST

Total your scores in each of the health dimension areas and compare them to the optimal score of 40. Which areas do you need to work on? How does your score compare with how you rated yourself in the first part of the assessment?

	Ideal Score	Your Score
Physical health	40	_____
Social health	40	_____
Intellectual health	40	_____
Emotional health	40	_____
Environmental health	40	_____
Spiritual health	40	_____
Personal health promotion/ disease prevention	40	_____

WHAT YOUR SCORES MEAN

Scores of 35–40: Outstanding! You are aware of the importance of these behaviors in your overall health. More important, you are putting your knowledge to work by practicing good health habits that should reduce your overall risks. Although you received a very high score on this part of the assessment, you may want to consider areas in which your scores could be improved.

Scores of 30–34: Your health practices in these areas are very good, but there is room for improvement. Look again at the items on which you scored one or two points. What changes could you make to improve your score? Even a small change in behavior can help you achieve better health.

Scores of 20–29: Your health risks are showing! Find information about the risks you are facing and why it is important to change these behaviors. If you need help in deciding how to

make the changes you desire, assistance is available from this book, your professor, and student health services at your school. Consider making a change by filling out the Behavior Change Contract at the end of this book.

Scores below 20: You may be taking unnecessary risks with your health. Perhaps you are not aware of the risks and what to do about them. Identify each risk area. As you read the associated chapter in this book, seek additional resources, either on your campus or through your local community health resources, and make a serious commitment to behavior change. If any area is causing you to be less than functional in your class work or personal life, seek professional help. In this book you will find the information you need to help you improve your scores and your health. Remember, these scores are only indicators, not diagnostic tools.

New Directions for Health

In 1990, in response to the indications that Americans were not as healthy as they should be, the U.S. Surgeon General proposed a national plan for promoting health among individuals and groups. Known as *Healthy People 2000*, the plan outlined a series of long-term objectives. Many communities worked toward achieving these goals; nevertheless, as a nation we still had a long way to go by the new millennium.

Healthy People 2000 and 2010

A new plan, *Healthy People 2010*, takes the original *Healthy People 2000* initiative to the next level. *Healthy People 2010* is a nationwide program with two broad goals: eliminate health disparities and increase the life span and quality of life. The plan includes 28 focus areas. Each area represents a public health priority, such as nutrition, tobacco use, substance abuse, and access to quality health services, and common health conditions, such as heart disease and stroke. In addition to these focus areas are a group of leading health indicators. These indicators are translated into rates or percentages that

Table 1.1
What Is *Healthy People 2010*?

Overarching Goals
1. Increase quality and years of healthy life
2. Eliminate health disparities

Focus Areas
1. Access to quality health services
2. Arthritis, osteoporosis, and chronic back conditions
3. Cancer
4. Chronic kidney disease
5. Diabetes
6. Disability and secondary conditions
7. Educational and community-based programs
8. Environmental health
9. Family planning
10. Food safety
11. Health communication
12. Heart disease and stroke
13. Human immunodeficiency virus (HIV)
14. Immunization and infectious diseases
15. Injury and violence prevention
16. Maternal, infant, and child health
17. Medical product safety
18. Mental health and mental disorders
19. Nutrition and overweight
20. Occupational safety and health
21. Oral health
22. Physical activity and fitness
23. Public health infrastructure
24. Respiratory disease
25. Sexually transmitted disease
26. Substance abuse
27. Tobacco use
28. Vision and hearing

Leading Health Indicators
1. Physical activity
2. Overweight and obesity
3. Tobacco use
4. Substance abuse
5. Responsible sexual behavior
6. Mental health
7. Injury and violence
8. Environmental quality
9. Immunization
10. Access to health care

Source: Office of Disease Prevention and Health Promotion, U.S. Department of Health and Human Services, "Healthy People 2010," 2000. www.health.gov/healthypeople/About/hpfact.htm

help public health professionals determine the nature and extent of the health problem and the degree to which they are achieving their goals in each of the focus areas (see Table 1.1)

For each focus area, the plan presents specific objectives for the nation to achieve during the next decade. For instance, nutrition data show that only 42 percent of Americans aged 20 and older are at their healthy weight; the goal is to raise that number to 60 percent. In the focus area of physical activity and fitness, 40 percent of Americans aged 18 and older do not engage in any leisure-time physical activity. The objective is to reduce this number to 20 percent by 2010.[5] As part of the goal to eliminate health disparities, *Healthy People 2010* also must address issues of social justice. Disparities in health care among various groups are often the result of disadvantages faced by minority groups, women, and children, whose health care suffers due to their race, ethnicity, gender, and/or socioeconomic status. The attention to social justice issues in the *Healthy People 2010* program is designed to address these disparities.

Steps to a HealthierUS and Other Initiatives

An ambitious five-year program, *Steps to a HealthierUS: Putting Prevention First* was launched in 2003. It is designed to improve the lives of Americans through innovative and effective community-based chronic disease prevention and control programs. Many of the goals are the same as those of *Healthy People 2010*, but *HealthierUS* comes with a healthy influx of funding for research grants and programs to reduce the dual epidemics of obesity and diabetes, to get people moving, and to provide support for school and community-based intervention. Government officials, community leaders, public health officials, and health educators are encouraged to work together to make effective programs happen. The official website (www.healthierus.gov/steps) provides key information, reports on annual summits, and links to specific aspects of *Healthy People 2010* that are being implemented.

In addition to the *Healthy People* and *HealthierUS* plans, other programs and agencies also offer recommendations for improving the health of Americans. The Agency for Health Care Research and Quality (AHRQ) offers additional direction for national health care efforts through its *AHRQ Guidelines*, a set of objectives for health care providers to meet in specific areas of practice. Other government agencies and research centers also address specific health concerns. An example is *Best Practices for Comprehensive Tobacco Control Programs*, which recommends budgets and treatment guidelines to curb smoking.[6]

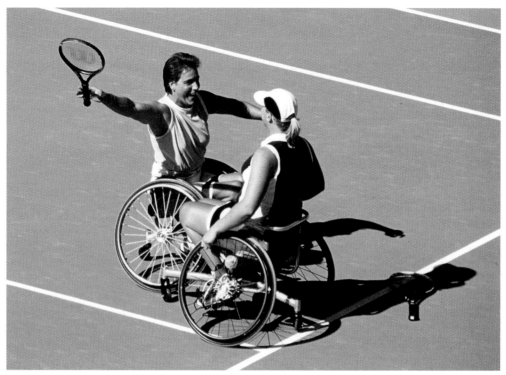

The motivation to improve quality of life within the framework of one's own unique capabilities is crucial to achieving health and wellness.

A New Focus on Health Promotion

The objectives of *Healthy People 2010* have prompted action to promote health and prevent premature disability through social, environmental, policy-related, and community-based programming. In addition, a new emphasis is emerging on assisting individuals in changing their healthy behaviors. However, changing behavior without help is not easy. The term **health promotion** describes the educational, organizational, procedural, environmental, social, and financial supports that help individuals and groups reduce negative health behaviors and promote positive change.

Health promotion programs identify healthy people who are engaging in **risk behaviors,** or actions that increase susceptibility to negative health outcomes, and motivate them to change their actions. Effective stop-smoking programs, for instance, don't simply say, "Just do it." Instead, they provide information about possible consequences to smokers and their sidestream smoke victims (educational

support); encourage smokers to participate in smoking cessation classes and allow time off for worker attendance or set up buddy systems to help them (organizational support); establish rules governing smokers' behaviors and supporting their decisions to change, such as banning smoking in the workplace and removing cigarettes from vending machines (environmental support); and provide monetary incentives to motivate people to participate (financial support).[7]

Health promotion programs also encourage those with sound health habits to maintain them. By attempting to modify behaviors, increase skills, change attitudes, increase knowledge, influence values, and improve health decision making, health promotion goes well beyond the simple information campaign. By basing programs and services in communities, organizations, schools, and other places where most people spend their time, health promotion increases the likelihood of long-term success on the road to health and wellness.

Whether we use the term *health* or *wellness,* we are talking about a person's overall responses to the challenges of living. Occasional dips into the ice cream bucket and other dietary indulgences, failures to exercise every day, flare-ups of anger, and other deviations from optimal behavior should not be viewed as major failures. Actually, the ability to recognize that each of us is an imperfect being attempting to adapt in an imperfect world signals individual well-being.

We must also remember to be tolerant of others. Rather than be warriors against pleasure in our zeal to change the health behaviors of others, we need to be supportive and nonjudgmental. We must avoid stigmatizing or ostracizing groups

Health promotion Combined educational, organizational, procedural, environmental, social, and financial supports that help people reduce negative health behaviors and promote positive change.

Risk behaviors Actions that increase susceptibility to negative health outcomes.

for being different. *Health bashing*—intolerance or negative feelings, words, or actions aimed at people who fail to meet our expectations of health—may indicate our own deficiencies in the emotional, social, and/or spiritual dimensions of health.

Disease Prevention

Most health promotion initiatives include **disease prevention.** Historically, the health literature describes three types of prevention: primary, secondary, and tertiary.

In a general sense, *prevention* means taking positive actions *now* to avoid becoming sick *later*. Getting immunized against diseases such as polio, deciding not to smoke cigarettes, and practicing safer sex constitute **primary prevention**—actions designed to reduce risk and avoid health problems before they start. **Secondary prevention** (also referred to as **intervention**) involves recognizing health risks or early problems and taking action (intervening) to stop them before they lead to actual illness. Getting a young smoker to quit is an example of secondary prevention. The third type of action, **tertiary prevention,** involves treatment and/or rehabilitation after a person is sick. Typically, health care professionals practice tertiary prevention.

In the United States, two of every three deaths and one of every three hospitalizations are linked to preventable lifestyle behaviors, such as tobacco use, sedentary lifestyle, alcohol consumption, and overeating. This means that primary and secondary prevention offer our best hope for reducing the **incidence** (number of new cases) and **prevalence** (number of existing cases) of disease and disability.

We need to move from a mind-set of tertiary prevention to a mind-set of early intervention designed to help individuals succeed in their behavior change strategies. Health educators in U.S. schools and communities offer an affordable and effective delivery of prevention and intervention programs. **Certified Health Education Specialists** make up a trained cadre of public health educators with special credentials and competencies in planning, implementing, and evaluating prevention programs that offer scientific, behaviorally based methods to help individuals and communities increase the likelihood of success in achieving good health. However, as a nation that historically spends little on prevention (less than 5 percent of our total national funding for health), such a shift in focus has been and will continue to be difficult.

Achievements in Public Health

To those of us in the field of public health, the saying "We've come a long way, baby" accurately reflects the health achievements of the past 100 years. According to the Centers for Disease Control and Prevention (CDC), here are the ten greatest public health achievements of the twentieth century:[8]

1. *Vaccinations.* Vaccinations have eradicated smallpox, eliminated poliomyelitis, and significantly controlled a number of infectious diseases, including measles, rubella, tetanus, diphtheria, and *Haemophilus influenzae* Type B, all of which killed large numbers of people in the early 1900s.

2. *Motor vehicle safety.* Improvements in motor vehicle safety have resulted from engineering efforts to make vehicles and highways safer and from successful efforts to change personal behavior, such as the use of safety belts, child safety seats, and motorcycle helmets, and the avoidance of drinking and driving.

3. *Workplace safety.* Work-related health risks common at the beginning of the century are now under better control or completely eliminated. Since 1980, the rate of fatal occupational injuries has fallen by 40 percent.

4. *Control of infectious diseases.* Clean water and improved sanitation have greatly reduced the development and transmission of infectious diseases. In addition, antimicrobial therapy, such as the use of antibiotics, has greatly reduced the risk of contracting diseases such as tuberculosis and sexually transmitted infections (STIs).

5. *Cardiovascular disease (CVD) and stroke deaths.* Efforts to educate the public on risk factors such as smoking and high blood pressure, coupled with improved access to early detection and better treatment, have reduced the rates of CVD and stroke.

6. *Safe and healthy foods.* Technology for eradicating microbial contaminants from foods has improved dramatically. In addition, the identification of essential micronutrients and establishment of food-fortification programs have almost eliminated major nutritional deficiencies such as rickets, goiter, and pellagra.

7. *Maternal and infant care.* Better hygiene and nutrition, improved availability of antibiotics, greater access to health care, and technological advances in medicine have greatly reduced the risks to infants and mothers. Since 1900, infant mortality has decreased by 90 percent, and maternal mortality has decreased by 99 percent.

Disease prevention Actions or behaviors designed to keep people from getting sick.

Primary prevention Actions designed to reduce risk and avoid health problems before they start.

Secondary prevention (intervention) Recognizing health risks and taking action to stop them before they lead to actual illness.

Tertiary prevention Treatment and/or rehabilitation after a person is sick.

Incidence The number of new cases.

Prevalence The number of existing cases.

Certified Health Education Specialists Academically trained health educators who have passed a national competency examination for prevention and intervention programming.

8. *Family planning.* Family planning and contraceptive services have altered social and economic roles of women. Family planning has decreased the number of infant, child, and maternal deaths; increased opportunities for preconceptional counseling and screening; and increased the use of barrier contraceptives to reduce unwanted pregnancies and transmission of sexually transmissible infections.

9. *Fluoridated drinking water.* Fluoridation of drinking water began in 1945. By 1999, an estimated 144 million persons in the United States drank fluoridated water. Fluoridation safely and inexpensively prevents tooth decay, regardless of socioeconomic status or access to health care. It has played an important role in reducing tooth decay in children and tooth loss in adults.

10. *Recognition of tobacco as a health hazard.* Public antismoking campaigns have changed social norms to prevent initiation of tobacco use, promote cessation, and reduce exposure to environmental tobacco smoke. Since the 1964 Surgeon General's report on the health risks of smoking, millions of smoking-related health problems have been prevented, and millions of lives have been saved.

While we have indeed come a long way, the possibilities for health and well-being in the future defy the imagination. Living longer, living more disease-free years, and injecting more quality into the extra years of life will be major goals. The more we learn about the remarkable resilience of the human body and spirit, and the more technology stretches our imagination and enlarges our possibilities, the more likely that the twenty-first century will surpass the twentieth in health-related breakthroughs.

> **What do you think?**
> *What do you consider the greatest achievements in public health in the twentieth century?* ✳ *What do you think would be the most important achievement that public health could make in the next 50 years?*

Gender Differences and Health Status

You don't have to be a health expert to know there are physiological differences between men and women. Although much of male and female anatomy is identical, major differences exist between the genders in such health factors as susceptibility to disease. Many diseases—osteoporosis, multiple sclerosis, and Alzheimer's disease, for example—are more common in women than in men. Finally, although women live longer than men, they don't necessarily enjoy better quality of life.[9]

Much of the current interest in exploring women's health came after 1990, when a highly publicized government study raised concern about the uneven numbers of women included in clinical trial research conducted by the National Institutes of Health (NIH). In response, the NIH established the Office of Research on Women's Health (ORWH) in 1990 to oversee the representation of women in NIH studies. According to Vivian Pinn, ORWH director, "For too long, medicine has viewed women as 'abnormal men' when considering health problems."[10]

Researchers exclude women of childbearing age from clinical trials of many new drugs for such reasons as concern about whether a medication might harm a fetus. Another concern is that women's menstrual cycles can influence the effects of a drug. Of course, men and women do vary physiologically, so the elimination of women from many studies means that the results from these studies cannot be applied to women directly.

To address these concerns, the government has specified that equal amounts of money and time must be spent on men's and women's health research.[11] The National Heart, Blood, and Lung Institute is conducting the **Women's Health Initiative (WHI).** This national 15-year, $625 million study focuses on the leading causes of death and disease in more than 160,000 postmenopausal women. WHI researchers hope to find out how a healthful lifestyle and increased medical attention can help prevent women's cancers, heart disease, and osteoporosis.[12]

> **What do you think?**
> *Do you think there are differences between men and women in their risks for certain diseases?* ✳ *Can you give examples?* ✳ *When you look at the leading causes of death in the U.S., how do men and women's rates differ?*

Improving Your Health

Factors Influencing Your Health Status

Table 1.2 summarizes by age the leading causes of death in the United States. Note that Americans aged 15 to 24 are most likely to die from unintentional injuries, followed by homicide and suicide. Unintentional injuries are also the major killer in the 25 to 44 age group, followed by cancer and heart disease.

Women's Health Initiative (WHI) National study focusing on the leading causes of death and disease in postmenopausal women, in conjunction with the NIH mandate for equal research priorities for women's health issues.

Table 1.2
Leading Causes of Death in the United States by Age (Years), 2001

Rank	All Ages	Under 1 Year	1–4	5–14	15–24	25–44	45–64	65+
1.	Diseases of heart 700,142	Congenital anomalies 5,513	Unintentional injuries 1,714	Unintentional injuries 2,836	Unintentional injuries 14,411	Unintentional injuries 27,784	Malignant neoplasms 139,785	Diseases of heart 582,730
2.	Malignant neoplasms 553,768	Short gestation or low birth weight 4,410	Congenital anomalies 558	Malignant neoplasms 1,008	Homicide 5,297	Malignant neoplasms 20,563	Diseases of heart 98,885	Malignant neoplasms 390,214
3.	Cerebrovascular diseases 163,538	Sudden infant death syndrome 2,234	Malignant neoplasms 420	Congenital anomalies 375	Suicide 3,971	Diseases of heart 16,486	Unintentional injuries 21,002	Cerebrovascular diseases 144,486
4.	Chronic lower respiratory diseases 123,013	Maternal complications 1,499	Homicide 415	Homicide 326	Malignant neoplasms 1,704	Suicide 11,705	Cerebrovascular diseases 15,518	Chronic lower respiratory diseases 106,904
5.	Unintentional injuries 101,537	Complications of placenta, cord, membranes 1,018	Diseases of heart 225	Suicide 279	Diseases of heart 999	Homicide 9,472	Diabetes mellitus 14,913	Influenza and pneumonia 55,518
6.	Diabetes mellitus 71,372	Respiratory distress 1,011	Influenza and pneumonia 112	Diseases of heart 272	Congenital anomalies 505	HIV disease 7,968	Chronic lower respiratory diseases 14,490	Diabetes mellitus 53,707
7.	Influenza and pneumonia 62,034	Unintentional injuries 976	Septicemia 108	In situ and benign neoplasms 105	HIV disease 225	Chronic liver disease and cirrhosis 3,723	Chronic liver disease and cirrhosis 13,009	Alzheimer's disease 53,245
8.	Alzheimer's disease 53,852	Bacterial sepsis 696	Conditions of perinatal period 72	Chronic lower respiratory diseases 104	Cerebrovascular diseases 196	Cerebrovascular diseases 3,092	Suicide 9,259	Nephritis, nephritic syndrome, and nephrosis 33,121
9.	Nephritis, nephritic syndrome, and nephrosis 39,480	Diseases of circulatory system 622	In situ and benign neoplasms 58	Influenza and pneumonia 92	Influenza and pneumonia 181	Diabetes mellitus 2,553	HIV disease 5,437	Unintentional injuries 32,694
10.	Septicemia 32,238	Intrauterine hypoxia/birth asphyxia 534	Cerebrovascular diseases 54	Cerebrovascular diseases 80	Chronic lower respiratory diseases 171	Influenza and pneumonia 1,322	Nephritis, nephritic syndrome, and nephrosis 5,106	Septicemia 25,418

Source: R. N. Anderson and B. L. Smith, "Deaths: Leading Causes for 2001," *National Vital Statistics Reports* 52 (Hyattsville, MD: National Center for Health Statistics, 2003).

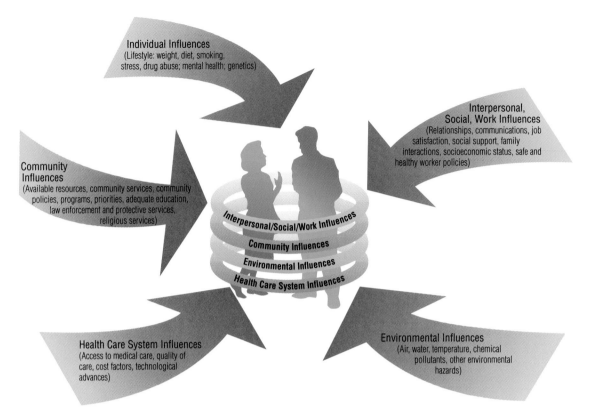

Figure 1.2
Factors That Influence Health Status

Individual behavior is a major determinant of good health. But health status can also be affected by interpersonal, social, and work influences; community influences; heredity; access to health care; and the environment (Figure 1.2). When these factors together form the basis of a person's lifestyle choices, the net effect on health can be great.

Healthy Behaviors

Most experts believe that several key behaviors will help people live longer, such as

- Getting a good night's sleep (minimum of seven hours)
- Maintaining healthy eating habits
- Managing weight
- Participating in physical recreational activities
- Avoiding tobacco products
- Practicing safer sex
- Limiting intake of alcohol
- Scheduling regular self-exams and medical checkups

Several other actions may not add years to your life, but they can add significant life to your years. They include:

- Controlling real and imaginary stressors
- Maintaining meaningful relationships with family and friends
- Making time for yourself
- Participating in at least one fun activity each day

- Respecting the environment and the people in it
- Considering alternatives when making decisions and assessing how actions affect others
- Valuing each day and making the best of opportunities
- Viewing mistakes as opportunities to learn and grow
- Being as kind to yourself as you are to others
- Understanding the health care system and using it wisely

Though it's easy to list things that one should do, change is not easy. All of us, no matter where we are on the health/wellness continuum, have to start somewhere. All people have faced personal and external challenges to their attempts to change health behaviors. Some have not done well, some have been successful, and some have made small changes that add up to significant improvements in how they feel and how they live.

Preparing for Behavior Change

As Mark Twain said, "Habit is habit, and not to be flung out the window by anyone, but coaxed downstairs a step at a time." The chances of successfully changing negative habits improve when you identify a key behavior that you want to change and develop a plan for gradual modification that allows you time to unlearn negative patterns and substitute positive ones.

Staging for Change

On any given morning, many of us get out of bed and resolve to change a given behavior that day. Whether it be losing weight, drinking less, exercising more, being nicer to others, or managing time better, we start out with enthusiasm and high expectations. Within a short time, however, a vast majority of people return to doing whatever it was they thought they shouldn't be doing.

Why do so many good intentions fail? According to Dr. James Prochaska, psychologist and head of the Health Promotion Partnership at the University of Rhode Island, and Dr. Carlos DiClemente, it's because we are going about things in the wrong way. According to Prochaska and DiClemente, fewer than 20% of us are really prepared to take action. Yet, health professionals continue to exhort us to "Just Do It! and do it now!" After considerable research, Prochaska and DiClemente believe that behavior changes usually do not succeed if they start with the change itself. Instead, we must go through a series of stages to adequately prepare ourselves for that eventual change. Our chances of keeping those New Year's resolutions will be greatly enhanced if we have proper reinforcement and help during each of the following stages.

1. *Precontemplation.* People in the precontemplation stage have no current intention of changing. They may have tried to change a behavior but gave up, or they may be in denial and unaware of any problem.
Strategies for Change: Sometimes a few frank yet kind words from friends may be enough to make precontemplators take a closer look at themselves. This is not to say that you should become a "warrior against pleasure" or tell precontemplators what to do when they haven't asked for advice. Recommending readings or giving tactful suggestions, however, can be useful in

helping precontemplators consider making a change.
2. *Contemplation.* In this phase, people recognize that they have a problem and begin to contemplate the need to change. Acknowledgment usually results from increased awareness often due to feedback from family and friends or access to information. Despite this acknowledgment, people can languish in this stage for years, realizing that they have a problem but lacking the time or energy to make the change.
Strategies for Change: Often, contemplators need a little push to get them started. This may come in the form of helping them set up a change plan (e.g., an exercise routine), buying a helpful gift (e.g., a low-fat cookbook), sharing articles about a particular problem, or inviting them to go with you to hear a speaker on a related topic. People often need time to think about a course of action or build skill. Your assistance can help them move off the point of indecision.
3. *Preparation.* Most people at this point are close to taking action. They've thought about what they might do and may even have come up with a plan. Rather than thinking about why they can't begin, they have started to focus on what they can do.
Strategies for Change: Those preparing for change need to follow a few standard guidelines: Set realistic goals (large and small), take small steps toward change, change only a few at once, reward small milestones, and seek support from friends. Identify those factors that have enabled success or served as a barrier to success in the past, and modify the latter where possible. Complete a Behavior Change Contract like the one at the end of this book to help commit to making these changes.
4. *Action.* In this stage, people begin to follow their action plans. Those who have prepared for change, thought about alternatives, engaged social sup-

port, and made a plan of action are more ready for action than those who have given it little thought. Unfortunately, too many people start behavior change here rather than going through the first three stages. Without a plan, without enlisting the help of others, or without a realistic goal, failure is likely.
Strategies for Change: Publicly stating the desire to change helps ensure success. Encourage friends who are making a change to share their plans with you. Offer to help, and try to remove potential obstacles from the person's intended action plan. Social support and the buddy system can motivate even the most reluctant person.
5. *Maintenance.* Maintenance requires vigilance, attention to detail, and long-term commitment. Many people reach their goals only to slip back into the undesired behavior. In this stage, it is important to be aware of the common causes of relapse, such as overconfidence, daily temptations, stress or emotional distractions, and self-deprecation, and develop strategies for dealing with them.
Strategies for Change: During maintenance, continue taking the same actions that led to success in the first place. Find fun and creative ways to maintain positive behaviors. This is where a willing and caring support group can be vital. Knowing where to turn on your campus for help when you don't have a close support network is also helpful.
6. *Termination.* By this point, the behavior is so ingrained that the current level of vigilance may be unnecessary. The new behavior has become an essential part of daily living. Can you think of someone you know who has succeeded in making a major behavior change?

Source: J. Prochaska, C. DiClemente, and J. Norcross, "In Search of How People Change: Application to Addictive Behaviors," *American Psychologist* 47, no. 9: 1102–1114.

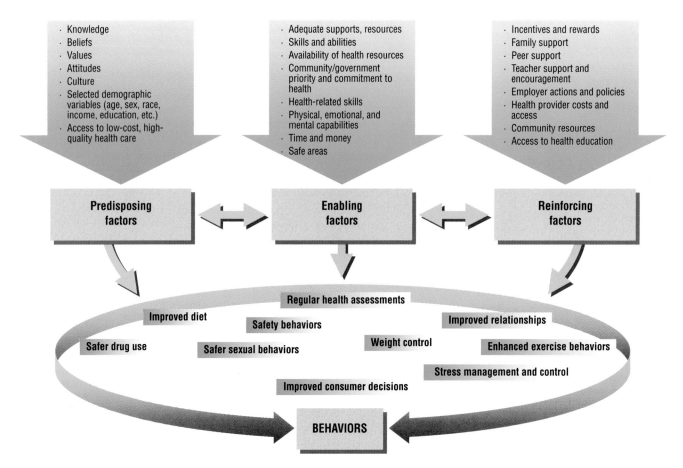

Figure 1.3
Factors That Influence Behavior-Change Decisions

Factors Influencing Behavior Change

Figure 1.3 identifies major factors that influence behavior and behavior-change decisions. They can be divided into three general categories: predisposing factors, enabling factors, and reinforcing factors.

Predisposing Factors Our life experiences, knowledge, cultural and ethnic heritage, and current beliefs and values are all *predisposing factors* that influence behavior. Factors that may predispose us to certain conditions include age, sex, race, income, family background, educational background, and access to health care. For example, if your parents smoked, you are 90 percent more likely to start smoking than someone whose parents didn't smoke. If your peers smoke, you are 80 percent more likely to smoke than someone whose friends don't smoke.

Enabling Factors Skills and abilities; physical, emotional, and mental capabilities; community and government priorities and commitment to health; and safe and convenient resources and facilities that make health decisions easy or difficult are *enabling factors.* Positive enablers encourage you to carry through on your intentions to change. Negative enablers work

against your intentions to change. For example, if you would like to join a local fitness center but discover that the closest one is four miles away and the membership fee is $500, those negative enablers may convince you to stay home. On the other hand, if your school's fitness center is two blocks away, stays open until midnight, and offers a special student membership, those positive enablers will probably convince you to join. Identifying positive and negative enabling factors and devising alternative plans when the negative factors outweigh the positive are part of planning for behavior change.

Reinforcing Factors *Reinforcing factors* include the presence or absence of support, encouragement, or discouragement that significant people in your life bring to a situation; employer actions and policies; health provider costs and access; community resources; and access to health education. For example, if you decide to stop smoking and your family and friends continue smoking in your presence, you may be tempted to start smoking again. In other words, your smoking behavior is reinforced. If, however, you are overweight and you lose a few pounds and all your friends tell you how terrific you look, your positive behavior is reinforced and you will likely continue your weight-loss plan.

Consumer Beware: Health Information on the Internet

Are you looking for health information? You should always consult your doctor first. But there also is a huge resource right at your fingertips: the Internet. Each year more than 100 million people seek health information on the Internet. Many of them end up frazzled, confused, and—worst of all—misinformed.

Clearly, not all health websites are created equal. Here are some tips to point you in the right direction.

- Websites sponsored by an official government agency, a university or college, or a hospital/medical center typically offer accurate, up-to-date information about a wide range of health topics. Government sites are easily identified by their .gov extensions (National Institute of Mental Health: www.nimh.nih. gov); college and university sites typically have .edu extensions (Johns Hopkins University is www.jhu.edu). Hospitals often have an .org extension (Mayo Clinic: www.mayoclinic.org). Major philanthropic foundations, such as the Robert Wood Johnson Foundation, the Legacy Foundation, and the Kellogg Foundation, also provide information about selected health topics.
- Links associated with well-established, professionally peer-reviewed journals such as *The New England Journal of Medicine* (http://content.nejm.org) or *The Journal of the American Medical Association (JAMA)* (http://jama.ama-assn.org) are good sources. While some of these sites require a fee for access, often you can locate basic abstracts and information such as a weekly table of contents that can help you conduct a search. Other times, you can pay a basic fee for a certain number of hours of unlimited searching.
- For consumer news and updates on health-related hoaxes, consult the Centers for Disease Control and Prevention (CDC). The CDC provides consumer alerts on topics such as buying antibiotics online and email health hoaxes. A sampler of recent email scares include poisonous perfume samples in the mail, underarm deodorants causing breast cancer, and transmission of human immunodeficiency virus (HIV) by contact with unused feminine (sanitary) pads. If you receive an email warning about a health topic, check the CDC hoax and rumor site (www.cdc.gov/hoax_rumors.htm) before giving it credibility.
- Use discretion, and don't believe everything you read. Cross-check information against reliable sources to see if facts and figures are consistent. Quackery runs rampant on the Internet, particularly on sites that are trying to sell you a quick fix for a health problem. Just because a source claims to be a physician or an expert does not mean that this is true. When in doubt, check with your own medical doctor, health education professor, or state health division website. There are many government and education sites that are independently sponsored and reliable. The following is just a sample. Others are provided in each chapter as we cover specific topics:

1. Aetna InteliHealth: www.intelihealth.com
2. drkoop.com: www.drkoop.com
3. WebMD Health: http://my.webmd.com
4. druginfonet.com: www.druginfonet.com
5. healthAtoZ.com: www.healthatoz.com

The American Accreditation HealthCare Commission (www.urac.org) has devised 50 criteria that health sites must meet to win its seal of approval, which makes it a little easier to determine a website's credibility. A rating scale and visible seal will tell you at a glance whether a site meets these rigorous standards. In addition to policing the accuracy of health claims, this accreditation will evaluate health information and provide a forum for reporting misinformation, privacy violations, and other complaints.

Source: Laura Landro, "Health Journal: Online Groups Step Up Attempts to Enforce Standards," *The Wall Street Journal,* July 20, 2001, B1.

The manner in which you reward or punish yourself in the process of change also plays a role. Accepting small failures and concentrating on your successes can foster further achievements. Berating yourself because you binged on ice cream or argued with a friend may create an internal environment in which failure becomes almost inevitable. Telling yourself that you're worth the extra effort and giving yourself a pat on the back for small accomplishments are often overlooked factors in positive behavior change. It is also important to invest time in your friendships. Not only is it rewarding to spend time with your friends, but when you need help making a change, you'll have the social support you need.

Motivation and Readiness

Your *motivation* to do something is your reason for doing it. For some people, motivation may come from an external reward or incentive, such as a bonus check. For others, it may be an internal reward such as a feeling of prestige or accomplishment. Finding the right motivator is key to making a positive change. Motivation must be combined with common sense, commitment, and a realistic understanding of how best to move from point A to point B.[13] *Readiness* is the state of being that precedes behavior change. People who are ready to change possess the attitudes, knowledge, skills, and internal and external resources that make change possible.

Beliefs and Attitudes

We often assume that when rational people realize their actions put them at risk, they will act to reduce that risk. But this is not necessarily true. Consider the number of health professionals who smoke, consume high-fat diets, and act in other unhealthy ways. They surely know better, but their knowledge is disconnected from their action. Why is this so? Two strong influences on behavior are at work: beliefs and attitudes.

A **belief** is an appraisal of the relationship between some object, action, or idea (for example, smoking) and some attribute of that object, action, or idea (for example, smoking is expensive, dirty, and causes cancer—or, it is relaxing). An **attitude** is a relatively stable set of beliefs, feelings, and behavioral tendencies in relation to something or someone.

Psychologists studying the relationship between beliefs and health habits have determined that although beliefs can subtly influence behavior, they may not actually cause people to behave differently. In 1966, psychologist I. Rosenstock developed a classic theory, the **Health Belief Model (HBM),** to show when beliefs affect behavior change.[14] Although many other models attempt to explain the influence of beliefs on behaviors, the HBM remains one of the most widely accepted. It holds that several factors must support a belief before change is likely.

- *Perceived seriousness of the health problem.* How severe would the medical and social consequences be if the health problem were to develop or to be left untreated? The more serious the perceived effects, the more likely that the person will take action.
- *Perceived susceptibility to the health problem.* What is the likelihood of developing the health problem? People who perceive themselves at high risk are more likely to take preventive action.
- *Cues to action.* Those who are reminded or alerted about a potential health problem are more likely to take action. For example, having your doctor tell you that your blood sugar levels indicate a prediabetic state may be the cue that pushes you to lose weight and exercise.

Three other factors are linked to perceived risk for health problems: *demographic variables,* including age, gender, race, and ethnic background; *sociopsychological variables,* including personality traits, social class, and social pressure; and *structural variables,* including knowledge about or prior contact with the health problem.

People follow the HBM many times every day. Take, for example, smokers. Older smokers are likely to know other smokers who have developed serious heart or lung problems. They are thus more likely to perceive tobacco as a threat to their health than a teenager will who has just begun smoking. The greater the perceived threat of health problems caused by smoking, the greater the chance a person will quit.

However, many chronic smokers know the risks yet continue to smoke. Why do they miss these cues to action? According to Rosenstock, some people do not believe that they will be affected by a problem—they act as if they have some kind of immunity to it—and are unlikely to change their behavior. In some cases, they may think that even if they get cancer or have a heart attack, the health care system will cure them. They also may feel that the immediate pleasure outweighs the long-range cost.

Intentions to Change

Our attitudes reflect our emotional responses to situations and follow from our beliefs. According to the **Theory of Reasoned Action,** our behaviors result from our intentions to perform actions. An intention is a product of our attitude toward an action and our beliefs about what others may want us to do.[15] A behavioral intention, then, is a written or stated commitment to perform an action.

In brief, the more consistent and powerful your attitudes about an action and the more you are influenced by others to take that action, the greater will be your stated intention to do so. The more you verbalize your commitment to change, the more likely you are to succeed. The more you have social support from family and friends to encourage you, the more your intentions will be bolstered.

Significant Others as Change Agents

Many of us are highly influenced by the approval or disapproval (real or imagined) of close friends, loved ones, and the social and cultural groups to which we belong. Such influences can support healthy behavior or interfere with even the best intentions.

Your Family From the time of your birth, your parents or other family members have given you strong cues about which actions are and are not socially acceptable. Brushing your teeth, bathing, wearing deodorant, and chewing food with your mouth closed are behaviors that your family probably instilled in you long ago. Your family culture influenced your food choices, religious and political beliefs, and all your other values and actions. If you deviated from your family's norms, your mother, father, or other family member probably

---

Belief Appraisal of the relationship between some object, action, or idea and some attribute of that object, action, or idea.

Attitude Relatively stable set of beliefs, feelings, and behavioral tendencies in relation to something or someone.

Health Belief Model (HBM) Model for explaining how beliefs may influence behaviors.

Theory of Reasoned Action Model for explaining the importance of our intentions in determining behaviors.

let you know fairly quickly. Good family units share unconditional trust, dedication to the healthful development of all family members, and commitment to work out difficulties.

When a loving family unit does not exist, when it does not provide for basic human needs, or when dysfunctional, irresponsible individuals try to build a family under the influence of drugs or alcohol, it becomes difficult for a child to learn positive health behaviors. Healthy behaviors get their start in healthy homes; unhealthy homes breed unhealthy habits. Healthy families provide the foundation for a clear and necessary understanding of what is right and wrong, what is positive and negative. Without this fundamental grounding, many young people have great difficulties.[16]

Your Social Bonds   Like family, personal environments also mold behaviors. If you deviated from the actions expected in your hometown, you probably suffered strange looks, ostracism by some high school cliques, and other negative social reactions. The more you value the opinions of other people, the more likely you are to change a behavior that offends them. If you couldn't care less what they think, you probably brush off their negative reactions. How often have you told yourself, "I don't care what so-and-so thinks; I'll do what I darn well please"? Although most of us have thought or said these words, often we care too much about what even the insignificant people in our lives think. In general, the lower your self-esteem and self-efficacy, the higher the chances that others will influence your actions.

Sometimes, the influence of others can be a powerful social support for positive behavior changes.[17] At other times, we are influenced to drink too much, party too hard, eat too much, or engage in some other negative action because we don't want to be left out or criticized. Learning to understand the subtle and not-so-subtle ways in which other people influence our actions is an important step toward changing our behaviors.

Choosing a Behavior-Change Strategy

Once you have analyzed all the factors that influence what you do, decide which behavior-change technique will work best for you. These techniques include shaping, visualization, modeling, controlling the situation, reinforcement, and changing self-talk.

Shaping

Regardless of how motivated you are, some behaviors are almost impossible to change immediately. To reach your goal, you may need to take a number of steps, each designed to change one small piece of the larger behavior. This process is known as **shaping.**

For example, suppose that you have not exercised for a while. You decide that you want to get into shape, and your goal is to jog three miles every other day. But you realize that you'd face a near-death experience if you tried to run even a few blocks in your current condition. So you decide to build up to your desired fitness level gradually. During week 1, you will walk for one hour every other day at a slow, relaxed pace. During week 2, you will walk for the same amount of time but speed up your pace and cover slightly more ground. During week 3, you will speed up even more and try to go even farther. You will continue taking such steps until you reach your goal.

Whatever the desired behavior change, all shaping involves the following actions:

- Start slowly, and try not to cause undue stress during the early stages of the program
- Keep the steps small and achievable
- Be flexible and ready to change if the original plan proves uncomfortable
- Refuse to skip steps or move to the next step until you have mastered the previous one

Behaviors don't develop overnight, so they won't change overnight.

Visualization

Mental practice can transform unhealthy behaviors into healthy ones. Athletes and others use a technique known as **imagined rehearsal** to reach their goals. By visualizing their planned action ahead of time, they are better prepared when they put themselves to the test.

For example, suppose you want to ask someone out on a date. Imagine the setting (walking together to class). Then practice exactly what you want to say ("Marcie, there's a great concert this Sunday, and I was wondering if. . . .") in your mind and aloud. Mentally anticipate different responses ("Oh, I'd love to, but I'm busy that evening. . . .") and what you will say in reaction ("How about if I call you sometime this week?"). Careful mental and verbal rehearsal—you could even try out your scenario on a friend—will greatly improve the likelihood of success.

Modeling

Modeling, or learning specific behaviors by watching others perform them, is one of the most effective strategies for

---

Shaping   Using a series of small steps to reach a particular goal gradually.

Imagined rehearsal   Practicing, through mental imagery, to become better able to perform an actual event.

Modeling   Learning specific behaviors by watching others perform them.

changing behavior. For example, suppose that you have trouble talking to people you don't know very well. One of the easiest ways to improve your communication skills is to select friends whose social skills you envy. Observe them. Do they talk more or listen more? How do people respond to them? Why are they such good communicators? If you observe behaviors you admire and isolate their components, you can model the steps of your behavior-change strategy on a proven success.

Controlling the Situation

Sometimes, the right setting or the right group of people will positively influence your behaviors. Many situations and occasions trigger certain actions. For example, in libraries, houses of worship, and museums, most people talk softly. Few people laugh at funerals. The term **situational inducement** refers to an attempt to influence a behavior by using occasions and social settings to control it.

For example, you may be more apt to stop smoking if you work in a smoke-free office, a positive situational inducement. But a smoke-filled bar, a negative situational inducement, may tempt you to resume or to keep smoking. Careful consideration of which settings will help and which will hurt your effort to change, and your decision to seek the first and avoid the second, will improve your chances for change.

Reinforcement

A **positive reinforcement** seeks to increase the likelihood that a behavior will occur by presenting a reward for it. Each of us is motivated by different reinforcers. Although a special t-shirt may be a positive reinforcer for young adults entering a race, for example, it would not be for a 40-year-old runner who dislikes message-bearing t-shirts.

Most positive reinforcers can be classified into five categories: consumable, activity, manipulative, possessional, and social.

- *Consumable reinforcers* are delicious edibles, such as candy, cookies, or gourmet meals.
- *Activity reinforcers* are opportunities to do something enjoyable, such as watching TV or going on a vacation.
- *Manipulative reinforcers* are incentives, such as getting a lower rent in exchange for mowing the lawn or the promise of a better grade for doing an extra-credit project.
- *Possessional reinforcers* are tangible rewards, such as a new TV or a sports car.
- *Social reinforcers* are signs of appreciation, approval, or love, such as loving looks, affectionate hugs, and praise.

Situational inducement   Attempt to influence a behavior through occasions and social settings that are structured to exert control over that behavior.

Positive reinforcement   Presenting a reward following a behavior to increase the likelihood that the behavior will be repeated.

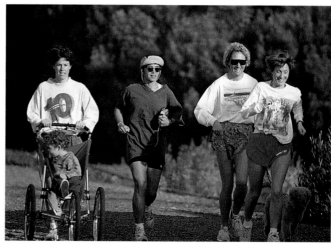

The support and encouragement of friends who have similar goals and interests will strengthen your commitment to develop and maintain positive health behaviors.

When choosing reinforcers, determine what would motivate you to act in a particular way. Research has shown that people can be motivated to change their behaviors, such as not smoking during pregnancy or abstaining from cocaine, if they set up a *token economy* system whereby they earn tokens or points that can be exchanged for meaningful rewards, such as financial incentives.[18] The difficulty often lies in determining *which* incentive will be most effective. Your reinforcers may initially come from others (extrinsic rewards), but as you see positive changes in yourself, you will begin to reward and reinforce yourself (intrinsic rewards). Although reinforcers should immediately follow a behavior, beware of overkill. If you reward yourself with a movie every time you go jogging, this reinforcer will soon lose its power. It would be better to give yourself this reward after, say, a full week of adhering to your jogging program.

What do you think?
What consumable reinforcers would be a healthy reward for your new behavior? ✱ *If you could choose one activity reinforcer with which to reward yourself after one week of success in your new behavior, what would it be?* ✱ *If you could obtain something (possessional reinforcer) after you reach your goal, what would it be?* ✱ *If you maintain your behavior for one week, what type of social reinforcer would you like to receive from your friends?*

Changing Self-Talk

Self-talk, or the way you think and talk to yourself, can also play a role in modifying health-related behaviors. Here are some cognitive procedures for changing self-talk.

Rational-Emotive Therapy   This form of cognitive therapy or self-directed behavior change is based on the premise that there is a close connection between what people say to themselves and how they feel. According to psychologist Albert Ellis, most emotional problems and related behaviors stem from irrational statements that people make to themselves when events in their lives are different from what they would like them to be.[19]

For example, suppose that after doing poorly on a test, you say to yourself, "I can't believe I flunked that easy exam. I'm so stupid." By changing this irrational, "catastrophic" self-talk into rational, positive statements about what is really going on, you increase the likelihood that positive behaviors will occur. Positive self-talk might be phrased as follows: "I really didn't study enough for that exam, and I'm not surprised I didn't do very well. I'm certainly not stupid. I just need to prepare better for the next test." Such self-talk will help you to recover quickly and take positive steps to correct the situation.

Meichenbaum's Self-Instructional Methods   Behavioral psychologist Donald Meichenbaum is perhaps best known for a process known as stress inoculation, which subjects clients to extreme stressors in a laboratory environment. Before a stressful event (e.g., going to the doctor), clients practice coping skills (e.g., deep breathing exercises) and self-instruction (e.g., "I'll feel better once I know what is causing my pain"). Meichenbaum's clients are also encouraged to give themselves "self-instructions" ("Slow down, don't rush") and "positive affirmations" ("My speech is going fine—I'm almost done!") instead of self-defeating thoughts ("I'm talking too fast—my speech is terrible"). Meichenbaum demonstrated that clients who practice coping techniques and self-instruction are less likely to resort to negative behaviors in difficult situations.

Blocking/Thought Stopping   By purposefully blocking or stopping negative thoughts, a person can concentrate on taking positive steps. For example, suppose you are preoccupied with your ex-partner, who has recently deserted you for someone else. You consciously stop dwelling on the situation and force yourself to think about something more pleasant (e.g., dinner tomorrow with your best friend). By refusing to dwell on negative images and forcing yourself to focus elsewhere, you can save wasted energy, time, and emotional resources and move on to positive change.

Changing Your Behavior

Self-Assessment: Antecedents and Consequences

Behaviors, thoughts, and feelings always occur in a context, that is, in a situation. Situations can be divided into two components: the events that come before and after. *Antecedents* are the setting events for a behavior; they stimulate a person to act in certain ways. Antecedents can be physical events, thoughts, emotions, or the actions of other people. *Consequences*—the results of behavior—affect whether a person will repeat that action.[20] Consequences also can consist of physical events, thoughts, emotions, or the actions of other people.

Suppose you are shy and must give a speech in front of a large class. The antecedents include walking into the class, feeling frightened, wondering whether you are capable of doing a good job, and being unable to remember a word of your speech. If the consequences are negative—if your classmates laugh and you get a low grade—your terror about speaking in public will be reinforced, and you will continue to dread this kind of event. In contrast, if you receive positive feedback from the class or instructor, you may actually learn to like speaking in public.

Learning to recognize the antecedents of a behavior and acting to modify them is one method of changing behavior. A diary noting your undesirable behaviors and identifying the settings in which they occur can be a useful tool. Figure 1.4 identifies several factors that can make behavior change more difficult.

Analyzing Personal Behavior

Successful behavior change requires determining what you want to change. All too often we berate ourselves by using generalities: "I'm lousy to my friends, I need to be a better person." Determining the specific behavior you would like to modify—in contrast to the general problem—will allow you to set clear goals. What are you doing that makes you a lousy friend? Are you gossiping or lying about your friends? Have you been a taker rather than a giver? Or are you really a good friend most of the time?

Let's say the problem is gossiping. You can analyze this behavior by examining the following components.

- *Frequency.* How often do you gossip—all the time or only once in a while?
- *Duration.* How long have you been doing this?
- *Seriousness.* Is your gossiping just idle chatter, or are you really trying to injure other people? What are the consequences for you? For your friends? For your relationships?
- *Basis for problem behavior.* Is your gossip based on facts, perceptions of facts, or deliberate embellishment of the truth?
- *Antecedents.* What kinds of situations trigger your gossiping? Do some settings or people bring it out in you more than others do? What triggers your feelings of dislike or irritation toward your friends? Why are you talking behind their backs?

Decision Making: Choices for Change

Now it is time to make a decision that will lead to positive health outcomes. Try to anticipate what might occur in a

OBSTACLE	STRATEGY
Stress (intrinsic and extrinsic)	Identify potential sources of stress. Find constructive ways to lower stress level.
Social pressures to repeat old habits	Enlist the support of friends. Identify specifics of these pressures.
Not expecting mistakes, perfectionist, hypercritical	Accept that slips are inevitable, but maintain control. Acknowledge that humans are imperfect beings.
Self-blame for poor coping or a weak personality	Blame pressures from the environment or lack of skills, rather than innate weakness.
Lack of effort, lack of motivation	Assess effort and make sure it is adequate. Provide rewards for successes.
Faulty beliefs, low self-efficacy	Develop new skills, focus on successes, and plan ahead for difficult situations. Change self-talk.

Figure 1.4
Obstacles to Behavior Change
Psychologists list a number of obstacles that might contribute to failing to change your behavior and strategies for overcoming these obstacles.
Source: From *Self-Directed Behavior: Self-Modification for Personal Adjustment, eighth edition* by D. L. Watson and R. G. Tharp. © 2002 by Wadsworth Publishing, a division of Thomson Publishing Inc. Reprinted by permission of the publisher.

given setting and think through all possible safe alternatives. For example, knowing that you are likely to be offered a drink when you go to a party, what response could you make that would be okay in your social group? If someone is flirting with you and the conversation takes on a distinct sexual overtone, what might you do to prevent the situation from turning bad? Advance preparation will help you stick to your behavior plan.

Remember that things typically don't just happen. By staying alert to potential problems, being aware of your alternatives, maintaining a good sense of your values, and sticking to your beliefs under pressure, you can gain control over many situations in your life.

Setting Realistic Goals

Changing behavior is not easy, but sometimes we make it even harder by setting unrealistic and unattainable goals. To start making positive changes, ask yourself these questions.

1. *What do I want?* What is your ultimate goal—to lose weight? Exercise more? Reduce stress? Have a lasting relationship? Whatever it is, you need a clear picture of the target outcome.

2. *Which change is the greatest priority at this time?* Often people decide to change several things all at once. Suppose that you are gaining unwanted weight. Rather than saying "I need to eat less, start jogging, and really get in shape," be specific about the current behavior you need to change. Are you eating too many sweets? Too many high-fat foods? Perhaps a realistic goal would be, "I am going to try to eat less fat during dinner every day." Choose the behavior that constitutes your greatest problem, and tackle that first. You can always work on something else later. Take small steps, experiment with alternatives, and find the best way to meet your goals.

3. *Why is this change important to me?* Think through why you want to change. Are you doing it because of your health? To look better? To win someone else's approval? Usually, doing something because it's right for you rather than to win others' approval is a sound strategy. If you are changing for someone else, what happens when that other person isn't around?

4. *What are the potential positive outcomes?* What do you hope to accomplish?

5. *What health-promoting programs and services can help me get started?* Nearly all campuses offer helpful resources.

You might buy a self-help book at the campus bookstore, speak to a counselor, or enroll in an aerobics class at the local fitness center.

6. *Are there family or friends whose help I can enlist?* Social support is one of your most powerful allies. Getting a friend to exercise with you, asking your partner to help you stop smoking by quitting at the same time you do, and making a commitment with a friend to never let each other drive if you've been drinking alcohol—these are all examples of how people can help each other make positive changes.

What do you think?

Why is it sometimes hard to make decisions? ✷
What factors influence your decision making? ✷
Select one behavior that you want to change and refer to the Behavior Change Contract at the end of this book. Using the goal-setting strategies discussed here, outline a plan for change.

Taking Charge

Make It Happen!

Assessment: The Assess Yourself box on page 6 gave you the chance to look at the status of your health in several dimensions. Now that you have considered these results, you can begin to take steps toward changing certain behaviors that may be detrimental to your health.

Making a Change: In order to change your behavior, you need to develop a plan. Follow these steps:

1. Evaluate your behavior, and identify patterns and specific things you are doing. What can you change now? What can you change in the near future?
2. Select one pattern of behavior that you want to change.
3. Fill out a Behavior Change Contract. It should include your long-term goal for change, your short-term goals, the rewards you'll give yourself for reaching these goals, potential obsta-

cles along the way, and strategies for overcoming these obstacles. For each goal, list the small steps and specific actions that you will take.

4. Chart your progress in a journal. At the end of a week, consider how successful you were in following your plan. What helped you be successful? What made change more difficult? What will you do differently next week?
5. Revise your plan as needed. Are the short-term goals attainable? Are the rewards satisfying?

Example: Felipe assessed his health and discovered that his score in the Personal Health Promotion section was low—25 points—because of some risky behaviors in which he was engaging. In particular, he realized that he had driven several times after drinking and that he was not performing monthly testicle self-examinations. Felipe decided to tackle one of these issues at a time. He completed a Behavior Change Contract to drive only

when he had had fewer than two drinks. Steps in his contract included finding out about designated driver programs, moderating his drinking so that he was sober and competent to drive at the end of a night out with friends, and finding concerts and other events to attend that did not involve drinking. The rewards he chose for these steps included tickets to a concert and a new computer game. After a few months, Felipe realized that he had been in several situations in which he might previously have driven under the influence. Instead, he had given himself alternatives such as designated drivers, budgeting for a taxi, and moderating his drinking, and thus had avoided unsafe situations.

Next month, Felipe will get a pamphlet from the health center on testicular self-exams and choose a day of the month to be his self-examination day. Every month that he does the exam, he'll sleep in an extra hour that weekend as a reward.

Summary

✷ Health encompasses the entire dynamic process of fulfilling one's potential in the physical, social, emotional, spiritual, intellectual, and environmental dimensions of life. Wellness means achieving the highest level of health possible in several dimensions.

✷ Although the average American life expectancy has increased over the past century, we need to increase the span of quality of life. Programs such as *Healthy People 2000* and *2010, HealthierUS,* and documents such as the *AHRQ Guidelines* have established national objectives for improving life span and quality of life for all Americans through health promotion and disease prevention.

☀ Gender continues to play a major role in health status and care. Women have longer lives but more medical problems than do men. To close the gender gap in health care, researchers have begun to include more women in medical research and training.

☀ For the U.S. population as a whole, the leading causes of death are heart disease, cancer, and stroke. But in the 15- to 24-year-old age group, the leading causes are unintentional injuries, homicide and legal intervention, and suicide. Many of the risks associated with heart disease, cancer, and stroke can be reduced through lifestyle changes. Many of the risks associated with accidents, homicide, and suicide can be reduced through preventive measures.

☀ Several factors contribute to a person's health status, and a number of them are within our control. Beliefs and attitudes, intentions to change, support from significant others, and readiness to change are factors over which individuals have some degree of control. Access to health care, genetic predisposition, health policies that support positive choices, and other factors are all potential reinforcing, predisposing, and enabling factors that may influence health decisions.

☀ Applying behavior-change techniques, such as shaping, visualization, modeling, controlling the situation, reinforcement, and changing self-talk help people succeed in making behavior changes.

☀ Decision making has several key components. Each person must explore his or her own problems, the reasons for change, and the expected outcomes. The next step is to plan a course of action best suited to the individual's needs.

Questions for Discussion and Reflection

1. How are the terms *health* and *wellness* similar? What, if any, are important distinctions between these terms? What is health promotion? Disease prevention? What does it really mean to be healthy?

2. How healthy are Americans today? How will health promotion and illness and accident prevention both increase life expectancy and improve quality of life right now? In the future?

3. What are some of the major differences in the way men and women are treated in the health care system? Why do you think these differences exist?

4. What are the leading causes of death across different ages and races? What are the leading causes of death for Americans aged 15 to 24? Why are these statistics so different? Explain why it is important to look at these statistics by age rather than just looking at them in total. What lifestyle changes can you make to lower your risks for contracting major diseases?

5. What is the HBM? What is the Theory of Reasoned Action? How may each of these models operate when a young woman decides to smoke her first cigarette? Her last cigarette?

6. Explain the predisposing, reinforcing, and enabling factors that might influence a young mother on welfare as she decides whether to sell drugs to support her children.

7. Using the Stages of Change model found in the Skills for Behavior Change box on page 17, discuss what you might do (in stages) to help a friend stop smoking. Why is it important that a person be ready to change before trying to change?

Accessing Your Health on the Internet

Visit the following Internet sites to explore further topics and issues related to personal health. To visit an organization's website, go to the Companion Website for *Health: The Basics, Sixth Edition* at www.aw-bc.com/donatelle, click on the book image, and select "Accessing Your Health on the Internet" from the navigation menu on the left.

1. *CDC Wonder.* Outstanding reference for comprehensive information from the CDC, including special reports, guidelines, and access to national health data.

2. *Mayo Clinic.* Reputable resource for specific information about health topics, diseases, and treatment options. Easy to navigate and consumer friendly.

3. *National Center for Health Statistics.* Outstanding place to start for information about health status in the United States. Links to key documents such as *Health United States* (published yearly); national survey information; and information on mortality by age, race, gender, geographic location, and other important data. Includes comprehensive information provided by the CDC as well as easy links to at least ten of the major health resources currently being used for policy and decision making about health in the United States.

4. *National Health Information Center.* Excellent resource for consumer information about health.

5. *Web MD.* Reputable and comprehensive overview of various diseases and conditions. Written for the public in an easy-to-understand format with links to more in-depth information.

Further Reading

Robins, Alexander, and Abby Wilner. *Quarterlife Crisis: The Unique Challenges of Life in Your 20s.* New York: JP Tarcher Paperbacks, 2001.

Overview of challenges facing young adults in America today.

U.S. Department of Health and Human Services. *Healthy People 2010: National Health Promotion and Disease Prevention Objectives for the Year 2010.* Washington, DC: Government Printing Office, 1998.

This plan constitutes the Surgeon General's long-range goals for increasing life expectancy for all Americans by three years and improving access to health for all Americans, regardless of sex, race, socioeconomic status, and other variables.

U.S. Department of Health and Human Services. *Health United States: 2003.* Centers for Disease Control and Prevention. Washington, DC: Government Printing Office, 2003.

Provides an up-to-date overview of U.S. health statistics, risk factors, and trends.

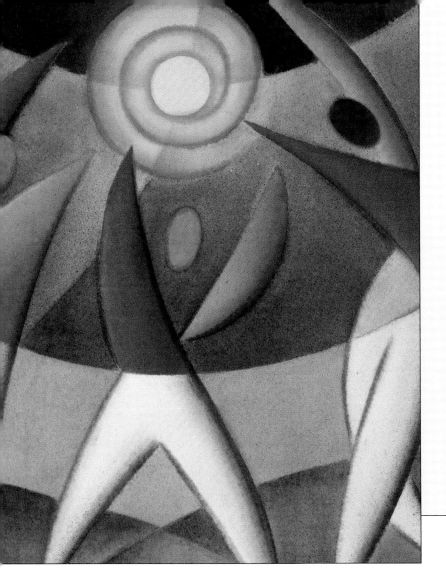

Psychosocial Health

Being Mentally, Emotionally, Socially, and Spiritually Well

Objectives

* Define psychosocial health in terms of its mental, emotional, social, and spiritual components, and identify the basic traits shared by psychosocially healthy people.

* Consider how each internal and external factor that influences psychosocial health may affect you.

* Discuss the positive steps you can take to enhance psychosocial health.

* Discuss the mind–body connection and show how emotions influence health status.

* Identify and describe common psychosocial problems of adulthood and explain their causes,

methods of prevention, and available treatments.

* Illustrate the warning signs of suicide and actions that can be taken to help a suicidal individual.

* Explain the goals and methods of different types of health professionals and therapies.

The New York Times
In the News

Debate Resumes on the Safety of Depression's Wonder Drugs

By Gardiner Harris

Warnings by drug regulators about the safety of Paxil, one of the world's most prescribed antidepressants, are reopening seemingly settled questions about a whole class of drugs that also includes Prozac and Zoloft.

Doctors are just beginning to react to the finding reported first by British drug authorities in June and then endorsed the next week by the Food and Drug Administration that unpublished studies about Paxil show that it carries a substantial risk of prompting teenagers and children to consider suicide.

Because the studies also found that Paxil was no more effective than a placebo in treating young people's depression, the regulators recommended that doctors write no new Paxil prescriptions for patients under 18. Experts say that the suicide risk is highest in the first few weeks young patients are on the drug.

The concern that Paxil and drugs like it could cause suicide had been weighed, and rejected, by regulators a dozen years ago, amid early concerns about the group of antidepressants known as selective serotonin reuptake inhibitors, or SSRIs.

Read the complete article online in the eThemes section of this book's website: www.aw-bc.com/donatelle.

A lthough often overlooked during the pursuit of a fit body, a fit mind can be equally important in determining not only the number of years we live, but also the quality of those years. All of us go through times when life seems difficult. Whatever the cause for the low points in our lives, they have the power to sap energy, drain emotions, and break the spirit. Over the long haul, they can even shorten life expectancy.

College students can be especially vulnerable to life's highs and lows. A study published in 2003 of the nearly 14,000 students who sought help from a Midwestern university counseling center over a 13-year period revealed that students frequently have more complex problems today than they did a decade ago. Issues included both the expected student problems—difficulties in relationships and developmental issues—as well as more severe problems, such as depression, effects of sexual assault, and thoughts of suicide. Some of these increases were dramatic. The number of students seen each year with depression doubled, the number of suicidal students tripled, and the number of students seen after a sexual assault quadrupled.[1]

However, human beings possess a resiliency that enables us to cope, adapt, and thrive, regardless of life's challenges. How we feel and think about ourselves, those around us, and our environment can tell us a lot about our psychosocial health and whether we are healthy emotionally, spiritu- ally, and mentally. Increasingly, health professionals recognize that having a solid social network, being emotionally and mentally healthy, and acknowledging and developing spiritual capacity may put life into years, as well as add years to life.

Defining Psychosocial Health

Psychosocial health encompasses the mental, emotional, social, and spiritual dimensions of health (Figure 2.1). It is the result of a complex interaction between a person's history

Psychosocial health   The mental, emotional, social, and spiritual dimensions of health.

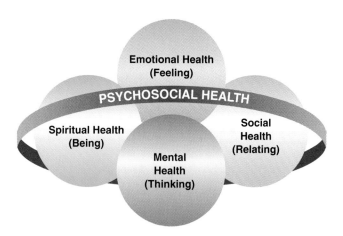

Figure 2.1
Psychosocial Health
Psychosocial health is a complex interaction of mental, emotional, social, and spiritual health.

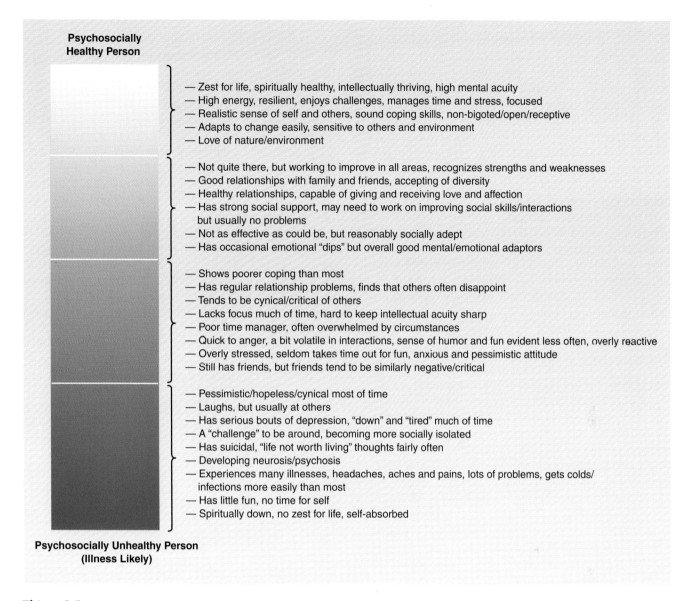

Psychosocially Healthy Person

— Zest for life, spiritually healthy, intellectually thriving, high mental acuity
— High energy, resilient, enjoys challenges, manages time and stress, focused
— Realistic sense of self and others, sound coping skills, non-bigoted/open/receptive
— Adapts to change easily, sensitive to others and environment
— Love of nature/environment

— Not quite there, but working to improve in all areas, recognizes strengths and weaknesses
— Good relationships with family and friends, accepting of diversity
— Healthy relationships, capable of giving and receiving love and affection
— Has strong social support, may need to work on improving social skills/interactions but usually no problems
— Not as effective as could be, but reasonably socially adept
— Has occasional emotional "dips" but overall good mental/emotional adaptors

— Shows poorer coping than most
— Has regular relationship problems, finds that others often disappoint
— Tends to be cynical/critical of others
— Lacks focus much of time, hard to keep intellectual acuity sharp
— Poor time manager, often overwhelmed by circumstances
— Quick to anger, a bit volatile in interactions, sense of humor and fun evident less often, overly reactive
— Overly stressed, seldom takes time out for fun, anxious and pessimistic attitude
— Still has friends, but friends tend to be similarly negative/critical

— Pessimistic/hopeless/cynical most of time
— Laughs, but usually at others
— Has serious bouts of depression, "down" and "tired" much of time
— A "challenge" to be around, becoming more socially isolated
— Has suicidal, "life not worth living" thoughts fairly often
— Developing neurosis/psychosis
— Experiences many illnesses, headaches, aches and pains, lots of problems, gets colds/infections more easily than most
— Has little fun, no time for self
— Spiritually down, no zest for life, self-absorbed

**Psychosocially Unhealthy Person
(Illness Likely)**

Figure 2.2
Characteristics of Psychosocially Healthy and Unhealthy People

and his or her conscious and unconscious thoughts about and interpretations of the past. Psychosocially healthy people are emotionally, mentally, socially, intellectually, and spiritually resilient. They respond to challenges and frustrations in appropriate ways most of the time, despite occasional slips. Most authorities identify several basic characteristics psychosocially healthy people share (Figure 2.2).[2]

- *They feel good about themselves.* They are not typically overwhelmed by fear, love, anger, jealousy, guilt, or worry. They know who they are, have a realistic sense of their capabilities, and respect themselves even though they realize they aren't perfect.
- *They feel comfortable with other people.* They enjoy satisfying and lasting personal relationships and do not take advantage of others or allow others to take advantage of

them. They can give love, consider others' interests, respect personal differences, and feel responsible for their fellow human beings.
- *They control tension and anxiety.* They recognize the underlying causes and symptoms of stress in their lives and consciously avoid irrational thoughts, hostility, excessive excuse making, and blaming others for their problems.
- *They are able to meet the demands of life.* They try to solve problems as they arise, accept responsibility, and plan ahead. They set realistic goals, think for themselves, and make independent decisions. Acknowledging that change is inevitable, they welcome new experiences. They use their natural abilities to control and fit themselves into their environment.

- *They curb hate and guilt.* They acknowledge and combat tendencies to respond with anger, thoughtlessness, selfishness, vengeful acts, or feelings of inadequacy. They do not try to knock others aside to get ahead but rather reach out to help others—even those they don't particularly like.
- *They maintain a positive outlook.* They approach each day with a presumption that things will go well. They block out most negative and cynical thoughts and give the good things in life star billing. They look to the future with enthusiasm rather than dread.
- *They enrich the lives of others.* They recognize that there are others whose needs are greater than their own.
- *They cherish the things that make them smile.* Reminders of good experiences brighten their day. Fun and making time for themselves are integral parts of their lives.
- *They value diversity.* They do not feel threatened by those of a different race, gender, religion, sexual orientation, ethnicity, or political party. They appreciate creativity in others as well as in themselves.
- *They appreciate and respect nature.* They take the time to enjoy their surroundings and are conscious of their place in the universe.

Of course, few of us ever achieve perfection in these areas. Attaining psychosocial health and wellness involves many complex processes. This chapter will help you understand not only what it means to be psychosocially well, but also why we may run into problems in our psychosocial health. In addition, learning how to assess your own health and help yourself or seek help from others are important parts of psychosocial health (see the Assess Yourself box on page 34).

> **What do you think?**
> *Which psychosocial qualities do you value most in your friends? ✻ Do you think that you are strong in these areas yourself? ✻ Explain your answer.*

Mental Health: The Thinking You

The term **mental health** is often used to describe the "thinking" part of psychosocial health. As a thinking being, you have the ability to reason, interpret, and remember events from a unique perspective; to sense, perceive, and evaluate

Mental health   The thinking part of psychosocial health that includes values, attitudes, and beliefs.

Emotional health   The feeling part of psychosocial health that includes emotional reactions to life.

Emotions   Intensified feelings or complex patterns of feelings we constantly experience.

what is happening; and to solve problems. In short, you are intellectually able to sort through the clutter of events, contradictory messages, and uncertainties of a situation and attach positive or negative meaning. (People often refer to this subset of mental health as *intellectual health.*) Your values, attitudes, and beliefs about your body, family, relationships, and life in general are usually—at least in part—a reflection of your mental health.

A mentally healthy person is likely to respond in a positive way even when things do not go as expected. For example, a mentally healthy student who receives a D on an exam may be disappointed but will try to assess why she did poorly. Did she study enough? Did she attend class and ask questions about the things she didn't understand? Even though the exam result may be very important to her, she will find a constructive way to deal with her frustration. She may talk to the instructor, spend more time studying, or hire a tutor. In contrast, a mentally unhealthy person may respond irrationally. She may believe that her instructor is out to get her or that other students cheated on the exam. She may allow her low grade to provoke a major crisis in her life. She may spend the next 24 hours getting wasted. Or she may decide to quit school, try to get back at her instructor, or blame her roommate for preventing her from studying.

When a person's mental health begins to deteriorate, he or she may experience sharp declines in rational thinking ability and increasingly distorted perceptions. The person may become cynical and distrustful, experience volatile mood swings, or choose to be isolated from others. Extreme negative reactions may even threaten the life and health of others. People who show such extreme behavior are classified as having mental illnesses, which is discussed later in this chapter.

Emotional Health: The Feeling You

The term **emotional health** is often used interchangeably with *mental health.* Although the two are closely intertwined, emotional health more accurately refers to the feeling, or subjective, side of psychosocial health that includes emotional reactions to life. **Emotions** are intensified feelings or complex patterns of feelings that we experience on a minute-by-minute, day-to-day basis. Love, hate, frustration, anxiety, and joy are only a few of the many emotions we feel. Typically, emotions are described as the interplay of four components: physiological arousal, feelings, cognitive (thought) processes, and behavioral reactions. Each time you are put in a stressful situation, you react physiologically while your mind tries to sort things out. You consciously or unconsciously react based on how rationally you interpret the situation.

Psychologist Richard Lazarus has indicated that there are four basic types of emotions: emotions resulting from harm, loss, or threats; emotions resulting from benefits; borderline emotions, such as hope and compassion; and more complex emotions, such as grief, disappointment, bewilderment, and curiosity.[3] Each of us may experience any of these feelings in any combination at any time. As rational beings, it is our responsibility to evaluate our individual emotional responses, the environment that is causing them, and the appropriateness of our actions.

Emotionally healthy people are usually able to respond appropriately to upsetting events. When they feel threatened, they are not likely to react in an extreme fashion, behave inconsistently, or adopt an offensive mode. Even when their feelings are trampled on or they suffer agonizing pain because of a lost love, they are able to express and show emotions in appropriate ways.

Emotionally unhealthy people are much more likely to let their feelings overpower them. They may be volatile and prone to unpredictable outbursts and inappropriate, sometimes frightening responses to events. An ex-boyfriend who is so jealous of your new relationship that he hits you is showing an extremely unhealthy and dangerous emotional reaction. Such violent responses have become a problem of epidemic proportions in the United States (see Chapter 4).

Emotional health also affects social health. Someone feeling hostile, withdrawn, or moody may become socially isolated. People in the midst of emotional turmoil may be irritable or overly quiet; they may cry easily or demonstrate disturbing emotional responses. Because they are not much fun to be around, their friends may avoid them at the very time they most need emotional support. Social isolation is just one of the many potential negative consequences of unstable emotional responses.

For students, a more immediate concern is the impact of emotional trauma on academic performance. Have you ever tried to study for an exam after a fight with a close friend or family member? Emotional turmoil may seriously affect your ability to think, reason, and act rationally. Many otherwise rational, mentally healthy people do ridiculous things when they are going through a major emotional upset. Mental functioning and emotional responses are intricately connected.

Social Health: Interactions with Others

Social health, an important part of the broader concept of psychosocial health, includes your interactions with others on an individual and group basis, your ability to use social resources and support in times of need, and your ability to adapt to a variety of social situations. Socially healthy individuals have a wide range of interactions with family, friends, and acquaintances, and are able to have a healthy interaction with an intimate partner. Typically, socially healthy individuals are able to listen, express themselves, form healthy attachments, act in socially acceptable and responsible ways, and find the best fit for themselves in society. Numerous studies have documented the importance of social health in promoting physical health, mental health, and enhanced longevity.[4]

As pack animals, we grow stronger in groups and learn valuable lessons through our social interactions. From the moment we are born, we rely on parents for our care. We are dependent on others for learning and skill development and develop much of our sense of self-worth as a result of our interactions with others. Our adult lives are spent working with others, developing relationships with family and friends, and participating in our community. Our value to society is measured by the number of connections we have and even by how many people come to our funerals. Few would disagree that **social bonds** are the very foundation of human life.

Social bonds reflect the level of closeness and attachment that we develop with individuals. They provide intimacy, feelings of belonging, opportunities for giving or receiving nurturance, reassurance of one's worth, assistance and guidance, and advice. Social bonds take multiple forms, the most common of which are **social support** and community engagements. Social support consists of networks of people and services with whom you share ties. These ties can provide tangible support, such as babysitting services or money to help pay the bills, or they can provide intangible support, such as understanding or allowing you to share intimate thoughts. Generally, the closer and the higher the quality of the social bond, the more likely a person may be to ask for and receive social support. If you were alone on a dark, country road in the middle of the night and your car broke down, for example, who would you call for help and know that they would do everything possible to get there? People who are socially isolated, estranged from their families, and have few social connections will have difficulty thinking of someone to count on when they are in trouble. Psychosocially healthy people work to create and maintain a network of friends and family with whom they can give and receive support, and they work hard to maintain these relationships in difficult times.

Social health also reflects the way we react to others. In its most extreme forms, a lack of social health may be represented by aggressive acts of **prejudice** toward other individuals or groups. In its most obvious manifestations, prejudice is reflected in acts of discrimination, hate, and bias, and in intent to harm individuals or groups.

There is also a flip side to social support. Just as supportive ties promote health and longevity, the loss of such relationships threatens health. For example, on average, widows and widowers are at increased risk of mental and physical ailments for up to two years after spousal death.

Social health   Aspect of psychosocial health that includes interactions with others, ability to use social supports, and ability to adapt to various situations.

Social bonds   Degree and nature of interpersonal contacts.

Social support   Network of people and services with whom you share ties and get support.

Prejudice   A negative evaluation of an entire group of people that is typically based on unfavorable and often wrong ideas about the group.

Assessing Your Psychosocial Health

Being psychosocially healthy requires both introspection and the willingness to work on areas that need improvement. Often it is difficult to assess one's own behaviors and actions. Ask someone who is close to you to take the same test and respond with his or her perceptions of you. Carefully assess areas where your responses differ from those of your friend or family member. Which areas might need some work? Which areas are in good shape?

	1 = Never describes me	2 = Describes me infrequently	3 = Describes me fairly frequently	4 = Describes me most of the time	5 = Describes me all of the time
1. My actions and interactions indicate that I am confident in my abilities.	1	2	3	4	5
2. I am quick to blame others for things that go wrong in my life.	1	2	3	4	5
3. I am spontaneous and like to have fun with others.	1	2	3	4	5
4. I am able to give love and affection to others and show my feelings.	1	2	3	4	5
5. I am able to receive love and signs of affection from others without feeling uneasy.	1	2	3	4	5
6. I am generally positive and upbeat about things in my life.	1	2	3	4	5
7. I am cynical and tend to be critical of others.	1	2	3	4	5
8. I have a large group of people whom I consider to be good friends.	1	2	3	4	5
9. I make time for others in my life.	1	2	3	4	5
10. I take time each day for myself for quiet introspection, having fun, or just doing nothing.					
11. I am compulsive and competitive in my actions.					
12. I handle stress well and am seldom upset or stressed out by others.	1	2	3	4	5
13. I try to look for the good in everyone and every situation before finding fault.	1	2	3	4	5
14. I am comfortable meeting new people and interact well in social settings.	1	2	3	4	5

Spiritual Health: An Inner Quest for Well-Being

Although mental health and emotional health are key factors in overall psychosocial functioning, it is possible to be mentally and emotionally healthy and still not achieve optimal well-being. For many people, the difficult-to-describe element that gives zest to life is the spiritual dimension.

Most experts agree that **spirituality** refers to a belief in a unifying force that gives meaning to life, a sense of belonging to a scheme of being that is greater than the purely physical or personal dimensions of existence. For some, this unifying force is nature; for others, it is a feeling of connection to other people; for others still, the unifying force is a god or other spiritual symbol. Dr. N. Lee Smith, internist and associate professor of medicine at the University of Utah, defines spiritual health in the following ways:[5]

- The quality of existence in which one is at peace with oneself and in good standing with the environment
- A sense of empowerment and personal control that includes feeling heard and valued and feeling in control over one's responses (but not necessarily in control of one's environment)
- A sense of connectedness to one's deepest self, to other people, and to all that is regarded as good
- A sense of meaning and purpose, which provides a sense of mission by finding meaning and wisdom in the here and now

Spirituality A belief in a unifying force that gives meaning to life and transcends the purely physical or personal dimensions of existence.

15. I would rather stay in and watch TV or read than go out with friends or interact with others.	1	2	3	4	5
16. I am flexible and can adapt to most situations, even if I don't like them.	1	2	3	4	5
17. Nature, the environment, and other living things are important aspects of my life.	1	2	3	4	5
18. I think before responding to my emotions	1	2	3	4	5
19. I tend to think of my own needs before thinking of the needs of others.	1	2	3	4	5
20. I am consciously trying to be a better person.	1	2	3	4	5
21. I like to set realistic goals for myself and others.	1	2	3	4	5
22. I accept others for who they are.					
23. I value diversity and respect others' rights, regardless of culture, race, sexual orientation, religion, or other differences.	1	2	3	4	5
24. I try to live each day as though it might be my last.	1	2	3	4	5
25. I appreciate the little things in life.	1	2	3	4	5
26. I cope with stress in appropriate ways.	1	2	3	4	5
27. I get enough sleep each day and seldom feel tired.	1	2	3	4	5
28. I have healthy relationships with my family.	1	2	3	4	5
29. I am confident that I can do most things if I put my mind to them.	1	2	3	4	5
30. I respect others' opinions and believe that others should be free to express their opinions, even when they differ from my own.	1	2	3	4	5

Look at items 2, 7, 11, 15, and 19. Add up your score for these five items and divide by 5. Is your average for these items above or below 3? Did you score a 5 on any of these items? Do you need to work on any of these areas?

Now look at your scores for the remaining 25 items. Total these scores and divide by 25. Is your average above or below 3? On which items did you score a 5? Obviously you're doing well in these areas. Now remove the items on which you scored a 5 from this grouping of 25, and add up your scores for the remaining items. Then divide your total by the number of items included. Now what is your average?

Do the same for the scores completed by your friend or family member. How do your scores compare? Which ones, if any, are different, and how do they differ? Which areas do you need to work on? What actions can you take now to improve your ratings in these areas?

- Enjoying the process of growth and having a vision of one's potential
- Having hope, which translates into positive expectations

On a day-to-day basis, many of us focus on acquiring material possessions and satisfying basic needs. But there comes a point when we discover that material possessions do not automatically bring happiness or a sense of self-worth. This realization may be triggered by a crisis. A failed relationship, a terrible accident, the death of a close friend or family member, or other loss often prompts a search for meaning, for the answer to the proverbial question, Is that all there is? Whatever the reason, this search brings new opportunities for understanding ourselves. As we develop into spiritually healthy beings, we recognize our identity as unique individuals. We gain a better appreciation of our strengths and shortcomings and our place in the universe. Perhaps most important, we gain an appreciation for the here-and-now rather than living for aspirations that we may never achieve.

In its purest sense, spirituality addresses four main themes: interconnectedness, the practice of mindfulness, spirituality as a part of everyday life, and living in harmony with the community.

- *Interconnectedness.* The term **interconnectedness** expresses a sense of belonging and connecting with oneself, with others, and with a larger meaning or purpose of life. Connecting with oneself involves exploring feelings, taking

> **Interconnectedness** A web of connections, including our relationship to ourselves, to others, and to a larger meaning or purpose in life.

time to consider how you feel in a given situation, assessing your reactions to people and experiences, and taking mental notes when things or people cause you to lose equilibrium. It also involves considering your values and achieving congruence between your goals and what you can do to achieve them without compromising your values.

- *Practice of mindfulness.* **Mindfulness** refers to the ability to be fully present in the moment. It has been described as a way of nurturing greater awareness and clarity. It is a form of inner flow—a holistic sensation you feel when you are totally involved in the present.[6] According to mindfulness experts, you can achieve this inner flow through an almost infinite range of opportunities for enjoyment and pleasure, either through the use of physical and sensory skills such as athletics, music, or yoga, or through the development of symbolic skills in areas such as poetry, philosophy, or mathematics.[7] The psychologist Abraham Maslow referred to these moments as peak experiences, during which a person feels integrated, synergistic, and at one with the world.

- *Spirituality as a part of daily life.* Spirituality is embodied in the ability to discover and articulate our own basic purpose in life; to learn how to experience love, joy, peace, and fulfillment; and to help ourselves and others achieve their full potential.[8] This ongoing process of growth fosters three convictions: faith, hope, and love. **Faith** is the belief that helps us realize our unique purpose in life; **hope** is the belief that allows us to look confidently and courageously to the future; and **love** involves accepting, affirming, and respecting self and others regardless of who they are.[9]

- *Living in harmony with our community.* Our values are an extension of our beliefs about the world and attitude toward life. They are formed over time through a series of life experiences, and they are reflected in our hopes, dreams, desires, goals, and ambitions.[10] Though most people have some idea of what is important to them, many spend life largely unaware of how their values impact them or those around them, until a life-altering event shakes up their perspective on life.

Spirituality: A Key to Health and Wellness Although many experts affirm the importance of spirituality in achieving health and wellness, the specific impact of this dimension remains elusive. Some researchers describe the spiritual dimension as a factor of well-being, which is achieved when four basic kinds of needs are satisfied:[11]

1. The need for having
2. The need for relating
3. The need for being
4. The need for *transcendence,* or that sense of well-being that is experienced when a person finds purpose and meaning in life. Nonphysical in nature, transcendence can best be described as spiritual.

A Spiritual Resurgence Over recent decades, studies have shown that most Americans believe in God and consider spirituality to be important in their lives, although not necessarily in the form of religion.[12] Many find spiritual fulfillment in music, poetry, literature, art, nature, and intimate relationships.[13] Many religious groups have spawned new philosophies that are more inclusive and often influenced by "New Age" ideas, such as using positive thought to achieve your goals and striving to find your rightful place in the world. An estimated 32 million baby boomers have turned to Eastern practices, New Age philosophies, 12-step programs, Greek mythology, shamanistic practices, massage, yoga, and a host of other traditions and practices.[14]

For some, spirituality means a quest for self and selflessness—a form of therapy and respite from a sometimes challenging personal environment. This quest for a life force, which helps people deeply experience the moments of their lives rather than just living through them, has received much scholarly and popular attention. Self-help books that focus on spirituality consistently top the bestseller lists. Television programs promote the virtues of a spiritual or natural existence. Writers and psychologists such as William James, Carl Jung, Gordon Allport, Erich Fromm, Viktor Frankl, Abraham Maslow, and Rollo May have made spirituality a major focus of their work.

Courses on spiritual health have emerged in public health and medical school training. For example, the Harvard Medical School of Continuing Education offers a course called "Spirituality and Healing in Medicine," which brings together scholars and medical professionals from around the world to discuss the role of spirituality in treating illness and chronic pain. Self-help workshops focusing on spiritual elements of health are popular throughout the world. The New Horizons in Health box describes some studies that may affirm the link between spirituality and health.

Mindfulness Awareness and acceptance of the reality of the present moment.

Faith Belief that helps each person realize a unique purpose in life.

Hope Belief that allows us to look confidently and courageously to the future.

Love Acceptance, affirmation, and respect for the self and others.

What do you think?
What do social, mental, emotional, and spiritual health mean to you? ✳ What are your strengths and weaknesses in each area of psychosocial health? ✳ What can you do to enhance your strengths? ✳ How can you improve areas that are not strong?

News from the World of Faith, Spirituality, and Healing Research

Dozens of studies are examining the effects of religion and spirituality on mental and physical health. Several of them provide interesting preliminary results in the following areas.

- *Mental health.* A review of articles published in the *The American Journal of Psychiatry* and the *Archives of General Psychiatry* during a 10-year period found that 80% showed a positive correlation between spirituality and better mental health.
- *Stress.* The Alameda County Study, which tracks nearly 7,000 Californians, showed that West Coast worshippers who participate in church-sponsored activities are markedly less stressed over finances, health, and other daily concerns than are nonreligious types.
- *Blood pressure.* Elderly people in a Duke University study who attended religious services, prayed, or read the Bible regularly had lower blood pressure than their nonpracticing peers did.
- *Recovery.* In another Duke University study, devout patients recovering from surgery spent an average of 11 days in the hospital, compared with nonreligious patients who spent an average of 25 days.
- *Mortality.* Research on 1,931 older adults indicates that those who attend religious services regularly have a lower mortality rate.
- *Immunity.* Research on 1,700 adults found that those who attend religious services are less likely to have elevated levels of interleukin-6, an immune substance prevalent in people with chronic diseases.
- *Lifestyle.* A recent review of several studies suggests that spirituality is linked with low suicide rates, less alcohol and drug abuse, less criminal behavior, fewer divorces, and higher marital satisfaction.
- *Depression.* A Duke University study of 577 men and women hospitalized for physical illness showed that the more patients used positive coping strategies (seeking spiritual support from friends and religious leaders, praying, meditating, etc.), the lower the level of their depressive symptoms and the higher their quality of life.

After reviewing a number of studies such as those listed above, researchers at Georgetown University School of Medicine concluded that at least 80% of them point to a positive link between spiritual and physical well-being. People who consider themselves spiritual tend to recover more quickly from illness, live longer, and enjoy better health throughout their lives.

Sources: MayoClinic.com, "Spirituality and Chronic Pain," February 4, 2002. www.mayoclinic.com; Susan S. Larson, *Oskar Pfister Address at the American Psychiatric Association,* Philadelphia: May 22, 2002; International Center for the Integration of Health & Spirituality. www.nihr.org; D. N. Elkins, "Spirituality," *Psychology Today,* September 1999, v. 32, Issue 5, p. 44. Reprinted with permission from *PsychologyToday* magazine © 1999 Sussex Publishers; W. J. Strawbridge et al., "Religiosity Buffers Effects of Some Stressors on Depression but Exacerbates Others," *Journal of Gerontology: Psychological Sciences* 53, no. 3 (1998).

Factors Influencing Psychosocial Health

Most of our mental, emotional, and social reactions to life are a direct outcome of our experiences and social and cultural expectations. Our psychosocial health is based, in part, on how we perceive life experiences.

External Factors

While some life experiences are under our control, others are not. External factors in life are those that we do not control, such as who raised us and where we live.

The Family Families have a significant influence on psychosocial development. Children raised in healthy, nurturing, happy families are more likely to become well-adjusted, productive adults. Children raised in **dysfunctional families** in which there is violence, negative behavior, distrust, anger, dietary deprivation, drug abuse, parental discord, or sexual, physical, or emotional abuse may have a harder time adapting to life. In dysfunctional families, love, security, and unconditional trust are so lacking that children often become confused and psychologically bruised. Yet, not all people raised in dysfunctional families become psychosocially unhealthy, and not all children from healthy environments become well adjusted. Obviously, more factors are involved in our "process of becoming" than just our family.

The Wider Environment Although isolated negative events may do little damage to psychosocial health, persistent stressors, uncertainties, and threats can cause significant problems. Children raised in environments where crime is rampant and daily safety is in question, for example, run an increased risk of psychosocial problems. Drugs, crime, violent acts, school failure, unemployment, and a host of other bad things can

Dysfunctional families Families in which there is violence; physical, emotional, or sexual abuse; parental discord; or other negative interactions and behaviors.

happen to good people. But it is believed that certain protective factors, such as having a positive role model in the midst of chaos, can help children from even the worst environments remain healthy and well adjusted.

Another important influence is access to health services and programs designed to enhance psychosocial health. Going to a support group or seeing a trained therapist is often a crucial first step in prevention and intervention efforts. Individuals from poor socioeconomic environments who cannot afford such services often find it difficult to secure help in improving their psychosocial health.

Social Bonds   Although often overlooked, a stable, loving support network of family and friends is key to psychosocial health. The social support of close relationships helps us get through even the most difficult times. Having those with whom we can talk, share thoughts, and practice good and bad behaviors without fear of losing their love is an essential part of growth.

> **What do you think?**
> *Over which external factors does an individual have the most control?* ✳ *Which factors had the greatest impact on making you who you are today?*

Internal Factors

Many internal factors also shape a person's development. These factors include hereditary traits, hormonal functioning, physical health (including neurological functioning), physical fitness level, and certain elements of mental and emotional health.

Self-Efficacy, Self-Esteem   During our formative years, successes and failures in school, athletics, friendships, intimate relationships, jobs, and every other aspect of life subtly shape our beliefs about our own personal worth and abilities. These beliefs become internal influences on our psychosocial health. Psychologist Albert Bandura used the term **self-efficacy** to describe a person's belief about whether he or she can successfully engage in and execute a specific behavior. Prior success in academics, athletics, or social events will lead to

Self-efficacy   Belief in one's own ability to engage in and execute a specific behavior successfully.

Personal control   Belief that one's own internal resources can control a situation.

Self-esteem   Sense of self-respect or self-worth.

Learned helplessness   Pattern of responding to situations by giving up because of repeated failure in the past.

expectations of success in the future. In general, the more self-efficacious a person is and the more positive his or her past experiences have been, the more likely the person will keep trying to execute a specific behavior successfully. Self-efficacious people are also more likely to feel a sense of **personal control** over situations, that their own internal resources allow them to control events. In contrast, someone with low self-efficacy may give up easily or never even try to change a behavior. Always being the last chosen to play basketball or having long-term difficulty in making friends, for example, may make failure seem inevitable.

Self-esteem refers to one's sense of self-respect or self-worth. It can be defined as one's evaluation of oneself and one's personal worth as an individual. People with high self-esteem tend to feel good about themselves and have a positive outlook on life. People with low self-esteem often do not like themselves, constantly demean themselves, and doubt their ability to succeed.

Our self-esteem is a result of the relationships we have with our parents and family during our formative years; with our friends as we grow older; with our significant others as we form intimate relationships; and with our teachers, co-workers, and others throughout our lives. If we felt loved and valued as children, our self-esteem allows us to believe that we are inherently lovable individuals. See the Skills for Behavior Change box for some strategies for increasing your self-esteem.

Learned Helplessness versus Learned Optimism   Psychologist Martin Seligman has proposed that people who continually experience failure may develop a pattern of responding known as **learned helplessness,** in which they give up and fail to take any action to help themselves. Seligman ascribes this in part to society's tendency toward victimology, blaming one's problems on other people and circumstances. Although viewing ourselves as victims may make us feel better temporarily, it does not address the underlying causes of a problem. Ultimately, it can erode self-efficacy and foster learned helplessness by making us feel that we cannot do anything to improve the situation.[15]

Countering this is Seligman's principle of *learned optimism.* Just as we learn to be helpless, so can we teach ourselves to be optimistic. His research provides growing evidence for the central place of mental health in overall positive development.[16]

In one study, university freshmen who had been identified as pessimistic on the basis of a questionnaire were randomly assigned to an experimental group or to a control group. The experimental group attended a 16-hour workshop in which they practiced social and study skills and learned to dispute chronic negative thoughts. The control group did not participate. Eighteen months later, 15 percent of the control group members were experiencing severe anxiety, and 32 percent were suffering from moderate to severe depression. In contrast, only 7 percent of workshop participants suffered from anxiety and 22 percent from depression. Seligman concluded

Tips for Building Self-Esteem

How can you build self-esteem? There are many things you can do in your day-to-day life that, when practiced regularly, can have a significant impact on the way you feel about yourself.

SQUELCH THAT INNER CRITIC

We are often our own worst enemies. We harp at ourselves continually about how we look and how we should have behaved in certain situations. Begin squelching that inner voice now.

- Examine your faults with a mirror rather than a magnifying glass. Instead of saying, "I'm stupid, and I'll never get through this class," say, "I didn't do so well on this last test, but I'm going to do better. I'm doing great in another class."
- View your mistakes as opportunities to know yourself better or as growth experiences that will teach you to do things differently next time. If you find that you made careless mistakes on a test because you rushed through it, allow more time on your next test to double-check your work.
- The next time someone compliments you, respond positively. Say thank you rather than mumbling a protest.

FOCUS ON THE POSITIVE

Don't wallow in self-pity. Although no one is upbeat all the time, you can do a great deal to shorten the interlude between positive thoughts.

- Don't sulk. When upset, allow yourself 15 minutes to worry, then force yourself to do or think of something else.
- Don't compare yourself with others. Concentrate on improving your own performance.
- Give yourself time to feel good. When you reach an objective, allow time for fun before starting another project.
- Spend time with a friend who cares about you and isn't afraid to let you know it. Friends are crucial to positive self-esteem, say experts, because they make up your psychic family—an important source of support and objectivity.
- Count your blessings. Make a list of the people, events, and things in your life for which you are grateful. Include your own accomplishments. Whenever you feel cheated by life, look at this list.

---

that even relatively brief interventions, such as this workshop, can produce measurable improvements in coping skills.[17]

Personality Your personality is the unique mix of characteristics that distinguish you from others. Heredity, environment, culture, and experience influence how each person develops. Personality determines how we react to the challenges of life, interpret our feelings, and resolve conflicts.

Most of the recent schools of psychosocial theory promote the idea that we have the power not only to understand our behavior, but also to change it and thus mold our own personalities. Although much has been written about the importance of a healthy personality, there is little consensus on what that concept really means. In general, however, people who possess the following traits often appear to be psychosocially healthy:[18]

- *Extroversion.* This refers to the ability to adapt to a social situation and demonstrate assertiveness as well as power or interpersonal involvement.
- *Agreeableness.* This refers to the ability to conform, to be likable, and to demonstrate friendly compliance as well as love.
- *Openness to experience.* This refers to the ability to demonstrate curiosity and independence (also referred to as *inquiring intellect*).
- *Emotional stability.* This refers to the ability to maintain social control.
- *Conscientiousness.* This refers to the ability to demonstrate self-control and be dependable. The conscientious person has a need to achieve.[19]

Our personalities are not static. Rather, they change as we move through the stages of our lives. Our temperaments also change as we grow. Consider, for example, the extreme emotions many early adolescents experience. Most of us learn to control our emotions as we advance toward adulthood.

Enhancing Psychosocial Health

Attaining self-fulfillment is a lifelong, conscious process that involves building self-esteem, understanding and controlling emotions, and learning to solve problems and make decisions.

Developing and Maintaining Self-Esteem and Self-Efficacy

There are several ways to build self-esteem and self-efficacy. These include finding a support group, completing required tasks, forming realistic expectations, making time for yourself, maintaining your physical health, and examining your problems and seeking help.

Find a Support Group The best way to promote self-esteem is through a support group—peers who share your values. The prime prerequisite for a support group is that it makes you feel good about yourself and forces you to take an honest look at your actions and choices. Although the idea of finding a support group seems to imply establishing a wholly new group, remember that old ties are often the strongest.

Keeping in contact with old friends and important family members can provide a foundation of unconditional love that will help you through the many life transitions ahead. Try to be a support for others, too. Join a discussion, political action, or recreational group. Write more postcards and "thinking of you" notes to people who matter. This will build your own self-esteem and that of your friends.

Complete Required Tasks A good way to boost your self-efficacy is to complete tasks well and develop a history of success. You are less likely to succeed in your studies if you leave term papers until the last minute or fail to ask about material that is confusing to you. Most college campuses provide study groups and learning centers that can help you manage time, understand assignments, deal with professors, and prepare for tests. Poor grades, or grades that do not meet expectations, are major contributors to emotional distress among college students.

Form Realistic Expectations Set realistic expectations for yourself. If you expect perfect grades, a steady stream of Saturday-night dates and soap-opera romances, and the perfect job, you may be setting yourself up for failure. Assess your current resources and the direction in which you are heading. Set small, incremental goals that are possible for you to meet.

Make Time for Yourself Taking time to enjoy yourself is another way to boost your self-esteem and psychosocial health. Try to view each new activity as something to look forward to and an opportunity to have fun. Anticipate and focus on the fun things you have to look forward to each day.

Maintain Physical Health Regular exercise fosters a sense of well-being. Nourishing meals can help you avoid the weight gain that many college students experience. (See Chapter 9 for information on nutrition and Chapter 10 for information on the role of exercise on health.)

Examine Problems, and Seek Help Knowing when to seek help from friends, support groups, family, or professionals is another important factor in boosting self-esteem. Sometimes you can handle life's problems alone; at other times, you need assistance. Recognizing your strengths and acting appropriately are keys to psychosocial health.

Sleep: The Great Restorer

Sleep serves at least two biological purposes in the body: *conservation* of energy so we are rested and ready to perform during high-performance daylight hours, and *restoration* so neurotransmitters depleted during waking hours can be replenished. This process clears the brain of daily minutiae to prepare for a new day. Getting enough sleep is a key factor in optimal physical and psychosocial health.

How much sleep do we need? The genetically based need for sleep is different for each species. Sleep duration also is controlled by *circadian rhythms,* which are linked to the hormone *melatonin*. People also may control sleep patterns by staying up late, drinking coffee, getting lots of physical exercise, eating a heavy meal, or using alarm clocks. The most important period of sleep is known as the time of *rapid eye movement (REM) sleep*. This is the period of deepest sleep during which we dream. Getting enough REM sleep is essential to feel rested and refreshed. If we miss this period of sleep, we feel groggy and sleep deprived.

Many people turn to over-the-counter sleeping pills, barbiturates, or tranquilizers to get some sleep. All of these are potentially harmful. Instead, try the following methods for conquering insomnia:[20]

- Establish a consistent sleep schedule. Go to bed and get up at about the same time every day.
- Evaluate your sleep environment, and change anything that could be keeping you awake. If it's noise, wear earplugs. If it's light, try room-darkening shades.
- Exercise regularly. It's hard to feel drowsy if you have been sedentary all day. However, don't exercise right before bedtime; activity speeds up your metabolism and makes it harder to go to sleep.
- Limit caffeine and alcohol. Caffeine can linger in your body for up to 12 hours and cause insomnia. Although alcohol may make you drowsy at first, it interferes with the normal sleep–wake cycle and can make you wake up early.
- Avoid eating a heavy meal, particularly at bedtime. Don't drink large amounts of liquid before bedtime.
- If you're unable to fall sleep in 30 minutes, get up and do something else. Read, play solitaire, or try other relaxing activities, and return to bed when you feel drowsy.
- If you nap, do so only during the afternoon, when circadian rhythms make you especially sleepy. Don't let naps interfere with your normal sleep schedule.
- Establish a relaxing nighttime ritual that puts you in the mood to sleep. Take a warm shower, relax in a comfortable chair, don your favorite robe. Doing this consistently will cue your mind and body that it's time to wind down.

Some people have difficulty getting a good night's sleep due to sleep apnea, an increasingly common and serious disorder. For more on this condition, see Chapter 14.

The Mind–Body Connection

Can negative emotions make us physically sick? Can positive feelings help us stay well? Researchers are exploring the interaction between emotions and health, especially in conditions of uncontrolled, persistent stress. According to one theory, the brain of an emotionally overwrought person sends signals to the adrenal glands, which respond by secreting cortisol and epinephrine (adrenaline), the hormones that activate the body's stress response. These chemicals are also known to suppress immune functioning, so a persistently overwrought person may undergo subtle immune changes. What remains to be shown is whether these changes affect overall health.

Happiness: A Key to Well-Being

Although we can list the actions that we should perform to become physically healthy, such as eating the right foods, getting enough rest, and exercising, it is less clear how to achieve that "feeling-good state" that researchers call **subjective well-being (SWB).** This refers to that uplifting feeling of inner peace and wonder that we call happiness. Psychologists David Myers and Ed Deiner completed a major study of happiness and noted that people experience it in many different ways, based on factors such as age, culture, and gender.[21] However, in spite of the differences in the way it is experienced, SWB is defined by three central components.[22]

1. *Satisfaction with present life.* People who are high in SWB tend to like their work and are satisfied with their current personal relationships. They are sociable, outgoing, and willing to open up to others. They also like themselves and enjoy good health and self-esteem.
2. *Relative presence of positive emotions.* People with high SWB more frequently feel pleasant emotions, mainly because they evaluate the world around them in a generally positive way. They have an optimistic outlook, and they expect success in what they undertake.
3. *Relative absence of negative emotions.* Individuals with a strong sense of subjective well-being experience fewer and less severe episodes of negative emotions, such as anxiety, depression, and anger.

You do not have to be happy all the time to achieve overall subjective well-being. Everyone experiences disappointments, unhappiness, and times when life seems unfair. However, people with SWB are typically resilient, able to look on the positive side, get themselves back on track fairly quickly, and less likely to fall into despair over setbacks. There are several myths about happiness: that it depends on age, gender, race, and socioeconomic status. Research and empirical evidence, however, have debunked these myths.[23]

- *There is no happiest age.* Age is not a predictor of SWB. Most age groups exhibit similar levels of life satisfaction, although the things that bring joy often change with age.
- *Happiness has no gender gap.* Women are more likely than men to suffer from anxiety and depression, and men are more at risk for alcoholism and personality disorders. However, an equal number of men and women report being fairly satisfied with life.
- *There are minimal racial differences in happiness.* For example, African Americans and European Americans report nearly the same levels of happiness, and African Americans are slightly less vulnerable to depression. Despite racism and discrimination, members of disadvantaged minority groups generally seem to think optimistically by making realistic self-comparisons and attributing problems less to themselves than to unfair circumstances.
- *Money does not buy happiness.* Wealthier societies report greater well-being. However, once the basic necessities of food, shelter, and safety are provided, there is a very weak correlation between income and happiness. Having no money is a cause of misery, but wealth itself does not guarantee happiness.

Humans are remarkably resourceful creatures. We respond to great loss, such as the death of a loved one or a traumatic event, with an initial period of grief, mourning, and sometimes rage. Yet, with time and the support of loving family and friends, we can brush off the bad times and find satisfaction and peace. Typically, humans learn from suffering and emerge even stronger and more ready to deal with the next crisis. Most find some measure of happiness after the initial shock and pain of loss. Those who are otherwise healthy, in good physical condition, and part of a strong social support network can adapt and cope effectively.

Does Laughter Enhance Health?

Remember the last time you laughed so hard that you cried? Remember how relaxed you felt afterward? Scientists are just beginning to understand the role of humor in our lives and health. For example, laughter has been shown to have the following effects.

- Stressed-out people with a strong sense of humor become less depressed and anxious than those whose sense of humor is less well developed.
- Students who use humor as a coping mechanism report that it predisposes them to a positive mood.
- In a study of depressed and suicidal senior citizens the patients who recovered were the ones who demonstrated a sense of humor.
- Telling a joke, particularly one that involves a shared experience, increases our sense of belonging and social cohesion.

Laughter helps us in many ways. People like to be around others who are fun-loving and laugh easily. Learning to laugh puts more joy into everyday experiences and increases the likelihood that fun-loving people will keep company with us.

Psychologist Barbara Fredrickson argues that positive emotions such as joy, interest, and contentment serve valuable life functions. Joy is associated with playfulness and creativity. Interest encourages us to explore our world, which enhances knowledge and cognitive ability. Contentment allows us to savor and integrate experiences, an important step in achieving mindfulness and insight. By building our physical, social, and mental resources, these positive feelings empower us to cope effectively with life's challenges. While the actual emotions may be transient, their effects can be permanent and provide lifelong enrichment.[24]

Laughter also seems to have positive physiological effects. A number of researchers, such as Lee Berk, M.D., and

---

Subjective well-being (SWB) That uplifting feeling of inner peace and wonder that we call happiness.

Stanley Tan, M.D., have noted that laughter sharpens our immune systems by activating T-cells and natural killer cells and increasing production of immunity-boosting interferon.[25] It also reduces levels of the stress hormone cortisol.

In one experiment, Fredrickson monitored the cardiovascular responses of human subjects who suffered fear and anxiety induced by an unsettling film clip. Some of them then viewed a humorous film clip, while others did not. Those who watched the humorous film returned more quickly to their baseline cardiovascular state, which indicates that laughter may counteract some of the physical effects of negative emotions.[26]

In another study, 50 women with advanced breast cancer who were randomly assigned to a weekly support group lived an average of 18 months longer than 36 cancer patients not in the support group. The implication of this finding is that the women in the support group cheered each other on, which allowed them to sleep and eat better and thus promoted their survival.[27] Other researchers have found that a fighting spirit and the determination to survive are vital adjuncts to standard cancer therapy.[28]

A large body of evidence points to an association between the emotions and physical health, although we still have much to learn about this relationship. Does an emotional state trigger negative behaviors that impair immune function? Or do emotions directly affect health by stimulating the production of hormones that tax the immune system? Whichever is true, it appears that happiness and an optimistic mind-set don't just feel good—they are also good for you.

When Psychosocial Health Deteriorates

Sometimes we are overwhelmed to such a degree that we need outside assistance to help us get back on track toward healthful living. Abusive relationships, traumatic events, unrelenting stress, anxiety at work or home, loneliness, financial upheavals, and a host of other things can sap our spirits, cause us to turn inward, or cause us to act in ways that are outside of what might be considered normal. Chemical imbalances, drug interactions, trauma, neurological disruptions, and other physical problems also may contribute to these behaviors. **Mental illnesses** are disorders that disrupt thinking, feeling, moods, and behaviors, and cause a varying

---

Mental illnesses   Disorders that disrupt thinking, feeling, moods, and behaviors and impair daily functioning.

Major depressive disorder   Severe depression that entails chronic mood disorder, physical effects such as sleep disturbance and exhaustion, and mental effects such as the inability to concentrate.

Chronic mood disorder   Experience of persistent sadness, despair, and hopelessness.

---

degree of impaired functioning in daily life. They are believed to be caused by life events in some instances and by actual biochemical and/or brain dysfunction in other instances.[29]

As with physical illnesses, mental illnesses can range from mild to severe and exact a heavy toll on the quality of life for those with the illnesses and those who come in contact with them. Although mental illness often is not discussed as openly as physical ailments are, mental illness is universal. Several recent reports by the World Health Organization, the World Bank, and Harvard University indicate that mental illness is the second leading cause of disability and premature death in developed countries. It is right behind cardiovascular disease and just ahead of cancer.[30] Or consider this from the Mayo Clinic:

> Imagine attending a 25th reunion at your local high school. Studies tell us that, on average, out of every 100 people on the dance floor, 28 have coped with a mental or substance abuse disorder in the past year. Of these, a dozen or so have had symptoms of an anxiety disorder, such as panic disorder or social phobia. Ten have struggled with an addiction, most likely to be alcohol, and about 10 have lived with a mood disorder, perhaps depression or bipolar disorder. These numbers add up to more than 28 because some people experience more than one illness at the same time, just as high blood pressure, diabetes and asthma may occur together. Although these conditions are common, fear of seeming weak or defective makes many people reluctant to acknowledge mental or emotional distress.[31]

Although there are many types of mental illnesses, we will only focus here on those most likely to be experienced by large numbers of college students. For more detailed information about other disorders, consult the websites at the end of this chapter or ask your instructor for local resources.

Depression: The Full-Scale Tumble

In a recent meeting of the American Psychological Association, the organization's president remarked, "Depression has been called the common cold of psychological disturbances, which underscores its prevalence, but trivializes its impact."[32] In any given one-year period, nearly 10 percent or 19 million American adults suffer from a depressive illness.[33] While the economic cost of this illness is staggering, the real toll in terms of human suffering, job problems, relationship disruptions, and sapping of one's energy and life, is impossible to calculate.

Major Depressive Disorder   It is normal to feel blue or depressed in response to certain experiences, such as death of a loved one, divorce, loss of a job, or an unhappy ending to a relationship. However, people with **major depressive disorder** experience a form of **chronic mood disorder** that involves, on a day-to-day basis, extreme and persistent sadness, despair, and hopelessness. Other typical symptoms may include the following:

- Loss of interest in hobbies, activities, and sexual intimacy
- Decreased energy, fatigue, feeling slowed down
- Difficulty concentrating, indecisiveness, memory lapses
- Insomnia, early-morning awakening, or oversleeping
- Disrupted eating patterns and weight gain or loss
- Restlessness, irritability, agitation
- Preoccupation with failures and inadequacies
- Withdrawal from friends and family
- Persistent physical symptoms that do not respond to treatment, such as headaches, digestive disorders, and chronic pain
- Thoughts of death or suicide; suicide attempts

People with major depression typically feel discouraged by life and circumstances and experience feelings of intense guilt and worthlessness. They may be hypercritical of others and feel disappointed by others most of the time. They may show some impairment of social and occupational functioning, although their behavior is not necessarily bizarre. Approximately 15 percent of them eventually attempt or succeed in committing suicide.[34] Untold numbers of others victimize their families, cause disruptions, or display outwardly violent acts.

Depression and Gender   According to the National Institutes of Mental Health (NIMH), women experience depression at nearly two times the rate of men. Between 8 and 11 percent of men experience depression, in contrast to between 19 and 23 percent of women. About 6 percent of women and 3 percent of men have experienced episodes severe enough to require hospitalization.[35] Many hormonal factors may contribute to the increased rates in women, particularly such events as the menstrual cycle changes, pregnancy, miscarriage, postpartum period, pre-menopause, and menopause. In fact, an NIMH study indicated that in the case of severe premenstrual syndrome (PMS), women with a preexisting vulnerability to PMS experienced relief from mood swings and physical symptoms when their sex hormones were suppressed. Shortly after the hormones were re-introduced, they again developed symptoms of PMS. Women with no history of PMS reported no effects of hormonal manipulation.[36]

Although adolescent and adult females have been found to experience depression at twice the rate of males, the college population seems to represent a notable exception, with equal rates experienced by males and females. Why? Several theories have been suggested.[37]

- The social institutions of the college campus provide more egalitarian roles for men and women.
- College women experience fewer negative events than do high school females. Men in college report more negative events than they experienced in high school.
- College women report smaller and more supportive social networks.

Depression is often preceded by a stressful event. Some psychologists therefore theorize that women are under more stress than are men and thus more prone to become depressed. However, women do not report more stressful events than men do.

Finally, researchers have observed gender differences in coping strategies, or the response to certain events or stimuli, and have proposed that women's strategies make them more vulnerable to depression. Presented with a list of things people do when depressed, college students were asked to indicate how likely they were to engage in each behavior. Men were more likely to assert that "I avoid thinking of reasons why I am depressed," "I do something physical," or "I play sports." Women were more likely to answer "I try to determine why I am depressed," "I talk to other people about my feelings," and "I cry to relieve the tension." In other words, the men tried to distract themselves from a depressed mood, whereas the women focused on it. If focusing on negative feelings intensifies them, women who do this may predispose themselves to depression. This hypothesis has not been directly tested, but some supporting evidence suggests its validity.[38]

Overall, the rate of depression among men may be increasing. Some factors, such as family history, undue stress, the loss of a loved one, or serious illnesses, seem to increase risks.[39] Men are less likely than women to admit to depression, and doctors are less likely to suspect it. Men's depression is also more likely to be hidden by alcohol or drug abuse, or by the socially acceptable habit of working excessively long hours. Depression typically shows up in men not as feeling hopeless and helpless, but as being irritable, angry, and discouraged. One marker of the problem is that the rate of suicide in men is four times that of women, though more women attempt suicide. In fact, after age 70, the rate of men's suicide rises, reaching a peak after age 85.[40] Interestingly, depression seems also to be more lethal for men than women in terms of physical health. Although depression is associated with an increased risk of coronary heart disease in both men and women, only men suffer a high death rate.[41] Because even men who realize they may be depressed are less likely to seek help than women will, encouragement and support from concerned friends and family members are important.

Depression in Selected Populations   There are a few exceptions to the findings on depression and gender. Among Jews, males are equally as likely as females to have major depressive episodes.[42] In recent years, there also has been a noteworthy increase in depression among children, the elderly, and adolescents (particularly adolescent girls), and perhaps in Native American and homosexual young people.[43] Writers, composers, and entertainers also seem to have higher than expected rates of major depression. People experiencing chronic, unrelenting pain have the highest rates of any group.[44]

Depression in older adults is often undiagnosed. Sufferers may be even less likely to report hopelessness, sadness, loss of interest in normally pleasurable activities, or prolonged grief than do their younger counterparts. Sometimes their depression is attributed to drug reactions or as a normal part of aging, rather than as part of an underlying problem. As the elderly person becomes more socially isolated and has fewer social contacts, it will be more difficult for anyone to recognize that depressed behaviors are unusual and the symptoms may become progressively worse without treatment.

Although depression can strike at any age, the first episode usually occurs before age 40. Some people experience one bout of depression and never have problems again, but others suffer recurrences throughout their lives. Stressful life events are often catalysts for these recurrences.

Risks for Depression
Major depressive disorders are caused by interaction between biology, learned behavioral responses, and cognitive factors. Chemical and genetic processes may predispose people to depression, and irrational ideas and beliefs can guide them to negative coping behaviors.[45] Some people, because of genetic history, environment, situational triggers and stressors, poor behavioral skills, and brain–body chemistry, may be particularly vulnerable.

Facts and Fallacies about Depression
Although it is one of the fastest-growing problems in U.S. culture, depression remains one of the most misunderstood mental disorders. Myths and misperceptions about the disease abound.[46]

- *True depression is not a natural reaction to crisis and loss.* It is a pervasive and systemic biological problem. Symptoms may come and go, and their severity will fluctuate, but they do not simply go away. Crisis and loss can lead an already depressed person over the edge to suicide or other problems, but crisis and loss do not inevitably result in depression.
- *People will not snap out of depression by using a little willpower.* Telling a depressed person to snap out of it is like telling a diabetic to produce more insulin. Medical intervention in the form of antidepressant drugs and therapy is often necessary for recovery. Understanding the seriousness of the disease and supporting people in their attempts to recover are key elements.
- *Frequent crying is not a hallmark of depression.* Some people who are depressed bear their burdens in silence or may even be the life of the party. Some depressed individuals don't cry at all. Rather, biochemists theorize that crying may actually ward off depression by releasing chemicals that the body produces as a positive response to stress.
- *Depression is not all in the mind.* Depression isn't a disease of weak-willed, powerless people. In fact, research suggests that depressive illnesses originate with an inherited chemical imbalance in the brain. In addition, some physiological conditions, such as thyroid disorders, multiple sclerosis, chronic fatigue syndrome, and certain cancers have depressive side effects. Certain medications also are known to prompt depressive-like symptoms.
- *In-depth psychotherapy is not the only cure for long-term clinical depression.* No single psychotherapy method works for all cases of depression.

Treating Depression
The best treatment involves determining the person's type and degree of depression and its possible causes. Both psychotherapeutic and pharmacological modes of treatment are recommended for clinical (severe and prolonged) depression. Drugs often relieve the symptoms of depression, such as loss of sleep or appetite, while psychotherapy can be equally helpful by improving the ability to function (Table 2.1).[47]

In some cases, psychotherapy alone may be the most successful treatment. The two most common psychotherapeutic therapies for depression are cognitive and interpersonal therapy.

Cognitive therapy helps a patient look at life rationally and correct habitually pessimistic thought patterns. It focuses on the here-and-now rather than on analyzing a patient's past. To pull a person out of depression, cognitive therapists usually need 6 to 18 months of weekly sessions that include reasoning and behavioral exercises. *Interpersonal therapy,* which is sometimes combined with cognitive therapy, also addresses the present but focuses on correcting chronic relationship problems. Interpersonal therapists focus on patients' relationships with their families and other people.

Antidepressant drugs relieve symptoms in nearly 80 percent of people with chronic depression. Several types of the medications known as *tricyclics* work by preventing excessive absorption of mood-lifting neurotransmitters. Tricyclics can take six weeks to three months to become effective. Newer antidepressant drugs called *tetracyclics* work in one or two weeks.

In recent years, Zoloft, Paxil, and Prozac have become such a common part of our vocabulary that it is not unusual to know someone taking an antidepressant. This could lead one to think that antidepressants can be taken like aspirin. However, countless emergency room visits occur when people misuse antidepressants, try to quit cold turkey, or suffer reactions to the drugs. The potency and dosage of each vary greatly.

Antidepressants should be prescribed only after a thorough psychological and physiological examination. If your doctor suggests an antidepressant, ask these questions first.

- What biological indicators are you using to determine whether I really need this drug? (Beware of the health professional who gives you a five-minute exam, asks you if you are feeling down, and prescribes an antidepressant to fix your problems.)
- What is the action of this drug? What will it do? When will I start to feel the benefits?
- What is your rationale for selecting this antidepressant over others?

Table 2.1
Drug Treatments for Depression

	SSRI (Selective Serotonin Reuptake Inhibitors)	TCA (Tricyclic Antidepressants)	MAOI (Monoamine Oxidase Inhibitors)
How They Work	An SSRI works by stabilizing levels of serotonin, an important neurotransmitter. Low levels of serotonin have been linked to depression and other mood disorders.	An earlier family of antidepressant drugs, TCAs increase the brain's levels of norepinephrine, a neurotransmitter.	MAOIs increase the levels of epinephrine, norepinephrine, and serotonin in the brain.
Commonly Prescribed Antidepressant Drugs	Zoloft, Prozac, Luvox, Paxil, Paxil CR, Celexa, Lexapro	Adapin, Endep, Norpramin, Pamelorf, Sinequan, Effexor	Nardil, Pamate, Remeron, Wellbutrin
Advantages	Relatively few side effects and no withdrawal symptoms. An SSRI is generally the first choice of most physicians.	Some patients respond better to TCA medication than they do to SSRIs.	May be used if other depression medications fail to treat the condition.
Disadvantages	Can be transferred in breast milk; may cause weight gain, reduced sexual desire.	More side effects than SSRIs. May cause sensitivity to heat, which makes it harder for the body to adapt to temperature changes. Must be discontinued slowly, or withdrawal symptoms may occur.	A strict dietary regime must be followed. Failure to do so can result in hypertensive crisis, which can be fatal. Many other medication react badly with MAOIs.

Source: "Selective Serotonin Reuptake Inhibitors" from Treatment-for-Depression.com. Copyright © NCER, LLC, Oceanside, CA. Reprinted by permission.

- What are the side effects of using this drug?
- How long can I be on this medication without significant risk to my health?
- What happens if I stop taking it?
- How will you follow up or monitor the levels of this drug in my body? How often will I need to be checked?

Electroconvulsive therapy (ECT) is another treatment for depression. A patient given ECT is sedated under light general anesthesia, and electric current is applied to the patient's temples for 5 seconds at a time, for 15 or 20 minutes. Between 10 and 20 percent of people with depression who do not respond to drug therapy respond to ECT. However, because it carries a risk of permanent memory loss, some therapists do not recommend ECT under any circumstances.

Clinics have been established in many metropolitan areas to offer group support for depressed people. Some clinics treat all types of depressed people; others restrict themselves to specific groups, such as widows, adolescents, or families and friends of people with depression.

Bipolar Disorder   Also known as manic-depressive illness, **bipolar disorder** is considered another form of depression. It is characterized by alternating emotional highs (mania) and lows (depression). Symptoms can vary from mild to disabling and severe. Bipolar disorder affects more than 2 million adult Americans, about 1 percent of the population. It often begins

in adolescence and may persist for life, and last for weeks or months at a time. In the depression phase, symptoms follow the same pattern as they do in a major depressive syndrome. In the manic phase, symptoms may include feelings of euphoria, extreme optimism, and inflated self esteem; rapid speech, racing thoughts, agitation, and increased physical activity; poor judgment and recklessness; difficulty sleeping; tendency to be easily distracted; inability to concentrate; and extreme irritability.[48]

Although the exact cause of bipolar disorder is unknown, biological, genetic, and environmental factors seem to be involved in causing episodes of the illness. Evidence indicates that neurotransmitters in people with the disorder differ from those without it. Bipolar disorder tends to run in families, with about 60 percent of cases showing a family history. Thus, a genetic predisposition to have abnormal genes regulating neurotransmitter action may be a risk factor.[49] Factors that are believed to trigger episodes include drug abuse and stressful or psychologically traumatic events. Once diagnosed, persons with bipolar disorder have a number of counseling and pharmaceutical options, and most will be able to live a healthy, functional life while being treated.

> **Bipolar disorder**   Form of depression characterized by alternating mania and depression.

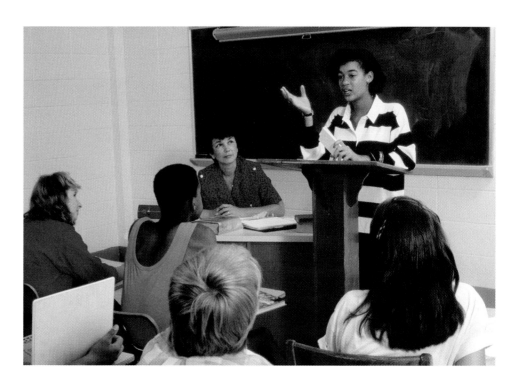

Panic attacks can be precipitated by stressful situations, such as public speaking.

Anxiety Disorders: Facing Your Fears

Anxiety disorders, which are characterized by persistent feelings of threat and anxiousness, are a little-understood yet common psychological problem. Consider John Madden, former head coach of the Oakland Raiders, and a true "man's man" who has outfitted his own bus and is driven every weekend across the country to serve as a commentator on NFL football games. What's the reason behind this exhausting schedule? Madden is terrified of getting on a plane.

Anxiety disorders are the number-one mental health problem in the United States. They affect more than 19 million people ages 18 to 54 each year, or about 13 percent of all adults.[50] Some sources place the number as high as 25 percent. Anxiety is also a leading mental health problem among adolescents; it affects 13 million youngsters ages 9 to 17. Costs associated with an overly anxious populace are growing rapidly; conservative estimates cite nearly $50 billion a year spent in doctor bills and workplace losses in America. According to a study by the World Health Organization, the odds of developing an anxiety disorder have doubled in the past four decades.[51] These numbers don't begin to address the human costs incurred when a person is too fearful to leave the house

Anxiety disorders   Disorders characterized by persistent feelings of threat and anxiousness in coping with everyday problems.

Generalized anxiety disorder (GAD)   A constant sense of worry that may cause restlessness, difficulty in concentrating, and tension

or talk to anyone outside the immediate family. Anxiety-related ailments include generalized anxiety disorders, panic disorder, specific phobias, and social phobias.

Generalized Anxiety Disorders   One common form of anxiety disorder, **generalized anxiety disorder (GAD),** is severe enough to significantly interfere with daily life. Generally, the person with this disorder is a consummate worrier who develops a debilitating level of anxiety. Often multiple sources of worry exist, and it is hard to pinpoint the root cause of the anxiety. A diagnosis of GAD depends on showing at least three of the following symptoms for more days than not during a period of six months:[52]

1. Restlessness or feeling keyed up or on edge
2. Being easily fatigued
3. Difficulty concentrating or mind going blank
4. Irritability
5. Muscle tension
6. Sleep disturbances (difficulty falling or staying asleep or restless sleep)

Often GAD runs in families and is readily treatable with benzodiazepines such as Librium, Valium, and Xanax, which calm the person for short periods. More effective long-term treatments are achieved through individual therapy.

Panic Disorders   It can happen at any time: while sleeping, while sitting in traffic, just before you deliver your class presentation. Suddenly and unexpectedly your heart starts to race, your face turns red, you can't catch your breath, you feel nauseated, you start to perspire, and you may feel like you are going to pass out.

What you are experiencing is probably a **panic attack,** a form of acute anxiety reaction that brings on an intense physical reaction. This reaction may be so severe that you think you are going to have a heart attack and die. Or you may dismiss it as the "jitters" from too much stress. Between 10 and 20 percent of Americans experience panic attacks at some time in their lives. Although it is a highly treatable mental disorder, it is also growing in incidence, particularly among young women. Panic attacks may become debilitating and destructive, particularly if they happen often and lead the person to avoid going out in public or interacting with others.

A panic attack typically starts abruptly, peaks within 10 minutes, lasts about 30 minutes, and leaves the victim tired and drained.[53] In addition to those just described, symptoms can include trembling, dizziness, increased respiration rate, chills, hot flashes, shortness of breath, stomach cramping, chest pain, difficulty swallowing, and a sense of doom or impending death.

Although researchers aren't sure of causation, heredity, stress, and certain biochemical factors may play a role. Your chance of having a panic attack increases if you have a close family member who has them. Some researchers believe that people who have panic attacks are experiencing an over-reactive "fight-or-flight" physical response. (See Chapter 3.)

As with other forms of anxiety-based disorders, medication and cognitive behavioral therapy are often the keys to treatment. Some individuals are given antidepressants, which often prevents future attacks. In some cases, a medication to relieve anxiety is effective given alone or with other drugs.[54] Cognitive therapy can help sufferers recognize and avoid triggers or deal with triggers through meditation, deep breathing, and other relaxation techniques. Patients usually show improvement within eight to ten sessions.

Specific Phobias   In contrast to panic disorders, **phobias,** or phobic disorders, involve a persistent and irrational fear of a specific object, activity, or situation, which is often out of proportion to the circumstances. Phobias result in a compelling desire to avoid the source of the fear. About 13 percent of Americans suffer from phobias, such as fear of spiders, snakes, and public speaking. Social phobias are perhaps the most common phobic response.[55]

Social Phobias   A **social phobia** is an anxiety disorder characterized by the persistent fear and avoidance of social situations. Essentially, the person dreads these situations for fear of being humiliated, embarrassed, or even looked at.[56] These disorders vary in scope. Some cause difficulty only in specific situations, such as speaking in front of a class. In more extreme cases, a person avoids all contact with others.

Sources of Anxiety Disorders   Because anxiety disorders vary in complexity and degree, scientists have yet to find clear reasons why one person develops them and another doesn't. The following factors are often cited as possible causes.

- *Biology.* Some scientists trace the origin of anxiety to the brain and brain functioning. Using sophisticated positron emission tomography scans (PET scans), scientists can analyze areas of the brain that react during anxiety-producing events. Families appear to display similar brain and physiological reactivity, so we may inherit our tendencies toward anxiety disorders.
- *Environment.* Anxiety also may be a learned response. Though genetic tendencies may exist, experiencing a repeated pattern of reaction to certain situations programs the brain to respond in a certain way. For example, monkeys separated from their mothers at an early age are more fearful, and their stress hormones fire more readily, than those that stayed with their mothers. If your mother (or father) screamed whenever a large spider crept into view, or if other anxiety-raising events occurred frequently, you might be predisposed to react with anxiety to similar events later in your life. Interestingly, animals also experience such anxieties—perhaps from being around their edgy owners.
- *Social and Cultural Roles.* Culture and social roles also may be a factor in risks for anxiety. Because men and women are taught to assume different roles in society (for example, man as protector, woman as victim), women may find it more acceptable to scream, shake, pass out, and otherwise express extreme anxiety. Men, on the other hand, have learned to stuff such anxieties rather than act upon them.

Seasonal Affective Disorder

An estimated 6 percent of Americans suffer from **seasonal affective disorder (SAD),** a type of depression, and an additional 14 percent experience a milder form of the disorder known as the winter blues. SAD strikes during the winter months and is associated with reduced exposure to sunlight. People with SAD suffer from irritability, apathy, carbohydrate craving and weight gain, increased sleep time, and general sadness. Researchers believe that SAD is caused by a malfunction in the hypothalamus, the gland that regulates responses to external stimuli. Stress also may play a role.

Certain factors seem to put people at risk for SAD. Women are four times more likely to suffer from it than

---

Panic attack   Severe anxiety attack in which a particular situation, often for unknown reasons, causes terror.

Phobia   A deep and persistent fear of a specific object, activity, or situation that results in a compelling desire to avoid the source of the fear.

Social phobia   A phobia characterized by persistent fear and avoidance of social situations.

Seasonal affective disorder (SAD)   A type of depression that occurs in the winter months, when sunlight levels are low.

men. Although SAD can occur at any age, people ages 20 to 40 appear to be most vulnerable. Certain families appear to be at risk. Residents of northern states, where there are fewer hours of sunlight during the winter, are more at risk than those living in the South. An estimated 10 percent of the population in Maine, Minnesota, and Wisconsin experience SAD, compared to fewer than 2 percent of those in Florida and New Mexico.

Therapies for SAD are simple but effective. The most beneficial is light therapy, in which patients are exposed to lamps that simulate sunlight. Eighty percent of patients experience relief from their symptoms within four days of treatment. Other treatments for SAD include diet change (eating more complex carbohydrates), increased exercise, stress management techniques, sleep restriction (limiting the number of hours slept in a 24-hour period), psychotherapy, and antidepressants.

Schizophrenia

Perhaps the most frightening of all mental disorders is **schizophrenia,** which affects about 1 percent of the U.S. population. Schizophrenia is characterized by alterations of the senses (including auditory and visual hallucinations); the inability to sort out incoming stimuli and make appropriate responses; an altered sense of self; and radical changes in emotions, movements, and behaviors. Victims of this disease often cannot function in society. Contrary to common misconception, schizophrenia is not the same as split personality, or multiple personality disorder.

For decades, scientists believed that schizophrenia was an environmentally provoked form of madness. They blamed abnormal family interactions or early childhood traumas. Since the mid-1980s, however, when magnetic resonance imaging (MRI) and positron emission tomography (PET) have allowed us to study brain function more closely, scientists have recognized that schizophrenia is a biological disease of the brain. The brain damage occurs early in life, possibly as early as the second trimester of fetal development. However, symptoms most commonly appear in late adolescence.

At present, schizophrenia is treatable but not curable. Treatments usually include some combination of hospitalization, medication, and supportive psychotherapy. Supportive psychotherapy, as opposed to more intensive psychoanalysis, can help the patient acquire skills for living in society.

Even though environmental theories on the causes of schizophrenia have been discarded in favor of biological theories, a stigma remains attached to the disease. Families of people with schizophrenia frequently experience anger and guilt.

Schizophrenia   A mental illness with biological origins that is characterized by irrational behavior, hallucinations, and, often, an inability to function in society.

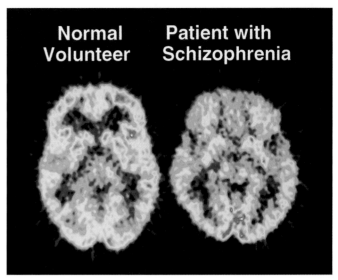

These brain images reveal significant differences between normal brain activity and that of a person with schizophrenia.

They often need information, family counseling, and advice on how to meet the schizophrenic person's needs for shelter, medical care, vocational training, and social interaction.

Gender Issues in Psychosocial Health

Unfortunately, gender bias can hinder the correct diagnosis of psychosocial disorders. In one study, for instance, 175 mental health professionals of both genders were asked to diagnose a patient based upon a summarized case history. Some of the professionals were told that the patient was male, others that the patient was female. The gender of the patient made a substantial difference in the diagnosis (though the gender of the clinician did not). When subjects thought the patient was female, they were more likely to diagnose hysterical personality, which is often thought of as a women's disorder. When they believed the patient to be male, the more likely diagnosis was antisocial personality, often thought of as a male disorder.

PMS: Physical or Mental Disorder?   A major controversy is the inclusion of a provisional diagnosis for premenstrual syndrome (PMS) in the American Psychiatric Association's *Diagnostic and Statistical Manual of Mental Disorders* (now in its fourth edition, known as DSM-IV). The provisional diagnosis, in an appendix to DSM-IV, signals that PMS merits further study and may be included as an approved diagnosis in future editions of the DSM. In other words, PMS could be considered a mental disorder in the future.

PMS is characterized by depression, irritability, and other symptoms of increased stress typically occurring just prior to menstruation and lasting for a day or two. A more severe case of PMS is known as *premenstrual dysphoric disorder* (PMDD). Whereas PMS is somewhat disruptive and

Cutting through the Pain

What is self-injury? Self-injury is an attempt to alter a mood state by inflicting physical harm on the body. This may include cutting (with razors, glass, knives, etc.), burning, hitting the body with an object or fists, or not allowing wounds to heal. People discover that hurting themselves brings relief from distress and turn to it as a primary coping mechanism.

Why does self-injury make some people feel better? Many factors or a combination of factors seem to be involved, including a biologic predisposition, a need to reduce tension, and a lack of experience in dealing with strong emotions. Some studies suggest that when people who self-injure feel emotionally overwhelmed, performing self-injury brings their levels of psychological and physiological tension and arousal back to a bearable level almost immediately. Simply stated, when they feel a strong uncomfortable emotion and don't know how to handle it, hurting themselves reduces the emotional discomfort quickly and calms them down.

Who is most likely to self-injure? The typical person in therapy for self-injury is a single, intelligent, well-educated female, and from a middle- to upper-middle-class family. She usually started self-injuring in middle to late adolescence. Often (but not always) she has a background of physical, emotional, and/or sexual abuse or has experienced chaotic family conditions. Eating disorders often are co-reported. However, focusing only on those receiving therapeutic treatment for self-injury may

vastly underreport the number of males and minorities who self-injure. One report estimates that males may account for as many as 40% of self-injurers, but their injuries are overlooked as a product of macho outbursts such as fighting or sports injuries.

How common is this behavior? It is difficult to accurately estimate the number of people who self-injure, because it is sometimes difficult to distinguish self-injurious behavior from suicide attempts. In some studies, no attempt is made to distinguish between the two behaviors. And, as the injuries are often purposely hidden, reports from hospitals, police, or social service agencies underreport the occurrence. In the general population of the United States, estimates of individuals engaging in self-injury range from 14 to 600 persons per 100,000 annually (.014 to .6%). The rates are higher in adolescents and young adults; estimates in the general college student population range from 1.8 to 12%.

Is treatment available? Treatments currently being explored range from talk therapy, to teaching problem-solving skills, to medications that help relieve underlying depression and anxiety that may contribute to the self-injury. What all of the treatments have in common is the aim to end the feelings that prompt the behavior, not just stop the behavior itself.

Are there signs and symptoms? Signs include scars or current cuts or abrasions and flimsy excuses for these wounds. A person may wear long sleeves and pants in warm weather to hide his or her wounds. Difficulty handling anger, social withdrawal,

sensitivity to rejection, or body alienation also may be symptoms of self-injury.

What do you do if a loved one self-injures?

✔ Educate yourself; read the books or visit the websites listed below.
✔ Don't avoid the subject of self-injury; let the person know that you're willing to talk.
✔ Let your friend know you understand that self-injury is helping the person to cope with strong negative emotions.
✔ Be available; it may be helpful to provide distractions when the person is tempted to self-injure.
✔ Show concern for the injuries. The injuries need to be treated to prevent scarring and infection.

Where can I get more information? Try these books and websites: Conterio, K. and Lader, W. *Bodily Harm: The Breakthrough Healing Program for Self-Injurers.* New York: Hyperion, 1998; Levenkron, S. *Cutting: Understanding and Overcoming Self-Mutilation.* New York: W.W. Norton and Company, 1998; "Self-Injury: You Are NOT the Only One." www.crystal.palace.net/~llama/selfinjury.

—Susan Dobie, Oregon State University

Sources: T. M. Edwards, "What Cutters Feel," *Time,* November 9, 1998; A. R. Favazza, *Bodies under Siege: Self-Mutilation and Body Modification in Culture and Psychiatry* (Baltimore, MD: The Johns Hopkins University Press, 1996); D. Martinson, "Self-Injury: A Quick Guide to the Basics," 1998. www.palace.net/~llama/psych/guide.html; K. L. Suyemoto and X. Kountz, "Self-Mutilation," *The Prevention Researcher* 7, no. 4 (2000): 1–4.

uncomfortable, it does not interfere with daily function; PMDD does. To be diagnosed with PMDD, a woman must have at least five symptoms of PMS for a week to ten days, with at least one symptom being serious enough to interfere with her ability to function at work or at home. In these more severe cases, antidepressants may be prescribed. The point of contention lies in whether administering this treatment indicates that PMDD is a mental disorder rather than a physical problem.[57] Is it legitimate to attach a label indicating dysfunction and disorder to symptoms experienced only once or twice a month? Further controversy stems from the

possible use (or misuse) of the diagnostic label to justify exclusion of women from certain desirable jobs.

Suicide: Giving Up on Life

There are more than 35,000 reported suicides each year in the United States. Experts estimate that there may be closer to 100,000 cases, given the difficulty in determining the causes of many suspicious deaths. More lives are lost to suicide than to any other single cause except cardiovascular

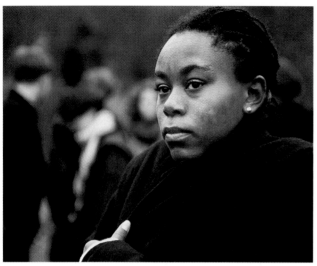

If you are experiencing problems such as depression or anxiety, don't try to go it alone. A qualified, caring therapist can help.

- Change in eating habits
- A direct statement about committing suicide, such as, "I might as well end it all."
- An indirect statement, such as, "You won't have to worry about me anymore."
- Final preparations, such as writing a will, repairing poor relationships with family or friends, giving away prized possessions, or writing revealing letters
- A preoccupation with themes of death
- A sudden and unexplained demonstration of happiness following a period of depression
- Marked changes in personal appearance
- Excessive risk taking and an "I don't care what happens to me" attitude

> **What do you think?**
>
> *If your roommate showed warning signs of suicide, what action would you take?* ❋ *Who would you contact first?* ❋ *Where on campus might your friend get help?* ❋ *What if someone in class whom you hardly know gave warning signs of suicide?* ❋ *What would you then do?*

disease and cancer. Suicide often results from poor coping skills, lack of social support, lack of self-esteem, and the inability to see one's way out of a bad situation.

College students are more likely than the general population to attempt suicide; suicide is the third leading cause of death in people between the ages of 15 and 24. In fact, this age group now accounts for nearly 20 percent of all suicides.[58] The pressures, joys, disappointments, challenges, and changes of the college environment are believed to be in part responsible for these rates. However, young adults who choose not to go to college but who are searching for direction in careers, relationships, and other life goals are also at risk.

Risk factors for suicide include a family history of suicide, previous suicide attempts, excessive drug and alcohol use, prolonged depression, financial difficulties, serious illness in the suicide contemplator or in his or her loved ones, and loss of a loved one through death or rejection. Societal pressures often serve as a catalyst.

In most cases, suicide does not occur unpredictably. In fact, between 75 and 80 percent of people who commit suicide give a warning of their intentions.

Warning Signs of Suicide

Common signs of possible suicide include:[59]

- Recent loss and a seeming inability to let go of grief
- Change in personality, such as sadness, withdrawal, irritability, anxiety, tiredness, indecisiveness, apathy
- Change in behavior, such as inability to concentrate, loss of interest in classes
- Diminished sexual interest, such as impotence, menstrual abnormalities
- Expressions of self-hatred
- Change in sleep patterns

Taking Action to Prevent Suicide

Most people who attempt suicide really want to live but see suicide as the only way out of an intolerable situation. Crisis counselors and suicide hotlines may help temporarily, but the best way to prevent suicide is to get rid of conditions and substances that may precipitate attempts, including alcoholism, drugs, loneliness, isolation, and access to guns.

If someone you know threatens or displays warning signs of suicide, take the following actions.

- Monitor the warning signals. Keep an eye on the person, or ensure there is someone around the person as much as possible.
- Take threats seriously. Don't brush them off.
- Let the person know how much you care about him or her. State that you are there if he or she needs help.
- Listen. Try not to discredit or be shocked by what the person says. Empathize, sympathize, and keep the person talking. Talk about stressors, and listen to the responses.
- Ask directly, "Are you thinking of hurting or killing yourself?"
- Do not belittle the person's feelings or say that he or she doesn't really mean it or couldn't succeed at suicide. To some people, these comments offer the challenge of proving you wrong.
- Help the person think about alternatives. Offer to go for help together. Call your local suicide hotline and use all available community and campus resources. Recommend a counselor or other person to talk to.
- Remember that your relationships with others involve responsibilities. Give of yourself by staying with the person,

taking the person to a health care facility, or providing support.

- Tell your friend's spouse, partner, relatives, or counselor. Do not keep your suspicions to yourself. Don't let a suicidal friend talk you into keeping your discussions confidential. If your friend succeeds in a suicide attempt because you kept a promise not to tell others of the danger, you may find that others will question your decision, just as you may blame yourself.

Seeking Professional Help

A physical ailment will readily send most of us to the nearest health professional, but many people view seeking professional help for psychosocial problems as an admission of personal failure. However, increasing numbers of Americans are turning to mental health professionals, and nearly one in five seeks such help. Researchers cite breakdown in support systems, high societal expectations of the individual, and dysfunctional families as three major reasons why more people are asking for assistance than ever before. You should consider seeking help if:

- You think you need help
- You experience wild mood swings
- A problem is interfering with your daily life
- Your fears or feelings of guilt frequently distract your attention
- You begin to withdraw from others
- You have hallucinations
- You feel that life is not worth living
- You feel inadequate or worthless
- Your emotional responses are inappropriate to various situations
- Your daily life seems to be nothing but repeated crises
- You feel you can't "get your act together"
- You are considering suicide
- You turn to drugs or alcohol to escape from your problems
- You feel out of control

Getting Evaluated for Treatment

If you are considering treatment for a psychosocial problem, schedule a complete evaluation first. Consult a credentialed health professional for a thorough examination, which should include three parts.

- A physical checkup, which will rule out thyroid disorders, viral infections, and anemia—all of which can result in depressive-like symptoms—and a neurological check of coordination, reflexes, and balance, to rule out brain disorders
- A psychiatric history, which will attempt to trace the course of the apparent disorder, genetic or family factors, and any past treatments

---

Table 2.2
Questions to Ask When Choosing a Therapist

A qualified mental health professional should be willing to answer all your questions during an initial consultation. Questions to ask include the following.

- Can you interview the therapist before starting treatment? An initial meeting will help you determine whether this person will be a good fit for you.
- Do you like the therapist as a person? Can you talk to him or her comfortably?
- Is the therapist watching the clock or easily distracted? *You* should be the main focus of the session.
- Does the therapist demonstrate professionalism? Be concerned if your therapist is frequently late or breaks appointments, suggests social interactions outside your therapy sessions, talks inappropriately about himself or herself, has questionable billing practices, or resists releasing you from therapy.
- Will the therapist help you set your own goals? A good professional should evaluate your general situation and help you set small goals to work on between sessions. The therapist should not tell you how to help yourself but help you discover the steps.

Remember, in most states, the use of the title *therapist* or *counselor* is unregulated. Make your choice carefully.

- A mental status examination, which will assess thoughts, speaking processes, and memory, and will include an in-depth interview with tests for other psychiatric symptoms[60]

Once physical factors have been ruled out, you may decide to consult a professional who specializes in psychosocial health.

Mental Health Professionals

Several types of mental health professionals are available to help you. The most important criterion is not how many degrees this person has, but whether you feel you can work together. Table 2.2 presents fundamental criteria to help you choose the best therapist for your needs.

Psychiatrist A **psychiatrist** is a medical doctor. After obtaining a medical doctor (M.D.) degree, a psychiatrist spends up to 12 years studying psychosocial health and disease. As a licensed M.D., a psychiatrist can prescribe medications for various mental or emotional problems and may have admitting privileges at a local hospital. Some psychiatrists are affiliated with hospitals, while others are in private practice.

Psychiatrist A licensed medical doctor who specializes in treating mental and emotional disorders.

Table 2.3
Traditional Forms of Psychotherapy: Assumptions, Goals, and Methods

Type of Therapy	Basic Assumptions	Goals and Methods
Psychoanalysis	Behavior is motivated by intrapsychic conflict and biological urges.	Discover the sources of conflict and resolve them through insight.
Psychodynamic therapy	Behavior is motivated by both unconscious forces and interpersonal experiences.	Understand and improve interpersonal skills by modifying the client's inappropriate schemas about interpersonal relationships.
Humanistic and Gestalt therapy	People are good and have innate worth.	Use techniques to enhance personal awareness and feelings of self-worth to promote personal growth and self-actualization and to enhance clients' awareness of bodily sensations and feelings.
Behavior and cognitive-behavior therapy	Behavior is largely controlled by environmental contingencies, people's perception of them, or a combination.	Change maladaptive behavior and thinking patterns by manipulating environmental variables, restructuring thinking patterns, and correcting faulty thinking or irrational beliefs.
Family/couples therapy	Problems in relationships entail everybody involved in them.	Analyze relationship patterns and others' roles in order to discover how interactions influence problems in individual functioning.

Source: Adapted from Neil R. Carson and William Buskist, *Psychology: The Science of Behavior, 5th ed.* (Boston: Allyn & Bacon, 1997), 629. Copyright © 1997 Pearson Education. Reprinted by permission of the publisher.

Psychologist   A **psychologist** usually has a doctor of philosophy (Ph.D.) degree in counseling or clinical psychology. In addition, many states require licensure. Psychologists are trained in various types of therapy, including behavior and insight therapy. Most can conduct both individual and group counseling sessions. Psychologists also may be trained in certain specialties, such as family counseling or sexual counseling.

Psychoanalyst   A **psychoanalyst** is a psychiatrist or psychologist with special training in psychoanalysis. This is a type of therapy that helps patients remember early traumas that have blocked personal growth. Facing these traumas helps them resolve conflicts and lead more productive lives.

Clinical/Psychiatric Social Worker   A **social worker** has at least a master's degree in social work (M.S.W.) and two years of experience in a clinical setting. Many states require an examination for accreditation. Some social workers work in clinical settings, whereas others have private practices.

Counselor   A **counselor** often has a master's degree in counseling, psychology, educational psychology, or related human service. Professional societies recommend at least two years of graduate course work or supervised practice as a minimal requirement. Many counselors are trained to do individual and group therapy. They often specialize in one type of counseling, such as family, marital, relationship, children, drug, divorce, behavioral, or personal counseling.

Psychiatric Nurse Specialist   Although all registered nurses can work in psychiatric settings, some continue their education and specialize in psychiatric practice. The psychiatric nurse specialist can be certified by the American Nursing Association in adult, child, or adolescent psychiatric nursing.

What to Expect in Therapy

Many different types of counseling exist, ranging from individual therapy, which involves one-on-one work between therapist and client, to group therapy, in which two or more clients meet with a therapist to discuss problems. Table 2.3 identifies traditional forms of psychotherapy.

The first trip to a therapist can be difficult. Most of us have misconceptions about what therapy is and about what it can do. That first visit is a verbal and mental sizing up between you and the therapist. You may not accomplish much in that first hour. If you decide that this professional is not

Psychologist   A person with a Ph.D. degree and training in counseling or clinical psychology.

Psychoanalyst   A psychiatrist or psychologist with special training in psychoanalysis.

Social worker   A person with an M.S.W. degree and clinical training.

Counselor   A person with a variety of academic and experiential training who deals with the treatment of emotional problems.

for you, you will at least have learned how to present your problem and what qualities you need in a therapist.

Before meeting, briefly explain your needs. Ask what the fee is. Arrive on time, wear comfortable clothing, and expect to spend about an hour during your first visit. The therapist will want to take down your history and details about the problems that have brought you to therapy. Answer as honestly as possible. Many will ask how you feel about aspects of your life. Do not be embarrassed to acknowledge your feelings. It is critical to the success of your treatment that you trust this person enough to be open and honest.

Do not expect the therapist to tell you what to do or how to behave. The responsibility for improved behavior lies with you. Ask if you can set your own therapeutic goals and timetables.

If after your first visit (or even after several visits) you feel you cannot work with this person, say so. You have the right to find a therapist with whom you feel comfortable.

Taking Charge

Make It Happen!

Assessment: The Assess Yourself box on page 34 gave you the chance to look at various aspects of your psychosocial health and to compare your self-assessment with a friend's perceptions. Now that you have considered these results, you can take steps toward changing certain behaviors that may be detrimental to your psychosocial health.

Making a Change: In order to change your behavior, you need to develop a plan. Follow these steps.

1. Evaluate your behavior, and identify patterns and specific things you are doing. What can you change now? What can you change in the near future?

2. Select one pattern of behavior that you want to change.

3. Fill out a Behavior Change Contract. It should include your long-term goal for change, your short-term goals, the rewards you'll give yourself for reaching these goals, potential obstacles along the way, and strategies for overcoming these obstacles. For each goal, list the small steps and specific actions that you will take.

4. Chart your progress in a journal. At the end of a week, consider how successful you were in following your plan. What helped you be successful? What made change more difficult? What will you do differently next week?

5. Revise your plan as needed. Are the short-term goals attainable? Are the rewards satisfying?

Example: John discovered that he assessed himself as a positive and upbeat person, while the assessment his friend gave him rated him as more impatient and cynical. John resolved to take steps that would help him slow down and be more appreciative of the good things around him. Among the changes that he made were to make an effort to listen to his sister without interrupting her and to be sure to pay a sincere compliment to a family member or friend every other day. John found that paying compliments made him stop to think about the qualities he appreciated in his friends and family. While he struggled to listen without interrupting, John found that he was learning a lot about his sister that he had never known before. After several weeks, John's friends commented on his calmer and happier demeanor.

Summary

☀ Psychosocial health is a complex phenomenon involving mental, emotional, social, and spiritual health.

☀ Many factors influence psychosocial health, including life experiences, family, the environment, other people, self-esteem, self-efficacy, and personality. Some of these are modifiable; others are not.

☀ Developing self-esteem and self-efficacy and getting enough sleep are key to enhancing psychosocial health.

☀ Many people believe spirituality is important to wellness. Though the exact reasons have not been established, many studies show a connection between the two.

☀ Happiness is a key factor in determining overall reaction to life's challenges. The mind–body connection is an important link in overall health and well-being.

☀ Indicators of deteriorating psychosocial health include depression. Identifying depression is the first step in treating this disorder.

☀ Common psychosocial problems include anxiety disorders, panic attacks, phobias, seasonal affective disorder, and schizophrenia.

☀ Suicide is a result of negative psychosocial reactions to life. People intending to commit suicide often give warning signs of their intentions. Such people often can be helped.

✱ Mental health professionals include psychiatrists, psychoanalysts, psychologists, clinical/psychiatric social workers, counselors, and psychiatric nurse specialists. Many therapy methods exist, including group and individual therapy. It is wise to interview a therapist carefully before beginning treatment.

Questions for Discussion and Reflection

1. What is psychosocial health? What indicates that you are or aren't psychosocially healthy? Why might the college environment provide a challenge to your psychosocial health?
2. Discuss the factors that influence your overall level of psychosocial health. Which factors can you change? Which ones may be more difficult to change?
3. What steps could you take today to improve your psychosocial health? Which steps require long-term effort?
4. What are four main themes of spirituality, and how are they expressed in daily life?
5. Why is laughter therapeutic? How can humor help you better achieve wellness?
6. What factors appear to contribute to psychosocial difficulties and illnesses? Which of the common psychosocial illnesses is likely to affect people in your age group?
7. What are the warning signs of suicide? Of depression? Why is depression so pervasive among young Americans today? Why are some groups more vulnerable to suicide and depression than are others? What would you do if you heard a friend in the cafeteria say to no one in particular that he was going to "do the world a favor and end it all"?
8. Discuss the different types of health professionals and therapies. If you felt depressed about breaking off a long-term relationship, which professional and therapy do you think would be most beneficial? Explain your answer. What services does your student health center provide? What fees are charged to students?
9. What psychosocial areas do you need to work on? Which are most important to you, and why? What actions can you take today?

Accessing Your Health on the Internet

Visit the following Internet sites to explore further topics and issues related to personal health. To visit an organization's website, go to the Companion Website for *Health: The Basics, Sixth Edition* at www.aw-bc.com/donatelle, click on the book image, and select "Accessing Your Health on the Internet" from the navigation menu on the left.

1. *American Psychological Association Help Center.* Includes information on psychology at work, the mind–body connection, psychological responses to war, and other topics.
2. *Anxiety Disorders Association of America.* Offers links to treatment resources, self-help tools, information on clinical trials, and other information.
3. *National Alliance for the Mentally Ill.* A support and advocacy organization of families and friends of people with severe mental illnesses. More than 1,200 state and local affiliates; local branches often can help with finding treatment.
4. *National Institute of Mental Health (NIMH).* Overview of mental health information and new research relating to mental health.
5. *National Mental Health Association.* Works to promote mental health through advocacy, education, research, and services.

Further Reading

Dalai Lama and H. C. Cutler. *The Art of Happiness: A Handbook for Living.* New York: Riverhead, 1998.

Through a series of interviews, the authors explore questions of meaning, motives, and the interconnectedness of life, including why so many people are unhappy, and offer strategies for becoming happy.

Norem, Julie. *The Positive Power of Negative Thinking.* New York: Basics Books, 2002.

Explores reasons for negative thinking and mechanisms for changing the way you think. Includes self-tests and analysis for helping you retrain your thinking processes.

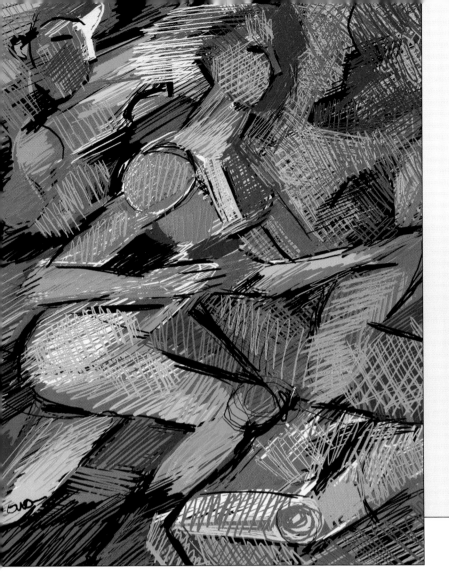

Managing Stress

Coping with Life's Challenges

3 **3** **3** **3** **3** **3**

Objectives

* Define stress and examine the potential impact of stress on health, relationships, and success in college.

* Explain the three phases of the general adaptation syndrome and describe what happens physiologically when we experience a real or perceived threat.

* Examine the health risks that may occur with chronic stress.

* Discuss psychosocial, environmental, and self-imposed sources of stress and examine ways in which you might reduce risks from these stressors or inoculate yourself against stressful situations.

* Examine the special stressors that affect college students and strategies for reducing risk.

* Discuss techniques for coping with unavoidable stress, reducing exposure to stress, and making optimum use of positive stressors to promote growth and enrich life experiences.

Hello to College Joys: Keep Stress Off Campus

By Jane E. Brody

Adults are often quick to tell college students: "Enjoy yourselves. This is the best time of your lives." But for an increasing number of students, the college experience is marred by chronic anxiety, stress and distress.

College counselors report a sharp increase in the need and demand for mental health services, and that can sometimes result in long waiting lists, making the troubled students' problems even worse.

In recent years more than 80 percent of campuses have noted significant increases in serious psychological problems, including severe stress, depression, anxiety and panic attacks, according to an annual survey of counseling centers by Dr. Robert P. Gallagher of the University of Pittsburgh.

Some of this emotional distress can be attributed to financial worries in these economically uncertain times. Looking at the dismal employment situation, many students with college loans fret about how they will be able to repay them.

Furthermore, family support systems are not what they used to be for students whose parents are separated, divorced or remarried.

Read the complete article online in the eThemes section of this book's website: www.aw-bc.com/donatelle.

Too much noise. Too many people. Long lines at the bookstore. Relationship problems. Financial worries. Not enough time. Pressure to get good grades. Too much to do. Technological overload. Terrorist threats. Stress! You can't run from it; there's no place to hide. It affects young and old, rich and poor, and people of all racial and ethnic groups. Stress is as much a part of daily life as is breathing. Whether it brings life and energy into our day or seems to crush the life out of us, stress is woven into the pattern of our lives.

Often, stress is insidious, and we don't even notice things that affect us. As we sleep, it encroaches on our psyche through noise or incessant worries. While we work at the computer, stress may interfere in the form of spam on our screens, noise from next door, strain on our eyes, and tension in our backs. The toll stress exacts from us during a lifetime is unknown, but it is increasingly believed to be much more than an annoyance. Rather, it is a significant health hazard that can rob the body of needed nutrients, damage the cardiovascular system, raise blood pressure, and dampen the immune system's defenses, all of which leave us vulnerable to infections and a host of diseases. In addition, it can drain our emotional reserves; contribute to depression, anxiety, and irritability; and cloud social interactions with hostility and anger. Stress is a major concern in the United States, and it appears to be getting worse: One-third of U.S. workers report an increase in job-related stress over the past year. Although much has been written about stress, we are only beginning to understand the multifaceted nature of the stress response and its tremendous potential for harm or benefit.

What Is Stress?

Often, we think of stress as an externally imposed factor. But for most of us, stress results from an internal state of emotional tension that occurs in response to the various demands of living. Most current definitions state that **stress** is the mental and physical response of our bodies to the changes and challenges in our lives. Inherent in these definitions is the idea that we sometimes take ourselves too seriously: that we should loosen up, worry less, and gain greater control over our minds as well as our bodies.

A **stressor** is any physical, social, or psychological event or condition that causes the body to adjust to a specific situation. Stressors may be tangible, such as an angry parent or a disgruntled roommate, or intangible, such as the mixed emotions associated with meeting your significant other's parents for the first time. **Adjustment** is the attempt to cope with a given situation. **Strain** is the wear and tear the body and mind sustain in adjusting to or resisting a stressor.

Stress   Mental and physical response of our bodies to the changes and challenges of our lives.

Stressor   A physical, social, or psychological event or condition that causes the body to adjust to a specific situation.

Adjustment   The attempt to cope with a given situation.

Stress and strain are associated with most daily activities. Generally, positive stress, or stress that presents the opportunity for personal growth and satisfaction, is called **eustress.** Getting married, starting school, beginning a career, developing new friendships, and learning a new physical skill all give rise to eustress. **Distress,** or negative stress, is caused by those events, such as financial problems, the death of a loved one, academic difficulties, and the breakup of a relationship, that result in debilitative stress and strain. Distress can have a negative effect on health.

We cannot get rid of distress entirely: like eustress, it is a part of life. However, we can train ourselves to recognize the events that cause distress and to anticipate our reactions to them. We can learn coping skills and strategies that will help us manage stress more effectively.

The Body's Response to Stress

Whenever we're surprised by a sudden stressor, such as someone swerving into our lane of traffic, the adrenal glands jump into action. Emotional reactions to a perceived life threatening event trigger these two almond-sized glands sitting atop the kidneys to secrete adrenaline and other hormones into the bloodstream. As a result, the heart speeds up, breathing rate increases, blood pressure elevates, and the flow of blood to the muscles increases with a rapid release of blood sugars into the bloodstream. This sudden burst of energy and strength is believed to provide the extra edge that has helped generations of humans survive during adversity. Known as the **fight-or-flight response,** this physiological reaction is one of our most basic, innate survival instincts. It is a point at which our bodies go on the alert either to fight danger or escape from it.

The General Adaptation Syndrome

What has just been described in very general terms is a complex physiological response to stress in which our bodies move from **homeostasis,** a level of functioning in which the body's systems operate smoothly and maintain equilibrium, to one of crisis in which the body attempts to return to homeostasis. This adjustment is referred to as an **adaptive response.** First characterized by Hans Selye in 1936, this internal fight to restore homeostasis is known as the **general adaptation syndrome (GAS)** (Figure 3.1). The GAS has three distinct phases: alarm, resistance, and exhaustion.[1]

Alarm Phase   When the body is exposed to a real or perceived stressor, the fight-or-flight response kicks into gear. Stress hormones flow into the body, and it prepares to do battle. The subconscious perceptions and appraisal of the stressor stimulate the areas in the brain responsible for emotions. Emotional stimulation, in turn, starts the physical reactions that we associate with stress (Figure 3.2 on page 58). This entire process takes only a few seconds.

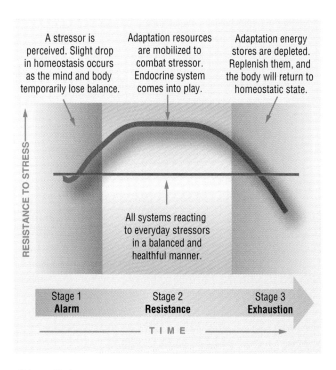

Figure 3.1
The General Adaptation Syndrome

Suppose that you are walking to your car after a night class on a dimly lit campus. As you pass a particularly dark area, you hear someone cough behind you and sense that this person is fairly close. You walk faster, only to hear the quickened footsteps of the other person. Your senses become increasingly alert, your breathing quickens, your heart races, and you begin to perspire. The stranger is getting closer and closer. In desperation you stop, clutching your

---

Strain   The wear and tear the body and mind sustain in adjusting to or resisting a stressor.

Eustress   Positive stress that presents opportunities for personal growth.

Distress   Negative stress that can have a negative effect on health.

Fight-or-flight response   Physiological reaction in which the body prepares to combat or escape a real or perceived threat.

Homeostasis   A balanced physical state in which all the body's systems function smoothly.

Adaptive response   Form of adjustment in which the body attempts to restore homeostasis.

General adaptation syndrome (GAS)   The pattern followed in the physiological response to stress, consisting of the alarm, resistance, and exhaustion phases.

book bag in your hands, determined to use force if necessary to protect yourself. You turn around quickly and let out a blood-curdling yell. To your surprise, the only person you see is Mrs. Fletcher, a woman in your class, who has been trying to stay close to you out of her own anxiety about walking alone in the dark. She screams and jumps back, only to trip and fall. You look at her in startled embarrassment, help her to her feet, and nervously laugh about your reaction. You have just experienced the alarm phase of GAS.

When the mind perceives a real or imaginary stressor, such as a potential attacker, the *cerebral cortex,* the region of the brain that interprets the nature of an event, is called to attention. If the cerebral cortex perceives a threat, it triggers an **autonomic nervous system (ANS)** response that prepares the body for action. The ANS is the portion of the central nervous system that regulates bodily functions that we do not normally consciously control, such as heart function, breathing, and glandular function. When we are stressed, the activity rate of all these bodily functions increases dramatically to give us the physical strength to protect ourselves or to make the physiological changes needed to respond and mobilize internal forces.

The ANS has two branches: sympathetic and parasympathetic. The **sympathetic nervous system** energizes the body for fight or flight by signaling the release of several stress hormones that speed the heart rate, increase the breathing rate, and trigger many other stress responses. The **parasympathetic nervous system** functions to slow all the systems stimulated by the stress response. Thus, the parasympathetic branch of the ANS serves as a system of checks and balances on the sympathetic branch. In a healthy person, these two branches work together in a balance that controls the negative effects of stress. However, long-term stress can strain this balance, and chronic physical problems can occur as stress reactions become the dominant forces in a person's body.

The responses of the sympathetic nervous system to stress involve a series of biochemical exchanges between

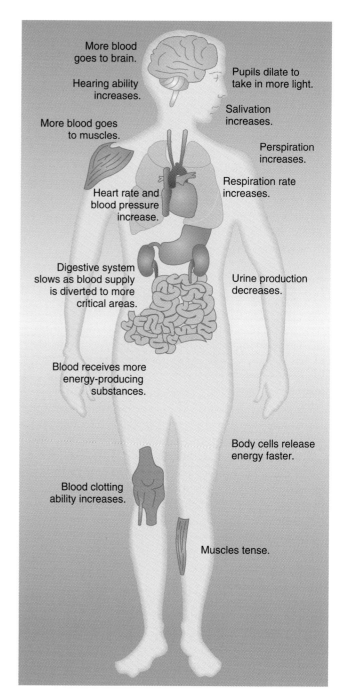

Figure 3.2
The General Adaptation Syndrome: Alarm Phase

More blood goes to brain.

Hearing ability increases.

More blood goes to muscles.

Heart rate and blood pressure increase.

Digestive system slows as blood supply is diverted to more critical areas.

Blood receives more energy-producing substances.

Blood clotting ability increases.

Pupils dilate to take in more light.

Salivation increases.

Perspiration increases.

Respiration rate increases.

Urine production decreases.

Body cells release energy faster.

Muscles tense.

Autonomic nervous system (ANS) The portion of the central nervous system that regulates bodily functions that a person does not normally consciously control.

Sympathetic nervous system Branch of the autonomic nervous system responsible for stress arousal.

Parasympathetic nervous system Part of the autonomic nervous system responsible for slowing systems stimulated by the stress response.

Hypothalamus A section of the brain that controls the sympathetic nervous system and directs the stress response.

Epinephrine Also called adrenaline, a hormone that stimulates body systems in response to stress.

---

different parts of the body. The **hypothalamus,** a structure in the brain, functions as the control center of the sympathetic nervous system and determines the overall reaction to stressors. This key player in the stress response is located above the pituitary gland. When the hypothalamus perceives that extra energy is needed to fight a stressor, it stimulates the adrenal glands, located near the top of the kidneys, to release the hormone **epinephrine,** also called adrenaline. Epinephrine causes more blood to be pumped with each beat of the heart, dilates the bronchioles (air sacs in the lungs) to increase oxygen intake, increases the breathing rate, stimulates the liver to release more glucose (which fuels muscular exertion), and dilates the pupils to improve visual sensitivity. The body is then poised to act immediately.

As epinephrine secretion increases, blood is diverted away from the digestive system, which might cause nausea and cramping if the distress occurs shortly after a meal, and drying of nasal and salivary tissues, which produces dry mouth. The alarm phase also provides for longer-term reaction to stress. The hypothalamus triggers the pituitary gland, which in turn releases another powerful hormone, **adrenocorticotrophic hormone (ACTH).** ACTH signals the adrenal glands to release **cortisol,** a hormone that makes stored nutrients more readily available to meet energy demands. Finally, other parts of the brain and body release endorphins, the body's naturally occurring opiates, which relieve pain that a stressor may cause.

Resistance Phase The resistance phase of the GAS begins almost immediately after the alarm phase starts. In this stage, the body has reacted to the stressor and adjusted in a way that allows the system to return to homeostasis. As the sympathetic nervous system energizes the body via the hormonal action of epinephrine, norepinephrine, cortisol, and other hormones, the parasympathetic nervous system helps control these energy levels and return the body to a normal level of functioning.

Exhaustion Phase In the exhaustion phase of the GAS, the physical and emotional energy used to fight a stressor has been depleted. The toll it takes on the body depends on the type of stress or the period of time spent under stress. Short-term stress probably would not deplete all of a person's energy reserves, but chronic stress experienced over a period of time can create continuous states of alarm and resistance, resulting in total depletion of energy and susceptibility to illness. The key to warding off the effects of stress lies in what many researchers refer to as *adaptation energy stores,* the physical and mental foundations of our ability to cope with stress.

Two levels of adaptation energy stores exist: deep and superficial. We apparently have little control over deep stores; their size appears to be preset by heredity. Superficial adaptation energy stores, however, are renewable and present the first line of defense against stress since they are tapped into initially when the body fights stress. Only when superficial stores are exhausted does the body tap into the deep energy stores. As our adaptation energy stores are depleted, we tire more quickly and require more rest. Without this replenishing sleep, the alarm and resistance phases eventually limit our ability to rebound properly.

As the body adjusts to chronic unresolved stress, the adrenal glands continue to release cortisol, which remains in the bloodstream for longer periods of time due to slower metabolic responsiveness. Over time, without relief, cortisol can reduce **immunocompetence,** or the ability of the immune system to respond to various assaults. Blood pressure can remain dangerously elevated, and our body systems can become unable to respond with the same vigor they once did. The net effect is a greater chance of minor illnesses at one end of the continuum and a greater risk of life-threatening disease at the other end.

Stress management, therefore, depends on the ability to replenish superficial stores and conserve deep stores. Besides getting replenished with adequate rest, adaptation energy stores also can be replenished by aerobic exercise, finding a balance between work and relaxation, practicing good nutritional habits, setting realistic goals, and maintaining supportive relationships.

Stress and Your Health

Although much has been written about the negative effects of stress, researchers have only recently begun to untangle the complex web of physical and emotional interactions that can break down the body over time. Stress is often described as a disease of prolonged arousal that leads to other negative health effects. Nearly all body systems become potential targets, and the long-term effects may be devastating.

Much of the initial impetus for studying the health effects of stress came from indirect observations. Cardiologists in the Framingham Heart Study and other research projects noted that highly stressed individuals seemed to experience significantly greater risks for cardiovascular disease (CVD) and hypertension.[2] Monkeys exposed to high levels of unpredictable stressors in studies showed significantly increased levels of disease and mortality.[3] In a landmark study, M. D. Jeremko observed that chronic stress activation can result in headaches, asthma, hypertension, ulcers, lower back pain, and other medical conditions, a finding substantiated by a meta-analysis of over 100 similar studies.[4] A Harvard study concluded that mental health was the most important predictor of physical health.[5] While the battle over the legitimacy of these observations continues to be waged in research labs across the country, the theory that chronic stress increases susceptibility to certain ailments has gained credibility.

Stress and Cardiovascular Disease Risks

Since Friedman and Rosenman's classic study of Type A and Type B personalities and heart disease (discussed later in this

---

Adrenocorticotrophic hormone (ACTH) A pituitary hormone that stimulates the adrenal glands to secrete cortisol.

Cortisol Hormone released by the adrenal glands that makes stored nutrients more readily available to meet energy demands.

Immunocompetence The ability of the immune system to respond to assaults.

Taming Technostress

Cell phones that ring constantly; email lists that grow on your desktop like an out-of-control fungus; laptop computers that somehow end up in your luggage when you go on vacation; electronic organizers that beep during dinner or at the movies; voice message systems that don't allow you to talk to a live person; busy signals as you try to get on the Internet; and slow, slow, slow downloading of information. Can you feel your heart rate speeding up just thinking about these situations?

If you are like millions of people today, you find that technology is often a daily terrorizer that raises your blood pressure, frustrates you, and prevents you from ever really getting away from it all. In short, you may unknowingly be a victim of stressors that previous generations only dreamed (or had nightmares) about. Known as *technostress*, this problem is defined as "personal stress generated by reliance on technological devices . . . a panicky feeling when they fail, and a state of near-constant stimulation, or being perpetually 'plugged in.'" When technostress grabs you, it may interact with other forms of stress to create a synergistic, never-ending form of stimulation that keeps your stress response reverberating all day.

Part of the problem, ironically, is that technology enables us to be so productive. Because it encourages polyphasic activity, or "multitasking," people are forced to juggle multiple thoughts and actions at the same time, such as driving and talking on cell phones or checking handheld devices for appointments. There is clear evidence that such multitasking contributes to auto accidents and other harmful consequences. What is less clear is what happens to someone who is always plugged in.

What are the symptoms of technology overload? It evokes typical stress responses by increasing heart rate and blood pressure, and causing irritability and memory disturbances. Over time, many stressed-out people lose the ability to relax and find that they feel nervous and anxious when they are supposed to be having fun. Headaches, stomach and digestive problems, skin irritations, more colds than usual, difficulty in wound healing, lack of sleep, ulcers, and a host of other problems may result. A study conducted by Yale University indicates that chronic stress may even thicken the waistline; increased secretions of cortisol caused even slender women to store more fat in the abdomen.

TIPS FOR FIGHTING TECHNOSTRESS

- Exercise. Get away from any form of technology. Quiet walks or runs away from the blare of music and the sound of machines (typical in fitness centers) are best. Try to find a place that has few people and little noise—that usually means outdoors.
- Become aware of what you are doing. Log the time you spend on email, voicemail, etc. Set up a schedule to limit your use of technology. For example, spend no more than a half-hour per day answering emails.
- Set up strict rules for when you can log on, and don't log on at other times.
- Give yourself more time for everything you do. If you are surfing the Web for resources for a term paper, start early rather than the night before the paper is due.
- Manage the telephone—don't let it manage you. Rather than interrupting what you're doing to answer, screen calls with an answering machine. Get rid of Call Waiting, which forces you to juggle multiple calls, and subscribe to a voicemail service that takes messages when you're on the phone.
- Set "time out" periods when you don't answer the phone, listen to the stereo, use the computer, or watch TV. Switch off email notification systems so you aren't beeped during these periods.
- Take regular breaks. Even when working, get up, walk around, stretch, do deep breathing, or get a glass of water, every hour.
- If you are working on the computer, look away from the screen and focus on something far away every 30 minutes. Stretch your shoulders and neck periodically as you work. Playing soft background music can help you relax.
- Resist the urge to buy the newest and fastest technology. Such purchases not only cause financial stress, but also add to stress levels with the typical glitches that occur when installing and adjusting to new technology.
- Do not take laptops, hand-held devices, or other technological gadgets on vacation. If you must take a cell phone for emergencies, turn it and your voice messaging system off, and use the phone only in true emergencies.
- Back up materials on your computer at regular intervals. Writing a term paper only to lose it during a power outage will send you into hyperstress very quickly.

Sources: Dr. Larry D. Rosen and Dr. Michelle M. Weil, *TechnoStress: Coping with Technology @Work@Home@Play* (New York: John Wiley & Sons, 1997). Copyright © 1997. Material used by permission of John Wiley & Sons; Yale University, "Stress May Cause Excess Abdominal Fat in Otherwise Slender Women, Study Conducted at Yale Shows," *ScienceDaily,* November 23, 2000. MayoClinic.com, "Are You a Slave to the Telephone?" (November 1, 2000). www.mayoclinic.com/

---

chapter), researchers have tried to definitively link personality, emotions, and a host of other variables to heart disease.[6] Results of numerous meta-analyses that summarize many studies have consistently pointed to a correlation between chronic, unresolved stress and prolonged elevations in heart rate and blood pressure. This increased pressure can cause turbulence in the blood flow and is believed to damage the inner lining of blood vessels. Once this damage occurs, fatty substances seem to stick to this site more readily, which leads to atherosclerotic plaque build-up. Recent studies point to increased risk of sudden myocardial infarction (heart attack) due to prolonged stress in the environment.[7] A large number of epidemiological studies have related the incidence of heart disease deaths to type of employment, particularly jobs in which a person is subject to many demands and has very little control in decision-making and daily tasks.[8]

Historically, the increased risk of CVD due to chronic stress has been linked to increased plaque buildup due to elevated cholesterol, hardening of the arteries, alterations in heart rhythms, increased and fluctuating blood pressure, and difficulties in cardiovascular responsiveness due to all of the above. While these continue to be considered major risks, recent research points to some type of inflammation in the vessels, perhaps due to lingering viral effects, as a major contributor to heart disease risks. (For more information about CVD risks, see Chapter 12.)

Stress and Impaired Immunity

A new area of scientific investigation known as **psychoneuroimmunology (PNI)** analyzes the intricate relationship between the mind's response to stress and the ability of the immune system to function effectively. An article in *The Journal of the American Medical Association* reviews the research linking stress to adverse health consequences.[9] According to the findings, too much stress, over a long period, can negatively regulate various aspects of the cellular immune response. In particular, stress disrupts bidirectional communication networks between the nervous, endocrine, and immune systems. When these networks fail, messenger systems that regulate hormones, blood cell formation, and a host of other health-regulating systems begin to falter or send faulty information.[10]

During prolonged stress, elevated levels of adrenal hormones destroy or reduce the ability of the white blood cells, known as natural killer T-cells, to aid the immune response. When killer T-cells are suppressed and other regulating systems aren't working correctly, illness may occur.

A study completed in 2003 of older people under chronic stress uncovered higher-than-normal levels of *interleukin-6 (IL-6),* an immune-system protein in the blood that promotes inflammation.[11] IL-6 has been linked with various age-related conditions, such as heart disease, diabetes, osteoporosis, frailty, and certain cancers. The researchers compared the health of 117 caregivers for patients suffering from dementia with a control group of 106 adults who had no care-giving role. Caregivers experienced consistently higher stress levels, worked longer hours, had less sleep, and reported more isolation and loneliness. Over the course of the six-year study, IL-6 levels increased an average of four times faster among caregivers. In cases where spouses died, IL-6 levels rose and, for many, remained elevated for several years. (These caregivers' immune systems did not rebound as quickly as expected, perhaps because of the dual effects of stress and depression.)

Earlier findings by this research team showed that stress levels had a detrimental effect on the effectiveness of certain vaccines, the speed of wound healing, and the impact of even short-term stress events, such as arguments and test-taking, on the immune response.

Other studies that link stress with infectious diseases include the following.

- Mice that are forced to live in crowded cages prior to and after infection with tuberculosis have much poorer outcomes than mice in less crowded situations. Social disruption in mice also seems to trigger outbreaks of herpes viruses.[12]
- Caregivers of Alzheimer's patients who were vaccinated against the flu still had a much greater chance of getting the flu or becoming ill than non-caregivers who received the same vaccine.[13]
- People with self-reported high stress levels were much more likely to develop upper respiratory infections than those who reported lower levels of stress.[14]
- People with high stress levels who skip breakfast and consume a high level of fats catch many more colds than those who eat healthily and have low stress levels.[15]
- Certain changes in lifestyle may increase resistance to infectious diseases. These changes include broadening one's social involvement (e.g., joining social or spiritual groups, having a confidant, spending time with supportive friends) and maintaining healthful practices, such as proper diet, exercise, and sleep.[16]
- Students' disease-fighting mechanisms are weaker during high-stress times, such as exam weeks and on days when they are upset. In one experiment, a stressful event increased the severity of symptoms in a group of volunteers who were knowingly infected with a cold virus. In another, 47 percent of subjects living high-stress lives developed colds after a virus was dropped into their noses, but only 27 percent of those living relatively stress-free lives caught these colds.[17]

Although strong indicators support the hypothesis of a relationship between high stress and increased risk for disease, we are only beginning to understand this link. Some research indicates that other factors, such as genetics and environmental stimuli, may be involved. However, in spite of questions, studies supporting the relationship between high stress and increased risk for disease outnumber those that don't.[18]

Stress and the Mind

Stress may be one of the single greatest contributors to mental disability and emotional dysfunction in the United States. Whether stress results in lost work productivity, difficulties in relationships, abuse of drugs and other substances, displaced anger and aggressive behavior, or a host of other problems,

> **Psychoneuroimmunology (PNI)** Science of the interaction between the mind's response to stress and the immune system.

the net toll is staggering. Clearly, stress does much more than cause the heart rate to soar and blood pressure to go up. Evidence suggests a strong relationship between stress and the potential for negative mental health reactions. Consider the following.[19]

- Numerous researchers have demonstrated that stressors that combine with low self-esteem and/or maladaptive coping styles predict depression and anxiety.
- Depression and drug abuse are highly correlated with excessive exposure to stress.
- Among college students, low self-esteem or depression, and concerns about stress and health, were identified as unresolved problems for 35 percent and 20 percent of the respondents, respectively.
- Mature coping styles predict happiness, occupational and social success, enjoyment, and absence of addictions.
- People with high nervous tension have increased risk for mental illness, suicide, and coronary heart disease.
- A recent national study of Americans ages 15 to 54 found that almost half will suffer a mental and addictive disorder during their lifetime. Many of these disorders are believed to be stress related.
- Mental illness is on the increase in almost all segments of U.S. society.

Sources of Stress

Both eustress and distress have many sources that include psychosocial factors, environmental stressors, and self-imposed stress.

Psychosocial Sources of Stress

Psychosocial stress refers to the factors in our daily lives that cause stress (see the Assess Yourself box on page 64). Interactions with others, the subtle and unsubtle expectations we and others have of ourselves, and the social conditions we live in force us to readjust constantly. Psychosocial stressors include change, hassles, pressure, inconsistent goals and behaviors, conflict, overload, burnout, and discrimination.

Change Anytime good or bad change occurs in your normal routine, you will experience stress. The more changes you experience and the more adjustments you must make, the greater the stress effects may be. In 1967, Drs. Thomas Holmes and Richard Rahe analyzed the social readjustments experienced by more than 5,000 patients and noted which events seemed to occur just prior to disease onset.[20] They determined that certain positive and negative events were predictive of increased risk for illness. They called their scale for predicting stress overload and the likelihood of illness the Social Readjustment Rating Scale (SRRS).[21] The SRRS since has served as the model for scales for certain groups, including college students, as shown in Table 3.1. Although many

other factors must be considered, in general, the more of these stressors you experience, the more you need to change your behaviors or situation before problems occur.

Hassles While Holmes and Rahe examined major stressors, psychologists such as Richard Lazarus have focused on petty annoyances and frustrations, collectively referred to as hassles.[22] Minor hassles—losing your keys, slipping and falling in front of everyone as you walk to your seat in a new class, finding that you went through a whole afternoon with spinach stuck in your front teeth—seem unimportant. However, their cumulative effects may be harmful in the long run.

Pressure Pressure occurs when we feel forced to speed up, intensify, or shift the direction of our behavior to meet a higher standard of performance.[23] Pressures can be based on our personal goals and expectations, concern about what others think, or on outside influences. Among the most significant outside influences are society's demands that we compete and be all that we can be. The forces that push us to compete for the best grades, nicest cars, most attractive significant others, and highest-paying jobs create significant pressure to personify American success.

Inconsistent Goals and Behaviors For many of us, the negative effects of stress are magnified when there is a disparity between our goals (what we value or hope to obtain in life) and our behaviors (actions that may or may not lead to these goals). For instance, you may want good grades, and your family may expect them. But if you party and procrastinate throughout the term, your behaviors are inconsistent with your goals; significant stress in the form of guilt, last-minute frenzy before exams, and disappointing grades may result. On the other hand, if you dig in, work, and remain committed to getting good grades, much of your negative stress may be eliminated. Thwarted goals can lead to frustration, and frustration has been shown to be a significant disrupter of homeostasis.

Determining whether behaviors are consistent with goals is an essential component of maintaining balance in life. If we consciously strive to attain our goals, we greatly improve our chances of success.

Here are several chronic stressors often experienced by college students. Each has the potential to cause serious health problems, particularly if experienced on a fairly regular basis (i.e., at least two or three times per week for the past month).

1. Roommate conflict	**13.** Uncertainty over the right major	**25.** Conflict with parents
2. Homesickness	**14.** Missing distant friends	**26.** Academic performance
3. Friend conflict	**15.** Family illness	**27.** Overweight
4. Writing major papers	**16.** Loneliness	**28.** Don't fit in; no friends
5. Dieting	**17.** Job pressures	**29.** Living/housing situations
6. Money/financial problems	**18.** Lack of privacy	**30.** Tuition bills/book costs
7. Long-distance relationship	**19.** Friends with problems	**31.** Health problems/not feeling well
8. Juggling school and job	**20.** Parental problems/family problems	**32.** Difficult class or instructor
9. Time management	**21.** Not enough sex/intimacy	**33.** Unsure of job future
10. Noisy dorm or apartment	**22.** Behind in schoolwork	**34.** Not enough sleep
11. No car or car not working	**23.** Problem with lover	**35.** Problem with drugs/alcohol
12. Underweight	**24.** Not enough exercise	

Source: Adapted from L. Towbes and L. Cohen, "Chronic Stress in the Lives of College Students: Scale Development and Prospective Predictions of Distress," *Journal of Youth and Adolescence* 25, no. 2 (1996): 202–203. By permission of Kluwer Academic/Plenum Publishers.

Conflict   Conflict occurs when we are forced to make difficult decisions between competing motives, behaviors, or impulses, or when we are forced to face incompatible demands, opportunities, needs, or goals.[24] What if your best friends all choose to smoke marijuana, and you don't want to smoke but fear rejection? Conflict often occurs as our values are tested. College students who are away from home for the first time often face conflict between parental values and their own set of developing beliefs.

Overload   Excessive time pressure, too much responsibility, high expectations of yourself and those around you, and lack of support can lead to **overload,** a state of being overburdened. Have you ever felt you had so many responsibilities that you couldn't possibly fulfill them all? Have you longed for a weekend when you could just take time out with friends and not feel guilty? These feelings are symptoms of overload. Students suffering from overload may experience anxiety about tests, poor self-concept, a desire to drop classes or drop out of school, and other problems. In severe cases where they are unable to see any solutions to their problems, students may suffer from depression or turn to substance abuse.

Burnout   People who regularly suffer from overload, frustration, and disappointment may eventually experience **burnout,** a state of physical and mental exhaustion caused by excessive stress. People involved in the helping professions, such as teaching, social work, drug counseling, nursing, and psychology, experience high levels of burnout, as do people who work in high-pressure, dangerous jobs.

"Isms"   Today's racially and ethnically diverse group of students, faculty members, and staff enriches everyone's educational experience yet also challenges us to deal with differences. Students come from vastly different contexts and life experiences. Often, those who act, speak, dress, or appear different face additional pressures that do not affect students considered more typical. Students perceived as different may become victims of subtle and not-so-subtle bigotry; insensitivity; and harassment, or hostility because of their race, ethnicity, religious affiliation, age, sexual orientation, or other "isms."[25]

Evidence of the health effects of excessive stress abound in the general population. African Americans suffer higher rates of hypertension, CVD, and most cancers than their white counterparts do. Gay men and lesbians have higher rates of suicide and are more likely to become victims of violence. Although poverty and socioeconomic status have been blamed for much of the spike in hypertension rates for African Americans and other marginalized groups, this chronic, physically debilitating stress may reflect real and perceived status in society more than it reflects actual poverty. Feeling that you occupy a position of low status due to living conditions, financial security, or job status can be a source of stress. The problem is exacerbated for those who are socially disadvantaged early in life and grow up without a nurturing environment.

Imagine what it would be like to find yourself isolated, lacking friends, and ridiculed on the basis of who you are or how you look. Even worse, consider the fate of Matthew Shepard, a young student in Wyoming who was brutally

(text continues on page 66)

Overload   A state in which a person feels overburdened by demands.

Burnout   A state of physical and mental exhaustion caused by excessive stress.

How Stressed Are You?

Each of us reacts differently to life's little challenges. Faced with a long line at the bookstore, most of us will get anxious for a few seconds before we start grumbling or shrug and move on. But for others—the one in five of us whom researchers call *hot reactors*—such incidents are part of a daily health assault. These individuals may get very angry outwardly, or they may appear calm and collected. It is what is going on under the surface that is what affects health. Surges in blood pressure, increases in heart rate, nausea, sweating, and a host of other hot reactor indicators may occur. Completing the following assessment will help you think about the nature and extent of stress in your life and how you respond to daily stressors. Although this survey is just an indicator of what stress levels might be, it will help you focus on areas that you may need to work on to reduce stress.

PART ONE: WHAT IS STRESSING YOU OUT?

For each statement, indicate how often the following stressful situations or feelings are a part of your daily life.

	Never	Rarely	Sometimes	Often	All the Time
1. I find that there are not enough hours in the day to finish everything I have to do.	1	2	3	4	5
2. I am anxious about how I am performing in my classes.	1	2	3	4	5
3. People don't seem to notice whether or not I do a good job.	1	2	3	4	5
4. I am tired and feel like I don't have the energy to do everything that I need to get done.	1	2	3	4	5
5. I seem to be easily irritated by things that people do.	1	2	3	4	5
6. I worry about what is happening in my family (health of a loved one, financial problems, relationship problems, etc.).	1	2	3	4	5
7. I'm worried about my finances and having enough money to pay my bills.	1	2	3	4	5
8. I don't have enough time for fun.	1	2	3	4	5
9. I am unhappy with my body (weight, fitness level, etc.).	1	2	3	4	5
10. My family and friends count on me to help them with their problems.	1	2	3	4	5
11. I am concerned about my current relationship (or a lack of a relationship).	1	2	3	4	5
12. I am impatient/intolerant of the weaknesses of others.	1	2	3	4	5
13. My house/apartment is a mess, and I'm embarrassed to have others see it.	1	2	3	4	5
14. I worry about whether I'll get a job and be able to support myself after graduation.	1	2	3	4	5
15. I worry that people don't like me.	1	2	3	4	5

Your Total Score: _____

ANALYZING THIS SECTION

Between 60–75: Your stress level is probably quite high. Prioritize the areas where you scored 5s, and list two to three things for each area that you could do to reduce your stress level. Note any increase in headaches, backaches, or insomnia; your body is telling you to lighten your load. Plan at least one fun thing to do for yourself each day. Make yourself more of a daily priority.

Between 45–60: Your stress level is moderate. Look at those areas that are 5s and list two to three things that you would like to change now to help yourself reduce stress. Practice at least one stress management technique each day. Make more time for yourself.

Between 30–45: You seem to have a lower level of stress. This is good. However, there are still areas that you could work on. Think about what these are and list things you could do now to reduce stress.

Less than 30: You seem to be doing a great job. Whatever your problems, stress isn't one of them. Even when stressful events do occur—and they will—your health probably won't suffer.

Remember, each of us has "stress slips" along the way. Think about your reactions to situations like those above. Whenever possible, make conscious choices to reduce stress.

PART TWO: HOW DO YOU RESPOND TO STRESS?

Respond to each of the following statements with a rating of how likely you are to react to a given stressful event.

1 = I would never respond like this	2 = I would occasionally respond like this	3 = I would respond like this a lot of the time	4 = I would almost always/always respond like this

SCENARIO 1

You've been waiting 20 minutes for a table in a crowded restaurant, and the hostess seats a group that arrived after you.

	1	2	3	4
a. You feel your anger rise as your face gets hot and your heart beats faster.	1	2	3	4
b. You yell "Hey! I was here first" in an irritated voice to the hostess.	1	2	3	4
c. You angrily confront the people who are being seated in front of you and tell them you were there first.	1	2	3	4
d. You say, "Excuse me" in a polite voice and inform the other group and/or the hostess that you were there first.	1	2	3	4
e. You note it, but don't react. It's no big deal, and the hostess obviously didn't notice the order of arrival.	1	2	3	4

SCENARIO 2

You get to a movie theater early so that you and a friend can get great seats. You strategically pick a seat that will give you a good view. Although the theater is nearly empty, a large, tall man plops himself in the seat directly in front of you. Try as you might, you cannot see the screen.

	1	2	3	4
a. You say in a very loud voice: "There's a whole theater, and he has to sit right in front of us!"	1	2	3	4
b. You yell directly at the man, saying, "Can't you sit somewhere else? I can't see!"	1	2	3	4
c. You tap the man on the shoulder and say, "Excuse me, I wonder if you could slide down a seat. I can't see."	1	2	3	4
d. You calmly nudge your friend and decide to move.	1	2	3	4
e. You aren't bothered by the person in front of you. This is just part of going to the movies, and it is no big deal.	1	2	3	4

(continued)

SCENARIO 3

How would you respond to the following?

a. Your sister calls out of the blue and starts to tell you how much you mean to her. Uncomfortable, you change the subject without expressing what you feel.	1	2	3	4
b. You come home to find the kitchen looking like a disaster area and your spouse/roommate lounging in front of the TV. You tense up and can't seem to shake your anger, but you decide not to bring it up.	1	2	3	4
c. Faced with a public speaking event, you get keyed up and lose sleep for a day or more, worrying about how you'll do.	1	2	3	4
d. Your boyfriend/girlfriend/partner is seen out with another person and appears to be acting quite close to the person. You are a trusting person and decide not to worry about it. If your significant other has anything to tell you, you know he/she will talk to you.	1	2	3	4
e. You aren't able to study as much as you'd like for an exam, yet you think that you really "nailed" the exam once you take it. When you get it back, you find that you did horribly. You make an appointment to talk with the professor and determine what you can do to improve on the next exam. You acknowledge that you are responsible for the low grade this time but vow to do better next time. You are disappointed but you don't let it bother you.	1	2	3	4

ANALYZING THIS SECTION

Look carefully at each of these scenarios. Obviously, none of us is perfect, and we sometimes react in ways that we later regret. The key here is to assess how you react the majority of the time.

If stressful events occur and you remain calm, do not experience increases in heart rate or blood pressure, or avoid outward displays or inner signs of anxiety, anger or frustration, you are probably a cool reactor who tends to roll with the punches when a situation is out of your control. This usually indicates a good level of coping; overall, you will suffer fewer health consequences when stressed. The key here is that you really are not stressed, and you really are calm and unworried about the situation.

If you fret and stew about a stressor, can't sleep, or tend to react with hostile confrontation, anger, or other negative physiological overreactions, you probably are a hot reactor who responds to mildly stressful situations with a fight-or-flight adrenaline rush that drives up blood pressure and can lead to heart rhythm disturbances, accelerated clotting, and damaged blood vessel linings. Some hot reactors can seem cool on the outside, but inside their bodies are silently killing them. They may be on edge or jumpy or unable to sleep, even though most people would never suspect that they are in trouble. Before you honk or make obscene gestures at the guy who cuts you off in rush hour traffic, remember that getting angry can destroy thousands of heart muscle cells within minutes. Robert S. Eliot, author of *From Stress to Strength,* says hot reactors have no choice but to calm themselves down with rational thought. Look at ways to change your perceptions and cope more effectively. Ponder the fact that the only thing you'll hasten by reacting is a decline in health. "You have to stop trying to change the world," Eliot advises, "and learn to change your response to it."

murdered for being gay, or of countless other students who have been victimized because of race, nationality, or religious affiliation. In addition to making the grade in classes, they must deal with hidden fears, suffering, and difficulties caused by intolerant factions on campus. (Chapter 4 focuses on violence and its incidence and prevalence on campus.)

> **What do you think?**
> *What are your greatest sources of stress right now?* ✳ *On a scale of 1 to 10, with 10 being the highest level, how stressed are you?* ✳ *Have you noticed any symptoms of stress?* ✳ *How can you reduce it?*

Environmental Stress

Environmental stress results from events occurring in the physical environment as opposed to social surroundings. Environmental stressors include natural disasters, such as floods and hurricanes, and human-made disasters, such as chemical spills and explosions. Often as damaging as one-time disasters are **background distressors,** such as noise, air, and water pollution, although we may be unaware of them and their effects may not become apparent for decades. As with other challenges, our bodies respond to environmental stressors with the GAS. People who cannot escape background distressors may exist in a constant resistance phase, which can contribute to stress-related disorders.

Self-Imposed Stress

Self-Concept and Stress   The **cognitive stress system** is the psychological system that governs our responses to stressors.[26] The cognitive stress system helps us recognize stressors; evaluate them on the basis of self-concept, past experiences, and emotions; and make decisions regarding how to cope with them.

Sensory organs serve as input channels for information reaching the brain. From that point on, the problem, memory, reasoning, and problem-solving processes are organized in various parts of the brain. This occurs before we act on the stressor. Because learning and memory involve the changing of various proteins in brain neurons, the emotions experienced during the stress response also "tickle" the memory storage neurons and contribute to responses. Behaviorally, we will respond to the stressor in ways consistent with our memories of similar situations.

Self-esteem is closely related to the emotions engendered by past experiences. Low self-esteem can lead to helpless anger. People suffering helpless anger usually have learned that they are wrong to feel anger, so instead of expressing it in healthy ways they turn it inward. They may swallow their rage in food, alcohol, or other drugs, or they may act in other self-destructive ways. Donna Shalala, former U.S. Secretary of Health and Human Services, has instituted "Girl Power," a program designed to improve the self-esteem of young women between the ages of 9 and 14, a time when low self-esteem is thought to trigger a host of negative health behaviors.

Research indicates that self-esteem significantly affects various disease processes. People with low self-esteem create a self-imposed stressor that can depress the immune system and increase the symptoms of illness such as acquired immune deficiency syndrome (AIDS), herpes, multiple sclerosis, and Epstein-Barr syndrome.

Personality Types and Hardiness   Personality may contribute to the kind and degree of self-imposed stress we experience. In 1974, physicians Meyer Friedman and Ray Rosenman identified two stress-related personality types:

Type A and Type B.[27] Type A personalities are hard-driving, competitive, anxious, time-driven, impatient, quick-tempered, and perfectionistic. Type B personalities are relaxed and noncompetitive. According to Rosenman and Friedman, people with Type A characteristics are more prone to heart attacks than are their Type B counterparts.

Researchers today believe that more needs to be discovered about personality types before we can say that all Type As have greater risks for heart disease. Most people are not one personality type all the time, and many other unexplained variables must be explored, such as why some Type A people seem to thrive in stress-filled environments.

Critics argue that these attempts to base ill health on personal behavioral patterns are crude. For example, researchers at Duke University contend that the Type A personality may be more complex than previously described. They have identified a toxic core in some Type A personalities. People who have this toxic core are angry, distrustful of others, and show above-average levels of cynicism. People who are angry and hostile often have below-average levels of social support and other increased risks for ill health. It may be this toxic core rather than the hard-driving nature of the Type A personality that makes people more vulnerable to self-imposed stress.[28]

According to psychologist Susanne Kobasa, **psychological hardiness** may negate self-imposed stress associated with Type A behavior. Psychologically hardy people are characterized by *control, commitment,* and *challenge.*[29] People with a sense of control are able to accept responsibility for their behaviors and change those that they discover to be debilitating. People with a sense of commitment have good self-esteem and understand their purpose in life. People with a sense of challenge see change as a stimulating opportunity for personal growth.

Because some Type A behavior is learned, it can be modified. Some Type As are able to slow down and become more tolerant and patient. Unfortunately, many people do not decide to modify their Type A habits until after they become ill or suffer a heart attack. Prevention of stress-related health problems entails recognizing and changing dangerous behaviors before damage is done.

Self-Efficacy   Whether people cope successfully with stressful situations often depends on their level of self-efficacy, or their belief in their skills and performance abilities.[30] If they have succeeded in mastering similar problems in the past,

---

Background distressors   Environmental stressors of which people are often unaware.

Cognitive stress system   The psychological system that governs emotional responses to stressors.

Psychological hardiness   A personality trait characterized by control, commitment, and challenge.

they will be more likely to believe in their own effectiveness. Similarly, people who have repeatedly tried and failed may lack confidence in their abilities to deal with life's problems. In some cases, this insecurity may prevent them from trying to cope.

External versus Internal Locus of Control   People who believe they lack control in a situation may become easily frustrated and give up. Those who feel they have no personal control tend to have an *external locus of control* and a low level of self-efficacy. People who are confident their behavior will influence the outcome tend to have an *internal locus of control*. Individuals who feel that they have limited control over their lives often show higher levels of stress.

Stress and the College Student

College students thrive under a certain amount of stress, but excessive stress can leave them overwhelmed and underenthused about their classes and social interactions. Some 29 percent of students surveyed for the National College Health Assessments reported that stress was the number one factor affecting their individual academic performance, followed closely by stress-related problems such as sleep difficulties (21.3 percent) and cold/flu/sore throats (21.2 percent).[31]

A recent study by UCLA's Higher Education Research Institute reported that current college freshmen are more stressed than any class of freshmen before them. These researchers define **psychological stress** as the relationship between a person and the environment that the person judges to be beyond his or her resources and jeopardizes his or her well-being.[32] Freshmen seem to be the most vulnerable to the negative effects of stress, with relationships, race relations, school events, physical assault (or being stalked), and feeling deviance from school norms noted as being particularly distressful. Not only did freshmen report more problems with these issues, they also reported more emotional reactivity in the form of anger/hostility/frustration and a greater sense of being out of control. Sophomores and juniors reported fewer problems with these issues. Seniors reported the fewest problems, which perhaps indicates progressive emotional growth through experience, maturity, increased awareness of support services, and more social connections.[33]

In a large study of chronic stressors, male and female college students differed significantly in the things they perceived to be significant stressors.[34] Women indicated that among their most frequent stressors were trying to diet, being overweight, having an overload of school work, and

> **Psychological stress**   Stress caused by being in an environment perceived to be beyond one's control and endangering one's well-being.

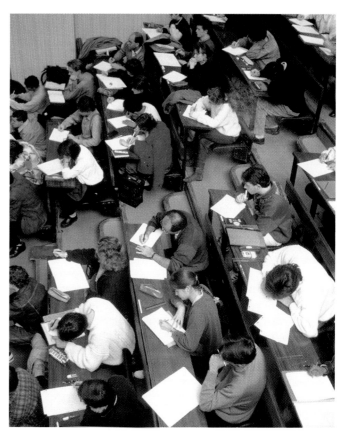

College can be a stressful time for students, whether they are young people choosing a career path or older adults returning to school to change directions later in life.

gaining weight. Men, in contrast, tended to list the following items as major stressors: being underweight, problems relating to commuting to school, not having someone to date, not having enough sex, being behind in schoolwork, not having enough friends, and concerns about drug or alcohol use.[35]

College students may be especially vulnerable because they are in a period of transition in which they are often away from home for the first time, striking out on their own, and forging new relationships. From the moment they start packing for school, these transitions cause them to face key developmental tasks as their lives begin to make dramatic changes, such as achieving emotional independence from family; choosing and preparing for a career; preparing for a major relationship, commitment, and/or family life; facing economic independence; and developing their own values and ethical system. These tasks require the college student to develop new social roles and modify old ones. Such changes can result in role strain as they attempt to form a new identity and lead to chronic stress responses.

If you experience any of the stressors listed in Table 3.1, act promptly to reduce their impact. Most colleges offer stress management workshops through health centers or student counseling departments. Do not ignore the symptoms of stress overload, which include a vague sense of anxiety or nervousness; changes in sleep, diet, or exercise patterns; headaches; dizziness; shortened temper; increased negativism, cynicism, anger, or frustration; recurring colds and minor illnesses; persistent time pressures; increased difficulty in completing tasks; inability to concentrate; wanting to get away from others; and less tolerance of petty annoyances.

Managing Your Stress

Realizing that you are having stress-related health problems or that stress is causing problems in your relationships is often the first step toward making positive changes. Being on your own in college poses many challenges. However, it also lets you evaluate your unique situation and take steps that fit your own schedule and lifestyle to reduce negative stressors in your life.

One of the most effective ways to combat stressors is to build skills and coping strategies that will help inoculate you against them. Such efforts are known collectively as *stress management techniques;* they may range from doing something as simple as taking 20 minutes each day to be alone, to developing an elaborate time management plan for eating, socializing, and exercising. Any strategy that you select should be developed in a series of steps; do not change too many things at once and cause your new stress management program to stress you out!

Building Skills to Reduce Stress

Dealing with stress involves assessing all aspects of a stressor, examining your response and how you can change it, and learning to cope. Often we cannot change the requirements at our college, assignments in class, or unexpected stressors. Inevitably, we will be stuck in classes that bore us and for which we find no application in real life. We feel powerless when a loved one dies. Although the facts cannot be changed, we can change our reactions to them.

Assessing Your Stressors   After recognizing a stressor, evaluate it. Can you alter the circumstances to reduce the amount of distress you are experiencing, or must you change your behavior and reactions to reduce stress levels? For example, you may have five term papers due for five different courses during the semester, but your professors are unlikely to drop such requirements. However, you can change your behavior by beginning the papers early and spacing them over time to avoid last-minute panic.

Changing Your Responses   Changing your responses requires practice and emotional control. If your roommate is habitually messy and this causes you stress, you can choose from among several responses. You can express your anger by yelling; you can pick up the mess and leave a nasty note; or you can defuse the situation with humor. The first reaction that comes to mind is not always the best. Stop before reacting to gain the time you need to find an appropriate response. Ask yourself, "What is to be gained from my response?"

Many people change their responses to potentially stressful events through *cognitive coping strategies.* These strategies help them prepare through gradual exposure to increasingly higher stress levels.

Learning to Cope   Everyone copes with stress in different ways. Some people drink or take drugs; others seek help from counselors; and still others try to forget about it or engage in positive activities, such as exercise. **Stress inoculation,** one of the newer techniques, helps people prepare for stressful events ahead of time. For example, suppose you are petrified about speaking in front of a class. Practicing in front of friends or in front of a video camera may inoculate you and prevent your freezing up on the day of the presentation. Some health experts compare stress inoculation to a vaccine given to protect against a disease. Regardless of how you cope with a situation, your conscious effort to deal with it is an important step in stress management.

Downshifting   Today's lifestyles are hectic and pressure-packed, and stress often comes from trying to keep up. Many people are questioning whether "having it all" is worth it, and they are taking a step back and simplifying their lives. This trend is known as **downshifting.** Moving from a large urban area to a smaller town, exchanging the expensive SUV for a modest four-door sedan, and a host of other changes in lifestyle typify downshifting. Some dedicated downshifters have given up television, phones, and even computers.

Downshifting involves a fundamental alteration in values and honest introspection about what is important in life. When you consider any form of downshift or perhaps even start your career this way, it's important to move slowly and consider the following.

- *Determine your ultimate goal.* What is most important to you, and what will you need to reach that goal? What can you do without? Where do you want to live?
- *Make a short-term and a long-term plan for simplifying your life.* Set up your plan in doable steps, and work slowly toward each step. Begin saying no to requests for your time, and determine those people with whom it is important for you to spend time.
- *Complete a financial inventory.* How much money will you need to do the things you want to do? Will you live alone or share costs with roommates? Do you need a car, or can you rely on public transportation? Pay off credit cards and eliminate existing debt, or consider debt consolidation. Get used to paying with cash. If you don't have the cash,

---

Stress inoculation   Newer stress management technique in which a person consciously tries to prepare ahead of time for potential stressors.

Downshifting   Conscious attempt to simplify life in an effort to reduce the stresses and strains of modern living.

Post-Traumatic Stress: The Aftermath of Terror

For many college students, war and other national threats were something studied in history classes, until the events of September 11, the grim specter of bioterrorism spread by anthrax in the mail, and war in Iraq. These were often our first brushes with threats to a secure world, and reactions such as fear, anxiety, anger, and depression were not uncommon. These reactions often are exacerbated in situations where individuals have suffered personal losses or may be separated from their families and loved ones due to impending threats.

It is important to know that each person, whether directly or indirectly affected by national disasters, will react differently and that a range of responses is normal. Emotional responses can appear immediately or sometimes develop months later. The National Mental Health Association has listed some common responses to disaster and its consequences, including:

- Disbelief and shock
- Fear and anxiety about the future

- Disorientation, difficulty making decisions or concentrating
- Inability to focus on schoolwork and extracurricular activities
- Irritability and anger
- Extreme mood swings
- Feelings of powerlessness
- Changes in eating patterns; loss of appetite
- Crying for no apparent reason
- Headaches and stomach problems
- Difficulty sleeping
- Excessive use of drugs or alcohol

TIPS FOR COPING

It is important to acknowledge the trauma and to address its effects. Ways to recover include:

- *Talking about it* and encouraging others to share their perspectives.
- *Taking care of yourself.* Get plenty of rest and exercise. Do things you find relaxing and soothing. Limit your exposure to media reports and images of the tragedy. As soon as possible, get back to normal routines.
- *Staying connected to friends and family.* Make plans to visit family or others who can offer reassurance and stability.

If you can't travel or are nervous about it, use phone or email contact.
- *Doing something positive* that will help you gain a greater sense of control, such as giving blood, taking a first aid class, or donating food or clothing. Get involved with campus activities planned in response to a disaster, such as candlelight vigils, benefits, or discussion groups and speakers.
- *Asking for help if you are feeling overwhelmed or out of control.* It's not a sign of weakness. Talk with a trusted friend or faith leader. Use on-campus resources such as the counseling center or student health center. If you don't know where to go, talk with your health professor about options. If your feelings of sadness and depression or excessive anxiety persist, seek professional help.

WHEN THE TRAUMA IS TOO GREAT

In severe cases, an individual's response to a national disaster may be considered **post-traumatic stress disorder (PTSD).** This acute stress disorder with extreme anxiety and behavioral disturbances develops within the first hours or days after a traumatic event. Typically, persons

don't buy. Remember, your lifestyle may be different as a student than when you were working or living at home.
- *Plan for health care costs.* Make sure that you budget for health insurance and basic preventive health services if you're not covered under your parents' plan. This should be a top priority. Be sure you understand your coverage so you're not caught off guard.
- *Select the right career.* Look for work that you enjoy and that isn't necessarily driven by salary. Can you be happy taking a lower-paying job that is less stressful and allows you the opportunity to have a life?
- *Consider options for saving money.* Downshifting doesn't mean you renounce money; it means you choose not to let money dictate your life. It's still important to save. If you're just getting started, you need to prepare for emergencies and for future plans.
- *Clear out/clean out.* A cluttered life can be distressing. Take an inventory of material items, and get rid of things you

haven't worn or used in the last year. Donate items to charity groups.

Managing Social Interactions

The importance of your social networks and social bonds with others should not be underestimated as you plan a stress management program. Consider the nature and extent of your friends. Do you have someone with whom you can share intimate thoughts and feelings? Is there someone you could call if you needed help in an emergency? Do you trust your friends to keep your confidences? To be supportive of you? To be honest with you if you are doing something risky or inappropriate? Having someone to give helpful advice when you are frustrated and need to vent is an invaluable stress reducer. It isn't necessary to have a large number of friends. However, different friends often serve

suffering from PTSD were soldiers returning from war, particularly those who saw friends killed or mangled or who experienced terrible suffering and pain themselves. Many of these soldiers continued to suffer from these experiences for decades afterward.

Other extreme traumatic events include rape or other severe physical attacks, near-death experiences in accidents, witnessing a murder or death, street crime or assault, being caught in a natural disaster, or falling victim to terrorist attacks such as the September 11 attacks. Typical symptoms of PTSD include the following.

- *Dissociation,* or perceived detachment of the mind from the emotional state or even the body. In dissociation, the person may have a sense of the world as a dreamlike or unreal place and have poor memory of the events—a form of *dissociative amnesia.*
- *Acute anxiety* or nervousness, in which the person is hyperaroused; may cry easily or experience mood swings; and experience flashbacks, nightmares, and recurrent thoughts or visual images. They may sense vague uneasiness or feel like the event is happening again and again. Some may experience

intense physiological reactions, such as shaking or nausea when something reminds them of the events. In some cases, they may have difficulty returning to areas that remind them of the trauma. For example, persons experiencing PTSD related to the Pentagon and World Trade Center attacks may be unable to work in tall buildings, have difficulty getting on a plane or traveling by air, or feel acutely afraid when they hear planes flying overhead.

- *Persistent stress symptoms.* Sufferers may have two or more of these symptoms:

  - Difficulty falling or staying asleep
  - Irritability or outbursts of anger or other emotions
  - Difficulty concentrating
  - Hypervigilance
  - Exaggerated startle response

If these symptoms last more than one month, PTSD may be diagnosed, either as an *acute form* (less than three months' duration), or a *chronic form* (longer than three months). A *delayed onset* form of PTSD may appear months after the event. In most people, symptoms disappear within six months.

Although exact figures for this illness are not available, the National Institutes of Health indicates that as many as 5–8% of the American public may have chronic forms of PTSD, with women having almost twice the prevalence of men. Rape victims and survivors of torture and concentration camps historically have been among those most likely to have PTSD.

Therapies designed to help trauma victims recover are increasingly effective as our knowledge about this disorder grows. Schools, communities, and workplaces now routinely bring in crisis experts immediately after an event to help survivors talk through their feelings and gain support from others. A supportive family, employer, and friends, and access to professional counseling are important in the recovery process. New generations of anti-anxiety drugs can help individuals who have difficulties. Sleep aids and other options are available to ease short-term symptoms.

Sources: National Mental Health Association, "Coping with Disaster," 2001. www.nmha.org/reassurance/collegetips.cfm; Posttraumatic Stress Disorder Society. www.mentalhealth.com/dis/p20-an06.html; *Mental Health: A Report of the SurgeonGeneral.* www.surgeongeneral.gov/library/mentalhealth/chapter4/sec2.html.

---

different needs, so having more than one is usually beneficial. Particularly for those who lack close ties with family, friends often serve as family away from home in college. As you work to develop and cultivate friendships, look for individuals who:

- Have values that are similar to your own
- Share common interests (as well as those with different interests that force you to stretch and grow in exploring new possibilities)
- Are good listeners, give and share freely, are tolerant, and do not rush to judgment
- Are trustworthy and have your best interests at heart
- Are not unusually critical, negative, selfish, or only bring you down. Avoid people who enjoy "stirring things up" and always seem to be in some crisis themselves; they often precipitate rather than reduce stress responses.
- Are responsible, value doing well in school, but also know when and how to have fun

- Have balance in their lives
- Are willing to be exercise and diet buddies or study partners with a mutual interest in a healthy lifestyle
- Know how to laugh, cry, engage in meaningful conversation, and listen to the silence

Just as it is important to find some or all of these characteristics in your friends, it is also important for you to bring these qualities to your friendships. Sometimes, focusing on others may help you get your own problems into better focus and control.

Learning to make and keep friends is an important aspect of inoculating yourself against harmful stressors. Studies have demonstrated the importance of social support in buffering individuals from the effects of stress.[36] Being well integrated socially seems to reduce all age-adjusted mortality by a factor of 2, about as much as being a nonsmoker versus a smoker. Researchers also have found that people are more likely to die right after, rather than before, their birthdays and

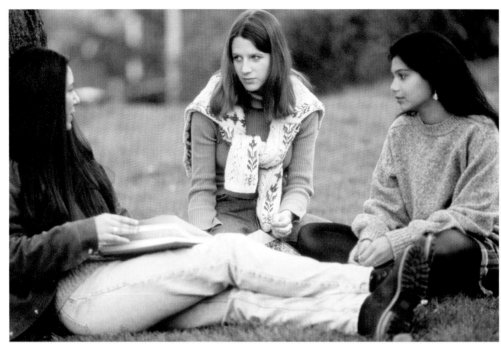
Spending time with friends is an important part of stress reduction.

important holidays, events that offer social interaction. Randomized trials also have provided evidence that psychosocial support is associated with longer survival for patients with breast cancer, malignant melanoma, and lymphoma. Finally, studies have found repeatedly that the death of a spouse is more strongly associated with depression among men than women. What could be the possible reasons for the final item? Though some argue that men depend more on women for daily activities of living, studies have shown that widowed men actually tend to cut off or reduce ties with surviving parents and adult children after such an event, presumably as they begin to search for a new partner. Women, in contrast, maintain and, in fact, increase their social connections during this time, which may serve as a stress buffer.

Managing Emotional Responses

Have you ever gotten all worked up about something only to find that your perceptions were totally wrong? We often get upset, not by realities but by our faulty perceptions. For example, suppose you found out that everyone except you is invited to a party. You might easily begin to wonder why you were excluded. Does someone dislike you? Have you offended someone? Such thoughts are typical. However, the reality of the situation may have absolutely nothing to do with your being liked or disliked. Perhaps you were sent an invitation, and it didn't get to you.

Stress management requires that you examine your *self-talk* and your emotional responses to interactions with others. With any emotional response to a stressor, you are responsible for the emotion and the resultant behaviors. Learning to tell the difference between normal emotions and those based on irrational beliefs can help you stop the emotion or express it in a healthy and appropriate way.

Fighting the Anger Urge Anger results when our wants, desires, and dreams differ from what we actually get in life. People who spend all their emotional energy in a quest for justice or grow frustrated over events that seem impossible to change can become driven by anger. Because anger triggers the fight-or-flight reaction, these people operate with the stress response turned on long after it should have dissipated.

Although much has been said about how hotheaded, short-fused people are at risk for health problems, recent research provides even more compelling reasons for chilling out. A study of nearly 13,000 people found that anger, even in the absence of high blood pressure, can increase the risk of heart attack by more than 2.5 times. Stress hormones released during anger may constrict blood vessels in the heart or actually promote clot formation, which can cause a heart attack.

Angry individuals typically display cynicism, a brooding, hypercritical view of their world. Like angry people, cynical individuals keep fight-or-flight reactions reverberating through their bodies indefinitely. Often labeled as hostile, these chronically stressed folks frequently have weakened immune responses and increased risk of disease. Counseling designed to determine the underlying cause of anger and deal with related issues can be effective. See Table 3.2 for strategies to control and redirect anger.

What do you think?

Do you know people who display the angry and cynical personality traits discussed here? ✳ *How do you feel when you are around them?* ✳ *How do others react to them?* ✳ *Do you regard yourself as a person whose "glass is half empty" or one whose "glass is half full"?* ✳ *What factors have been most important in molding your own anger/hostility profile?* ✳ *What actions would you recommend for someone trying to be more positive, less hostile, and less critical of others?*

Taking Mental Action

Stress management calls for mental action in two areas. First, positive self-esteem, which can help you cope with stressful situations, comes from learned habits and responses to people and events. Successful stress management involves mentally developing and practicing self-esteem skills, focusing on positive thinking about yourself, and examining self-talk to reduce irrational responses. Focus on the here and now rather than on past problems.

Second, because you can't always anticipate what the next stressor will be, you need to develop the mental skills necessary to manage your reactions after it has occurred. The ability to react productively and appropriately comes with time, practice, patience, and experience with a variety of stressful situations.

Changing the Way You Think   Once you realize that some of your thoughts may be irrational or overreactive, make a conscious effort to adjust your thinking. Focus on more positive patterns. Here are specific actions you can take to develop these mental skills.

- *Worry constructively.* Don't waste time and energy worrying about things you can't change or events that may never happen.
- *Look at life as being fluid.* If you accept that change is a natural part of living and growing, the jolt of changes will become less stressful.
- *Consider alternatives.* Remember, there is seldom only one appropriate action. Anticipating options will help you plan for change and adjust more rapidly.
- *Moderate your expectations.* Aim high, but be realistic about your circumstances and motivation.
- *Weed out trivia.* Cardiologist Robert Eliot offers two rules for coping with life's challenges: "Don't sweat the small stuff," and remember that "it's all small stuff."
- *Don't rush into action.* Think before you act.
- *Tolerate mistakes by yourself and others.* Rather than getting angry or frustrated by mishaps, evaluate what happened and learn from them.
- *Live simply.* Eliminate unnecessary things and obligations. Prioritize. Commitments should be to things you have to and want to do.

Table 3.2
Strategies for Anger Control

Get over it.
Try honestly to forgive and forget. Become more accepting of human weaknesses. Set a statute of limitations on how much time you can allow yourself to stay angry. Don't let yourself dredge up old hurts and disappointments again and again.

Learn problem-solving techniques.
Think of viable options. Rather than complaining, suggest possible solutions. Seek opportunities rather than problems. Try to adopt a more optimistic reframing of your situation.

Develop a support system.
Find a trusted friend to confide in and with whom you can simply vent. Listen to what others have to say. Try to get objective opinions rather than persuading others to agree with you. Use such input as you determine realistic solutions to problems.

Plan ahead.
You'll learn from your journal which situations trip you up. It it's traffic, plan ahead or take alternate routes. If it's your parents, think about how you'll respond to get the results you want.

Learn to express feelings comfortably and constructively.
Don't avoid, ignore, or repress them permanently. Deal with the situation after the initial rage reaction has cooled. Express yourself openly and honestly. Learning to confront people with your disappointments and still remain friends is a real gift.

Learn to deescalate.
Count to 10, take a walk, take some deep breaths, get a drink of water. Take time out to validate your feelings, assess consequences of possible actions, and regroup. Try to rechannel anger. Punch a pillow, weed the yard, vacuum your room.

Know your anger style.
Do you hold anger in, or are you the kind of person who explodes? Know what trips your triggers. Keep a journal of such times, places, people, and patterns. Avoid these if possible.

Source: Adapted from Brian L. Seaward., *Managing Stress* (Sudbury, MA: Jones and Bartlett, 1999), www.jbpub.com. Reprinted with permission.

Once you have improved your mental outlook and gained a more positive perspective on life, you will find it easier to cope with stressors.

Taking Physical Action

Physical activities can complement the emotional and mental strategies of stress management.

Exercising   Exercise reduces stress by raising levels of endorphins—mood-elevating, pain-killing hormones—in the bloodstream. Exercise increases energy, reduces hostility, and improves mental alertness. It also can be a source of social interaction, which further reduces stressor effects.

Most of us have relieved stress by engaging in aggressive physical activity: chopping wood when angry is one example. Exercise performed as an immediate response can help alleviate stress symptoms. However, a regular exercise program yields even more substantial benefits. Try to engage in at least 25 minutes of aerobic exercise three or four times a week. But simply walking up stairs, parking farther away from your destination, or standing rather than sitting helps to conserve and replenish your adaptation energy stores. Although it may not improve your aerobic capacity, a quiet walk can refresh your mind and calm your stress response. Plan walking breaks alone or with friends. Stretch after prolonged periods of study at your desk. A short period of physical exercise may provide the break you really need. For more information on the beneficial effects of exercise, see Chapter 11.

Relaxing   Like exercise, relaxation can help you cope with stressful feelings, preserve adaptation energy stores, dissipate excess hormones associated with GAS, and refocus your energies. Relaxation techniques that involve both the mind and body are great stress reducers for college students.[37] Yoga and other exercises that increase flexibility also aid in relaxation (see Chapter 11). Practice relaxation daily until it becomes a habit. You probably will find that you enjoy it.

Once you have learned simple relaxation techniques, you can use them at any time—before or during a tough exam or when faced with a stressful confrontation or assignment, for example. As your body relaxes, your heart rate slows, your blood pressure and metabolic rate decrease, and many other body-calming effects occur, all of which allow you to channel energy appropriately. (See the Skills for Behavior Change box on page 76 on relaxation techniques.)

Eating Right   Is food really a de-stressor? Whether foods can calm us and nourish our psyches is a controversial question. Much of what has been published about hyperactivity and its relation to the consumption of sweets has been shown to be scientifically invalid. High-potency supplements that are supposed to boost resistance against stress-related ailments are nothing more than gimmicks. But it is clear that eating a balanced, healthful diet will help provide the stamina you need to get through problems and will stress-proof you in ways that are not fully understood. It also is known that undereating, overeating, and eating the wrong kinds of foods can create distress in the body. For more information about the benefits of sound nutrition, see Chapter 9.

Managing Your Time

Time. Everybody needs more of it, especially students trying to balance the demands of classes, social life, earning money for school, and family obligations. Include the following time management tips in your stress management program.

- *Take on only one thing at a time.* Don't try to pay bills, clean the bathroom, wash clothes, and write your term paper all at once. Stay focused.

- *Clean off your desk.* According to Jeffrey Mayer, author of *Winning the Fight between You and Your Desk,* most of us spend many stressful minutes each day looking for things that are lost on our desks or in our homes. Go through the things on your desk, toss the unnecessary papers, and put into folders the papers for tasks that you must do.

- *Find a clean, comfortable place to work.* Go someplace where you won't be distracted.

- *Never handle papers more than once.* When bills and other papers come in, take care of them immediately. Write a check and hold it for mailing. Read your mail, and file it or toss it. If you haven't looked at something in over a year, toss it.

- *Prioritize your tasks.* Make a daily "to do" list, and try to stick to it. Categorize the things you must do today, the things that you have to do but not immediately, and the things that it would be nice to do. Prioritize the *Must Do Now* and *Have to Do Later* items, and put deadlines next to each. Only consider the *Nice to Do* items if you finish the others or if the *Nice to Do* list includes something fun. Give yourself a reward as you finish each task.

- *Don't be afraid to say no.* All too often, we do things out of fear of what someone may think. Set your school and personal priorities.

- *Avoid interruptions.* When you've got a project that requires total concentration, schedule uninterrupted time. Unplug the phone, or let your answering machine get it. Close your door and post a *Do Not Disturb* sign. Go to a quiet room in the library or student union where no one will find you.

- *Reward yourself for being efficient.* Did you finish a task early? Take some time for yourself. Enjoy a cup of coffee or hot chocolate. Go for a walk. Start reading something you've wanted to read but haven't had time for. Differentiate between rest breaks and work breaks. Work breaks simply mean switching tasks for awhile. Rest breaks give you time to yourself. Make sure that your rest breaks help you recharge and refresh your energy levels.

- *Become aware of your own time patterns.* We all have 168 hours in a week; how do you spend yours? Keep a time journal for one week (see Figure 3.3). Note the time that was wasted and the time spent in productive work or restorative pleasure. Assess how you could be more productive, and make more time for yourself.

- *Use time to your advantage.* If you're a morning person, schedule activities to coincide with the time when you're at your best. Study and write papers in the morning, and take breaks when you start to slow down. Take a short nap when you need it.

- *Break overwhelming tasks into small pieces, and allocate a certain amount of time to each.* If you are floundering in a task, move on and come back to it when you're refreshed.

- *Remember that time is precious.* Many people learn to value their time only when they face a terminal illness. Try to value each day. Time spent not enjoying life is a tremendous waste of potential.

Activity	Monday	Tuesday	Wednesday	Thursday	Friday	Saturday	Sunday	Total Hours
Getting ready								
On the road								
In class								
Working for pay								
Exercising								
Eating (meals & snacks)								
Studying								
Watching TV, videos								
Using computer (school-related)								
Using computer (recreational)								
Spending time with friends								
Leisure activities								
Other (specify)								
Total Hours								

Figure 3.3

How Do You Spend Your Time?

Fill in your daily activities for a week and assess where you spend time. Are there any activities you could cut back or that you would like to increase?

Alternative Stress Management Techniques

Popular stress fighters include hypnosis, massage therapy, meditation, and biofeedback. Recently, herbal supplements such as St. John's wort (SJW) have also become popular for stress management. See Chapter 18 for more on the pros and cons of SJW.

Hypnosis   Hypnosis is a process that requires a person to focus on one thought, object, or voice, thereby freeing the right hemisphere of the brain to become more active. The person then becomes unusually responsive to suggestion. Whether self-induced or induced by someone else, hypnosis can reduce certain types of stress.

Massage Therapy   If you have ever had someone massage your stiff neck or aching feet, you know that massage is an excellent way to relax. Massage techniques vary from vigorous Swedish massage to the gentler acupressure and Esalen

massage. Before selecting a massage therapist, check his or her credentials carefully. The therapist should have training from a reputable program that teaches scientific principles for anatomic manipulation and should be certified through the American Massage Therapy Association.

Meditation   There are many different forms of **meditation**. Most involve sitting quietly for 15 to 20 minutes, focusing on a particular word or symbol, controlling breathing, and getting in touch with the inner self. Practiced by Eastern religions for centuries, meditation is believed to be an important

Hypnosis   A process that allows people to become unusually responsive to suggestion.

Meditation   A relaxation technique that involves focusing on a word or symbol, controlling breathing, and getting in touch with the inner self.

Relaxation Techniques for Stress Management

Although relaxation techniques for stress reduction have been practiced for centuries, finding the one that works best for you takes time and effort. You may find that what calms and renews your friends makes you tense and nervous. Among the most common strategies are diaphragmatic or deep breathing and progressive muscle relaxation.

DIAPHRAGMATIC BREATHING

Typically, we breathe only using the upper chest and thoracic region rather than involving the abdominal region. Simply stated, diaphragmatic breathing is deep breathing that maximally expands the chest by involving the movement of the lower abdomen. This technique is commonly used in yoga exercises. The diaphragmatic breathing process occurs in three stages.

- *Stage 1: Assume a comfortable position.* Whether sitting or lying down on your back, find the most natural position to be in. Close your eyes, unbutton your shirt or binding clothes, remove your belt, or unbutton your pants. Often it works best to fold your hands over your abdomen and get used to feeling the rise and fall of your stomach.
- *Stage 2: Concentrate on the act of breathing.* Shut out external noise. Stay focused on inhaling, exhaling, and the route the air is following. Try saying to yourself, "Feel the warm air coming into your nose, warming your windpipe, and flowing into your lungs. Feel your stomach rise and fall as you inhale slowly and exhale slowly, noting the air flowing out of your nose or mouth." Repeat this action several times.
- *Stage 3: Visualize.* The above stages seem to work best when combined with visualization. A common example is to visualize clean, fresh, invigorating air slowly entering the nose and being exhaled as gray, stale air that has accumulated in the body. Such processes, particularly when they involve the whole body, seem to help deep breathers become more refreshed from their experience.

PROGRESSIVE MUSCLE RELAXATION

Progressive muscle relaxation is another common form of relaxation technique. Each of several muscle groups is systematically contracted and relaxed; proper breathing and concentration are part of this process. Again, find a comfortable position similar to that discussed in the deep breathing section above, and begin a deep breathing cycle.

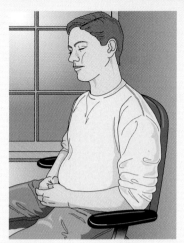

Finding a comfortable position is important for relaxation techniques.

The difference from diaphragmatic breathing is that, as you concentrate on inhaling, you also contract a particular muscle group (for example, the hand and fingers). Hold that position for a short period and then, as you exhale, slowly release the muscles that you have been contracting. Repeat and add more muscle groups. You might start with a hand, then move to the forearm, the entire arm, the neck, to the shoulders, back, buttocks, foot, and thigh. You can add components of other relaxation techniques to this experience by saying, "My hands are getting warmer, my arm is getting warmer," and so on as you work to gain maximum control of blood flow and muscle tension in a region.

form of introspection and personal renewal. As a stress management tool, it can calm the body and quiet the mind, creating a sense of peace.

Biofeedback Biofeedback involves self-monitoring by machine of physical responses to stress and attempts to control these responses. The machine records perspiration, heart rate, respiration, blood pressure, surface body temperature, muscle tension, and other stress responses. Then, by trial and error, the person using biofeedback techniques learns to lower his or her stress responses through conscious effort.

> **Biofeedback** A technique that involves self-monitoring by machine of physical responses to stress and attempts to control the responses.

Eventually, the person develops the ability to lower stress responses at will, without using the machines.

Making the Most of Support Groups

Support groups are an important part of stress management. Friends, family members, and co-workers can provide emotional and physical support. Although the ideal support group differs for each of us, you should have one or two close friends in whom you are able to confide and neighbors with whom you can trade favors. Try to participate in community activities at least once a week. A healthy committed relationship also can provide vital support.

If you do not have a close support group, find out where to turn when the pressures of life seem overwhelming. Family members are often a steady base of support on which you can rely. But if friends or family are unavailable, most colleges and universities offer counseling services at no cost for short-term crises. Clergy, instructors, and dorm supervisors also may be excellent resources. If university services are unavailable or if you are concerned about confidentiality, most communities offer low-cost counseling through mental health clinics.

Developing Your Spiritual Side: Mindfulness

In discussions of spirituality, the concept of mindfulness often emerges. As a meditative technique, **mindfulness**—the ability to be fully present in the moment—can aid relaxation; reduce emotional and physical pain; and help us connect more effectively with ourselves, with others, and with nature. The practice of mindfulness includes strategies and activities that contribute to overall health and wellness. In fact, mindfulness and wellness are interconnected and can be developed concurrently, each reinforcing the other. We can think of spirituality as encompassing four dimensions: physical, emotional, social, and intellectual.

The Physical Dimension: Moving in Nature

A delightful way to strengthen the body, build endurance, and bring peace of mind is to interact with the natural environment. Activities such as walking, jogging, biking, and swimming foster this interaction, providing sensory experience (feeling, smelling, touching, listening, and hearing) while strengthening muscles and the cardiovascular system. By focusing on the birdsong or the crunch of your shoes on freshly fallen snow, you can free yourself of worry or anxious thoughts. Appreciating and absorbing the beauty of nature allow us to unwind emotionally even as our bodies are at work.

The Emotional Dimension: Dealing with Negative Feelings

Each of us has positive and negative emotions that govern moods and behaviors throughout the day. We often take joy, happiness, and contentment for granted since we tend not to notice the *absence* of stress and distress. However, we typically are aware of negative emotions, such as jealousy, hatred, and anger, because they deplete our energy reserves and cause us problems in interacting with others.

To improve our emotional health and access our spiritual side, we must take notice of the situations that trigger negative feelings such as anger. (Refer to Table 3.2, "Strategies for Anger Control"). By stopping in the midst of anger and concentrating on physical reactions, we begin to realize the full extent of the damage we inflict upon ourselves when we allow

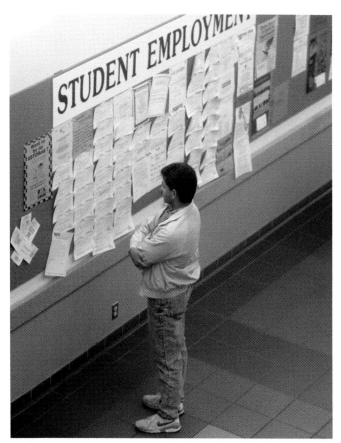

Many college students are dealing with financial responsibilities for the first time. Juggling work and school, pursuing financial aid, and keeping to a budget all can contribute to stress.

negativity to get the best of us. We might ask ourselves, "Is it worth it?" And probably we will conclude, "I don't like allowing this kind of hit on my body. I've got to get a handle on this before I hurt myself or someone else." By practicing thought-stopping, blocking negative thoughts, and focusing on positive emotions via self-talk and other methods of diversion, we can help ourselves through a negative experience.

The Social Dimension: Interacting, Listening, and Communicating

Developing the spiritual side is not just an internal process. It is also a social process that enhances relationships with others. The ability to give and take, speak and listen, forgive and move on are all integral to spiritual development.

Today, life is busier than ever. While constantly juggling responsibilities, it is easy to get so caught up in the stresses of our own lives that we find it difficult to give to others. Here again, we need to stop and think about how being too self-enmeshed can affect relationships and the ability to

> **Mindfulness** The ability to be fully present in the moment.

communicate with others. Communication is a two-way process in which listening is every bit as important as speaking. Learning to *listen actively* is a potent asset. Active listeners take note of content, intent, and feelings being expressed. They listen to all levels of the communication. Sensitivity and honesty are also essential to the give and take of communication. Ask questions, rephrase the speaker's ideas, and focus genuine attention on the speaker. Through such active participation, we gain a greater insight into the other person, who in turn will be encouraged to share more. Sharing becomes more intimate and relationships more connected when people feel that others care and are genuinely interested in their well-being. Both parties benefit from such an interchange.

The Intellectual Dimension: Sharpening Intuition

Take the time to assess events in life, their causes, and your own involvement in them. This often involves putting aside our emotional dimension for a moment to reflect, read, and ponder. Sometimes this process leads to startling new insights—"Ah-ha! . . . Now I get it; this all makes sense!" Such moments mean so much, but few people include this mental activity in daily rituals. Examining the past, how we've gotten to where we are in the present, and what actions might have changed the course of events is a critical element of spiritual growth. By using our minds for objective reasoning, we develop the intellectual dimension of spiritual health.

Taking Charge

3   3   3

Make It Happen!

Assessment: The Assess Yourself box on page 64 gave you the chance to look at your stress levels and identify certain situations in your life that particularly cause stress. Now that you are aware of these patterns, you can change a behavior that leads to increased stress.

Making a Change: In order to change your behavior, you need to develop a plan. Follow these steps.

1. Evaluate your behavior, and identify patterns and specific things you are doing. What can you change now? What can you change in the near future?
2. Select one pattern of behavior that you want to change.

3. Fill out a Behavior Change Contract. It should include your long-term goal for change, your short-term goals, the rewards you'll give yourself for reaching these goals, potential obstacles along the way, and strategies for overcoming these obstacles.
4. Chart your progress in a journal. At the end of a week, consider how successful you were in following your plan. What helped you be successful? What made change more difficult? What will you do differently next week?
5. Revise your plan as needed. Are the short-term goals attainable? Are the rewards satisfying?

Example: Kim discovered that much of her stress was caused by school

deadlines. She wanted to take steps to manage her time more efficiently. She filled out a Behavior Change Contract, with a goal of finishing her History term paper five days before its due date in order to give herself enough time to study for her Biology final. She broke the paper-writing process into manageable steps of research, writing, revising, and proofreading. Each time she finished a stage, she rewarded herself with a movie or a trip to the local coffeehouse. She fell behind when her sister unexpectedly visited her for two days, but she got back on schedule when she worked on her paper instead of watching her afternoon soap opera. Kim completed her paper in plenty of time, was able to study efficiently for her Biology exam, and didn't come down with her usual end-of-term cold.

Summary

✸ Stress is an inevitable part of our lives. Eustress refers to stress associated with positive events, distress to negative events.
✸ The alarm, resistance, and exhaustion phases of the general adaptation syndrome involve physiological responses to both real and imagined stressors and cause a complex cascade of hormones to rush through the body. Prolonged arousal due to stress may be detrimental to health.

✸ Undue stress for extended periods of time can compromise the immune system and result in serious health consequences. Psychoneuroimmunology is the science that analyzes the relationship between the mind's reaction to stress and the function of the immune system. While increasing evidence links disease susceptibility to stress, much of this research remains controversial. However, stress has been linked to numerous health problems, including CVD, cancer, and increased susceptibility to infectious diseases.

✳ Multiple factors contribute to stress and the stress response. Psychosocial factors include change, hassles, pressure, inconsistent goals and behaviors, conflict, overload, and burnout. Other factors are environmental stressors and self-imposed stress. Persons subjected to discrimination or bias due to "isms" may face unusually high levels of stress.

✳ College can be especially stressful. Recognizing the signs of stress is the first step toward better health. Learning to reduce test anxiety and cope with multiple stressors is also important.

✳ Managing stress begins with learning simple coping mechanisms: assessing stressors, changing responses, and learning to cope. Finding out what works best for you—probably some combination of managing emotional responses, taking mental or physical action, downshifting, learning time management, or using alternative stress management techniques—will help you better cope with stress in the long run.

✳ Developing the spiritual side involves practicing mindfulness and its many dimensions. These include the physical dimension (moving in nature); the emotional dimension (identifying and controlling negative feelings); the social dimension (interacting, listening, and communicating); and the intellectual dimension (sharpening intuition).

Questions for Discussion and Reflection

1. Compare and contrast distress and eustress. Are both types of stress potentially harmful?
2. Describe the alarm, resistance, and exhaustion phases of the general adaptation syndrome and the body's physiological response to stress. Does stress lead to more irritability or emotionality, or does emotionality lead to stress? Provide examples.
3. What are some of the health risks that result from chronic stress? How does the study of PNI link stress and illness?
4. What major factors seem to influence the nature and extent of a person's susceptibility to stress? Explain how social support, self-esteem, and personality may make a person more or less susceptible.

5. Why are some students more vulnerable to stress than others? What services are available on your campus to help you deal with excessive stress?
6. What can college students do to inoculate themselves against negative stress effects? What actions can you take to manage your stressors? How can you help others manage their stressors more effectively?
7. How does anger affect the body? Discuss the steps you can take to fight your own anger urge and help your friends control theirs.

Accessing Your Health on the Internet

Visit the following Internet sites to explore further topics and issues related to personal health. To visit an organization's website, go to the Companion Website for *Health: The Basics, Sixth Edition* at www.aw-bc.com/donatelle, click on the book image, and select "Accessing Your Health on the Internet" from the navigation menu on the left.

1. **American College Counseling Association**. This website of the professional organization for college counselors offers useful links and articles.
2. **American College Health Association.** Provides information and data from the National College Health Assessment survey.

3. **Center for Anxiety and Stress Treatment**. Provides resources and services regarding a broad range of stress-related topics.
4. **Hampden-Sydney College.** Provides links to helpful tips for dealing with stressful issues college students commonly experience.
5. **Mind Tools.** Focuses on all aspects of stress and stress management.
6. **National Institute of Mental Health.** A resource for information on all aspects of mental health, including the effects of stress.

Further Reading

Coffey, R. *Unspeakable Truths and Happy Endings*. Veritas, 1998. www.sover.net/ ~ schwcof

An outstanding resource focusing on survivors of trauma/stress and recovery from human cruelty. Reports on survivors of war, rape, sexual assault, street crime, terrorism, and domestic violence; covers all major stressors in contemporary life.

Health and Stress: The Newsletter of the American Institute of Stress. www.stress.org/news.htm

Excellent monthly resource on stress. Reports on latest developments in all areas of stress research. Each issue contains a listing of meetings of interest and a book review.

Greenberg, J. S. *Comprehensive Stress Management*, 9th ed. New York: McGraw-Hill, 2004.

An overview of current perspectives on stress and the influence of personal control and behavior on health. Discusses stress management as a factor in controlling pain, anxiety, and depression. An excellent resource for health professionals.

Romas, J. A. and M. Sharma. *Practical Stress Management, 3rd ed.* San Francisco: Benjamin Cummings, 2004.

An accessible text that combines theory and principles with hands-on exercises to manage stress. Includes an audio CD with guided relaxation techniques such as progressive muscle relaxation, deep breathing, and visual imaging.

Weil, A. *Ask Dr. Weil.* New York: Random House, 1998.

A holistic doctor who provides an overview of mind–body health and alternative strategies for coping with life's challenges.

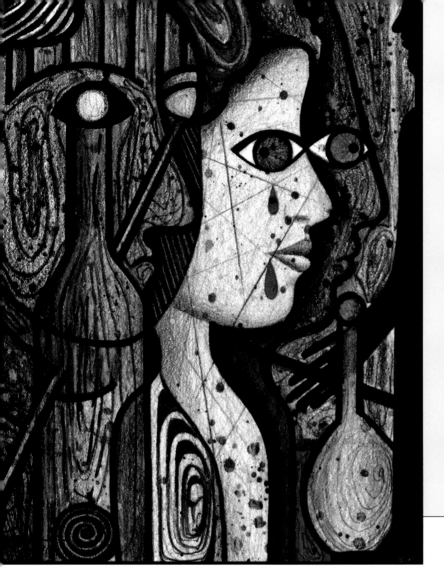

Violence and Abuse

Creating Healthy Environments

4 4 4 4 4 4

Objectives

* Differentiate between intentional and unintentional injuries, and discuss societal and personal factors that contribute to violence in American society.

* Discuss factors that contribute to homicide, domestic violence, sexual victimization, and other intentional acts of violence.

* Explain how terrorism can affect individuals and populations, and summarize practical steps to lower your risk from terrorist attacks.

* Discuss strategies to prevent intentional injuries and reduce their risk of occurrence.

* Explain how the campus community, law enforcement officials, and individuals can prevent crimes that are common on campuses.

* Discuss the impact of unintentional injuries on American society, and explain actions that might contribute to personal risk of injuries of all types.

When Campus Violence Flares

By Jeremy Pearce

NEW BRUNSWICK These days, on college campuses across New Jersey, the familiar and once-reassuring progress of freshman orientation, homecoming, mid-term exams and winter break has seemingly been shattered by a new rite of passage.

Incidences of murder, rape, arson and other violent crimes are shaking the inner sanctum—most recently in two shootings last month at Rider University in Lawrenceville and a melee that occurred here at Rutgers only a week earlier. At Rutgers, the baseball bat beatings of two students in front of a College

Avenue social house startled the university by their savageness and public location, within sight of the New Brunswick campus's student center.

"It's the level of brutality," said Abeed Hossain, a history major from Somerset. At 20 years old, Mr. Hossain is the same age as the victims, both members of the Squam club. The two men sustained severe head injuries that left them in critical condition.

"I was shocked, and the people I know were shocked," said Mr. Hossain, making a gesture of frustration with his hand. "It creates an image that blows the reputation of this school."

Read the complete article online in the eThemes section of this book's website: www.aw-bc.com/donatelle.

The September 11, 2001 terrorist attack on the United States galvanized the country in a burst of patriotic fervor. For many, this horrendous act of violence was incomprehensible, something that had previously seemed possible only on television or in the movies. While reactions of generosity, heroism, goodwill, and other positive behaviors persisted for months after the incident, there was also a darker side to how some Americans reacted. Reports of racist attacks, beatings, and human rights violations became widespread. Some political leaders called for American schools to ban all students from Iran, Afghanistan, Pakistan, and other countries in the Middle East. Many compared the treatment of Muslim groups to that of Japanese Americans during World War II.

What do you think are the major reasons why violent incidents occur? Can you think of other examples in which certain segments of society have been the victims of hate crimes and discrimination? What underlying beliefs and philosophies ignite such behaviors? Do you believe that violence is really worse now than it was back in the good old days? What actions could we take as a society to reduce violence?

> *"Across the land, waves of violence seem to crest and break, terrorizing Americans in cities and suburbs, in prairie towns and mountain hollows."*

> *"To millions of Americans few things are more pervasive, more frightening, more real today than violent crime. . . . The fear of being victimized by criminal attack has touched us all in some way."*

> *"Among urban children ages 10–14, homicides are up 150 percent, robberies are up 192 percent, assaults are up 290 percent."*

You might think these statements are from today's newspapers or television news. But they're not. The first quotation comes from President Herbert Hoover's 1929 inauguration speech, the second from the 1860 Senate report on crime, and the third from a 1967 report on children's violence.[1] Clearly, violence and our concern over its rising rates are not new concepts.

The term **violence** indicates a set of behaviors that produce injuries, regardless of whether they are **intentional injuries** (committed with intent to harm) or **unintentional injuries** (committed without intent to harm, often accidentally). Any definition of *violence* implicitly includes the use of force, regardless of the intent, but as you'll see, some forms of violence are also extremely subtle.

Violence   A set of behaviors that produce injuries, as well as the outcomes of these behaviors (the injuries themselves).

Intentional injuries   Injuries committed with intent to harm.

Unintentional injuries   Injuries committed without intent to harm, often accidentally.

In this chapter, we focus on the various types of intentional and unintentional injuries, the underlying causes of or contributors to these problems, strategies to reduce risk of encountering violence, and possible methods for preventing violence. Although certain indicators of violence, such as murders and deadly assaults, seem to be on the decline, other forms of violence, such as rape and hate crimes, are on the increase. Even more important is that for all we know about the incidence and prevalence of violence, a great deal remains unknown. Just how many people suffer in silence, failing to report violent acts because of fear of repercussions or because they accept violence as the way life is, remains unknown.

Violence in the United States

Even though violence has long been a concern in American society, not until 1985 did the U.S. Public Health Service formally identify violence as a leading public health problem that contributed significantly to death and disability rates. The Centers for Disease Control and Prevention (CDC) created the Division of Violence Prevention and considers violence a chronic disease that is pervasive at all levels of American society. Vulnerable populations, such as children, women, black males, and the elderly, were listed as being at high risk.

Recent numbers indicate that we have made dramatic improvements in certain areas. Since 1973, Federal Bureau of Investigation (FBI) statistics show that overall crime and certain types of violent crime actually have decreased each year (Figure 4.1). In addition, a recent Department of Justice report suggests that colleges and universities are relatively safe.[2] However, many question the accuracy of such reports, since petty theft, date rape, fighting, and other common campus incidents are not always reported to police. Although a person's chances of being murdered or violently assaulted may have declined, the odds of being a victim of burglary, theft, and minor assault in general are on the increase.[3]

Violence affects everyone directly or indirectly. Although the direct victims of violence and those close to them obviously suffer the most, others suffer in various ways because of the climate of fear that violence generates. Women are afraid to walk alone at night. The elderly are often afraid to go out even in the daytime. Since terrorist episodes such as the 2001 World Trade Center attack, some people are afraid to fly, to work in tall buildings, or to live in heavily populated areas. The cost of homeland security is staggering. International travelers often fear coming to the United States just as Americans fear traveling to other regions of the world where U.S. citizens have been attacked. The news media broadcast stories of children dodging bullets in city neighborhoods or drivers being carjacked. Even people who live in supposedly safe areas can become victims of violence within their own homes or at the hands of family members.

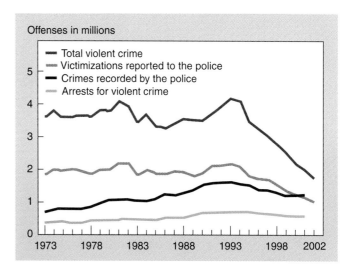

Figure 4.1
Changes in Crime Rates, 1973–2002
Note: Total serious violent crime is the number of homicides recorded by police plus the number of rapes, robberies, and aggravated assaults reported in the National Crime Victimization Survey. Victimization is the number of homicides recorded by police plus other serious crimes that respondents to the survey said were reported to police. Crimes recorded by police and arrests are based on law enforcement reports to the FBI.

Source: Bureau of Justice Statistics, "Key Crime and Justice Facts at a Glance," August 2003. www.ojp.usdoj.gov/bjs/glance.htm

Societal Causes of Violence

Several social, cultural, and individual factors increase the likelihood of violent acts (Figure 4.2), including the following.[4]

- *Poverty.* Low socioeconomic status and poor living conditions can create an environment of hopelessness, leaving people feeling trapped and seeing violence as the only way to obtain what they want.
- *Unemployment.* It is a well-documented fact that when the economy goes sour, violent crime, suicide, assault, and other crimes increase.
- *Parental influence.* Violence is cyclical. Children raised in environments in which shouting, slapping, hitting, and other forms of violence are commonplace are more apt to act out these behaviors as adults. Reports in recent years of abused children who grow up to commit horrifying crimes have made this pattern impossible to ignore.
- *Cultural beliefs.* Cultures that objectify women and empower men to be tough and aggressive show higher rates of violence in the home.
- *The media.* A daily dose of murder and mayhem can take a toll on even resistant minds.
- *Discrimination/oppression.* Whenever one group is oppressed by another, seeds of discontent are sown, and hate crimes arise.

8	Lack of Understanding and Community	• May result from intermixed cultures, fear, misunderstanding, distrust, or competition; focus on self-gratification rather than concern for others
7	Community Deterioration	• Decline of funding for community services, mental health, etc. • Poverty, hopelessness, helplessness
6	Incarceration	• Often a training ground and a communication center for criminals • Ineffective programs for rehabilitation
5	Witnessing Acts of Violence	• May cause posttraumatic stress • May make violence seem normal • Learn poor coping/anger management
4	Alcohol and Other Drugs	• Often associated with violence
3	Media Portrayal of Violence	• Frequent portrayal of violence (by age 16, most Americans have seen over 200,000 acts of violence on TV) • Images related to race, gender, or ethnicity may lead to violence
2	Guns	• Involved in the vast majority of homicides and suicides
1	Negative Home/ Family Influences	• Learned lack of respect, lack of responsibility, poor models for relationships, low self-esteem, low self-worth, spiritual bankruptcy

Figure 4.2
Correlates to Violence

- *Religious differences.* Religious persecution has been a part of the human experience since earliest times.
- *Political differences.* Civil unrest and differences in political party affiliations and beliefs have historically been triggers for violent acts.
- *Breakdowns in the criminal justice system.* Overcrowded prisons, lenient sentences, early releases from prison, and trial errors subtly encourage violence in a number of ways.
- *Stress.* People who are in crisis or under stress are apt to be highly reactive, striking out at others or acting irrationally.
- *Heavy use of alcohol and other substances.* Alcohol and drug abuse are often catalysts for violence, and risk

---

Primary aggression Goal-directed, hostile self-assertion that is destructive in character.

Reactive aggression Emotional reaction brought about by frustrating life experiences.

---

factors for domestic violence, rape, child abuse, homicide, and other crimes.[5]

In addition to these broad, societally based factors, many personal factors also can lead to violence.

> **What do you think?**
> *Why do you think there is so much violent behavior in the United States?* ✳ *Why do you think the rate of violent crime decreased in the six months following the September 11 terrorist attacks?* ✳ *What actions can you take personally to prevent violence from occurring?* ✳ *What could be done to reduce risk on your campus?* ✳ *In your community?*

Personal Precipitators of Violence

If you are like most people, you probably acted out your anger more readily as a child than you do today. However, even the worst-behaved children mature. And as we mature, we learn to control outbursts of anger and approach conflict rationally.

Yet, others go through life acting out their aggressive tendencies in much the same ways they did as children or as their families did. Why do two children from the same neighborhood, or even from the same family, go in different directions when it comes to violence? There are several predictors of future aggressive behavior.

Anger Anger is a spontaneous, usually temporary, biological feeling or emotional state of displeasure that occurs most frequently during times of personal frustration. Because life is stressful, anger becomes a part of daily experience. Anger can range from slight irritation to rage, a violent and extreme form of anger.[6] When it is acted out at home or on the road, the consequences can be deadly.

What makes some people flare at the slightest provocation? Often, people who anger quickly have a low tolerance for frustration and believe that they should not have to put up with inconvenience or petty annoyances. The cause may be genetic or physiological; there is evidence that some people are born unstable, touchy, or easily angered.[7] Another cause of anger is sociocultural. Because many people are taught not to express anger in public, many do not know how to handle it when it reaches a level that cannot be hidden. Family background may be the most important factor. Typically, anger-prone people come from families that are disruptive, chaotic, and unskilled in emotional expression.[8] In fact, the single largest predictor of future violence is past violence.[9]

Aggressive behavior is often a key aspect of violent interactions. **Primary aggression** is goal-directed, hostile self-assertion that is destructive in nature. **Reactive aggression** is more often part of an emotional reaction brought about by frustrating life experiences. Whether aggression is

Road Rage!

We pulled out into traffic and immediately were serenaded by a blaring horn from a car speeding by us in the next lane. Apparently we had pulled out in front of the car, causing the driver to swerve quickly to avoid hitting us. We felt bad and were thankful that nothing serious had happened, but the other driver wasn't so quick to forgive. For several miles she maneuvered to make us pull over, or slowed down in the neighboring lane in order to pull alongside our car. I wanted nothing to do with this and slowed down as well to avoid facing her. Finally, she pulled over as she approached a right-hand turn, and as we went by, she stuck her head out the window and screamed venomous slurs our way. I'll never forget the expression on the woman's face as we went by. It was filled with such hatred, such rage.

—From the author's files

If you drive at all, you have probably encountered road rage. While drunk driving remains a critical problem, the facts about aggressive driving are surely as ominous. According to the National Highway Transportation Safety Association,

41,907 people died on the highways last year. An estimated two-thirds of these fatalities were caused at least in part by aggressive driving behavior.

Why is road rage becoming more common? One reason is sheer overcrowding. In the last decade, the number of cars on the roads has increased by more than 11%, and the number of miles driven has increased by 35%; however, the number of new road miles has only increased by 1%. That means more cars in the same amount of space; and the problem is magnified in urban areas. Also, people have less time and more things to do. When people try to fit more activities into the day, stress levels rise. Stress creates anxiety, which leads to short tempers and road rage.

ARE YOU IMMUNE TO ROAD RAGE?

You may think you are the last person who would drive aggressively, but you might be surprised. Have you ever tailgated a slow driver, honked long and hard at another car, or sped up to keep another driver from passing? If you recognize yourself in any of these situations, watch out!

AVOID THE RAGE (YOURS AND OTHER DRIVERS')

Whether you are getting angry at other drivers, or another driver is visibly upset with you, there are things you can do to avoid major confrontations. The key is to discharge your emotion in a healthy way. If you are the target of another driver's rage, do everything possible to get away safely.

- Avoid eye contact!
- If you need to use your horn, do it sparingly.
- Get out of the way. Even if the other guy is speeding, it's safest to not make a point by staying in your lane.
- If someone is following you after an on-the-road encounter, drive to a public place or the nearest police station.
- Report any aggressive driving incidents to the police department immediately. You may be able to prevent further occurrences by the same driver.
- Above all, always buckle your seat belt! Seat belts save 9,500 lives annually.

Source: Allstate Insurance. "Don't Be Blinded by Road Rage." www.allstate.com/safety/auto/rage.html.

---

primary or reactive, it is most likely to flare in times of acute stress, during relationship difficulties or loss, or when a person is so frustrated that the only recourse is to strike out at others.

What do you think?

What are some examples of primary aggression? ✳ *Reactive aggression?* ✳ *Can both of them result in the same degree of harm?* ✳ *Do you think our laws are more lenient when violent acts result from reactive aggression?* ✳ *Why?*

Substance Abuse Although much has been written about a strong link between substance abuse and violence, we have yet to show that substance abuse actually causes violence. In fact, many violent episodes are carefully planned actions that involve no alcohol or drug abuse. In some situations,

however, psychoactive substances appear to be a form of ignition for violence.

- Consumption of alcohol—by perpetrators of the crime, the victim, or both—immediately preceded over half of all violent crimes, including murder.[10]
- Chronic drinkers are more likely than others to have histories of violent behavior.[11]
- Criminals using illegal drugs commit robberies and assaults more frequently than nonusing criminals and do so especially during periods of heavy drug use.[12]
- In domestic assault cases, more than 86 percent of the assailants and 42 percent of victims reported using alcohol at the time of the attack. Nearly 15 percent of victims and assailants reported using cocaine at the time of the attack.[13]
- Ninety-two percent of assailants and 42 percent of victims reported having used alcohol or other drugs on the day of the assault.[14]

- Mentally ill patients who fail to adhere to prescription drug regimens and abuse alcohol and/or other drugs are significantly more likely to be involved in a serious violent act.[15]
- Substance abuse increases markedly the risk of both homicide and suicide. Problems at work due to drinking, hospitalization for a drinking problem, use of illicit drugs, and arrest for use of illicit drugs all place subjects at risk for violent death by homicide. The combination of depression and use of alcohol or other drugs increases homicide and suicide rates threefold.[16]

Intentional Injuries

Any time someone sets out to harm other people or their property, the incident may be referred to as intentional violence. Such incidents often result in intentional injuries, which come in many forms. Whether the situation entails a simple outburst of anger or a fatal attack with a weapon, the resulting intentional injuries cause pain and suffering at the very least, and death and disability at the worst.

Gratuitous Violence

Violence can manifest itself in many ways. Often the most shocking or gratuitous crimes gain the greatest attention, such as stories of innocent victims of drive-by shootings or young students who turn their rage on family, classmates, and teachers.

Assault/Homicide Homicide, death that results from intent to injure or kill, accounts for nearly 17,000 premature deaths in the United States.[17] These numbers are down slightly from 1997 but still represent a significant contributor to life lost in certain segments of the population. Although homicide was the fifteenth leading cause of death in the United States among all age groups in 2000, it was the second leading cause of death for persons age 15 to 24 (Figure 4.3). Homicide is the leading cause of death for African American males age 15 to 24 and the second leading cause of death for young Hispanic males. In 2000 the homicide rate for young African American males was 17 times the rate for young non-Hispanic white males. The rate for young Hispanic males was 7 times the rate for young non-Hispanic males.[18] As measured by Years of Potential Life Lost, homicide exacts a heavy toll (Table 4.1).

For every violent death, at least 100 nonfatal injuries are caused by violence. In 1999, an estimated 28,874 firearm-related deaths occurred, including large numbers of homicides and suicides.[19] For every person shot and killed by a firearm, almost three others were treated annually for nonfatal shootings, many of them children under age ten.[20] Data

Homicide Death that results from intent to injure or kill.

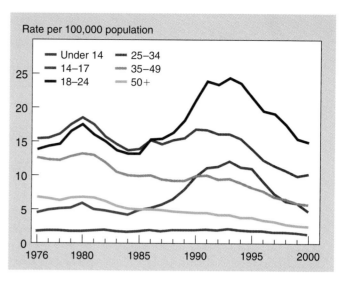

Figure 4.3
Rate of Homicide Victimization by Age, 1976–2000

Source: Bureau of Justice Statistics, "Homicide Trends in the U.S.," 2002. www.ojp.usdoj.gov/bjs/homicide/teens.htm

from a 1998 study showed that 12 women used a handgun to kill an assailant in self-defense, while 1,209 women were murdered with a handgun, a ratio of over 100 to 1.[21]

For an American, the average lifetime probability of being murdered is 1 in 153—but the average masks large differences for specific segments of the population. For white women, the risk of murder is 1 in 450; for African American men, it is 1 in 28. For an African American man in the 20- to 22-year age group, the risk is 1 in 3. Combined across races, males represent 77 percent of all murder and nonnegligent manslaughter victims. African American males are 1.14 times more likely than are white males to be murder victims; white females are 1.5 times more likely than are African American females to be victims.[22] More than half of all homicides occur among people who know one another. In two-thirds of these cases, the perpetrator and the victim are friends or acquaintances; in one-third, they belong to the same family.[23]

Bias and Hate Crimes In spite of national efforts in workplaces, schools, and communities to promote understanding and diversity, intolerance continues to smolder in many parts of U.S. society. The killings of James Byrd and Matthew Shepard and the arson attacks on several U.S. synagogues remind Americans that violence as a result of racism and other "isms" still occurs. International terrorist acts often reflect the hatred of one religious or political group for another that is considered to be of less value due to differences in religion, language, or other characteristics. Recent acts of violence against different racial groups by police, beatings in public schools and on the streets that are racially motivated gang events, and other hate crimes are common events on the nightly news.

Table 4.1
Years of Potential Life Lost (per 100,000)

Years of Potential Life Lost (YPLL) is a rough measure of the impact of a specific disease or societal event/condition on a given population. It is calculated by subtracting the age at death of a person from the expected life expectancy for this person. In this table, the total years are those lost before age 75 per 100,000 population under the age of 75. It provides a glimpse of the overall impact of a problem on the lives of particular populations.

Some questions to consider: Where are the greatest disparities in YPLL among males? Among females? What factors do you think contribute to the low rates of suicide in some groups? High rates of assault?

	Unintentional Injury	Suicide	Assault (Homicide)
Male			
White	1,475.9	624.7	253.9
African American	1,888.7	388.1	1,753.5
American Indian/Alaska Native	2,771.7	850.8	568.3
Asian/Pacific Islander	637.1	308.8	210.2
Hispanic	1,536.8	346.6	676.8
White, non-Hispanic	1,440.8	657.6	167.1
Female			
White	586.8	154.4	95.0
African American	676.9	67.0	370.2
American Indian/Alaska Native	1,276.8	219.7	205.8
Asian/Pacific Islander	309.6	102.5	80.2
Hispanic	461.8	306.3	121.9
White, non-Hispanic	599.1	164.4	88.2

Note: The groups of white, African American, Asian/Pacific Islander, and American Indian/Alaska Native include persons of Hispanic and non-Hispanic origin. Conversely, persons of Hispanic origin may be of any race.

Source: Department of Health and Human Services, National Institutes of Health, Centers for Disease Control and Prevention, Health U.S. 2001. www.cdc.gov

According to the FBI's most recent Hate Crime Statistics Report, nearly 8,000 bias-motivated crimes were reported in 1999, compared to 7,700 in 1998. Of the total reported incidents, 4,300 were motivated by racial bias, 1,400 by religious bias, 1,300 by sexual orientation bias, and over 800 were related to ethnicity/national origin.[24]

Since the September 11 terrorist attack in the United States, reports of hate-related incidents, beatings, and other physical and verbal assaults have escalated, even as other rates of violent crime decreased. In particular, persons of the Muslim faith or of Middle-Eastern descent report civil rights violations at work, in public transit, and in communities throughout the United States. Many believe that the reported incidents are but the tip of the iceberg and that actual numbers of bias- and hate-related crimes are much higher, but people do not report them out of fear of possible retaliation.

Hate crimes vary along two dimensions: (1) the way they are carried out and (2) their effects on victims. Vicious gossip, nasty comments, and pranks may not make campus headlines, but they can hurt nonetheless. Generally, about 30 percent of all hate crimes are against property; the other 70 percent are against the person. Recent studies have identified three additional characteristics of hate crimes. They are:[25]

- Excessively brutal
- Perpetrated at random on total strangers
- Perpetrated by multiple offenders

In addition, the perpetrators tend to be motivated by thrill, defensive feelings, or a hate-mongering mission.

Academic settings are not immune to hatred and bias. Students bring with them attitudes and beliefs from past family and life experiences. According to a report in the *Chronicle of Higher Education*, nearly one-third of our nation's campuses have reported hate crimes. Another study of four campuses found that victimization rates varied widely throughout the student population, from 12 percent of Jewish students

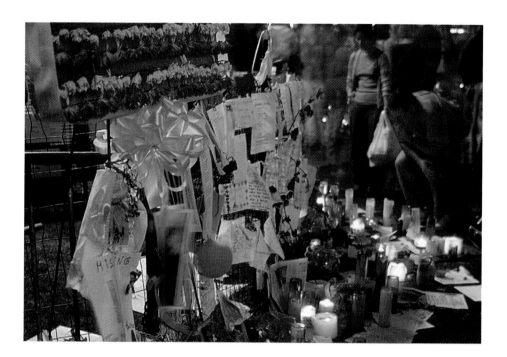

The events of September 11, 2001, were a grim reminder of the power and senselessness of hatred.

victimized to as high as 60 percent of Hispanic students. White students were victimized at rates ranging from 5 to 15 percent.[26] The sad truth is, however, that many minor assaults go unreported, so this may be only part of the picture.

The tendency toward violent acts on campus that are based on prejudice and discrimination might best be defined as campus **ethnoviolence,** a term that reflects relationships among groups in the larger society. Although ethnoviolence often is randomly directed at persons affiliated with a particular group, the group itself is specifically targeted apart from other people, and that differentiation is usually based on ethnicity. Typically, the perpetrators agree that "the group is an acceptable target." For example, in a largely Christian community, Jews and Muslims may be considered acceptable targets.[27]

Prejudice and discrimination are always at the base of ethnoviolence. **Prejudice** is a set of negative attitudes toward a group of people. To say that a person is prejudiced against some group is to say that the person holds a set of beliefs about the group, has an emotional reaction to or way of thinking about the group, and is motivated to behave in a certain way toward the group. **Discrimination** constitutes

---

Ethnoviolence Violence directed randomly at persons affiliated with a particular group.

Prejudice A set of negative attitudes and beliefs or an emotional reaction or way of thinking about a group of people.

Discrimination Actions often based on bias and prejudice that deny equal treatment or opportunities to a group.

---

actions often based on bias and prejudice that deny equal treatment or opportunities to a group of people.

What do you think?

Think about the bias and hate crimes that you have heard about. Who were the victims? ✳ *Did you know any of them?* ✳ *Why do you think people are motivated to initiate such crimes against strangers?* ✳ *What can you do to reduce the risk of such crimes in your area?* ✳ *What should be done nationally?*

Gang Violence The growing influence of street gangs has had a harmful impact on our country. Drug abuse, gang shootings, beatings, thefts, carjackings, and the possibility of being caught in the crossfire have caused entire neighborhoods to be held hostage by gang members. Once thought to occur only in inner-city areas, gang violence now also appears in rural and suburban communities, particularly in the Southeast, Southwest, and in the West.

Why do young people join gangs? Although the reasons are complex, gangs seem to meet many of their needs. Gangs provide a sense of belonging to a family that gives them self-worth, companionship, security, and excitement. In other cases, gangs provide economic security through criminal activity, drug sales, or prostitution. Once young people become involved in the gang subculture, it is difficult for them to leave. Threats of violence or fear of not making it on their own dissuade even those who are most seriously trying to get out.

Who is at risk for gang membership? Membership varies considerably from region to region. The age range of gang members is typically 12 to 22 years. Risk factors include low self-esteem, academic problems, low socioeconomic status, alienation from family and society, a history of family violence, and living in gang-controlled neighborhoods.

Terrorism: Increased Risks from Multiple Sources

Not so long ago, Americans considered acts of terrorism to be isolated events in distant cities that seldom amount to more than a blip on the evening news. The bombing of the Oklahoma City Federal Building in 1995 briefly focused national attention on terrorism. Most of us, however, went about our daily business after the event, acknowledged that it was the act of a madman, and sympathized with the victims.

On September 11, 2001, Americans got a huge wake-up call. Terrorist attacks on the World Trade Center and the Pentagon revealed the vulnerability of our nation to domestic and international threats. The terms *terrorist attack, bioterrorism,* and *biological weapons* catapulted us into the new millennium with an emotional reaction unlike any ever seen. America had lost its innocence and its illusion of invisibility as a terrorist target. An undercurrent of fear and anxiety about potential threats from faceless strangers shook many of us in ways that we never had considered.

What Is Terrorism? According to the FBI, terrorism is the use of unlawful force or violence against persons or property to intimidate or coerce a government, the civilian population, or any segment thereof, in furtherance of political or social objectives. Typically, there are two major types of terrorism. *Domestic terrorism* involves groups or individuals whose terrorist activities are directed at elements of our government or population without foreign direction. *International terrorism* involves groups or individuals whose terrorist activities are foreign-based, transcend national boundaries, and are directed by countries or groups outside the United States.

Clearly, terrorist activities may have immediate impact in terms of loss of lives and resources. However, the September 2001 attacks also had far-reaching effects on the U.S. economy, the airline industry, and transportation systems. Perhaps most damaging in the aftermath of the attacks were the fear, anxiety, and altered behavior of countless Americans. How many people will fear working in skyscrapers for years to come? How many will fear traveling on a plane, crossing a bridge, or getting on the subway? How many will worry excessively about biological weapons? Will worry about future terrorist attacks disrupt our lives and our interactions with others?

As the media spurs our anxieties about germ, chemical, and nuclear warfare, and the multitude of ways that terrorists can breach our defenses, is it any wonder that an already stressed American public is demonstrating increasing concern? What can we do to reduce our risk of terrorist attack?

Be assured that the U.S. Department of Health and Human Services CDC has a wide range of ongoing programs and services designed to help Americans respond to terrorist threats and prepare for possible attacks. Information on programs and services is available on the CDC website and is updated regularly. See the New Horizons in Health box on page 90 for information on bioterrorism. A new government entity, the Department of Homeland Security, has been established to prevent future attacks. The FBI and other government agencies also have prepared a sweeping set of procedures and guidelines for ensuring citizen safety. Here are some things you can do to help reduce anxiety about and actual harm related to terrorist attacks.

- *Be aware of your own reactions to stress, anxiety, and fear.* Try to assess how much of your fear is justifiable and how much is a product of media sensationalism. Practice stress-reduction techniques, try to determine the source of your stressors, and react as prudently as possible.
- *Be conscious of your surroundings.* If you note suspicious activities or irregularities, report them to a person in authority. Being a passive observer and not speaking up when warranted may put you and others at risk.
- *Stay informed.* Try to stay on top of the news and understand the underlying roots of violent activity. Persistent poverty, pervasive religious or political fanaticism, and political situations in which there is an imbalance of power can provide fodder for violent acts. Consider when a self-righteous contempt for others may lead to persecution and violation of human rights. Be skeptical of acts perpetrated in the name of some cause, and intervene if possible to defuse violence.
- *Seek understanding.* Whenever two opposing groups mentally stop engaging with each other or communication breaks down, hate, bigotry, and anger may occur. Knowing about other's customs, cultures, and beliefs, and keeping a line of communication open are good steps to avoiding separation.
- *Seek information.* When political parties fight for power in election years, know your candidates. What are their underlying beliefs regarding national defense, spending for consumer protection, policies on immigration, human rights violations, diversity issues, hate crimes, gun control, etc.? Which candidates are aligned with which ideology? What is their stance on government interference and control, punishment of offenders, and other key issues?
- *Know what to do in an emergency.* Whom would you call? How would you access local and regional assistance? Do you have the necessary provisions for basic survival—food, water, first aid—in case of an attack? What happens when your electricity is off, your phone and communication systems are down, and your access to health care is limited?

Bioterrorism: Pandora's Box

For many, the threat of any kind of viable attack on the United States was incomprehensible until the World Trade Center and Pentagon attacks on September 11, 2001. As shocking as those events were, they may pale in comparison to the unleashing of a Pandora's box of biological killers, which could threaten the entire global population. Before the 2001 terrorist attacks, many people had never heard of diseases such as anthrax, but within a few days Americans watched as endless newscasts discussed the potential horrors of biological warfare.

As chilling as these threats might be, the actual potential for bioterrorism is more far-reaching than any of us might imagine. Included are a wide range of threats from both biological diseases and chemical agents, as indicated below. You can find a complete overview of each of these, plus national initiatives for preventing bioterrorism attacks, on the CDC website, www.bt.cdc.gov.

BIOLOGICAL AGENTS/DISEASES

Category A diseases are pathogens rarely seen in the United States. They pose a risk to national security because they (a) can be easily disseminated or transmitted person-to-person; (b) cause high mortality, with potential for major public health impact; (c) might cause widespread panic and social disruption; and (d) require special action for public health preparedness. The category A threats of greatest concern are highlighted below; you can find information on others on the CDC website.

- *Bacillus anthracis* (**anthrax**). An acute infectious disease caused by a bacterium, anthrax typically occurs in host animals but also can infect humans. Three major forms of anthrax may occur: inhalation, cutaneous (skin), and intestinal anthrax, all with symptoms that usually appear within seven days after infection. Early symptoms of inhalation anthrax resemble a common cold, followed by respiratory symptoms and shock, which is often fatal. The intestinal form appears initially as nausea, vomiting, loss of appetite, and fever, followed by abdominal pain, bloody vomit, and severe diarrhea. It is believed that direct person-to-person spread of anthrax is very rare; thus, immunization and treatment of contacts are not recommended. If exposed, antibiotics are effective treatments in the early stages. Vaccination is also effective.

- *Clostridium botulinum* toxin (**botulism**). Botulism is an acute, muscle-paralyzing disease caused by a toxin that a bacterium produces. There are three major forms of botulism. Food-borne, the most common strain, leads to illness within hours. Infant botulism affects babies who harbor the organism in their intestines. Wound botulism occurs when cuts are infected. Fortunately, botulism is not spread from person to person. Symptoms include double vision, blurred vision, slurred speech, difficulty swallowing; and muscle weakness that descends through the body, eventually paralyzes the ability to breathe, and kills the person.

- *Versinia pestis* (**plague**). An infectious disease of animals and humans that is found in many parts of the world, plague is caused by a bacterium carried by rodents and their fleas. The plague organism infects the lungs. Fever, headache, weakness, and a watery, blood-laden cough are frequent symptoms. Pneumonia follows quickly, and over two to four days may cause septic shock. Without treatment, plague

Domestic Violence

Domestic violence refers to the use of force to control and maintain power over another person in the home environment. It can involve emotional abuse, verbal abuse, threats of physical harm, and actual physical violence ranging from slapping and shoving to beating, rape, and homicide.

Women as Victims   While young men are more apt to become victims of violence from strangers, women are much more likely to become victims of violent acts perpetrated by spouses, lovers, ex-spouses, and ex-lovers. In 2000, more than 6 million women were victims of assault. In fact, 6 of every 10 women in the United States will be assaulted at some time in their lives by someone they know.[28] Every year, approximately 12 percent of married women are the victims of physical aggression perpetrated by their husbands, according to a national survey.[29] This aggression often includes pushing, slapping, and shoving, but can take more severe forms.

Each year about 4 percent of married women are beaten, threatened, or actually injured by knives or guns.[30] Acts of aggression by a husband or boyfriend are a common cause of death for young women; roughly 2,200 women in the United States are killed each year by their partners or ex-partners.[31] Over a recent ten-year period, according to the National Crime Survey, on average more than 2 million assaults on women occurred each year. More than two-thirds of these assaults were committed by someone the woman knew.[32]

Domestic violence   The use of force to control and maintain power over another person in the home environment, including both actual harm and the threat of harm.

can be fatal. Person-to-person contact with transfer of respiratory droplets spreads the disease. A vaccine has not been developed, but several antibiotics are effective if given early.

- Variola major (**smallpox**). Although smallpox was eliminated from the world in 1977, stockpiling of the virus that causes this disease has occurred in many regions of the world. Smallpox spreads from person to person by infected saliva droplets and is most contagious during the first week of illness. Initial symptoms include high fever, fatigue, headaches, and backaches. In two to three days, a characteristic rash develops with flat red lesions that evolve into pustules most prominent on the face, arms, and legs. Lesions crust early in the second week. Scabs develop, separate, and fall off after about three to four weeks. Most people who get smallpox recover, but death occurs in up to 30% of cases. Although most Americans were vaccinated prior to 1972, it is uncertain whether these shots conferred lasting immunity. Although vaccines are effective, the current supply is limited. Treatment for smallpox focuses on relieving symp-toms, but new antiviral agents are being tested.

Category B diseases are of concern but are not transmitted as easily or have as a high of a mortality rate as those in Category A. Examples include *Coxiella burnetii* (Q fever), *Brucella* species (Brucellosis), *Burkholderia Mallei* (Glanders), Ricin toxin from *Ricinus Communis* (castor beans), Epsilon toxin of *Clostridium perfringens,* and Staphylococcal enterotoxin B.

Category C diseases are emerging pathogens that could be engineered for bioterrorism in the future because they have the potential for high morbidity and mortality rates and could be easily produced and disseminated. Examples include Nipah virus, hantavirus, tickborne hemorrhagic fever, tickborne encephalitis viruses, yellow fever, and multidrug-resistant tuberculosis.

CHEMICAL AGENTS

These agents are classified by the body system they damage or by the effect that they produce in victims. See the CDC website for a complete listing.

Blister/Vesicants
Distilled Mustard (HD)
Lewisite
Various forms of nitrogen mustard and Lewisite combinations

Blood
Arsine
Cyanogen chloride
Hydrogen chloride
Hydrogen cyanide

Choking/Lung/Pulmonary damage
Chlorine
Diphosgene
Nitrogen oxide
Zinc oxide

Incapacitating
Agent 15
BZ
Canniboids
Fentanyls
LSD
Phenothiazines

Nervous system
Cyclohexyl sarin
Sarin

Riot control/tearing

Vomiting

Source: Centers for Disease Control and Prevention, Public Health Emergency Preparedness and Response, 2002. www.bt.cdc.gov

---

The following U.S. statistics indicate the seriousness of this long-hidden problem:[33]

- The most vulnerable women are African American and Hispanic, live in large cities far from their families, and are young and unmarried.
- Every 15 seconds, someone batters a woman.
- Only 1 in every 250 such assaults is reported to the police.
- More than one-third of female victims of domestic violence are severely abused on a regular basis.
- About five women are killed every day in domestic violence incidents.
- Three of every four women murdered are killed by their husbands.
- Domestic violence is the single greatest cause of injury to women; it surpasses rape, mugging, and auto accidents combined.

- About 25 to 45 percent of all women who are battered sustain such attacks during pregnancy.
- One-quarter of suicide attempts by women occur as a result of domestic violence.

How many times have you heard of a woman who is beaten repeatedly by her partner and wondered, "Why doesn't she just leave him?" There are many reasons why some women find it difficult to break their ties with their abusers. Many women, particularly those with small children, are financially dependent on their partners. Others fear retaliation against themselves or their children. Some women hope that the situation will change with time (it rarely does); others stay because their cultural or religious beliefs forbid divorce. Finally, some women still love the abusive partner and are concerned about what will happen to him if they leave.[34]

Psychologist Lenore Walker developed a theory known as the "cycle of violence" to explain how women can get

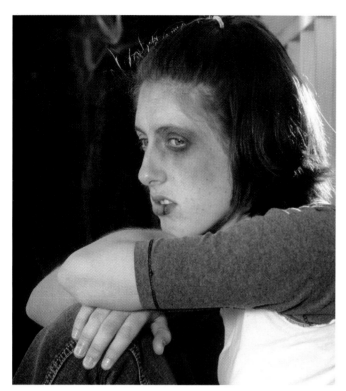

Despite obvious physical and psychological injury, it can be difficult for a person to leave an abusive partner.

caught in a downward spiral without knowing what is happening to them.[35] The cycle has three phases.

1. *Tension building.* In this phase, minor battering occurs, and the woman may become more nurturant, more pleasing, and more intent on anticipating the spouse's needs in order to forestall more violence. She assumes guilt for doing something to provoke him and tries hard to avoid doing it again.
2. *Acute battering.* At this stage, pleasing her man doesn't help, and she can no longer control or predict the abuse. Usually, the spouse is trying to "teach her a lesson," and when he feels he has inflicted enough pain, he'll stop. When the acute attack is over, he may respond with shock and denial about his own behavior. Both batterer and victim may soft-pedal the seriousness of the attacks.
3. *Remorse/reconciliation.* During this "honeymoon" period, the batterer may be kind, loving, and apologetic, swearing he will never act violently again. He may stop his violent behavior for several weeks or months, and the woman may come to question whether she overreacted.

When the tension that precipitated past abuse resurfaces, the man beats the woman again. Unless some form of inter-

Child abuse The systematic harming of a child by a caregiver, typically a parent.

vention breaks this downward cycle of abuse that consists of contrition, further abuse, denial, and contrition, it will repeat itself again and again and perhaps end only with the woman's or, rarely, the man's death.

It is very hard for most women who get caught in this cycle of violence (which may include forced sexual relations and psychological and economic abuse as well as beatings) to summon the resolution to extricate themselves. Most need effective outside intervention.

Men as Victims Are men also victims of domestic violence? Some women do abuse and even kill their partners. Approximately 12 percent of men reported that their wives had engaged in physically aggressive behavior against them in the past year—nearly the same percentage of claims reported from women. The difference between male and female batterers is twofold. First, although the frequency may be similar, the impact is drastically different: women are typically injured in domestic incidents two to three times more often than are men.[36] These injuries tend to be more severe and have resulted in significantly more deaths. Women do engage in moderate aggression, such as pushing and shoving, at rates almost equal to those of men. But severe aggression that is likely to land a victim in the hospital is almost always male against female. Second, a woman who is physically abused by a man is generally intimidated by him: she fears that he will use his power and control over her in some fashion. Men, however, generally report that they do not live in fear of their wives.

Causes of Domestic Violence There is no single explanation for why people tend to be abusive in relationships. Although alcohol abuse often is associated with such violence, marital dissatisfaction is also a predictor.[37] Numerous studies also point to differences in the communication patterns between abusive and nonabusive relationships.[38] While some argue that the hormone testosterone causes male aggression, studies have failed to show a strong association between this hormone and physical abuse in relationships.[39] Many experts believe that men who engage in severe violence are more likely than other men to suffer from personality disorders.[40]

Regardless of the cause, the dynamics that *both* people bring to a relationship result in violence and allow it to continue. Community support and counseling services can help determine underlying problems and allow the victim and the batterer to break the cycle. The Assess Yourself box may help you determine if you are a victim of abuse.

Child Abuse Children raised in families in which domestic violence and/or sexual abuse occur are at great risk for damage to personal health and well-being. The effects of such violent acts are powerful and long-lasting. **Child abuse** refers to the systematic harm of a child by a caregiver, generally a parent.[41] The abuse may be sexual, psychological, physical, or any combination of these. Although exact figures are lacking, many experts believe that more than 2 million cases of

Relationship Violence: Are You at Risk?

Although we all want to have healthy relationships, many of us get caught in patterns of behavior that are a direct result of things we've learned or haven't learned in our past. Sometimes we don't even recognize that we are acting inappropriately; other times we know we should act in a particular way, but we get caught up in our own emotions and act out in ways that are physically or emotionally abusive to others. If you have been a victim of emotional or physical violence, you may have become so used to certain behaviors that you might not recognize them as inappropriate. To prevent violence, we have to be able to recognize it, deal with it in appropriate ways, and/or take action to avoid it. One place to start is to examine our intimate interpersonal relationships. Answer the following questions about your current or past relationships.

HOW OFTEN DOES YOUR PARTNER

1. Criticize you for your appearance (weight, dress, hair, etc.)?	Never	Sometimes	Often
2. Embarrass you in front of others by putting you down?	Never	Sometimes	Often
3. Blame you or others for his or her mistakes?	Never	Sometimes	Often
4. Curse at you, say mean things, or mock you?	Never	Sometimes	Often
5. Demonstrate uncontrollable anger?	Never	Sometimes	Often
6. Criticize your friends, family, or others who are close to you?	Never	Sometimes	Often
7. Threaten to leave you if you don't behave in a certain way?	Never	Sometimes	Often
8. Manipulate you to prevent you from spending time with friends or family?	Never	Sometimes	Often
9. Express jealousy, distrust, and anger when you spend time with other people?	Never	Sometimes	Often
10. Tell you that you are crazy, irrational, or paranoid?	Never	Sometimes	Often
11. Call you names to make you lose confidence in yourself?	Never	Sometimes	Often
12. Make all the significant decisions in your relationship?	Never	Sometimes	Often
13. Intimidate or threaten you, making you fearful or anxious?	Never	Sometimes	Often
14. Make threats to harm others you care about?	Never	Sometimes	Often
15. Prevent you from going out by taking your car keys?	Never	Sometimes	Often
16. Control your telephone calls, listen in on your messages, or read your email?	Never	Sometimes	Often
17. Punch, hit, slap, or kick you?	Never	Sometimes	Often
18. Gossip about you to turn others against you or make them think bad things about you?	Never	Sometimes	Often
19. Make you feel guilty about something?	Never	Sometimes	Often
20. Use money or possessions to control you?	Never	Sometimes	Often
21. Force you to have sex or perform sexual acts that make you uncomfortable?	Never	Sometimes	Often
22. Threaten to kill himself or herself if you leave?	Never	Sometimes	Often
23. Control your money and make you ask for what you need?	Never	Sometimes	Often
24. Set many rules that you must abide by?	Never	Sometimes	Often
25. Follow you, call to check on you, or demonstrate a constant obsession with what you are doing?	Never	Sometimes	Often

Now look at your responses to the above questions. If you answered "sometimes" to one or more of these questions, you may be at risk for emotional or physical abuse. If you answered "often" to any question, you may need to talk with someone about immediate threats to your emotional or physical health. Typically, such potentially abusive patterns only get worse over time as a person gains control and power in a relationship. If you are nervous or anxious about talking to your partner, seek counseling through your campus counseling center, student health center, or community services. If you don't know where to go, ask your professor for possible options.

After you have completed the test about your partner's behavior, you should ask the same questions about your own behavior. If any of the questions describe your actions in a relationship, you should seek help to change these behavioral patterns. These actions are not conducive to healthy relationships and may result in harm to you or your loved ones. Seek help now to insure healthier relationships in the future.

child abuse occur every year in the United States involving severe injury, permanent disability, or death. The psychological effects may be equally damaging: being abused or neglected as a child increases the likelihood of arrest as a juvenile by 53 percent and of arrest for a violent crime as an adult by 38 percent.[42]

Child abusers exist in both genders and in all social, ethnic, religious, and racial groups, but they tend to share certain characteristics: a history of abuse as a child, a poor self-image, feelings of isolation, extreme frustration with life, higher stress or anxiety levels than normal, a tendency to abuse drugs and/or alcohol, and unrealistic expectations of the child. It is estimated that one-half to three-quarters of men who batter their female partners also batter children. In fact, spouse abuse is the single most identifiable risk factor for predicting child abuse. Children with handicaps or other differences from the norm are more likely to be abused.

Child Sexual Abuse   Sexual abuse of children by adults or older children includes sexually suggestive conversations; inappropriate kissing; touching; petting; oral, anal, or vaginal intercourse; and other kinds of sexual interaction. The most frequent abusers are a child's parents or their companions or spouses. The next most frequent abusers are grandfathers and siblings. Girls are more commonly abused than boys, although young boys are also frequent victims, usually of male family members. Between 20 and 30 percent of all adult women report an unwanted childhood sexual encounter with an adult male, usually a father, uncle, brother, or grandfather. It is a myth that male deviance or mental illness accounts for most of these incidents: "Stories of retrospective incest patients typically involved perpetrators who are 'Everyman'— attorneys, mental health practitioners, businessmen, farmers, teachers, doctors, and clergy."[43]

Most sexual abuse occurs in the child's home. The risk is higher in the following situations:[44]

1. The child lives without one of his or her biological parents.
2. The mother is unavailable because she is disabled, ill, or working outside the home.
3. The parents' marriage is unhappy.
4. The child has a poor relationship with his or her parents or is subjected to extremely punitive discipline.
5. The child lives with a stepfather.

Sexual abuse of children   Sexual interaction between a child and an adult or older child. Includes, but is not limited to, sexually suggestive conversations; inappropriate kissing; touching; petting; and oral, anal, or vaginal intercourse.

Sexual assault   Any act in which one person is sexually intimate with another person without that other person's consent.

Consider only two points about the impact of child abuse in later life. Ninety-nine percent of the inmates in the maximum security prison at San Quentin were either abused or raised in abusive households. Three hundred thousand children between the ages of 8 and 15 are living on the nation's streets, willing to prostitute themselves to survive rather than return to their abusive households.[45]

Although most people who were abused as children do not end up as convicts or prostitutes, many do bear spiritual, psychological, and/or physical scars. Clinical psychologist Marjorie Whittaker has found that "of all forms of violence, incest and childhood sexual abuse are considered among the most 'toxic' because of their violations of trust, the confusion of affection and coercion, the splitting of family alignments, and serious psychological and physical consequences."[46]

Not all child violence is physical. Health can be affected severely by psychological violence—that is, assaults on personality, character, competence, independence, or general dignity as a human being. The negative consequences of this kind of victimization can be harder to discern and therefore harder to combat. They include depression, low self-esteem, and a pervasive fear of doing something that will offend the abuser.

> **What do you think?**
> *What factors in society lead to child abuse and neglect?* * *What are common characteristics of children's abusers?* * *Why are family members often the perpetrators of child abuse and child sexual abuse?* * *What actions can be taken to prevent such behaviors?*

Sexual Victimization

As with all forms of violence, men and women alike are susceptible to sexual victimization. However, sexual violence against women is of epidemic proportions, so we will focus on women. Sexual battering is the single greatest cause of injury to women in the United States; it occurs more frequently than car accidents, muggings, and rapes combined.[47] Physical battering and emotional abuse often leave psychological as well as physical scars. One-quarter to one-third of high school and college students report involvement in dating violence, either as perpetrators, victims, or both.[48]

Sexual Assault and Rape   Sexual assault is any act in which one person is sexually intimate with another person without that other person's consent. This may range from simple touching to forceful penetration. It may include such acts as ignoring indications that intimacy is not wanted, threatening force or other negative consequences, and actually using force.

Rape, the most extreme form of sexual assault, is defined as "penetration without the victim's consent."[49] Whether committed by an acquaintance, a date, or a stranger, rape is a criminal activity that usually has serious emotional, psychological, social, and physical consequences for the victim. Typically, victims are young females; 29 percent are under 11 years of age, 32 percent are between the ages of 11 and 17, and 22 percent are between the ages of 18 and 24.[50]

Rape is thought to be the most underreported of all violent crimes in the United States. However, while as many as two-thirds of all rapes are never reported, there were more than 261,000 reported cases of rape, attempted rape, or sexual assault in 2001.[51]

Incidents of rape generally fall into one of two types: aggravated or simple. An **aggravated rape** involves multiple attackers, strangers, weapons, or physical beatings. A **simple rape** is perpetrated by one person, whom the victim often knows, and does not involve a physical beating or use of a weapon. Most incidents are classified as simple rapes. One report suggests that 82 percent of female rape victims have been victimized by acquaintances (53 percent), current or former boyfriends (16 percent), current or former spouses (10 percent), or other relatives (3 percent). Almost half of all rape charges are dismissed before the cases reach trial. Combined with a perception that men may lack understanding of how rape affects women, it's easy to understand why experts feel that so-called simple rape is seriously underreported and ignored.

Acquaintance or Date Rape

Although the terms *date rape, friendship rape,* and *acquaintance rape* have become standard terminology, they typically are misused. Not all rapes occur on dates, not all the relationships are friendships, and sometimes the term *acquaintance* is used all too loosely. Many acquaintance rapes occur as the result of incidental contact at a party or when people congregate at one person's house. These are crimes of opportunity, not necessarily the result of a prearranged date. This is an important distinction because the term *date* suggests some type of reciprocal interaction arranged in advance. While most date or acquaintance rapes happen to women aged 15 to 21 years, the 18-year-old new college student is the most likely victim.[52]

In a study of 6,000 college students from 32 different universities, researchers uncovered the following data:[53]

- More than 50 percent of the college women surveyed had endured some form of sexual abuse.
- More than 25 percent had been the victims of rape or attempted rape.
- Eighty-four percent of the assault victims knew their assailants.
- Fifty-seven percent of the assaults occurred on dates.
- Forty-one percent of the women raped were virgins at the time of the assault.

- Seventy-three percent of the assailants and 55 percent of the victims had used alcohol or drugs prior to the assault.
- Forty-two percent of the victims indicated that they had sex with the offender again (it is unknown whether the subsequent sex was voluntary).
- Twenty-five percent of the men admitted to some degree of aggressive sexual behavior.
- Men were most likely to commit sexual assaults during their senior year in high school or first year in college.

Marital Rape

Marital rape is any unwanted intercourse or penetration (vaginal, anal, or oral) obtained by force, threat of force, or when the wife is unable to consent.[54] Some researchers estimate that marital rape may account for 25 percent of all rapes; rape in marriage may be an extremely prevalent form of sexual violence. Although this problem has undoubtedly been common since the earliest origins of marriage as a social institution, it is noteworthy that marital rape did not become a crime in all 50 states until 1993. Even more noteworthy is the fact that in 33 states, there are still exemptions from rape prosecution, which means that the judicial system may treat it as a lesser crime.

Who is most vulnerable to marital rape? In general, women under the age of 25 and those who are from lower socioeconomic groups are at highest risk. Women from homes where other forms of domestic violence are common and where there is a high rate of alcoholism and/or substance abuse also tend to be victimized at greater rates than others. Women who are subjected to marital rape often report multiple offenses over a period of time; these events are likely to be forced anal and oral experiences.[55]

Again, abuse of power and a need to control and dominate seem to be key factors in the husband–rapist profile. Marital rape can have devastating short- and long-term consequences for women, including injuries to the vaginal and anal areas, lacerations, soreness, bruising, torn muscles, fatigue, panic attacks, sexually transmitted infections, broken bones, wounds, and other emotional and physical scars.

Sexual Harassment

If we think of violence as including verbal abuse and the threat of coercion, then sexual harassment is a form of violence. Under Title VII of the Civil Rights Act, **sexual harassment** is defined as "unwelcomed sexual advances, requests for sexual favors, and other verbal or

---

Rape   Sexual penetration without the victim's consent.

Aggravated rape   Rape that involves multiple attackers, strangers, weapons, or a physical beating.

Simple rape   Rape by one person usually known to the victim that does not involve a physical beating or use of a weapon.

Sexual harassment   Any form of unwanted sexual attention.

Violence: A Global Health Problem

A 2002 report from the World Health Organization (WHO) revealed that violence kills more than 1.6 million people every year. Such statistics on violence are just the tip of the iceberg, with the majority of violent acts being committed behind closed doors and going largely unreported. In addition to the deaths, millions of people are left injured as a result of violence and suffer from physical, sexual, reproductive, and mental health problems.

The death and disability caused by violence make it one of the leading public health issues of our time, says the report. Violence is among the leading causes of death for people aged 15 to 44 years of age, accounting for 14% of deaths among males and 7% of deaths among females. On an average day, 1,424 people are killed in acts of homicide (almost one person every minute), one person commits suicide roughly every 40 seconds, and about 35 people are killed every hour as a direct result of armed conflict. In the twentieth century, an estimated 191 million people lost their lives directly or indirectly as a result of conflict (well over half of them civilians). Studies have shown that in some countries, health care expenditures due to violence account for up to 5% of the Gross Domestic Product.

The data on youth violence show that youth homicide rates have increased in many parts of the world. For every young person killed by violence, an estimated 20 to 40 receive injuries that require treatment. Fighting and bullying are common among young people and drunkenness is one of the situational factors found to precipitate violence. Data from selected countries also suggests that about 20% of women and 5 to 10% of men suffered sexual abuse as children.

Women often face the greatest risk at home and in familiar settings, says the report. Almost half the women who die due to homicide are killed by their current or former husbands or boyfriends; in some countries the rate is as high as 70%. While exact numbers are hard to come by due to lack of reporting, available data suggest that nearly one in four women will experience sexual violence by an intimate partner in their lifetime. Most female victims of physical aggression are subjected to multiple acts of violence over extended periods of time. One-third to more than one-half of these cases are accompanied by sexual violence. In some countries, up to one-third of adolescent girls report forced sexual initiation.

Abuse of the elderly is one of the most hidden faces of violence, according to the report, and one that is likely to grow given the rapidly aging populations in many countries. Up to 6% of the elderly report having been abused. As for suicide or self-inflicted violence, it is recognized as one of the leading causes of death in the world. Among those ages 15 to 44 years, suicide is the fourth leading cause of death and the sixth leading cause of disability and ill-health.

Although the statistics are chilling, the situation is far from hopeless. Dr Etienne Krug, Director, WHO Department of Injuries and Violence Prevention, points to evidence which suggests that violence can be prevented by a variety of measures aimed at individuals, families, and communities. The report calls for a public health understanding of the complex social, psychological, economic, and community underpinnings of violence. While biological and other individual factors may explain some of the predisposition to aggression, these factors more often interact with family, community, cultural, and other external factors to create a situation where violence is likely to occur. Understanding these situations and these causes creates opportunities to intervene before violent acts occur and provides policy-makers with a variety of concrete options to prevent violence. Among the recommendations are preschool and social development programs for children and adolescents, parent training and support programs, and measures to reduce firearm injuries and improve firearm safety. Other recommendations include strengthening responses for victims of violence, promoting adherence to international treaties and laws, and improving data collection on violence.

Source: World Health Organization, "First Ever Global Report on Violence and Health Released," October 2002. www.who.int/mediacentre/releases/pr73/en/print.html

---

physical contact of a sexual nature." Despite what might appear to be a clear definition, sexual harassment is often difficult to identify. Although many people would say that sexual harassment is anything the offended person *believes* is harassment, others will say that this definition is too nebulous.

The issue of sexual harassment was brought to our collective consciousness in the early 1990s when Anita Hill charged Supreme Court justice nominee Clarence Thomas with sexual harassment in a previous employment environment. The alleged harassment was partly in the form of sexually offensive humor, not all directed at Hill. What had long been dismissed as harmless behavior became a cause for concern in business, academia, and government. More recently, the Paula Jones and Monica Lewinsky scandals have kept sexual harassment issues in the news and have focused attention on additional aspects, such as improper touching, improper suggestions, and inappropriate uses of power.

Most colleges and universities now offer courses on identifying and preventing sexual harassment, and most companies have established sexual harassment policies and procedures for dealing with it.

If you feel you are being harassed, the most important thing you can do is to be assertive. The following are steps to help you deal with harrassment.

- *Tell the harasser to stop.* Be clear and direct about what is bothering you and why you are upset.
- *Document the harassment.* Make a record of the incident. If the harassment becomes intolerable, a record of exactly what occurred (and when and where) will help make your case.
- *Complain to a higher authority.* Talk to your manager about what happened. If the manager or supervisor doesn't take you seriously, investigate the internal grievance procedures for your organization.
- *Remember that you have not done anything wrong.* You will likely feel awful after being harassed (especially if you have to complain to superiors). However, feel proud that you are not keeping silent.

What do you think?
Why do you think women are often reluctant to report sexual harassment? ✳ *Why do you think so many men report that they were unaware of their own sexually harassing behaviors?* ✳ *What can be done to increase awareness in this area?*

Social Contributors to Sexual Assault According to many experts, certain common assumptions in our society prevent both the perpetrator and the public from recognizing the true nature of sexual assault.[56] These assumptions include the following.[57]

- *Minimization.* It is often assumed that sexual assault of women is rare because official crime statistics, including the Uniform Crime Reports of the FBI, show very few rapes per thousand population. However, rape is the most underreported of all serious crimes. Researchers have found that nearly 25 percent of women in the United States have been raped.
- *Trivialization.* Incredibly enough, sexual assault is still often viewed as a jocular matter. During a gubernatorial election in Texas a few years back, one of the candidates reportedly compared a bad patch of weather to rape: "If there's nothing you can do about it, just lie back and enjoy it." (He lost the election—to a woman.)
- *Blaming the victim.* Many discussions of sexual violence against women display a sometimes unconscious assumption that the woman did something to provoke the attack—that she dressed revealingly or flirted outrageously, for example.
- *"Boys will be boys."* According to this assumption, men just can't control themselves once they become aroused.

Over the years, psychologists and others have proposed several theories to explain why many males sexually victimize women. In one of the first major studies to explore this issue, almost two-thirds of the male respondents had engaged in intercourse unwanted by the woman, primarily because of male peer pressure.[58] By all indicators, these trends continue today. Peer pressure is certainly a strong factor, but a growing body of research suggests that sexual assault is encouraged by the socialization processes that males experience daily.[59]

- *Male socialization.* Throughout our lives, we are exposed to social norms that objectify women—make them appear as objects that can be used. Media portrayals of half-dressed and undressed women in seductive poses promoting products, for instance, contribute to sex-role stereotyping. These portrayals often show males as aggressors and females as targets. In addition, men are exposed from an early age to anti-female jokes and vulgar and obscene terms for women. These reinforce the idea that females are lesser beings who may be pushed around with impunity.[60] Males also are discouraged from acting in ways that society views as feminine. They are told to act tough and unemotional; to strive for power, status, and control; and to be aggressive and take risks.
- *Male attitudes.* Several studies have confirmed a greater tolerance of rape among men who accept the myth that rape is something women secretly desire, who believe in adversarial relationships between men and women, who condone violence against women, or who hold traditional attitudes toward sex roles. Such men are more apt to blame the victim and more likely to commit rape themselves if they think they can get away with it.[61]
- *Male sexual history and hostility.* Most rapists do not look abnormal or appear to be psychologically disturbed. They typically are employed, often married and have families, and have a history of multiple sexual experiences (both forced and voluntary) during childhood. Many feel hostility toward women.[62]
- *Male misperceptions.* Men who are convinced that women really want sex even if they say they don't are more likely to perpetrate sexual assaults. They more readily misinterpret a woman's words and behavior and act on their misperceptions—only to be surprised later when the woman claims that she has been assaulted.[63]
- *Situational factors.* Several factors increase the likelihood of sexual assault. Dates in which the male makes all the decisions, pays, drives, and in general controls what happens are more likely to end in aggression. Alcohol and drug use increase the risk and severity of assault. Length of relationship is another important situational factor: the more long-standing the relationship, the greater the chance of aggression. Finally, males who belong to a close-knit social group involving intense interaction are more prone to engage in a peer-pleasing assault.

What do you think?
What factors make men likely to commit sexual assault or rape? ✳ *What measures might be effective in preventing such behaviors?*

Crime on Campus: A Safe Haven?

Though the majority of crimes on campus still consist of nonviolent crimes—larceny, vandalism, and setting off fire alarms illegally—the rate of violent crime is increasing. Traditionally, most campus crimes were handled internally. This procedure has changed as more states have passed legislation requiring colleges and universities to warn their students about crime and danger both on campus and in off-campus housing that they recommend.[64] In 1992, Congress passed the Campus Sexual Assault Victim's Bill of Rights known as the Ramstad Act. The act gives victims the right to call in off-campus authorities to investigate serious campus crimes. In addition, universities must set up educational programs and notify students of available counseling.

Sexual Assault on Campus   Most studies of sexual assault among college students indicate that 25 percent to 60 percent of college men have engaged in some form of sexually coercive behavior.[65] This is consistent with the 27 percent of college women who have reported experiencing rape or attempted rape since they were 14 years old, and the 54 percent who claim to have been sexually victimized (forced to endure unwanted petting, kisses, and other advances).[66] In one survey, only 39 percent of the men sampled denied coercive involvement, 28 percent admitted to having used a coercive method at least once, and 15 percent admitted that they had forced a woman to have intercourse at least once.[67] According to a large, nationally representative sample of college and university students, 25 percent of the male respondents had been involved in some form of sexual assault since age 14.[68] Since this early national study, many smaller studies have reported similar statistics.

As it is among the general public, the incidence of sexual assault on campuses is believed to be seriously underreported. In a recent report, one major university familiar to the author claimed there were no rapes on campus. But based on national averages, it seems highly unlikely that no forcible sexual encounters would occur in a setting where nearly 16,000 students date, drink, and socialize every week. The fact is that coercive sex or date rape is seldom reported to campus police. When a rape victim seeks help at the campus health center, the center is not compelled to report the crime. In one study, 20 percent of female respondents at a Midwestern university said they had been raped by someone they knew, but only 8 percent had reported it to the police. At another Midwestern university, 20 percent of 247 women interviewed said they had experienced date rape, but few had reported it.[69] Other sexual violations, such as obscene phone calls, stalking, sexual molestation that does not result in penetration, exhibitionism, voyeurism, and attempted rape, go equally unreported.[70]

Sexual Harassment on Campus   According to a national study by the American Association of University Women, four out of five students attending public schools have been sexually harassed by other students. More than one-third of these incidents are reported to occur before the seventh grade. Another study indicates that 90 percent of undergraduate women and 52 percent of graduate women report at least one negative experience from male students. According to the study, the students most likely to harass these women are members of fraternities, athletic teams, and all-male groups and cliques; men who are defiant or angry at women; and those who have been abused themselves.[71]

While peers pose a threat of harassment, a study by the Institute of Social and Economic Research at Cornell University found that 61 percent of upperclass and graduate students experienced "unwanted sexual attention from someone of authority within the University."[72] Typically, this attention comes from male professors and may include affairs with married and unmarried female students; demands for sex, with threats of lower grades for noncompliance; and sexually offensive and hostile environments in the classroom.[73] Many universities have strict codes of conduct relating to faculty–student consensual as well as nonconsensual relationships. Many of these policies stem from reported difficulties with power and control between faculty and students and the potential for negative consequences.

What do you think?
What policies does your school have regarding consensual relationships between faculty members and students? ✳ Should consenting adults have the right to interact, regardless of their positions within a system or workplace? ✳ What are the potential dangers of such interactions?

Reducing Your Risk

After a violent act is committed against someone we know, we acknowledge the horror of the event, express sympathy, and go on with our lives. But the person who has been brutalized may take months or years to recover. It is far better to prevent a violent act than to recover from it.

Self-Defense against Rape

Rape can occur no matter what preventive actions you take, but commonsense self-defense tactics can lower the risk. Self-defense is a process that includes learning increased awareness, self-defense techniques, reasonable precautions, and the self-confidence and judgment needed to determine appropriate responses to different situations.[74] Figure 4.4 identifies practical tips for preventing personal assaults.

Taking Control   Most rapes by unknown assailants are planned in advance. They are frequently preceded by a casual, friendly conversation. Although many women have said that they started to feel uneasy during such a conversation, they denied the possibility of an attack until it was too late.

Listen to your feelings, and trust your intuition. Be assertive and direct to someone who is getting out of line or threatening—this may convince the would-be rapist to back off. Stifle your tendency to be nice, and don't fear making a scene. Let him know that you mean what you say and are prepared to defend yourself. Consider the following.

- *Speak in a strong voice.* Use statements such as "Leave me alone" rather than questions such as "Will you please leave me alone?" Avoid apologies and excuses. Sound as if you mean what you say.
- *Maintain eye contact with the would-be attacker.* This keeps you aware of the person's movements and conveys an aura of strength and confidence.
- *Stand up straight, act confident, and remain alert.* Walk as if you own the sidewalk.

Many rapists use certain ploys to initiate their attacks. Among the most common are the following:

- *Request for help.* This allows him to get close—to enter your house to use the phone, for instance.
- *Offer of help.* This also can help him gain entrance to your home: "Let me help you carry that package."
- *Guilt trip.* "Gee, no one is friendly nowadays. . . . I can't believe you won't talk with me for just a little while."
- *Purposeful accident.* He may bump into the back of your car and then assault you when you get out to see the damage. Don't stop unless you have to in these situations; if you do stop, stay in your car with the doors locked.
- *Authority.* Many women fall for the old "policeman at the door" ruse. If anyone comes to your door dressed in uniform, ask him to show his ID before you unlock the door. You also can call the police department to confirm his ID.

If you are attacked, act immediately. Don't worry about causing a scene. Draw attention to yourself and your assailant. Scream "fire!" loudly. Research has shown that passersby are much more likely to help if they hear the word *fire* rather than just a scream. Your attacker also may be caught off-balance by the action.

To prevent an attack, remember the following points.

- *Always be vigilant.* Even the safest communities have rapes. Don't be fooled by a sleepy-little-town atmosphere.
- *Use campus escort services whenever possible.*
- *Be assertive in demanding a well-lit campus.*
- *Don't use the same route all the time.* Vary your movement patterns.
- *Don't leave a bar alone with a friendly stranger.* Stay with your friends, and let the stranger come along. Don't give your address to anyone you don't know.
- *Let friends and family know where you are going, what route you'll take, and when to expect your return.*
- *Stay close to others.* Avoid shortcuts through dark or unlit paths. Don't be the last one to leave the lab or library late at night.
- *Keep your windows and doors locked.* Don't open the door to strangers.

In Your Car

- Always keep your doors and windows locked.
- Purchase cars with an alarm system and remote entry.
- Don't stop for vehicles in distress; call for help.
- If your car breaks down, lock the doors and wait for help from the police.
- If you think someone is following you, do not drive to your home; drive to a busy place and attract attention.
- Stick to well-traveled routes.
- Keep your car in good running order and always filled with gas.
- On long trips, don't make it obvious you're traveling alone.
- Do not sleep in your car along interstate highways.
- Carry a cell phone with programmed emergency numbers.

On the Street

- Walk or jog at a steady pace.
- Walk or jog with others.
- At night, avoid dark parking lots, wooded areas, and any place that offers an assailant good cover.
- Listen for footsteps and voices.
- Be aware of cars that keep driving around in your area.
- Vary your running or walking routes.
- Carry pepper spray or other deterrents, or walk or jog with a dog . . . the bigger, the better!
- Carry a cell phone or change to make a phone call.
- Tell others where you are going, your route, and when you'll return.

Figure 4.4
Preventing Personal Assaults

What to Do if a Rape Occurs

If you are a rape victim, report the attack. This gives you a sense of control. Follow these steps.

- Call 911 (if a phone is available).
- Do not bathe, shower, douche, clean up, or touch anything the attacker may have touched.
- Do not throw away or launder the clothes you were wearing. They will be needed as evidence.
- Bring a clean change of clothes to the clinic or hospital.
- Contact the rape assistance hotline in your area, and ask for advice on therapists or counseling if you need additional help.

If a friend is raped, here's how you can help.

- Believe her, and don't ask questions that may appear to implicate her in the assault.
- Recognize that rape is a violent act and the victim was not looking for this to happen.
- Encourage her to see a doctor immediately, because she may have medical needs but feel too embarrassed to seek help on her own. Offer to go with her.
- Encourage her to report the crime.
- Be understanding, and let her know you will be there for her.
- Recognize that this is an emotional recovery, and it may take six months to a year for her to bounce back.
- Encourage her to seek counseling.

A Campus-wide Response to Violence

Increasingly, campuses have become microcosms of the greater society, complete with the risks, hazards, and dangers people face in the world. Many college administrators have been proactive in establishing violence prevention policies, programs, and services.[75]

Changing Roles   To increase student protection, campus law enforcement has changed over the years in both numbers and authority to prosecute student offenders. Campus police are responsible for emergency responses to situations that threaten safety, human resources, the general campus environment, traffic and bicycle safety, and other dangers. They have the power to enforce laws with students in the same way they are handled in the general community. In fact, many campuses now hire state troopers or local law enforcement officers to deal with campus issues rather than maintain a separate police staff.

Many of these law enforcement groups follow a *community policing model* in which officers have specific responsibilities for certain areas of campus, departments, or events. By narrowing the scope of each officer's territory, officers get to know people in the area and are better able to anticipate and prevent risks. This differs from earlier safety policies in which campus security typically swooped down only in times of trouble.

Prevention Efforts   Many universities now hire crime prevention and safety specialists. They commonly recommend the following activities:

- A rape awareness and education program for members of the campus community
- A crime prevention orientation program for new faculty and staff as well as students
- Specialized safety workshops for particular groups, such as commuters, international students, athletes, and students with disabilities
- Printed and electronic educational messages about personal safety
- A notification process to distribute information about special hazards

- Alcohol and drug programs dealing with policy, awareness, education, and enforcement
- A grounds safety program, including measures such as providing good lighting and removing shrubs from dark areas
- Emergency call boxes or telephones across campus
- Escort services for students who must be out after dark
- Motorist assistance programs for persons with car trouble
- Antitheft programs, including regular patrols of parking lots and other areas
- Victim advocacy programs, such as rape or abuse counseling

The Role of Student Affairs   Although there may be some overlap with law enforcement activities, student affairs offices need to play a vital role in all on-campus programs, both to prevent trouble and to resolve problems that do occur. Student groups should monitor progress, identify potential threats, and advocate for improvements in any areas found to be deficient. A student affairs office can play a key role in making sure that mental health services, student assistance programs, and other services are high quality, easily accessible, and meet student needs. A human services or student affairs office should seek to involve the wider student body and ensure that all are acutely aware of its services. If these programs are not visible or proactive in ensuring campus safety, their roles and responsibilities should be carefully assessed. Student leaders can play a major role in shaping such services and advocating for the campus population.

Community Strategies for Preventing Violence

Because the causes of homicide and assaultive violence are complex, community strategies for prevention must be multidimensional. Successful strategies include the following.[76]

- Developing and implementing educational programs to teach communication, conflict resolution, and coping skills
- Working with individuals to help them develop self-esteem and respect for others
- Rewarding youngsters for good behavior and never spanking them when angry. (Children need to know that anger is sometimes acceptable, but violence never is. Use family meetings to resolve conflicts.)
- Establishing and enforcing policies that forbid discrimination on the basis of gender, religious affiliation, race, sexual orientation, marital status, and age
- Increasing and enriching educational programs for family planning
- Increasing efforts by health care and social service programs to identify victims of violence
- Improving treatment and support for victims
- Treating the psychological as well as the physical consequences of violence

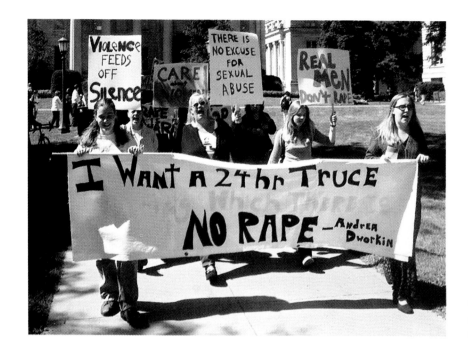

College students can organize vigils, marches, and educational programs to raise awareness about violence against women.

Unintentional Injuries

As stated previously, unintentional injuries occur without planning or intending to harm. Examples of unintentional injuries include car accidents, falls, water accidents, accidental gunshots, recreational accidents, and workplace accidents. None of them happen on purpose, yet they may result in pain, suffering, and possibly even death. Most efforts to prevent unintentional injuries focus on changing something about the *person,* the *environment,* or the *circumstances* (policies, procedures) that put people in harm's way.

Residential Safety

Injuries within the home typically occur in the form of falls, burns, or intrusions by others. Some populations, such as the elderly, are particularly vulnerable. However, older adults are not the only victims; each year, hundreds of children suffer severe burns or die from accidental fires, falls, and other home-based injuries. To reduce the risk of accidents, consider the following.

Fall-Proof Your Home

- Eliminate clutter, particularly objects you may stumble over in the dark. Leave nothing lying around on the floor.
- Fasten all rugs securely to the floor so they don't slide. Inexpensive rubberized mats or strips will hold rugs in place.
- Train your pets to stay away from your feet. Many an unsuspecting person has ended up on the floor while trying to avoid a pet.

- Make sure handrails are secure and within easy reach. All stairs should have slip-proof treads.
- Install slip-proof mats or decals in showers and tubs. Add handrails for stability in tubs and showers.

Avoid Burns

- Extinguish all cigarettes in ashtrays before bed. Don't smoke and drink before bed. Don't smoke in bed at any time! Sparks can smolder in mattresses or upholstered furniture, then flare into flames. Don't throw spent matches in the trash with paper and other combustibles. Soak matches in water before discarding.
- Set all lamps away from drapes, linens, and paper.
- Keep hotpads and kitchen cloths away from stove burners. When not using a cloth, set it on a counter far from the stove.
- Keep candles under control and away from combustibles. Although it may seem romantic to sleep by candlelight, it is highly risky. Don't do it.
- Purchase ovens with controls in front so you can avoid reaching over hot pans to change burner temperatures.
- Use caution when lighting barbecue grills and other home-based fires. Never spray combustible fluids directly onto the fire.
- Check chimneys and fireplaces regularly for buildup of flammable soot.
- Service furnaces annually, and be sure to change the filters.
- Avoid overloading electrical circuits with appliances and cords. Older buildings are at particular risk for fire from such overloads.
- Program phones with emergency numbers for speed dialing, and keep these numbers in clear sight near phones as well.

- Replace batteries in fire alarms periodically, and test them regularly to make sure the batteries are working.
- Have the proper fire extinguishers ready in case of fire.

Prevent Intruders

- Close blinds and drapes whenever you are away and in the evening when you are home. Remove large bushes and obstructions from around your windows and doors so that anyone lurking outside will be visible.
- Install dead-bolt locks on all doors and locks on windows. Put a peephole in the main entryway to your home, and do not let anyone in without checking to see who it is.
- If you have a screen door, lock it. If an unfamiliar visitor comes to the door, the screen door serves as a barrier.
- If possible, install a low-cost home alarm system.
- Rent apartments that require a security code or clearance to gain entry.
- Avoid easily accessible apartments such as first-floor units with large patio doors.
- Don't give information about your home or schedule to telephone solicitors. Try to vary the times of day that you come home for lunch or run errands.
- Don't let repair people in without asking for their identification. Preferably, landlords should inform you about such visits well in advance. Have someone else with you when repairs are being made in your home or apartment. Just because a person is licensed to fix refrigerators does not mean he or she can be trusted.
- Avoid dark parking structures, laundry rooms, etc. Try to use these areas only when others are around.
- Use initials for first names on mailboxes and in phone listings. Keep your address out of phone books.
- Keep a cell phone near your bed and program it to dial 911. Unlike the scenarios you see on TV, many intruders do not cut phone lines. More commonly, they simply pick up the receiver in another room as they walk through, thereby disabling a bedroom phone.
- Get to know your neighbors. Organize a neighborhood watch.
- Be careful of "doggy doors." Some thieves let their smallest associate crawl through them and unlock a door to the house.
- Be careful of skylights and other areas that open up from the outside. Keep them locked and bolted.
- When you are away, put the lights in different rooms on timers set to come on and go off at different times. Stop your mail and newspaper.

Although no amount of security will prevent all threats of intrusion, following these precautions, as well as actively searching for well-maintained housing in low-crime areas, are good steps toward preventing break-ins. Usually intruders enter searching for items to sell. If you encounter an intruder, it is far better to give up your money than to fight.

> ### What do you think?
> *Do a spot check of your home. What areas might pose a risk for home accidents or forced entry?*
> ✳ *Do you have a fire extinguisher in your house?*
> ✳ *Do you know the numbers of your local fire and police departments?* ✳ *What would you do if the house caught fire and you needed to escape immediately?*

Workplace Safety

American adults spend most of their waking hours on the job. While most job situations are pleasant and productive, others pose physical and emotional hazards. Stress, burnout, hostile or abusive interactions, discrimination, power struggles, sexual harassment, and a host of other threats are possible whenever people are cloistered together for prolonged periods of time. The nature of the job itself, the corporate culture, and the policies and procedures that characterize certain professions can add to workplace stress.

Fatal Work Injuries Certain industries are inherently more hazardous than others; outdoor occupations show the highest fatality and injury rates. Although workplaces have instituted programs and services to reduce risks, the following statistics indicate a continuing problem.[77]

- In 1999, job-related fatalities reached their highest levels since record keeping began. Rates have decreased slightly since then but continue to surpass most previous fatality reports.
- Highway crashes were the leading cause of on-the-job fatalities and accounted for 27 percent of fatal work injury totals in 2000. Most involved truck drivers.
- Sixteen percent of worker fatalities resulted from other types of transportation-related incidents, such as tractors and forklifts overturning, workers being struck by vehicles, aircraft and railway crashes, and water vessels crashing or capsizing.
- Workplace homicides have declined in recent years but continue to be a major cause of workplace danger, accounting for more than 13 percent of all occupational injuries. Current and former coworker disputes and shootings during the course of robbery led the list. In addition, homicides occur at workplaces as a carryover of domestic violence, when a violent spouse or partner comes to seek revenge.
- Falls, being struck by objects, and electrocutions are also significant causes of worker fatalities.
- On average, about 17 workers were fatally injured each day in 2000. Hundreds more were permanently or temporarily disabled. Overall, there were 2,576,000 workdays lost to injury that year.
- Most fatally injured workers under age 16 were killed while doing farm work.

Nonfatal Work Injuries Although workplace deaths capture media attention, nonfatal work injuries, which are seldom publicized, can result in serious injury or disability. Chronic, debilitating pain and other injuries can cause great economic strain on organizations as a result of workers' compensation claims and days lost from work. Injuries that cause the greatest number of lost work days include carpal tunnel syndrome, hernia, amputation of a limb, fractures, sprains and strains (often of the back), cuts or lacerations, and chemical burns.[78] For example, nearly half of the employees with carpal tunnel syndrome miss 30 days or more of work each year. Because so many work injuries are due to repetitive motion, overexertion, or inappropriate motion, they are largely preventable through training and techniques designed to reduce employees' risks.

> ### What do you think?
> *What can be done to prevent injuries?* ✳ *Are students on your campus at risk from any of the problems discussed?* ✳ *Does your school have programs in place to prevent injuries?* ✳ *Do you think more can be done, and if so, what?*

Taking Charge

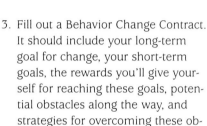

Make It Happen!

Assessment: The Assess Yourself box on page 93 gave you a chance to consider symptoms of abuse. If any of the symptoms describe a relationship experienced by you or someone you know, you should consider taking action.

Making a Change: In order to change your behavior, you need to develop a plan. Follow these steps.

1. Evaluate your behavior, and identify patterns and specific things you are doing. What can you change now? What can you change in the near future?
2. Select one pattern of behavior that you want to change.

3. Fill out a Behavior Change Contract. It should include your long-term goal for change, your short-term goals, the rewards you'll give yourself for reaching these goals, potential obstacles along the way, and strategies for overcoming these obstacles. For each goal, list the small steps and specific actions that you will take.
4. Chart your progress in a journal. At the end of a week, consider how successful you were in following your plan. What helped you be successful? What made change more difficult? What will you do differently next week?
5. Revise your plan as needed. Are the short-term goals attainable? Are the rewards satisfying?

Example: Sondra thought that her roommate Jessie was experiencing several symptoms of abuse. Jessie's boyfriend Carl sometimes belittled her in front of her friends. He once broke her cell phone by throwing it against a wall toward Jessie and seemed resentful when she spent time with anyone but him. When Sondra talked to Jessie about her perceptions, Jessie was surprised and very defensive at first. The more she thought about it, though, she realized that sometimes she was afraid of Carl's actions. She started to consider what she could do about the situation. As a first step, Sondra helped Jessie make immediate appointments at the school counseling center, one for herself and one for her and Carl together.

Summary

✳ Intentional injuries result from actions committed with intent to harm. Unintentional injuries are the result of actions involving no intent to harm. Violence is at epidemic levels in the United States. Many factors lead people to be violent. Among them are anger; substance abuse; and root causes of oppression, mental health, and economic difficulties.

✳ Acts of terrorism are becoming more common in the United States. In addition to their immediate impact, terrorist activities can exert damaging long-term effects by fostering an atmosphere of fear and anxiety.

✳ Violence affects everyone in society—from the direct victims, to those who live in fear, to those who pay higher taxes and insurance premiums. Over half of all homicides are committed by people who know their victims. Bias and hate crimes divide people, but teaching tolerance can reduce risks. Gang violence continues to grow but can be combated by programs that reduce the problems that lead to gang membership. Violence on campus may be increasing, but victims' rights also have increased as a result of major legislation.

☀ Prevention begins with avoiding situations in which harm may occur. There are several avenues available for reducing risks, including community, school, workplace, and individual strategies. Many crimes committed in general society are now commonplace at universities and colleges, including personal assaults, harassment, hate crimes, and even murder.

☀ Unintentional injuries frequently occur in homes and at worksites and can produce serious consequences, including death. By following common-sense guidelines, you can significantly reduce your risk of falls, burns, and other injuries.

Questions for Discussion and Reflection

1. What major types of crimes are committed in the United States? What is the difference between primary and re-active aggression?
2. What major factors lead to violent acts?
3. Who tends to be susceptible to the appeal of gang membership?
4. What is terrorism, and why does it occur? What can you do to protect yourself against terrorist attacks?
5. Compare domestic violence against men and against women. What are the differences? What are the similarities? What causes domestic violence?
6. What conditions put a child at risk for abuse? What can be done to prevent or decrease child abuse?
7. What is sexual harassment, and what factors contribute to it in the workplace?
8. What factors increase risk for sexual assault?
9. What are the most effective violence prevention strategies on your campus?
10. What steps can you take to lower your risk of injury from unintentional violence?

Accessing Your Health on the Internet

Visit the following Internet sites to explore further topics and issues related to personal health. To visit an organization's website, go to the Companion Website for *Health: The Basics, Sixth Edition* at www.aw-bc.com/donatelle, click on the book image, and select "Accessing Your Health on the Internet" from the navigation menu on the left.

1. *Communities against Violence Network.* An extensive, searchable database for information about violence against women, with articles, legal information, and statistics.
2. *Crimes on College Campuses.* Comprehensive source of information and statistics of colleges and universities across America.
3. *National Center for Injury Prevention and Control.* The WISQARS database of this Centers for Disease Control and Prevention (CDC) section provides statistics and information on fatal and nonfatal injuries, both intentional and unintentional.
4. *National Center for Victims of Crime.* Provides information and resources for victims of crimes ranging from hate crimes to sexual assault.
5. *National Criminal Justice Reference Service.* A federally funded resource for information on crime, criminal justice, and substance abuse.
6. *National Institute for Occupational Safety and Health.* Excellent reference for national statistics on injury and violence, both in the community and in the workplace.

Further Reading

Hoffman, A., J. Schuh, and R. Fenske. *Violence on Campus.* Gaithersburg, MD: Aspen, 1998.

Overview of violence on campus, unique factors that lead to violence and abuse on college campuses, and current programs and policies designed to reduce risk.

Ottens, A., and K. Hotelling, eds. *Sexual Violence on Campus: Policies, Programs, and Perspectives.* New York: Springer Publishing, 2001.

Overview of trends, causes, and contributors to violence on campus, as well as policies and programs designed to prevent violence.

U.S. Department of Health and Human Services. "Inventory of Federal Data Systems for Injury, Surveillance, Research and Prevention Activities." Washington, DC: Government Printing Office, 2001.

Excellent reference for data, reporting mechanisms, and instruments used in assessing U.S. violence statistics.

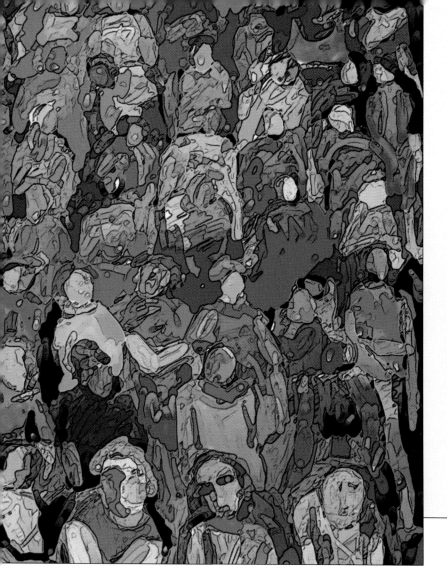

Healthy Relationships and Sexuality

Making Commitments

Objectives

* Discuss ways to improve communication skills and interpersonal interactions.

* Explain the characteristics of intimate relationships, the purposes they serve, types of intimacy, and how to maintain effective relationships.

* Discuss similarities and differences between men and women in communication styles.

* Discuss the importance of commitment, honesty, and mutual respect in relationships.

* Examine factors that affect life decisions, such as whether to remain single and whether to have children.

* Discuss the warning signs of relationship decline and where to get help with relationship problems.

* Define sexual identity, and discuss the role of gender identity.

* Identify major features and functions of sexual anatomy and physiology.

* Classify sexual dysfunctions, and describe major disorders.

For Better or Worse: Marriage's Stormy Future

By Tamar Lewin

Traditionally, the idea of being a little bit married made no more sense than being a little bit pregnant: you either were or you weren't.

But that isn't so black and white anymore. As the courts deal with the issue of same-sex unions, they are reconsidering a fundamental question: What is marriage? And the ruling Tuesday by the Massachusetts Supreme Judicial Court that the state constitution gives gay couples the right to marry opens the way for more litigation over the shades of gray.

For more than a decade, European countries have experimented with different forms of Marriage Lite from the registered partnerships that started in Norway and Denmark, to France's "civil solidarity pacts," which can be dissolved by either party on three months' notice.

The United States, too, has gradually recognized more nontraditional unions, gay or straight: Many employers, including some state and local governments, extend some benefits to domestic partners. And Vermont recognizes "civil unions" between same-sex couples.

Read the complete article online in the eThemes section of this book's website: www.aw-bc.com/donatelle.

Humans are social animals—we have a basic need to belong and to feel loved, appreciated, and wanted.[1] We can't live without relating to others in some way. In fact, a study done by researchers at the Harvard School of Public Health shows that the ability to relate well with people throughout your life can have almost as much impact on your health as do exercise and good nutrition.[2]

All relationships involve a degree of risk. However, only by taking these risks can we grow and truly experience all that life has to offer. By looking at our intimate and nonintimate relationships, components of sexual identity, gender roles, and sexual orientation, we will come to better understand who we are.

Communicating: A Key to Good Relationships

From the moment of birth, we struggle to be understood. We flail our arms, cry, scream, smile, frown, belch, and make sounds and gestures to attract attention, get a reaction from someone we care about, or have someone understand what we want or need from them.

By the time we enter adulthood, each of us has developed a unique way of communicating to others with gestures, words, expressions, and body positions. No two of us communicate in the exact same way or have the same need for connecting with others. Some of us are outgoing and quick to express our emotions and thoughts. Others of us are quiet, withdrawn, and reluctant to talk about our feelings.

Different cultures not only have different languages and dialects, but also have different ways of expressing themselves and using body language to communicate information.[3] Some cultures gesture wildly; others maintain a closed and rigid means of speaking. Some cultures are offended by apparent "fixed and dilated" staring; others welcome a steady look in the eyes.

Although it is well established that people differ in the way they communicate, this doesn't mean that one sex, culture, or group is better or should be a model for the others. We have to be willing to accept differences and work to keep communication lines open and fluid. Appearing interested, actively engaged in the interaction, and open and willing to exchange ideas and thoughts is something that we typically learn with practice and hard work.

Communicating How You Feel

Do you find it easy to convey how much you care about friends and family members with hugs and verbal expressions of appreciation and love? If you are comfortable telling them you love them and that they mean a lot to you, chances are that you also will be able to tell them when you are feeling bad, disappointed, angry, or frustrated. However, it's important to realize that some people were not raised in affectionate families, that they do not readily discuss feelings or emotions, and that sometimes these individuals may struggle to find the right words for expressing what they feel.

When two people begin a relationship, they bring their past communication styles with them.[4] How often have you heard someone say, "We just can't communicate," or "You're sending mixed messages"? These exchanges occur regularly as people start relationships or work through ongoing communication problems in an existing relationship. Because communication is a process, our every action, word, facial expression, gesture, or body posture becomes a part of our shared history and part of the evolving impression we make on others. If we are angry in our responses, others will be reluctant to interact with us. If we bring "baggage" from past bad interactions to new relationships, we may be cynical, distrustful, and guarded in our exchanges with others. If we are positive, happy, and share openly with others, they may be more likely to communicate openly with us. Being able to communicate assertively is also an important skill in relationships (see the Assess Yourself box on page 108).

Improving Communication/ Improving Relationships

Because people have such different ways of communicating, there is no recipe for how to communicate best in a given situation. At times, silence may be the best approach. However, there are things that each of us can do to become better communicators and to encourage and assist others in their attempts to interact with us.

Learning to Share/Self-Disclose   Learning when to share, how much to share, and who you can trust in sharing information is never an easy task. We've all experienced frustrations and disappointments by sharing too much when we probably should have stopped earlier; whenever you self-disclose, you take a risk. Sharing personal feelings and thoughts makes you vulnerable, so move cautiously in self-disclosing. Get to know a person better before you "tell all." Remember, you can't take back things you have said, so consider why you are sharing and what the consequences of sharing might be. If a person seems to be pushing you to share information that you would rather not share, ask why it is important to them.

However, if you have really thought about what you believe in and have analyzed your feelings, it is often easier to self-disclose because you know that you have relayed information that you believe is important and honest. Remember, too, that disclosing information about past sexual partners, drug histories, and so forth, is now often done as part of responsible sexual behavior. Although you may feel uncomfortable in asking about sexual history, you have a responsibility to disclose information that might put a prospective partner at risk.

Learning to Listen   All of us have tried to talk with someone who won't let us get a word in edgewise. We listen to them to be polite or to avoid conflict. But how did it make you feel? Frustrated? Angry? Wanting to run? Unfortunately, these nonstop talkers often don't have a clue that they are driving people away. They may see themselves as charming and

entertaining, and it is hard to steer them to listen more and talk less. However, for comfortable interactions to occur, a gentle prod about listening more and talking less may be in order. Nearly everyone could benefit from working on their listening and speaking skills. Here are a few key pointers.

- *Focus on the speaker.* Maintain eye contact, nod, ask questions, and use body language to let the speaker know you are listening.
- *Avoid interruptions.* Let the speaker finish a thought before you cut in.
- *Avoid focusing on speaker quirks.* Sometimes we get so focused on a speaker's habits that they consume all our attention.
- *Demonstrate understanding.* Try to avoid constant philosophizing or moralizing to the person who is pouring his or her heart out.
- *Avoid challenging the speaker or becoming defensive.* Listen objectively, and try to get a sense of what the person is really saying or feeling.
- *Try using "I" messages when you respond, particularly in potentially volatile situations.* This means communicating your own feelings and emotions, such as "I feel frustrated when this happens" instead of "You frustrate me when do you do that!"
- *Avoid generalities.* Be specific in what you are telling a person you want from them, and tune in when they respond.

Although there are no foolproof communicating strategies, it is important to speak honestly, respectfully, and to pay attention to how your listener responds. Sometimes the real message lies not in what is actually being said, but in the nonverbal message of what is *not* said. Rolling your eyes in reaction to the speaker's comments, looking at your watch, or other such actions can send signals that ignite responses that you were not looking for. Getting a handle on these behaviors and learning to interact more effectively with friends, family members, and romantic partners can make a huge difference in the quality of your relationships.

Characteristics of Intimate Relationships

We can define **intimate relationships** in terms of four characteristics: *behavioral interdependence, need fulfillment, emotional attachment,* and *emotional availability.* Each of these characteristics may be related to interactions with family, close friends, and romantic partners.[5]

> **Intimate relationships**   Relationships with family members, friends, and romantic partners, characterized by behavioral interdependence, need fulfillment, emotional attachment, and emotional availability.

Standing Up for Yourself

You know that sinking feeling. Someone asks you to do something, and your stomach lurches. You don't want to go along, but you can't come up with a good excuse not to do so. It's hard to say no. How often are you caught in the "I can't say no" trap? Read the following situations and assess your response according to the following 5-point scale:

1 = Never, 2 = Seldom, 3 = Sometimes, 4 = Frequently, 5 = Always.

	1	2	3	4	5
1. Friends ask you to ride home with them after they've all been drinking. You know you shouldn't go. But you think one of them is cute, and you don't want to seem like a prude. You take the ride.	1	2	3	4	5
2. Your decisions can be easily swayed by a strong argument from someone else pushing you in the opposite direction.	1	2	3	4	5
3. You feel strongly about a political issue, but it is the opposite of the opinion your parents hold. You remain silent rather than getting into an argument.	1	2	3	4	5
4. You start out by saying no to something but get talked into doing it after a short time.	1	2	3	4	5
5. You're stressed out with too much to do and too little time, but you can't seem to say no when someone asks for a favor.	1	2	3	4	5
6. Someone says something really nasty about a person you like. You jump to the defense of the person being criticized, even though you are in the minority opinion.	1	2	3	4	5
7. You would describe yourself as assertive and tend to quickly let others know your thoughts about certain issues.	1	2	3	4	5
8. Someone is critical of something you do. You quickly defend your actions by explaining why you did what you did.	1	2	3	4	5

Think about your responses to each statement. Do your responses indicate an assertive communication style in which you stand up for your feelings or beliefs? What factors cause you to hold back when you should probably speak up? How can you work to improve your communication behaviors in this area? For statements 1 through 5, do you have several "5" responses? If yes, you should consider what skills you could develop to help you communicate more assertively.

Behavioral interdependence refers to the mutual impact that people have on each other as their lives and daily activities intertwine. What one person does influences what the other person wants to do and can do. Behavioral interdependence may become stronger over time to the point that each person would find a great void if the other were gone.

Intimate relationships also fulfill psychological needs and so are a means of *need fulfillment*. Through relationships with others, we fulfill our needs for:

• Intimacy—someone with whom we can share our feelings freely
• Social integration—someone with whom we can share our worries and concerns
• Being nurturant—someone whom we can take care of and be supportive of
• Assistance—someone to help us in times of need
• Affirmation—someone who will reassure us of our own worth and tell us that we matter

In rewarding, intimate relationships, partners and friends meet each other's needs. They disclose feelings, share confidences, and provide support and reassurance. Each person comes away from interactions feeling better for the experience and validated by the other person.

In addition to behavioral interdependence and need fulfillment, intimate relationships involve strong bonds of *emotional attachment*, or feelings of love. When we hear the word *intimacy*, we often think of a sexual relationship. Although sex can play an important role in emotional attachment, a relationship can be very intimate and yet not sexual. Two people can be emotionally intimate (they share feelings) or spiritually intimate (they share spiritual beliefs and meanings). Or they can be intimate friends. The intimacy level two people experience cannot be judged easily by those outside the relationship.

Emotional availability, the ability to give to and receive from others emotionally without fear of being hurt or rejected, is the fourth characteristic of intimate relationships.

At times, all of us may limit our emotional availability. For example, after a painful breakup we may decide not to jump into another relationship immediately, or we may decide not to talk about it with every friend. Holding back can offer time for introspection and healing as well as for considering the lessons learned. However, because of intense trauma, some people find it difficult ever to be fully available emotionally. This limits their ability to experience intimate relationships.

Forming Intimate Relationships

In the early years of life, families provide the most significant relationships. Gradually, the circle widens to include friends, coworkers, and acquaintances. Ultimately, most of us develop romantic or sexual relationships with significant others. Each of these relationships plays a significant role in psychological, social, spiritual, and physical health.

Families: The Ties That Bind

The United Nations defines seven basic types of families, including single-parent families, communal families (unrelated people living together for ideological, economic, or other reasons), and extended families. But most Americans think of family in terms of the "family of origin" or the "nuclear family." The **family of origin** includes the people present in the household during a child's first years of life—usually parents and siblings. However, the family of origin also may include stepparents, grandparents, aunts and uncles, partners, and friends. The family of origin has a tremendous impact on the child's psychological and social development. The **nuclear family** consists of parents (usually married, but not necessarily) and their offspring.

The modern American family looks quite different from families of previous generations. Over half of today's moms work outside the home, and large numbers of children are cared for by single parents, grandparents, relatives, stepparents, friends, nannies, day care centers, and other caregivers. No particular family structure is inherently good or bad. Families that promote the most positive health outcomes for all members appear to be those that offer a sense of security, safety, love, and the opportunity for members to grow through positive interactions.

If parents are not afraid to share feelings, affection, and love with each other and their offspring, their children are likely to become emotionally connected adults. If the home environment provides stability and safety, it is likely that the children will learn to express feelings and develop intimacy skills. Sibling interactions provide a way to learn and practice interpersonal skills. When the family itself is healthy, people can practice positive behaviors and learn the consequences of negative behaviors in a safe and nonjudgmental environment. However, if the family is psychologically or physically unhealthy, it may pose significant barriers to later relationships, as we will discuss later in this chapter.

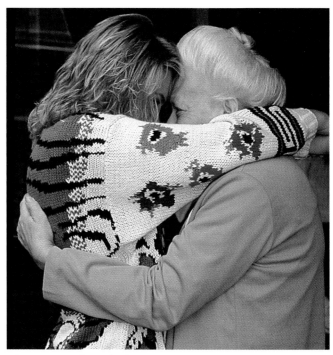

The emotional bonds that characterize intimate relationships often span the generations and help individuals gain insight and understanding into each other's worlds.

Establishing Friendships

A Friend is one who knows you as you are
understands where you've been
accepts who you've become
and still gently invites you to grow.

—Author Unknown

Good friends can make a boring day fun, a cold day warm, or a gut-wrenching worry disappear. They can make us feel that we have the strength to get through just about anything and give us perspective on the craziest of situations. They also can make us angry or seriously jolt our comfortable ideas about right and wrong. No friendship is perfect, and most friendships need careful attention if they are to remain stable over time. Psychologists believe that people are attracted to and form relationships with people who give them positive reinforcement and they dislike those who punish or overcriticize them. The basic idea is simple: You like the people who like you. Another factor that affects the

---

Family of origin People present in the household during a child's first years of life—usually parents and siblings.

Nuclear family Parents (usually married, but not necessarily) and their offspring.

development of a friendship is a real or perceived similarity in attitudes, opinions, and background.[6] In addition, true friends have a sense of *equity* that allows them to share confidences, contribute fairly and equally to maintaining the friendship, and consistently try to give as much as they get back from the interactions.[7]

Though we all know that friends enrich our lives, most people don't realize that real health benefits result from strong social bonds. Social support has been shown to boost the immune system, improve the quality and possibly the length of life, and even reduce the risks of heart disease.[8]

Although most of us have a fairly clear idea of the distinction between a friend and a lover, this difference is not always easy to verbalize. Some people believe that the major difference is that no intimate physical involvement exists between friends. Others have suggested that intimacy levels are much lower between friends than between lovers. But as we have stated, people can be intimate without being sexually involved. Also, some people have sex with others as friends or as "one-night stands," not as true lovers and partners. So sex, per se, is not necessarily intimate. Confused? You are not alone. Surprisingly, little research has been done to clarify the terms *friend* and *lover*. Psychologists Jeffrey Turner and Laura Rubinson have described the characteristics that make a good friendship.[9]

- *Enjoyment.* Friends enjoy each other's company most of the time, although temporary states of anger, disappointment, or mutual annoyance may occur.
- *Acceptance.* Friends accept each other as they are, without trying to change or make the other into a different person.
- *Mutual trust.* Each assumes that the other will act in his or her friend's best interest.
- *Respect.* Friends respect each other in the sense that each assumes the other exercises good judgment in making life choices.
- *Mutual assistance.* Friends are inclined to assist, support, and count on each other in times of need, trouble, or personal distress.
- *Confiding.* Friends share experiences and feelings with each other that they don't share with other people.
- *Understanding.* Friends have a sense of what each person values. They are not puzzled or mystified by each other's actions.
- *Spontaneity.* Friends feel free to be themselves in the relationship, without being required to play a role or inhibit revelation of personal traits.

Significant Others, Partners, Couples

Most people choose at some point to enter into an intimate sexual relationship with another person. Numerous studies have analyzed the ways in which couples form significant partnering relationships. Most partners fit into one of four categories: married heterosexual couples, cohabiting heterosexual couples, lesbian couples, and gay male couples.

These groups are discussed in greater detail later in this chapter.

Love relationships in each of these four groups typically include all the characteristics of friendship as well as the following characteristics related to passion and caring.[10]

- *Fascination.* Lovers tend to pay attention to the other person even when they should be involved in other activities. They are preoccupied with the other and want to think about, look at, talk to, or merely be with the other.
- *Exclusiveness.* Lovers have a special relationship that usually precludes having the same relationship with a third party. The love relationship takes priority over all others.
- *Sexual desire.* Lovers desire physical intimacy and want to touch, hold, and engage in sexual activities with the other.
- *Giving the utmost.* Lovers care enough to give the utmost when the other is in need, sometimes to the point of extreme sacrifice.
- *Being a champion or advocate.* Lovers actively champion each other's interests and attempt to ensure that the other succeeds.

What do you think?

Is sex the only difference between a friend and someone you would select as a partner? ✳ *Can you have a good relationship with a partner and not have sex?* ✳ *Can you have sex with a friend and be just friends?* ✳ *Can you have sex with someone you love and not be friends?* ✳ *What issues are at stake in each instance?*

This Thing Called Love

What is love? Defining it may be more difficult than listing the characteristics of a loving relationship. The term *love* has more entries in *Bartlett's Familiar Quotations* than any other word except *man*.[11] This four-letter word has been written about and engraved on walls; it has been the theme of countless novels, movies, and plays. There is no one definition of *love*, and the word may mean different things to people, depending on cultural values, age, gender, and situation. Yet, we all know what it is when it strikes (Figure 5.1).

Many social scientists maintain that love may be of two kinds: *companionate* and *passionate*. Companionate love is a secure, trusting attachment, similar to what we may feel for family members or close friends. In companionate love, two people are attracted, have much in common, care about each other's well-being, and express reciprocal liking and respect. Passionate love, in contrast, is a state of high arousal filled with the ecstasy of being loved and the agony of being rejected.[12] The person experiencing passionate love tends to be preoccupied with his or her partner and to perceive the love object as perfect.[13] According to researchers Hatfield and Walster, passionate love will not occur unless three

Is it love?

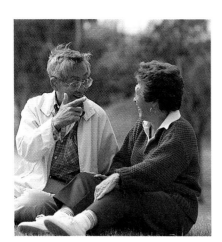

— **Verbally expressing affection,** such as saying "I love you"

— **Offering self-disclosure,** such as revealing intimate facts about oneself

— **Giving nonmaterial evidence,** such as emotional and moral support in times of need, and respecting the other's opinion

— **Expressing nonverbal feelings,** such as feeling happy, more content, more secure when the person is present

— **Giving material evidence,** such as gifts, flowers, small favors, or doing more than one's own share of a task

— **Physically expressing love,** such as hugging, kissing, making love

— **Tolerating the other,** such as accepting his or her idiosyncrasies, peculiar routines, or forgetfulness

— **Wanting to promote** the partner's welfare

— **Feeling happiness** with the partner

— **Holding the partner** in high regard

— **Being able to count on the partner** in time of need

— **Being able to understand** each other

— **Sharing oneself and one's possessions** with the partner

— **Giving emotional support** to the partner

— **Being able to communicate** about intimate things.

— **Valuing the partner's presence** in one's own life

Figure 5.1
Common Experiences of Love

Source: From B. Strong, C. DeVault, and B. Sayad, *Human Sexuality* (Mountain View, CA: Mayfield, 1999). Reprinted by permission of McGraw-Hill Education, a division of the McGraw-Hill Companies.

conditions are met.[14] First, the person must live in a culture in which the concept of "falling in love" is idealized. Second, a "suitable" love object must be present. If someone has been taught by parents, movies, books, and peers to seek partners of a certain appearance, socioeconomic status, or racial background, and if no such partner is available, the person may find it difficult to become involved. Finally, there must be some type of physiological arousal that occurs when a person is in the presence of the beloved. Often this arousal takes the form of sexual excitement.

In his article "The Triangular Theory of Love," researcher Robert Sternberg attempts to clarify love further by isolating three key ingredients:[15]

- *Intimacy:* the emotional component, which involves feelings of closeness
- *Passion:* the motivational component, which reflects romantic, sexual attraction
- *Decision/commitment:* the cognitive component, which includes the decisions you make about being in love and the degree of commitment to your partner

According to Sternberg's model, the higher the levels of intimacy, passion, and commitment, the more likely a person is to be involved in a healthy, positive love relationship.

According to anthropologist Helen Fisher (and others), attraction and falling in love follow a fairly predictable pattern based on (1) *imprinting,* in which our evolutionary patterns, genetic predispositions, and past experiences trigger romantic reaction; (2) *attraction,* in which neurochemicals produce feelings of euphoria and elation; (3) *attachment,* in which endorphins—natural opiates—cause lovers to feel peaceful, secure, and calm; and (4) *production of a cuddle chemical,* in which the brain secretes the chemical *oxytocin,* thereby stimulating sensations during lovemaking and eliciting feelings of satisfaction and attachment.[16]

Lovers who claim that they are swept away by passion may not, therefore, be far from the truth.

> A meeting of the eyes, a touch of the hands or a whiff of scent may set off a flood that starts in the brain and races along the nerves and through the blood. The familiar results—flushed skin, sweaty palms, heavy breathing—are identical to those experienced when under stress. Why? Because the love-smitten person is secreting chemical substances such as dopamine, norepinephrine, and phenylethylamine (PEA) that are chemical cousins of amphetamines.[17]

Although attraction may in fact be a "natural high," with PEA levels soaring, this hit of passion loses effectiveness over time as the body builds up a tolerance. Needing a continual fix of passion, many people may become attraction junkies, seeking the intoxication of love much as the drug user seeks a chemical high.[18]

Fisher speculates that PEA levels drop significantly over a three- to four-year period, which leads to the "four-year itch" that shows up in the peaking fourth-year divorce rates present in more than 60 cultures. Romances that last beyond the four-year decline of PEA are influenced by another set of chemicals, known as endorphins, which are soothing substances that give lovers a sense of security, peace, and calm.[19]

Oxytocin also is being studied for its role in the love formula. Produced by the brain, it sensitizes nerves and

Men and Women Really Are Different: Recognizing and Acknowledging Uniqueness

Make no mistake about it, men and women learn very different patterns of behavior and communication from their earliest years and carry these patterns with them throughout their lives. Sometimes this makes understanding each other difficult, such as when we are bothered by mannerisms or habits but don't know why. Recognizing that these differences make us unique is a good first step in anticipating and preventing potential problems in communication. Note that these characteristics are not absolute. No doubt you know men who demonstrate traits that are more like those of their female counterparts and vice versa.

Sources: Kings Communications, "Men and Women are Different!" 2002. www.Kings Communications.com. Used by permission; Mark L. Knapp and Anita L. Vangelisti, *Interpersonal Communication and Human Relationships,* (Boston: Allyn & Bacon, 2000).

	Men	Women
Body Language	Occupy more space; gesture away from the body; lean back when listening; less feedback through body language; more forceful gestures (backslapping, stronger handshakes); overt fidgeting	Take up less space; movement is light and easy; gesture toward the body; lean forward when listening; provide feedback via body language; less likely to invade another's space; more gentle when touching others
Facial Expressions	Often avoid eye contact; show less warmth in facial expression; frown more often	Maintain better eye contact; smile and nod more often
Speech Patterns	More likely to interrupt, mumble, and use fewer speech tones (approximately three); voices are lower and usually louder; sound more abrupt; talk less personally about selves; make more direct statements than feeling statements; use fewer adjectives and descriptive statements; use fewer terms of endearment; tendency to lecture	Interrupt less often; articulate more clearly; use more speech tones (approximately five); may sound more emotional; voices are higher pitched and softer; more likely to discuss feelings and disclose more personal information; make more tentative statements ("kind of," "isn't it?")
Behavioral Differences	More inclined to be analytical; give fewer compliments; use more sarcasm and teasing to show affection; cry less often; more argumentative; difficulty in expressing intimate feelings; hold fewer grudges; gossip less; less likely to ask for help; tend to take rejection less personally; apologize less often	More emotional approach to issues; give more compliments; show more expression; express feelings more readily; greater tendency to hold grudges; inclined to gossip more; more likely to ask for help; take rejection more personally; apologize more frequently

stimulates muscle contractions, the production of breast milk, and the desire for physical closeness between mother and infant. Scientists speculate that oxytocin may encourage similar cuddling between men and women. Oxytocin levels also have been shown to increase dramatically during orgasm for both men and women.[20]

In addition to such possible chemical influences, past experiences significantly affect our attractions for others. Our parents' modeling of traits we believe are desirable or undesirable may play a role in drawing us to people with similar traits. Many researchers have investigated the possible link between males seeking their mothers and females seeking their fathers in partners. To date, research on chemical

attractions and parent-seeking tendencies is inconclusive and should be viewed only as preliminary. Much more research is needed to confirm these provocative theories.

Gender Issues in Relationships

When it comes to relationships, are men really from Mars and women from Venus? If they are not planets apart, how far apart are they, and what are the implications of the disparities?

Differences in Communication Styles

Psychologist Deborah Tannen has described several basic differences in conversational styles between men and women that can make communication between genders challenging.[21] In her book *You Just Don't Understand: Women and Men in Conversation,* Tannen coins the term **genderlect**

Genderlect The "dialect," or individual speech pattern and communication style, of each gender.

to characterize differences in word choices, interruption patterns, questioning patterns, language interpretations and misinterpretations, and vocal inflections based on gender. Recent research validates much of Tannen's work and indicates that women are more expressive, relationship oriented, and concerned with creating and maintaining intimacy; men tend to be more instrumental, task oriented, and concerned with gathering information or with establishing and maintaining social status or power.[22] Unlike women, many men believe that they are not supposed to show emotions and are brought up to believe that "being strong" is often more important than having close friendships. As a result, according to research, only one male in ten has a close male friend to whom he divulges his innermost thoughts.[23] Although these are generalizations, the conclusions have been validated repeatedly in research focused on such patterns.

Although men often are perceived as less emotional than women, the question remains whether they really feel less or just express their feelings differently. In one study in which men and women were shown scenes of people in distress, the men exhibited little outward emotion, whereas the women communicated feelings of concern. However, physiological measures of emotional arousal (such as heart rate and blood pressure) indicated that the male subjects were actually as affected emotionally as the female subjects. In other studies, men and women responded very differently to the same test,[24] so definite conclusions cannot be drawn. Researchers continue to investigate emotional responsiveness in men and women.

Understanding gender differences in communication patterns, rather than casting blame at each other, is an important step toward bettering communication between men and women. Don't expect members of the other sex to change their style of communication. Instead, learn to interpret their messages while you explain your own unique way of communicating. Both men and women want to be heard and understood in their relationships. Understanding the different ways in which we use language will help us all achieve this goal. See the Women's Health/Men's Health box for more on the unique qualities of male and female communication.

What do you think?
Who are the people with whom you feel most comfortable talking about very personal issues? * *Do you talk with both males and females about these issues, or do you tend to gravitate toward just one sex?* * *Why do you think you do this?*

Picking Partners

For both males and females, the choice of partners is influenced by more than just chemical and psychological processes.

One important factor is *proximity,* or being in the same place at the same time. The more you see a person in your hometown, at social gatherings, or at work, the more likely that interaction will occur. Thus, if you live in New York, you'll probably end up with another New Yorker. If you live in northern Wisconsin, you'll probably end up with another Wisconsinite. (With the advent of the Internet, however, geographic proximity is not always important. See the Reality Check box on page 114.)

You also pick a partner based on *similarities* (attitudes, values, intellect, interests); the old adage that "opposites attract" usually isn't true. If your potential partner expresses interest or liking, you may react with mutual regard known as *reciprocity.* The more you express interest, the safer it is for someone else to return the regard, and the cycle spirals onward.

A final factor that apparently plays a significant role in selecting a partner is *physical attraction.* Whether such attraction is caused by a chemical reaction or a socially learned behavior, males and females appear to have different attraction criteria. Men tend to select their mates primarily on the basis of youth and physical attractiveness. Although physical attractiveness is an important criterion for women in mate selection, they tend to place higher emphasis on partners who are somewhat older, have good financial prospects, and are dependable and industrious.

What do you think?
What factors do you consider the most important in a potential partner? * *Which are absolute musts?* * *Are there any differences between what you believe to be important in a relationship and the things your parents feel are important?*

Overcoming Barriers to Intimacy

Obstacles to intimacy include lack of personal identity, emotional immaturity, and a poorly developed sense of responsibility. The fear of being hurt, low self-esteem, mishandled hostility, chronic busyness (and its attendant lack of emotional presence), a tendency to "parentify" loved ones, and a conflict of role expectations may be equally detrimental. In addition, individual insecurities and difficulties in recognizing and expressing emotional needs can create obstacles. These barriers to intimacy may have many causes, including a dysfunctional family background and jealousy.

Dysfunctional Families

As noted earlier, the ability to sustain genuine intimacy is largely developed in the family of origin. If you were to examine even the most pristine family under a microscope, you would likely find some problems. No group of people

Computer Dating: Issues for the Communication Age

Ten years ago, the thought of sharing intimate details with a faceless stranger in cyberspace would have been unthinkable. Today, such meetings may lead to excitement, intrigue, or "happy-ever-after" encounters. In increasingly large numbers, however, they also may lead to disappointment as the computer persona turns out to be an ordinary person in real life.

Occasionally, as recent newspaper headlines point out, chance computer relationships can lead to victimization and death. In one such instance, a woman had been communicating daily with her "computer friend" for several months. When her friend began to use increasingly vivid and kinky sexual references and seemed to know more about her than she wished, she became uncomfortable and tried to back off. She was relentlessly stalked via her home and work computers, and it became evident that her online stalker knew her address and much about her personal life. Eventually, she was found dead, the result of a vicious attack by the person she knew only via computer.

Though this incident is a dramatic example of computer interactions gone wrong, it is important to remember that there are inherent risks in communicating with people you don't know in any traditional sense. Remembering these key points of computerized communication may save you many hours of worry and frustration.

- Never give your real name or vital information (e.g., credit card numbers) to a computer chat partner. Use a screen name only, and avoid giving information that may help chat partners home in on you personally.
- If your conversations become suggestive, threatening, or make you uncomfortable in any way, terminate the session. Report such violations to your Internet service provider.
- Never arrange to meet strangers at your home or their homes. Pick a safe public meeting place, and bring a friend. Do not give specific identifying information until you know much more about the person. Keep job location and employment information out of the conversation, except in generic terms.
- Ask yourself why you are seeking intimacy from strangers via the computer rather than interacting with people you know, particularly if the computer seems to be taking up a disproportionate amount of your time. If your hours online are excessive, consider talking to a counselor or friend about your situation.

---

can interact perfectly all the time, but this does not necessarily make them dysfunctional. In a truly **dysfunctional family,** interaction between family members inhibits psychological growth, self-love, emotional expression, and individual development. Negative interactions are the norm rather than the exception. It is important to note that dysfunctional families are found in every social, ethnic, religious, economic, and racial group.

Children raised in dysfunctional settings tend to face tremendous obstacles to growing up healthy. Coming to terms with past hurts may take years. However, with careful planning and introspection, support from loved ones, and counseling when needed, children from even the most dysfunctional homes have proved to be remarkably resilient. Many are able to forget the past, focus on the future, and develop into healthy, well-adjusted adults. But some have problems throughout their lives.[25] For example, adults who grew up with alcoholic parents may have serious problems creating and maintaining intimate relationships. The family messages that these children receive are typically contradictory, since the family usually tries to hide the presence of alcohol abuse in the home.

Many adult children of alcoholics (ACOAs) claim that they become involved in unhealthy relationships and have difficulty trusting others, communicating with partners, and defining a healthy relationship.[26] Research supporting this theory is conflicted, and many questions remain concerning how past experiences affect relationships for ACOAs. Another tragically large group of people struggling with intimacy problems that originated in the family of origin are survivors of childhood emotional, physical, or sexual abuse (see Chapter 4).

Jealousy in Relationships

"Jealousy is like a San Andreas fault running beneath the smooth surface of an intimate relationship. Most of the time, its eruptive potential lies hidden. But when it begins to rumble, the destruction can be enormous."[27] **Jealousy** has been described as an aversive reaction evoked by a real or imagined relationship involving one's partner and a third person.

Contrary to what many of us may believe, jealousy is not a sign of intense devotion. Instead, jealousy often

---

Dysfunctional family   A family in which the interaction between family members inhibits rather than enhances psychological growth, self-love, emotional expression, and individual development.

Jealousy   An aversive reaction evoked by a real or imagined relationship involving one's partner and a third person.

News from the World of Marriage, Divorce, and Cohabitation Studies

Are you considering marriage? Consider these facts: By age 30, about three-fourths of women in the U.S. have been married and about half have cohabited outside of marriage, according to a comprehensive new report by the Centers for Disease Control and Prevention. The study was based on interviews with nearly 11,000 women 15 to 44 years of age and examined individual and community factors that influence whether a person marries, divorces, cohabits, or chooses to remain single. Points of interest from this study include the following.

- Divorce rates are up, but so are the number of second marriages. Divorcees who remarry usually wait three years before saying "I do" again.
- More women are choosing to remain single. In 1963, 83% of women in the age group studied were married; today, just over 66% of all women will marry.
- The pre-1950s family pattern of Mom, Dad, and kids living under the same roof is no longer the norm.

- Roughly half of all first marriages for people younger than 45 end in divorce. First marriages that end in divorce typically last about eight years. (This is only a statistical average and does not necessarily prove the existence of the "seven-year itch.")
- Younger generations of Americans are delaying marriage until later in life. Most people are spending more of their lives unmarried.
- People who are more educated are more likely to marry and stay married, perhaps because they are more mature and/or financially stable when they tie the knot.
- Overall, unmarried cohabitations are less stable than marriages. The probability of a premarital cohabitation breaking up within five years is 49%. The probability of a first marriage ending in separation or divorce within five years is 20%. After ten years, the probability of a first marriage ending is 33%, compared with 62% for cohabitations.
- Cohabitations and marriages tend to last longer under certain conditions that include a woman's age at the time the cohabitation or marriage began (older is better); whether she was raised throughout childhood in an intact two-parent family that seemed to be happy; whether religion plays an

important role in her life; and whether she had a higher family income or lived in a community with high median family income, low male unemployment, and low poverty.
- Marriages that end do not always end in divorce; many end in separation and do not go through divorce. Separated white women are much more likely (91%) to divorce after three years, compared with separated Hispanic women (77%) and separated African American women (67%).
- The probability of remarriage among divorced women is 54% in five years overall: 58% for white women, 44% for Hispanic women, and 32% for African American women. However, there is also a strong probability that second marriages will end in separation or divorce (23% after five years and 39% after ten years.)
- In the 1950s if a woman divorced, there was a 65% chance that she would remarry. Today, only about 50% of divorced women choose to remarry.

Source: National Center for Health Statistics, Centers for Disease Control and Prevention, "New Report Sheds Light on Trends and Patterns in Marriage, Divorce, and Cohabitation," July 24, 2002. www.cdc.gov/nchs/releases/02news/div_mar_cohab.htm.

indicates underlying problems that may prove to be a significant barrier to a healthy intimate relationship. Causes of jealousy typically include the following.

- *Overdependence on the relationship.* People who have few social ties and rely exclusively on their significant others tend to be fearful of losing them.
- *High value on sexual exclusivity.* People who believe that sexual exclusivity is a crucial indicator of love are more likely to become jealous.
- *Severity of the threat.* People may feel uneasy if someone with stunning good looks and a great personality appears interested in their partners. But they may brush off the threat if they appraise their rival "unworthy" in terms of appearance or other characteristics.
- *Low self-esteem.* The underlying question that torments people with low self-esteem is "Why would anyone want

me?" People who feel good about themselves are less likely to feel unworthy and to fear that someone else is going to snatch their partners.
- *Fear of losing control.* Some people need to feel in control of the situation. Feeling that they may be losing the attachment of or control over a partner can cause jealousy.

In both sexes, jealousy is related to the expectation that it would be difficult to find another relationship if the current one ends. For men, jealousy is positively correlated with self-evaluative dependency, the degree to which the man's self-esteem is affected by his partner's judgments. Though a certain amount of jealousy can be expected in any loving relationship, it doesn't have to threaten a relationship as long as partners communicate openly about it.[28]

Committed Relationships

Commitment in a relationship means that there is an intent to act over time in a way that perpetuates the well-being of the other person, oneself, and the relationship. Polls show that the majority of Americans—as many as 96 percent—strive to develop a committed relationship, even though many have difficulty maintaining them. These relationships can take several forms, including marriage, cohabitation, and gay and lesbian partnerships.

Marriage

In many societies around the world, traditional committed relationships take the form of marriage. In the United States, marriage means entering into a legal agreement that includes shared financial plans, property, and responsibility for raising children. Many Americans also view marriage as a religious sacrament that emphasizes certain rights and obligations for each spouse.

Close to 90 percent of all Americans marry at least once. U.S. Census Bureau data show that we are marrying later in life than ever before. In 1970, the median age for first marriage was 22.5 years for men and 20.6 years for women; by 2002, this had risen to 26.9 years for men and 25.3 years for women.[29] This trend appears to be continuing.

Many Americans believe that marriage involves **monogamy,** or exclusive sexual involvement with one partner. In fact, the lifetime pattern for many Americans appears to be **serial monogamy,** which means that a person has a monogamous sexual relationship with one partner before moving on to another monogamous relationship. However, some people prefer to have an **open relationship,** or open

Monogamy   Exclusive sexual involvement with one partner.

Serial monogamy   A series of monogamous sexual relationships.

Open relationship   A relationship in which partners agree that sexual involvement can occur outside the relationship.

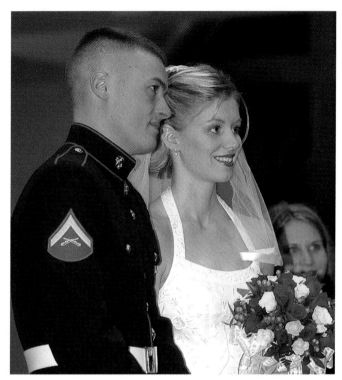

For many people, marriage or commitment ceremonies serve as the ultimate symbol of commitment between two people and validate their love for each other.

marriage, in which the partners agree that there may be sexual involvement for each person outside their relationship.

Humans are not naturally monogamous; most of us are capable of being sexually and/or emotionally involved with more than one person at a time. Sexual infidelity is an extremely common factor in divorces and breakups. So why do we continue to get married?

Certainly marriage is socially sanctioned and highly celebrated in our culture, so there are numerous incentives for couples to formalize their relationship with a wedding ceremony. A healthy marriage provides emotional support by combining the benefits of friendship and a loving committed relationship. A happy marriage also provides stability for both the couple and for those involved in the couple's life. Considerable research indicates that married people live longer, feel happier, remain mentally alert longer, engage in less risky behavior, take better care of themselves, engage in sex more often, have higher incomes and better health insurance, and suffer fewer physical and mental health problems.[30] Even people who divorce seem to miss being married; nearly 80 percent of them remarry.

While a successful marriage can bring much satisfaction, traditional marriage does not work for everyone. Some research suggests that today's women who choose marriage may not be as happy as their mothers were.[31] This may reflect increasing pressure on women to perform multiple roles, such as taking care of a family while working outside the home. Other studies suggest that the happiness of men who have never married has increased. Traditional marriage is not the only path to a successful committed relationship.

Cohabitation

Cohabitation is defined as two unmarried people with an intimate connection who live together in the same household. For a variety of reasons, increasing numbers of Americans are choosing cohabitation. These relationships can be stable and happy, with a high level of commitment between the partners. In some states, cohabitation that lasts a designated number of years (usually seven) legally constitutes a **common-law marriage** for purposes of purchasing real estate and sharing other financial obligations.

Cohabitation can offer many of the same benefits that marriage does: love, sex, companionship, and the ongoing opportunity to know a partner better over time. In addition to enjoying emotional and physical benefits, some people may cohabit for practical reasons, such as the opportunity to share bills and housing costs. Although many cohabitors are young, some older adults choose this lifestyle because they would lose income, such as Social Security or a late spouse's pension, if they were to marry.

Successful cohabitations also can offer benefits not found in marriage. Partners may feel greater autonomy and independence than they might find in a traditional arrangement. Furthermore, if they decide to separate, they do not experience the legal problems and expense of a divorce.

Although cohabitation has its advantages, it also has some drawbacks. Perhaps the greatest disadvantage is the lack of societal validation for the relationship. Many cohabitors must deal with pressures from parents and friends, difficulties in obtaining insurance and tax benefits, and legal issues over property. In 1996, Congress reaffirmed tax advantages for married couples and effectively blocked cohabiting heterosexual and homosexual couples from these benefits through the "Defense of Marriage Bill." Today, controversy continues over whether traditional marriage should remain the only means of eligibility for tax deductions, health insurance, and other benefits. In general, there appears to be a trend toward recognizing the validity of unmarried relationships. The state of Vermont, for example, has passed a law that allows partners to form "civil unions."[32] Also, some companies now offer insurance benefits to employees' unmarried partners.

Gay and Lesbian Partnerships

Most adults want intimate, committed relationships, whether they are gay or straight, men or women. Lesbians and gay men seek the same things in primary relationships that heterosexual partners do: friendship, communication, validation, companionship, and a sense of stability.

The 2000 U.S. Census revealed a significant increase in the number of same-sex partner households across the country—more than three times the total reported in the 1990 Census. The states with the most reported same-sex households are California, New York, Florida, Illinois, and Georgia. According to Lee Badgett, research director of the Institute for Gay and Lesbian Strategic Studies, the actual number of households is probably much higher. Many gay and lesbian partners hesitate to report their relationship because of concerns about discrimination.[33]

Studies of lesbian couples indicate high levels of attachment and satisfaction and a tendency toward monogamous, long-term relationships. Gay men, too, tend to form committed, long-term relationships, especially as they age, much like their heterosexual counterparts.

Challenges to successful lesbian and gay male relationships often stem from discrimination and from difficulties dealing with social, legal, and religious doctrines. For lesbian and gay couples, obtaining the same level of marriage benefits, such as tax deductions, power-of-attorney, and other rights, continues to be a challenge. However, commitment ceremonies and marriage ceremonies are becoming more frequent in the United States and in several foreign countries. As mentioned above, Vermont now recognizes same-sex civil unions.[34]

Staying Single

Increasing numbers of adults of all ages are electing to remain single. In 1970, 18.9 percent of adult men and 13.7 percent of adult women had decided that marriage wasn't for them. By the year 2000, the proportion of adult Americans who were single by choice or by chance (sometimes after failed marriages) had increased significantly to more than 44 percent of men and over 48 percent of women.[35] According to most figures from the Census Bureau and National Center for Health Statistics, the number of unmarried women aged 15 and older soon will surpass the number of married women.[36] The number of unmarried men also is increasing. Other changes are reflected in the following facts:

- More than 10 percent of all people say they would never marry.
- People marrying today have more than a 50 percent chance of divorcing.
- As more women enjoy financial independence, they are less likely to remarry after divorce.
- Increasing numbers of widows and widowers are opting not to remarry.

Cohabitation Living together without being married.

Common-law marriage Cohabitation lasting a designated period of time (usually seven years) that is considered legally binding in some states.

- The number of households composed of unmarried couples is steadily increasing
- The percentage of children living with one parent has increased from 9 percent in 1960 to 28 percent in 2002.[37]

Today, large numbers of people prefer to remain single. Singles clubs, social outings arranged by communities and religious groups, extended family environments, and a large number of social services support the single lifestyle. Many singles live rich, rewarding lives and maintain a large network of close friends and families. Although sexual intimacy may or may not be present, the intimacy achieved through other interactions with loved ones is a key aspect of the single lifestyle.

Some research indicates that single people live shorter lives, are more unhappy, and are more likely to experience financial and health problems than are their married peers. However, other studies refute these conclusions. Few research studies to date have controlled for other confounding variables, such as environmental conditions, past histories, and other factors that may carry more weight than the married or single state.

What do you think?

Although there are advantages and disadvantages in marriage, many people feel that marriage is a desirable option. Are there advantages in remaining single? ❋ *Are there potential disadvantages?* ❋ *Are there any societal or organizational supports for the single lifestyle?*

Success in Relationships

Most people's definition of success in a relationship tends to be based on whether a couple stays together over the years. Learning to communicate, respecting each other, and sharing a genuine fondness are crucial to relationship success. Many social scientists agree that the happiest committed relationships are flexible enough to allow the partners to grow throughout their lives.

Partnering Scripts

Parents often believe that their children will achieve happiness by living much as they have. Accordingly, most children

---

Accountability Accepting responsibility for personal decisions, choices, and actions.

Self-nurturance Developing individual potential through a balanced and realistic appreciation of self-worth and ability.

---

are reared with a very strong script for what is expected of them as adults. Each group in society has its own partnering script that prescribes standards regarding sex, age, social class, race, religion, physical attributes, and personality types. By adolescence, people generally know exactly what type of person they are expected to befriend or date. By which partnering script were you raised? Just picture whom you could or couldn't bring home to meet your family.

Society provides constant reinforcement for traditional couples, but it may withhold this reinforcement from couples of the same sex, mixed race, mixed religion, or mixed age. People who have not chosen an "appropriate" partner are subject to a great deal of external stress. In addition to denying recognition to such couples, friends and family often blame the "inappropriateness" of the couple if the relationship fails.

Nonetheless, many nontraditional relationships survive and flourish. For example, the number of interracial marriages has quadrupled since the late 1960s, and the number of same-sex partner households has grown from 145,130 to almost a half-million over the past ten years.[38] Recognizing that this stress is external to the relationship can help alleviate criticism and distancing between the partners.

Being Self-Nurturant

It is often stated that you must love yourself before you can love someone else. What does this mean? Learning how you function emotionally and how to nurture yourself through all life's situations is a lifelong task. You should certainly not postpone intimate connections with others until you have achieved this state. However, a certain level of individual maturity helps in maintaining a committed relationship. For example, divorce rates are much higher for couples under age 30 than for older couples.

Two concepts that are especially important to a good relationship are accountability and self-nurturance. **Accountability** means that both partners in a relationship see themselves as responsible for their own decisions, choices, and actions. They don't hold the other person responsible for positive or negative experiences.

Self-nurturance, which goes hand in hand with accountability, means developing individual potential through a balanced and realistic appreciation of self-worth and ability. In order to make good choices in life, a person needs to balance many physical and emotional needs, including sleeping, eating, exercising, working, relaxing, and socializing. When the balance is disrupted, as it will inevitably be, self-nurturing people are patient with themselves and try to put things back on course. It is a lifelong process to learn to live in a balanced and healthy way. Two people who are on a path of accountability and self-nurturance together have a much better chance of maintaining a satisfying relationship.

Table 5.1
The Emerging Twenty-First-Century American Family

	Percentage of Children in Various Types of Families				
	One Single Parent	Two Parents, Continuing	Two Parents, Remarried	Two Adults, Ex-Married	Adults, Never married
1972	4.7	73.0	9.9	3.8	8.6
1978	10.2	65.3	13.6	4.0	6.9
1982	14.3	59.3	13.7	5.2	7.3
1988	18.6	54.7	13.0	5.0	8.7
1990	14.9	56.1	17.9	5.1	6.0
1994	18.4	52.8	14.7	7.1	7.0
1998	18.2	51.7	12.3	8.6	9.2

Note: Single parent = only one adult in household; *two parents, continuing* = married couple, never divorced; *two parents, remarried* = married couple, at least one remarried (unknown whether children came before or after remarriage); *two adults, ex-married* = two or more adults, previously but not currently married; *adults, never married* = two or more adults, never married (this category also included some other family structures).
Source: General Social Survey News, no. 13, August 1999. Published by the National Opinion Research Center.

Having Children . . . or Not?

When a couple decides to raise children, their relationship changes. Resources of time, energy, and money are split many ways, and the partners no longer have each other's undivided attention. Babies and young children do not time their requests for food, sleep, and care to the convenience of adults. Therefore, individuals or couples whose own basic needs for security, love, and purpose already are met make better parents. Any stresses that already exist in a relationship will be further accentuated when parenting is added to the list of responsibilities. Having a child does not save a bad relationship—in fact, it only seems to compound the problems that already exist. A child cannot and should not be expected to provide the parents with self-esteem and security.

Changing patterns in family life affect the way children are raised. In modern society, it is not always clear which partner will adjust his or her work schedule to provide the primary care of children. Nearly a half-million children each year become part of a blended family when their parents remarry; remarriage creates a new family of stepparents and stepsiblings. In addition, an increasing number of individuals are choosing to have children in a family structure other than a heterosexual marriage. Single women can choose adoption or alternative (formerly called "artificial") insemination as a way to create a family. Single men can choose to adopt or to obtain the services of a surrogate mother. According to the 2000 census more than 9 percent of all U.S. households were headed by a man or woman raising a child alone, which reflects a growing trend in America and in the international community (see Table 5.1).[39] Regardless of the structure of the family, certain factors remain important to the well-being

of the unit: consistency, communication, affection, and mutual respect.

Some people become parents without a lot of forethought. Some children are born into a relationship that was supposed to last and didn't. This does not mean it is too late to do a good job of parenting. Children are amazingly resilient and forgiving if parents show respect and communicate about household activities that affect their lives. Even children who grow up in a household of conflict can feel loved and respected if the parents treat them fairly. This means that parents must take responsibility for their own conflicts and make it clear to children that they are not the reason for the conflict.

Today, many families discover that two incomes are needed just to make ends meet. That's why more than 80 percent of all mothers with children under the age of five work outside the home. Day care, extended family and friends, grandparents, neighbors, and nannies "mind the kids." Some employers offer family leave arrangements that allow parents more latitude in taking time from work. Consider the financial implications of deciding to have a child: It is estimated that a low-income family that had a child in 2002 will spend about $169,750 to raise the child over the next 17 years; this does not take into account the costs of college.[40]

What do you think?

What characteristics of a healthy family environment are important to you? ✳ *Do you think that day care centers, extended family units, and full-time baby-sitters can provide a positive environment for children?* ✳ *Why or why not?*

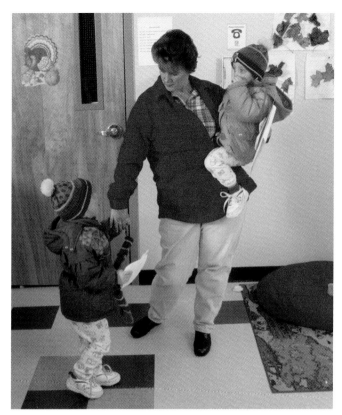

Single parents face additional challenges in juggling their work and family responsibilities. Many use community resources such as after-school day care centers.

When Relationships Falter

Breakdowns in relationships usually begin with a change in communication, however subtle. Either partner may stop listening and cease to be emotionally present for the other. In turn, the other feels ignored, unappreciated, or unwanted. Unresolved conflicts increase, and unresolved anger can cause problems in sexual relations.

When a couple who previously enjoyed spending time alone together find themselves continually in the company of others, spending time apart, or preferring to stay home alone, it may be a sign that the relationship is in trouble. Of course, the need for individual privacy is not a cause for worry—it's essential to health. If, however, a partner decides to change the amount and quality of time spent together without the input or understanding of the other, it may be a sign of hidden problems.

College students, particularly those who are socially isolated and far from family and hometown friends, may be particularly vulnerable to staying in unhealthy relationships. They may become emotionally dependent on a partner for everything from eating meals to recreational and study time; mutual obligations such as shared rental arrangements, transportation, and child care can make it tough to leave.

It's also easy to mistake unwanted sexual advances for physical attraction or love. Without a network of friends and supporters with whom a student can talk, obtain validation for feelings, or share concerns, he or she may feel stuck in a relationship that is headed nowhere.

Honesty and verbal affection are usually positive aspects of a relationship. In a troubled relationship, however, they can be used to cover up irresponsible or hurtful behavior. "At least I was honest" is not an acceptable substitute for acting in a trustworthy way. "But I really do love you" is not a license for acting inconsiderate or rude.

Most communities have trained therapists who specialize in relationship difficulties, and most student health centers offer these services at reduced fees for students. If you are unaware of such services, ask your instructor for suggestions.

When and Why Relationships End

Based on recent statistics, it has been predicted that 20 percent of those who marry today will divorce within five years; one-third may divorce within ten years; and 40 percent will divorce before their fifteenth anniversary. Ultimately, half of all marriages will end in divorce.[41] While these numbers may seem alarming, the actual number of failed relationships is probably much higher. Many people never go through a legal divorce process and therefore are not counted in these statistics. Cohabitors and unmarried partners who raise children, own homes together, and exhibit all the outward appearances of marriage without the license also are not included.

Relationships end for many reasons, including illness, financial concerns, and career problems. Other breakups arise from unmet expectations. Many people enter a relationship with certain expectations about how they and their partner will behave. Failure to communicate these beliefs to a partner can lead to resentment and disappointment. Differences in sexual needs also may contribute to the demise of a relationship.

Under stress, communication and cooperation between partners can break down. One of the greatest predictors of divorce appears to be husband dissatisfaction in the first five years of marriage.

> **What do you think?**
> *What factors do you think contribute to the U.S. divorce rate? ✳ How would you explain Americans' attitudes about marriage and divorce to a friend from another country?*

Coping with Loneliness

When a relationship ends, it is normal to experience painful emotions of anger, guilt, rejection, and unworthiness. No matter how miserable the relationship was, feelings of failure are common. Counselors estimate that it takes at least a year

Table 5.2
Key Factors Predicting Success and Failure in Marriages and Relationships

Traits that Predict Success

Individual
- High self-esteem
- Flexibility
- Assertiveness
- Sociability

Couple
- Similarity
- Long acquaintanceship
- Good communication skills
- Good conflict-resolution skills

Context
- Older age
- Healthy family-of-origin experiences
- Happy parental marriage
- Parents' and friends' approval
- Significant educational career preparation

Traits that Predict Failure

Individual
- Neurotic characteristics
- Anxiety, depression, impulsiveness, anger/hostility
- Self-consciousness
- Vulnerability to stress
- Dysfunctional beliefs

Couple
- Dissimilarity
- Short acquaintanceship Premarital sex with many partners
- Premarital pregnancy
- Cohabitation
- Poor communication and conflict-resolution skills

Context
- Younger age
- Unhealthy family-of-origin experiences
- Parental divorce or chronic conflict
- Parents' and friends' disapproval
- Pressure to marry
- Little education or career preparation

Common Reasons for Marriage and Relationship Failure
- Poor communication
- Financial problems
- Lack of commitment to the marriage
- Dramatic change in priorities
- Infidelity
- Failed expectations or unmet needs
- Addictions and substance abuse
- Physical, sexual, or emotional abuse
- Lack of conflict-resolution skills

Source: American Academy of Matrimonial Lawyers, 2000. "Making Marriage Last." www.aaml.org/Marriage_Last/MarriageMain.htm

and often longer to recover from the loss of a major relationship, whether by death or separation.

Although it may be painful, reflecting on the past relationship can help prevent similar mistakes in the future. Concentrating on the negative aspects of an ex-partner is a natural tendency, but it is equally important to remember what you loved in the other person and what is lovable about you. When we accept the risk and challenge of close relationships, we accept one of the greatest gifts life has to offer. With time, support from others, and community or professional help, most people recover and establish rewarding new relationships.

Building Better Relationships

Most relationships start with great optimism and true love. So why do so many run into trouble? "We just don't know how to handle the negative feelings that are the unavoidable by-product of the differences between two people, the very differences that attract them to each other in the first place. Think of it as the friction any two bodies would generate rubbing against each other countless times each day," says Howard Markman, Ph.D., professor of psychology at the

University of Denver.[42] According to Markman, most unhappy couples don't need therapy; they need education in how relationships work and the special skills that make them work well. Markman and others promote **psychoeducation,** the teaching of crucial psychological skills that give people knowledge so they can help themselves. Psychoeducation courses aren't therapy per se, but they typically have a therapeutic effect on couples.

Elements of Healthy Relationships

Satisfying and stable relationships are characterized by good communication, intimacy, friendship, and other factors discussed in this chapter. In addition, they share certain identifiable traits (Table 5.2). A key ingredient is **trust,** the degree of

Psychoeducation   The teaching of crucial psychological skills that give people knowledge so they can help themselves.

Trust   The degree of confidence partners feel in a relationship.

confidence partners feel in a relationship. Without trust, intimacy will not develop, and the relationship could fail. Trust includes three fundamental elements.

- *Predictability* means that you can predict your partner's behavior, based on the knowledge that your partner acts in consistently positive ways.
- *Dependability* means that you can rely on your partner to give support in all situations, particularly those in which you feel threatened with hurt or rejection.
- *Faith* means that you feel absolutely certain about your partner's intentions and behavior.

Trust can develop even when it is initially lacking. This requires opening yourself to others, which carries the risk of hurt or rejection.

Other characteristics of happy relationships include:

- Partners interpret each other's behavior in the context of their own relationship, without overreacting to behaviors that remind them of past relationships.
- Partners who like each other and find each other interesting are happier than those who don't. Although most relationships have their share of ups and downs, members of successful couples are able to talk, listen, and touch each other in an atmosphere of caring.
- Sexual intimacy is a major component of healthy relationships, but sex is not a major reason for the existence of the relationship. Some couples admit to sexual dissatisfaction but find the relationship more important than sexual satisfaction. Many couples report that as communication and trust increase, the sexual relationship also improves.
- Another important quality is a shared and cherished history, including private jokes, special places where key events have occurred, nicknames, rituals, emotions, and significant shared time and activities.

Sexual identity   Acknowledgement of oneself as a sexual being; a composite of biological sex, gender roles, gender identity, and sexual orientation.

Gonads   The reproductive organs in a male (testes) or female (ovaries).

Puberty   The period of sexual maturation.

Pituitary gland   The endocrine gland controlling the release of hormones from the gonads.

Secondary sex characteristics   Characteristics associated with gender but not directly related to reproduction, such as vocal pitch, degree of body hair, and location of fat deposits.

Gender   The psychological condition of being feminine or masculine as defined by the society in which one lives.

Socialization   Process by which a society communicates behavioral expectations to its individual members.

Your Sexual Identity

Sexual identity, the acknowledgment of oneself as a sexual being, is determined by a complex interaction of genetic, physiological, environmental, and social factors. The beginning of sexual identity occurs at conception with the combining of chromosomes that determine sex. The biological father determines whether a baby will be a boy or a girl. All eggs (ova) carry an X sex chromosome; sperm may carry either an X or a Y chromosome. If a sperm carrying an X chromosome fertilizes an egg, the resulting combination of sex chromosomes (XX) provides the blueprint to produce a female. If a sperm carrying a Y chromosome fertilizes an egg, the XY combination produces a male.

The genetic instructions included in the sex chromosomes lead to the differential development of male and female **gonads** (reproductive organs) at about the eighth week of fetal life. Once the male gonads (testes) and the female gonads (ovaries) are developed, they play a key role in all future sexual development because the gonads are responsible for the production of sex hormones. The primary sex hormones produced by females are estrogen and progesterone. In males, the sex hormone of primary importance is testosterone. The release of testosterone in a maturing fetus signals the development of a penis and other male genitals. If no testosterone is produced, female genitals form.

At the time of **puberty,** the period of sexual maturation, sex hormones again play major roles in development. Hormones released by the **pituitary gland,** called gonadotropins, stimulate the testes and ovaries to make appropriate sex hormones. The increase of estrogen production in females and testosterone production in males leads to the development of **secondary sex characteristics.** Male secondary sex characteristics include deepening of the voice, development of facial and body hair, and growth of the skeleton and musculature. Female secondary sex characteristics include growth of the breasts, widening of the hips, and the development of pubic and underarm hair.

Thus far, we have described sexual identity only in terms of a person's biology. While biology is an important facet of sexual identity, the relationship of biology and culture is much more complicated than the popular notion of sex as biology and gender as social. Biological facts are always understood and interpreted within the cultural framework that gives meaning to those facts. Sex simply refers to the biological condition of being male or female based on physiological and hormonal differences.

Gender is the practice of behaving in masculine or feminine ways as defined by the society in which one lives. It is a component of our identity, while sex is more related to physical form and function. In this sense, gender is a performance, something we do rather than something we have. We learn gender through the process of **socialization** in which society communicates behavioral expectations to its members. Through interactions with family, peers, teachers, media, and other social organizations, we learn to act in ways that society deems appropriate. Think about the television shows you watch. Do the characters play out traditional gender roles?

Each of us expresses our maleness or femaleness to others on a daily basis by the **gender roles** we play. **Gender identity** refers to the personal sense or awareness of being masculine or feminine, a male or a female. It sometimes may be difficult to express one's true sexual identity because of the bounds established by **gender-role stereotypes,** or generalizations about how males and females should express themselves and the characteristics each possesses. Our traditional sex roles are an example of gender-role stereotyping. Men are thought to be independent, aggressive, better in math and science, logical, and always in control of their emotions. Women, on the other hand, traditionally are expected to be passive, nurturing, intuitive, sensitive, and emotional. Many of these stereotypes have been refuted in recent years.

Androgyny is the combination of traditional masculine and feminine traits in a single person. Androgynous people do not always follow traditional sex roles but rather try to act appropriately based on the given situation.

Transsexuality, also known as *gender dysphoria,* refers to a condition in which a person is in a state of conflict between gender identity and physical sex. Transsexuals have the sex-related structures in their brains of one sex, but the physical sex organs of the other sex. Simply stated, a transsexual is a mind physically trapped in the body of the opposite sex. The condition is not related to sexual orientation, nor should it be confused with transvestism or cross-dressing.

Another variation in identity is **intersexuality.** This refers to a medical condition in which a person is born with sex chromosomes, external genitalia, and/or an internal reproductive system that has both male and female components. Some of these individuals may not even be aware that their internal reproductive organs are unusual, while others may have external evidence. There is great variation in the manifestations of the condition.

What transsexuals and intersexed persons have in common are their experiences of stigma and misunderstanding from others, which often leads to social isolation. With treatment, support, and understanding, transsexual and intersexed individuals can lead normal, healthy lives.

By now you can see that defining sexual identity is not a simple matter. It is a lifelong process of growing and learning. Your sexual identity is made up of the unique combination of your sex, gender identity, chosen gender roles, sexual orientation, and personal experiences. No other person on this earth is exactly like you, and it is up to you to take every opportunity to get to know and like yourself so that you may enjoy your life to the fullest.

> **What do you think?**
>
> *How often do you challenge existing gender-role stereotypes?* ✳ *What is the outcome?* ✳ *Do you think men and women have the same degree of freedom in gender-role expression?*

Sexual Anatomy and Physiology

An understanding of the functions of the male and female reproductive systems will help you derive pleasure and satisfaction from your sexual relationships, be sensitive to your partner's wants and needs, and make responsible choices regarding your own sexual health.

Female Sexual Anatomy and Physiology

The female reproductive system includes two major groups of structures, the external genitals (Figure 5.2 on page 124) and the internal genitals. The **external female genitals** include all structures that are outwardly visible; they are referred to as the vulva. Specifically, the **vulva,** or external genitalia, includes the mons pubis, the labia minora and majora, the clitoris, the urethral and vaginal openings, and the vestibule of the vagina and its glands. The **mons pubis** is a pad of fatty tissue covering the pubic bone. The mons protects the pubic bone, and after puberty it becomes covered with coarse hair. The **labia minora** are inner lips or folds of mucus membrane, and the **labia majora** are folds of skin and erectile tissue that enclose the urethral and vaginal openings. The labia minora are found just inside the labia majora.

Gender roles   Expression of maleness or femaleness in everyday life.

Gender identity   Personal sense or awareness of being masculine or feminine, a male or a female.

Gender-role stereotypes   Generalizations about how males and females should express themselves and the characteristics each possesses.

Androgyny   Combination of traditional masculine and feminine traits in a single person.

Transsexuality   Condition in which a person is psychologically of one sex but physically of the other; also called gender dysphoria.

Intersexuality   Not exhibiting exclusively male or female secondary sex characteristics.

External female genitals   The mons pubis, labia majora and minora, clitoris, urethral and vaginal openings, and the vestibule of the vagina and its glands.

Vulva   The female's external genitalia.

Mons pubis   Fatty tissue covering the pubic bone in females; in physically mature women, the mons is covered with coarse hair.

Labia minora   "Inner lips," or folds of mucus membrane just inside the labia majora.

Labia majora   "Outer lips," or folds of skin and erectile tissue that cover the female sexual organs.

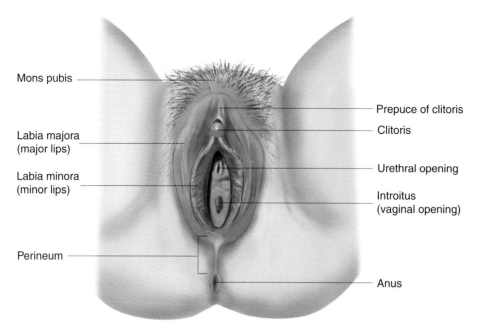

Figure 5.2
External Female Genital Structures
Source: From R. D. McAnulty and M. M. Burnette, *Exploring Human Sexuality: Making Healthy Decisions* (Boston: Allyn & Bacon, 2001). Copyright © 2001 by Pearson Education.

The **clitoris** is the female sexual organ whose only known function is sexual pleasure. It is located at the upper end of the labia minora and beneath the mons pubis. Directly below the clitoris is the urethral opening through which urine is expelled from the body. Below the **urethral opening** is the vaginal opening, or opening to the vagina. In some women, the vaginal opening is covered by a thin membrane called the **hymen.** It is a myth that an intact hymen is proof of virginity. The **perineum** is the tissue between the vulva and the anus. Although not technically part of the external genitalia, the tissue in this area has many nerve endings and is sensitive to touch; it can play a part in sexual excitement.

The **internal female genitals** of the reproductive system include the vagina, uterus, fallopian tubes, and ovaries (Figure 5.3). The **vagina** is a tubular organ that serves as a passageway from the uterus to the outside of a female's body. This passageway allows menstrual flow to exit from the uterus during a woman's monthly cycle and serves as the birth canal during childbirth. The vagina also receives the penis during intercourse. The **uterus,** also known as the **womb,** is a hollow, muscular, pear-shaped organ. Hormones acting on the soft, spongy matter that makes up the inner lining of the uterus, called the **endometrium,** either prepare the uterus for implantation and development of a fertilized egg or signal that no fertilization has taken place, in which case the endometrium deteriorates and becomes menstrual flow.

The lower end of the uterus, the **cervix,** extends down into the vagina. The **ovaries** are almond-sized structures suspended on either side of the uterus. The ovaries produce the hormones estrogen and progesterone and are also the reservoir for developing eggs. All the eggs a female will ever have are present in the ovaries at birth. Eggs mature and are released from the ovaries in response to hormone levels. Extending from the upper end of the uterus are two thin,

Clitoris   A pea-sized nodule of tissue located at the top of the labia minora.

Urethral opening   The opening through which urine is expelled.

Hymen   Thin membrane covering the vaginal opening.

Perineum   Tissue between the vulva to the anus.

Internal female genitals   The vagina, uterus, fallopian tubes, and ovaries.

Vagina   The passageway in females that leads from the uterus to the vulva.

Uterus (womb)   Hollow, muscular, pear-shaped organ whose function is to contain the developing fetus.

Endometrium   Soft, spongy matter that makes up the uterine lining.

Cervix   Lower end of the uterus, which extends into the vagina.

Ovaries   Almond-sized organs suspended on either side of the uterus that house developing eggs and produce hormones.

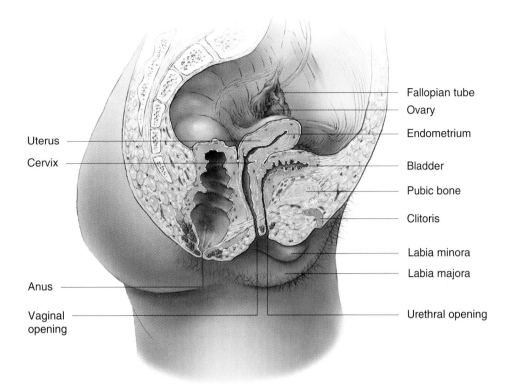

Figure 5.3
Side View of the Female Reproductive Organs

flexible tubes called the **fallopian tubes.** The fallopian tubes are where sperm and egg meet and fertilization takes place. Following fertilization, the fallopian tubes serve as the passageway to the uterus, where the fertilized egg becomes implanted and development continues.

The Onset of Puberty and the Menstrual Cycle With the onset of puberty, the female reproductive system matures, and the development of secondary sex characteristics transforms young girls into young women. The first sign of puberty is the development of breast buds, which occurs around age 11. Under the direction of the endocrine system, the pituitary gland, the **hypothalamus,** and the ovaries all secrete hormones that act as chemical messengers among them. Working in a feedback system, hormonal levels in the bloodstream act as the trigger mechanism for release of more or different hormones.

Around age 9½ to 11½, the hypothalamus receives the message to begin secreting **gonadotropin-releasing hormone (GnRH).** The release of GnRH in turn signals the pituitary gland to release hormones called gonadotropins. Two gonadotropins, **follicle-stimulating hormone (FSH)** and **luteinizing hormone (LH),** signal the ovaries to start producing **estrogens** and **progesterone.** Increased estrogen levels assist in the development of female secondary sex characteristics. In addition, estrogens regulate the menstrual cycle. Progesterone helps keep the endometrium developing in order to nourish a fertilized egg; it also helps maintain pregnancy.

The normal age range for the onset of the first menstrual period, the **menarche,** is 9 to 17 years, with the average age being 11½ to 13½ years. Body fat heavily influences

Fallopian tubes Two thin, flexible tubes that extend from the ovaries to the uterus; the sperm and the egg meet here and fertilization takes place.

Hypothalamus An area of the brain located near the pituitary gland; works in conjunction with the pituitary gland to control reproductive functions.

Gonadotropin-releasing hormone (GnRH) Hormone that signals the pituitary gland to release gonadotropins.

Follicle-stimulating hormone (FSH) Hormone that signals the ovaries to prepare to release eggs and to begin producing estrogens.

Luteinizing hormone (LH) Hormone that signals the ovaries to release an egg and to begin producing progesterone.

Estrogens Hormones that control the menstrual cycle.

Progesterone Hormone secreted by the ovaries; helps keep the endometrium developing in order to nourish a fertilized egg; also helps maintain pregnancy.

Menarche The first menstrual period.

the onset of puberty, and increasing rates of obesity in children may account for the fact that girls here and in other countries seem to be reaching puberty much earlier than they used to.[43] Very thin girls, such as young athletes, tend to start menstruating later.

The average menstrual cycle is 28 days and consists of two phases: the *menstrual/proliferative* (also known as the follicular) phase, and the *secretory* or *luteal* phase. During the proliferative phase, the pituitary gland releases FSH and LH. The FSH acts on the ovaries to stimulate the maturation process of several **ovarian follicles (egg sacs),** areas within the ovaries in which individual eggs develop. These follicles secrete estrogens. In response to this estrogen stimulation, the lining of the uterus, the endometrium, begins to grow and develop. The inner walls of the uterus become coated with a thick, spongy lining composed of blood and mucus. In the event of fertilization, this endometrial tissue will become a nesting place for the developing embryo. The increased estrogen level also signals the pituitary to slow down FSH production but increase LH secretion. Of the several follicles developing in the ovaries, only one each month normally reaches complete maturity. Under the influence of LH, this follicle rapidly matures; about the fourteenth day of the proliferative phase, it releases an ovum into the fallopian tube—a process called **ovulation.** Just prior to ovulation, the mature egg's follicle begins to increase secretion of progesterone, the first function of which is to spur the addition of further nutrients to the developing endometrium.

After ovulation, the secretory phase begins. The ovarian follicle is converted into the *corpus luteum,* or yellow body, which continues to secrete estrogen and progesterone but in decreasing amounts. In addition, FSH also falls back to preproliferative levels. Essentially, the woman's body is waiting to see whether fertilization will occur. During this time, LH declines and progesterone levels begin to rise, which causes additional tissue growth in the endometrium.

Ovarian follicles (egg sacs)   Areas within the ovaries in which individual eggs develop.

Ovulation   The point of the menstrual cycle at which a mature egg is released into the fallopian tube.

Human chorionic gonadotropin (HCG)   Hormone that increases estrogen and progesterone secretion if fertilization has taken place.

Menopause   The permanent cessation of menstruation.

Hormone replacement therapy (HRT)   Use of synthetic or animal estrogen and progesterone to compensate for decreases in hormones in a woman's body.

External male genitals   The penis and scrotum.

Internal male genitals   The testes, epididymides, vasa deferentia, ejaculatory ducts, urethra, and accessory glands.

If fertilization takes place, cells surrounding the developing embryo release a hormone called **human chorionic gonadotropin (HCG).** HCG increases estrogen and progesterone secretion, which maintains the endometrium while signaling the pituitary gland not to start a new menstrual cycle.

When fertilization does not occur, the egg disintegrates within approximately 72 hours. The corpus luteum gradually becomes nonfunctional, which causes levels of progesterone and estrogen to decline. As hormonal levels decrease, the endometrial lining of the uterus loses its nourishment, dies, and is sloughed off as menstrual flow.

For more information on issues associated with menstruation such as premenstrual syndrome, toxic shock syndrome, and dysmenorrhea (painful menstruation), see Chapter 14.

Menopause   Just as menarche signals the beginning of a woman's reproductive years, **menopause**—the permanent cessation of menstruation—signals the end. Generally occurring between the ages of 40 and 60, and at age 51 on average, menopause results in decreased estrogen levels, which may produce troublesome symptoms in some women. Decreased vaginal lubrication, hot flashes, headaches, dizziness, and joint pains all have been associated with the onset of menopause. Hormones, such as synthetic or animal estrogen and progesterone through **hormone replacement therapy (HRT),** have long been prescribed to compensate for decreases of hormones in a woman's body, relieve menopausal symptoms, and reduce the risk of heart disease and osteoporosis. (In 2002 the National Institutes of Health adopted the term *menopausal hormone therapy* because hormone treatment is not a replacement and does not restore the physiology of youth.) However, recent studies indicate that HRT actually may increase the risk of cardiovascular problems, blood clots, and breast cancer.

Other studies continue to support HRT for osteoporosis benefits and reductions in menopausal symptoms.[44] All women need to discuss the risks and benefits of HRT with their health care provider and come to an informed decision. It is crucial to find a doctor who specializes in women's health and keeps up to date with the latest research findings. Certainly lifestyle changes, such as regular exercise, a healthy diet, and adequate calcium, also can help protect postmenopausal women from heart disease and osteoporosis.

Male Sexual Anatomy and Physiology

The structures of the male reproductive system may be divided into external and internal genitals (Figure 5.4). The penis and the scrotum make up the **external male genitals.** The **internal male genitals** include the testes, epididymides, vasa deferentia, ejaculatory ducts, and urethra, and three other structures—the seminal vesicles, the prostate gland,

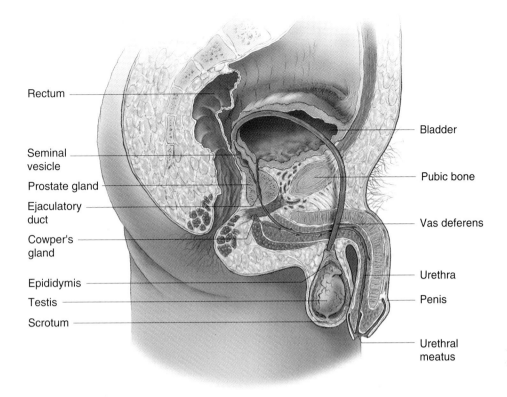

Rectum

Seminal vesicle

Prostate gland

Ejaculatory duct

Cowper's gland

Epididymis

Testis

Scrotum

Bladder

Pubic bone

Vas deferens

Urethra

Penis

Urethral meatus

Figure 5.4
Side View of the Male Reproductive Organs

and the Cowper's glands—that secrete components which, with sperm, make up semen. These three structures are sometimes referred to as the **accessory glands.**

The **penis** serves as the organ that deposits sperm in the vagina during intercourse. The urethra, which passes through the center of the penis, acts as the passageway for both semen and urine to exit the body. During sexual arousal, the spongy tissue in the penis becomes filled with blood, which makes the organ stiff, or erect. Further sexual excitement leads to **ejaculation,** a series of rapid spasmodic contractions that propel semen out of the penis.

Situated behind the penis and also outside the body is a sac called the **scrotum.** The scrotum protects the testes and also helps control the temperature within the testes, which is vital to proper sperm production. The **testes** (singular: *testis*) are egg-shaped structures in which sperm are manufactured. The testes also contain cells that manufacture **testosterone,** the hormone responsible for the development of male secondary sex characteristics.

The development of sperm is referred to as **spermatogenesis.** Like the maturation of eggs in the female, this process is governed by the pituitary gland. FSH is secreted into the bloodstream to stimulate the testes to manufacture sperm. Immature sperm are released into a comma-shaped structure on the back of the testis called the **epididymis** (plural: *epididymides*), where they ripen and reach full maturity.

The epididymis contains coiled tubules that gradually straighten out to become the **vas deferens.** The two vasa deferentia, which is plural for vas deferens, make up the tubular

Accessory glands   The seminal vesicles, prostate gland, and Cowper's glands.

Penis   Male sexual organ that releases sperm into the vagina during intercourse.

Ejaculation   The propulsion of semen from the penis.

Scrotum   Sac of tissue behind the penis and outside the body that encloses the testes.

Testes   Two organs, located in the scrotum, that manufacture sperm and produce hormones.

Testosterone   The male sex hormone manufactured in the testes.

Spermatogenesis   The development of sperm.

Epididymis   A comma-shaped structure on the back of the testis where sperm mature.

Vas deferens   A tube that transports sperm toward the penis.

Ritual Genital Mutilation

Despite hundreds of years of tradition, Hajia Zuwera Kassindja would not let it happen to her 17-year-old daughter, Fauziya. Hajia's own sister had died from it. So Hajia gave her daughter all her savings, which amounted to only $3,500, and left Hajia a pauper. Fauziya used the money to flee from the African country of Togo. Upon arrival in the United States, Fauziya requested asylum from persecution. After she spent a year in prison, government officials finally agreed that Fauziya was fleeing persecution, and she was allowed to remain in the United States, where she now lives. From what had Hajia's sister died? From what was Fauziya escaping? Ritual genital mutilation. This report is only an example of a surprisingly common problem.

Cultures in some parts of Africa and the Middle East ritually mutilate or remove the entire clitoris or, in some cases, just the clitoral hood. Removal of the clitoris, called a clitoridectomy, is a rite of initiation into womanhood in many of these predominantly Islamic cultures. It often is performed as a puberty ritual in late childhood or early adolescence.

The clitoris gives rise to feelings of sexual pleasure in women. A reason given for its removal or mutilation is to ensure the girl's chastity, because it is assumed that uncircumcised girls are consumed with sexual desires. Some groups in rural Egypt and in the northern Sudan perform clitoridectomies primarily because it is a social custom that has been passed down from ancient times. Some perceive it as part of their faith in Islam. However, neither Islam nor any other religion requires it. Ironically, many young women do not grasp that they are victims. They assume that clitoridectomy is part of being female.

Clitoridectomies are performed under unsanitary conditions without benefit of anesthesia. Medical complications are common, including infections, bleeding, tissue scarring, painful menstruation, and obstructed labor. The procedure is psychologically traumatizing. An even more radical form of clitoridectomy, called infibulation or pharaonic circumcision, is practiced widely in the Sudan. Pharaonic circumcision involves complete removal of the clitoris along with the labia minora and the inner layers of the labia majora. After removal of the skin tissue, the raw edges of the labia majora are sewn together. Only a tiny opening is left to allow passage of urine and menstrual discharge. The sewing together of the vulva may be intended to ensure girls' chastity until marriage. Medical complications are common, including menstrual and urinary problems, and even death. After marriage, the opening is enlarged to permit intercourse. Enlargement is a gradual process that often is made difficult by scar tissue from the circumcision. Hemorrhaging and tearing of surrounding tissues are common consequences. It may take three months or longer before the opening is large enough to allow penile penetration. (Do not confuse male circumcision with the maiming inflicted on girls. Former representative Patricia Schroeder of Colorado depicts the male equivalent of female genital mutilation as cutting off the penis.)

Millions of women in Africa and the Middle East—130 million by some estimates—have undergone ritual genital mutilation. Mutilation of the labia is now illegal in the Sudan, although the law continues to allow removal of the clitoris. Some African countries have outlawed clitoridectomies, although such laws are rarely enforced. The procedure remains common or even universal in nearly 30 African countries; in many Middle Eastern countries; and in parts of Malaysia, Yemen, Oman, Indonesia, and the India–Pakistan subcontinent. Thousands of African immigrant girls living in European countries and the United States also have been mutilated.

In 1996, the United States outlawed ritual genital mutilation within its borders. The government also directed U.S. representatives to world financial institutions to deny aid to countries that have not established educational programs to end the practice. Yet, calls from Westerners to ban the practice in parts of Africa and the Middle East have sparked controversy on grounds of "cultural condescension"—that people in one culture cannot dictate the cultural traditions of another. As the debate continues, some 2 million African girls continue to undergo ritual genital mutilations each year.

Sources: Adapted from A. R. Rathus, J. S. Nevid, and L. Fichner-Rathus, *Essentials of Human Sexuality* (Boston: Allyn and Bacon, 1998), 30–31; Population Council, "Women's Health— Female Genital Mutilation: Common, Controversial, and Bad for Women's Health," *Population Briefs* 3, no. 2 (1997); www.popcouncil.org/ publications/popbriefs/pbs(2).html. See also www.who.int/inf-fs/en/fact241.html (World Health Organization website on genital mutilation) and www.fgm.org (the FGM, or Female Genital Mutilation, Information Page).

Seminal vesicles   Storage areas for sperm where nutrients and other fluids are added to them.

Semen   Fluid containing sperm and nutrient fluids that increase sperm viability and neutralize vaginal acid.

Prostate gland   Gland that secretes nutrients and neutralizing fluids into the semen.

transportation system whose sole function is to store and move sperm. Along the way, the **seminal vesicles** provide sperm with nutrients and other fluids that compose **semen.**

The vasa deferentia eventually connect each epididymis to the ejaculatory ducts, which pass through the prostate gland and empty into the urethra. The **prostate gland** contributes more fluids to the semen, including chemicals to aid the sperm in fertilizing an ovum, and neutralize the acidic environment of the vagina to make it more conducive to sperm motility (ability to move) and potency (potential for fertilizing an ovum).

Just below the prostate gland are two pea-shaped nodules called the **Cowper's glands.** The Cowper's glands secrete a fluid that lubricates the urethra and neutralizes any acid that may remain in the urethra after urination. Urine and semen do not come into contact with each other because during ejaculation, a small valve closes off the tube to the urinary bladder.

Debate continues over the practice of **circumcision,** the surgical removal of a fold of skin covering the end of the penis known as the foreskin. Most circumcisions are performed for religious or cultural reasons or because of concerns of hygiene. (Uncircumcised males must regularly clean the area under the foreskin.) Some studies suggest that penile cancer is more prevalent among uncircumcised men. However, the rate of penile cancer is so low that an equal number of deaths occur from complications due to circumcision as from penile cancer. The American Academy of Pediatrics does not consider the procedure medically necessary; if it is performed, the infant should be given pain relief.[45]

Human Sexual Response

Psychological traits greatly influence sexual response and sexual desire. Thus, you may find a relationship with one partner vastly different from that you might experience with other partners.

Sexual response is a physiological process that generally follows a pattern. Both males' and females' sexual responses are somewhat arbitrarily divided into four stages: excitement/arousal, plateau, orgasm, and resolution. Researchers agree that each individual has a personal response pattern that may or may not conform to these phases. Regardless of the type of sexual activity (stimulation by a partner or self-stimulation), the response stages are the same.

During the first stage, *excitement/arousal,* **vasocongestion,** or increased blood flow in the genital region, stimulates male and female genital responses. Increased blood flow to these organs causes them to swell. The vagina begins to lubricate in preparation for penile penetration, and the penis becomes partially erect. Both sexes may exhibit a "sex flush," or light blush all over their bodies. Excitement/arousal can be generated by touching other parts of the body, by kissing, through fantasy, by viewing films or videos, or by reading erotic literature.

During the *plateau phase,* the initial responses intensify. Voluntary and involuntary muscle tensions increase. The female's nipples and the male's penis become erect. The penis secretes a few drops of *pre-ejaculatory fluid,* which may contain sperm.

During the *orgasmic phase,* vasocongestion and muscle tensions reach their peak, and rhythmic contractions occur through the genital regions. In females, these contractions are centered in the uterus, outer vagina, and anal sphincter.

In males, the contractions occur in two stages. First, contractions within the prostate gland begin propelling semen through the urethra. In the second stage, the muscles of the pelvic floor, urethra, and anal sphincter contract. Semen usually, but not always, is ejaculated from the penis. In both sexes, spasms in other major muscle groups also occur, particularly in the buttocks and abdomen. Feet and hands may also contract, and facial features often contort.

Muscle tension and congested blood subside in the *resolution phase,* as the genital organs return to their pre-arousal states. Both sexes usually experience deep feelings of well-being and profound relaxation. Following orgasm and resolution, many females can become aroused again and experience additional orgasms. However, some men experience a *refractory period,* during which their systems are incapable of subsequent arousal. This refractory period may last from a few minutes to several hours and tends to lengthen with age.

Men and women experience the same stages in the sexual response cycle; however, the length of time spent in any one stage varies. Thus, one partner may be in the plateau phase while the other is in the excitement or orgasmic phase. Such variations in response rates are entirely normal. Some couples believe that simultaneous orgasm is desirable for sexual satisfaction. Although simultaneous orgasm is pleasant, so are orgasms achieved at different times.

Sexual pleasure and satisfaction are also possible without orgasm or even intercourse. Expressing sexual feelings for another person involves many pleasurable activities, of which intercourse and orgasm may be only a part.

What do you think?

Why do we place so much importance on orgasm?
* *Can sexual pleasure and satisfaction be achieved without orgasm?* * *What is the role of desire in sexual response?*

Expressing Your Sexuality

Finding healthy ways to express your sexuality is an important part of developing sexual maturity. Many avenues of sexual expression are available.

Cowper's glands The pea-shaped glands that secrete a fluid that lubricates the urethra and neutralizes any acid remaining in the urethra after urination.

Circumcision Surgical removal of the foreskin from the tip of the penis.

Vasocongestion The engorgement of the genital organs with blood.

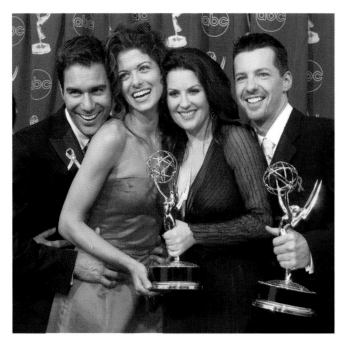

The presence of gay and lesbian characters and their friends, such as those portrayed by these actors on the TV program *Will and Grace,* contributes to increasing acceptance of gay relationships in everyday life.

Sexual Orientation

Sexual orientation refers to a person's enduring emotional, romantic, sexual, or affectionate attraction to other persons. You may be primarily attracted to members of the other sex (**heterosexual**), your same sex (**homosexual**), or both sexes (**bisexual**).

Many homosexuals prefer the terms *gay* and *lesbian* to describe their sexual orientations, since these terms go beyond the exclusively sexual connotation of the term *homosexual.* The term *gay* applies to both men and women, but *lesbian* refers only to women.

Throughout history, scientists and laypersons alike have debated the mental health status of gays and lesbians. In 1973, the American Psychiatric Association's board of

---

Sexual orientation   A person's enduring emotional, romantic, sexual, or affectionate attraction to other persons.

Heterosexual   Experiencing primary attraction to and preference for sexual activity with people of the other sex.

Homosexual   Experiencing primary attraction to and preference for sexual activity with people of the same sex.

Bisexual   Experiencing attraction to and preference for sexual activity with people of both sexes.

Homophobia   Irrational hatred or fear of homosexuals or homosexuality.

---

trustees unanimously voted that homosexuality was not a mental illness or psychiatric disorder. This position was affirmed by the American Psychological Association and the Sexuality Information and Education Council of the United States (SIECUS). Recently, the issue of homosexuality as a treatable disease has been resurrected. Treatments labeled as conversion or reparative therapies are advertised through magazines, TV, and the Internet. Mental health professionals have found these ads so troubling that the American Psychological Association passed a resolution reaffirming that homosexuality is *not* a disease in need of a "cure."[46]

Most researchers today agree that sexual orientation is best understood using a multifactorial model, which incorporates biological, psychological, and socioenvironmental factors.[47] Biological explanations focus on research into genetics, hormones (perinatal and postpubertal), and differences in brain anatomy, while psychological and socioenvironmental explanations examine parent–child interactions, sex roles, and early sexual and interpersonal interactions. Collectively, this growing body of research suggests that the origins of homosexuality, like heterosexuality, are complex. To diminish the complexity of sexual orientation to "a choice" is a clear misrepresentation of current research. Homosexuals do not choose their sexual orientation any more than heterosexuals do.

Irrational fear or hatred of homosexuality creates antigay prejudice and is expressed as **homophobia.** Homophobic behaviors range from avoiding hugging same-sex friends to name-calling and physical attacks. Herek and colleagues surveyed 2,259 gay and lesbian people and found that 1 in 5 women and 1 in 4 men had been victimized in the preceding five years because of their sexual orientation.[48]

Sexual Behavior: What Is Normal?

Most of us want to fit in and be identified as normal, but how do we know which sexual behaviors are considered normal? What or whose criteria should we use? These are not easy questions.

Every society sets standards and attempts to regulate sexual behavior. Boundaries arise that distinguish good from bad, acceptable from unacceptable, and result in criteria used to establish what is viewed as normal or abnormal. Common sociocultural standards for sexual behavior in Western culture today include the following.

- *The heterosexual standard.* Sexual attraction should be limited to members of the other sex.
- *The coital standard.* Penile/vaginal intercourse (coitus) is viewed as the ultimate sex act.
- *The orgasmic standard.* All sexual interaction should lead to orgasm.
- *The two-person standard.* Sex is an activity to be experienced by two.
- *The romantic standard.* Sex should be related to love.
- *The safer sex standard.* If we choose to be sexually active, we should act to prevent unintended pregnancy or disease transmission.[49]

These are not laws or rules, but rather social scripts that have been adopted over time. Sexual standards often shift through the years, and many people choose not to follow them. We are a pluralistic nation, and that pluralism extends to our sexual practices. Rather than making blanket judgments about normal versus abnormal, we might ask the following questions:[50]

- Is a sexual behavior healthy and fulfilling for a particular person?
- Is it safe?
- Does it lead to the exploitation of others?
- Does it take place between responsible, consenting adults?

In this way, we can view behavior along a continuum that takes into account many individual factors. As you read about the options for sexual expression in the pages ahead, use these questions to explore your feelings about what is normal for you.

Options for Sexual Expression

The range of human sexual expression is virtually infinite. What you find enjoyable may not be an option for someone else. The ways you choose to meet your sexual needs today may have been very different two weeks ago or will be different two years from now. Accepting yourself as a sexual person with individual desires and preferences is the first step in achieving sexual satisfaction.

Celibacy Celibacy is avoidance of or abstention from sexual activities with others. Some individuals choose celibacy for religious or moral reasons. Others may be celibate for a period of time because of illness, the breakup of a long-term relationship, or lack of an acceptable partner. For some, celibacy is a lonely, agonizing state, but others find it an opportunity for introspection, values assessment, and personal growth.

Autoerotic Behaviors Autoerotic behaviors involve sexual self-stimulation. The two most common are sexual fantasy and masturbation.

Sexual fantasies are sexually arousing thoughts and dreams. Fantasies may reflect real-life experiences, forbidden desires, or the opportunity to practice new or anticipated sexual experiences. The fact that you may fantasize about a particular sexual experience does not mean that you want to, or have to, act that experience out. Sexual fantasies are just that—fantasy.

Masturbation is self-stimulation of the genitals. Although many people feel uncomfortable discussing masturbation, it is a common sexual practice across the life span. Masturbation is a natural, pleasure-seeking behavior in infants and children. It is a valuable and important means for adolescent males and females, as well as adults, to explore sexual feelings and responsiveness.

Kissing and Erotic Touching Kissing and erotic touching are two very common forms of nonverbal sexual communication. Both males and females have **erogenous zones,** areas of the body that when touched lead to sexual arousal. Erogenous zones may include genital as well as nongenital areas, such as the earlobes, mouth, breasts, and inner thighs. Almost any area of the body can be conditioned to respond erotically to touch. Spending time with your partner to explore and learn about his or her erogenous areas is another pleasurable, safe, and satisfying means of sexual expression.

Oral–Genital Stimulation Cunnilingus refers to oral stimulation of a female's genitals, and **fellatio** to oral stimulation of a male's genitals. Many partners find oral–genital stimulation intensely pleasurable. Seventy percent of college-aged men and women have had oral sex.[51] For some people, oral sex is not an option because of moral or religious beliefs. Remember, HIV (human immunodeficiency virus) and other sexually transmitted infections (STIs) can be transmitted via unprotected oral–genital sex just as they can through intercourse. Use of an appropriate barrier device is strongly recommended if either partner's health status is in question.

Vaginal Intercourse The term *intercourse* generally refers to **vaginal intercourse** (*coitus,* or insertion of the penis into the vagina), which is the most often practiced form of sexual expression. Coitus can involve a variety of positions, including the missionary position (man on top facing the woman), woman on top, side by side, or man behind (rear entry). Many partners enjoy experimenting with different positions. Knowledge of yourself and your body, along with your ability to communicate effectively, will play a large part in determining the enjoyment or meaning of intercourse for you and your partner. Whatever your circumstance, you should practice safer sex to avoid disease and unwanted pregnancy.

Celibacy Avoidance or abstention from sexual activities with others.

Autoerotic behaviors Sexual self-stimulation.

Sexual fantasies Sexually arousing thoughts and dreams.

Masturbation Self-stimulation of genitals.

Erogenous zones Areas of both the male and female body that, when touched, lead to sexual arousal.

Cunnilingus Oral stimulation of a female's genitals.

Fellatio Oral stimulation of a male's genitals.

Vaginal intercourse The insertion of the penis into the vagina; also called coitus.

Anal Intercourse   The anal area is highly sensitive to touch, and some couples find pleasure in the stimulation of this area. **Anal intercourse** is insertion of the penis into the anus. Sixteen percent of college-aged men and women have had anal sex.[52] Stimulation of the anus by mouth or with the fingers also is practiced. As with all forms of sexual expression, anal stimulation or intercourse is not for everyone. If you do enjoy this form of sexual expression, remember to use condoms to avoid transmitting disease. Also, anything inserted into the anus should not be directly inserted into the vagina, since bacteria commonly found in the anus can cause vaginal infections.

Variant Sexual Behavior

Although attitudes toward sexuality have changed radically since the Victorian era, some people still believe that any sexual behavior other than heterosexual intercourse is abnormal or perverted. People who study sexuality prefer the neutral term **variant sexual behavior** to describe sexual activities such as the following that are not engaged in by most people.

- *Group sex*. Sexual activity involving more than two people. Participants in group sex run a higher risk of exposure to HIV and other STIs.
- *Transvestism*. Wearing the clothing of the opposite sex. Most transvestites are male, heterosexual, and married.
- *Fetishism*. Sexual arousal achieved by looking at or touching inanimate objects, such as underclothing or shoes.

Some variant sexual behaviors can be harmful to the individual, to others, or to both. Many of the following activities are illegal in at least some states.

- *Exhibitionism*. Exposing one's genitals to strangers in public places. Most exhibitionists are seeking a reaction of shock or fear from their victims. Exhibitionism is a minor felony in most states.

Anal intercourse   The insertion of the penis into the anus.

Variant sexual behavior   A sexual activity that is not engaged in by most people.

Sexual dysfunction   Problems that can hinder sexual functioning.

Inhibited sexual desire (ISD)   Lack of interest and pleasure in sexual activity.

Sexual aversion disorder   Type of desire dysfunction characterized by sexual phobias and anxiety about sexual contact.

- *Voyeurism*. Observing other people for sexual gratification. Most voyeurs are men who attempt to watch women undressing or bathing. Voyeurism is an invasion of privacy and illegal in most states.
- *Sadomasochism*. Sexual activities in which gratification is received by inflicting pain (verbal or physical abuse) on a partner or by being the object of such infliction. A sadist is a person who enjoys inflicting pain, and a masochist is a person who enjoys experiencing it.
- *Pedophilia*. Sexual activity or attraction between an adult and a child. Any sexual activity involving a minor, including possession of child pornography, is illegal.
- *Autoerotic asphyxiation*. The practice of reducing or eliminating oxygen to the brain, usually by tying a cord around one's neck, while masturbating to orgasm. Tragically, asphyxiation usually is discovered when people accidentally hang themselves.

What do you think?

How does our society define normal sexual behavior? ✳ *What behaviors do you consider normal or abnormal?* ✳ *Do you consider your own preferred forms of sexual expression to be normal?* ✳ *Why or why not?*

Difficulties That Can Hinder Sexual Functioning

Research indicates that **sexual dysfunction,** the problems that can hinder sexual functioning, are quite common. Don't feel embarrassed if you experience sexual problems at some point in your life. The sexual part of you does not come with a lifetime warranty. You can have breakdowns involving your sexual function just as in any other body system. Sexual dysfunction is divided into five major classes: disorders of sexual desire, sexual arousal, orgasm, sexual performance, and sexual pain. All of them can be treated successfully.

Sexual Desire Disorders

The most frequent reason why people seek out a sex therapist is **ISD,** or **inhibited sexual desire.**[53] ISD is the lack of interest and pleasure in sexual activity. In some instances, it can result from stress or boredom. **Sexual aversion disorder** is another type of desire dysfunction characterized by sexual phobias (unreasonable fears) and anxiety about sexual contact. The psychological stress of a punitive upbringing, a rigid religious background, or a history of physical or sexual abuse may be sources of these desire disorders.

Sexual Arousal Disorders

The most common sexual arousal disorder is **erectile dysfunction (impotence)**—difficulty in achieving or maintaining a penile erection sufficient for intercourse. At some time in his life, every man experiences impotence. Causes are varied and include underlying diseases, such as diabetes or prostate problems; reactions to some medications (for example, medication for high blood pressure); depression; fatigue; stress; alcohol use; performance anxiety; and guilt over real or imaginary problems (such as when a man compares himself to his partner's past lovers).

Some 30 million men in this country, half of them under age 65, suffer from impotence. Impotence generally becomes more of a problem as men age; it affects one in four men over the age of 65. The Food and Drug Administration has approved the drug Viagra (sildenafil citrate) to treat impotence. Taken by mouth one hour before sexual activity, Viagra is reported to manage erectile dysfunction successfully in 60 to 80 percent of cases.[54] However, the medication is not without risk. The most commonly reported side effects include headache, flushing, stomachache, urinary tract infection, diarrhea, dizziness, rash, and mild and temporary visual changes. In addition, there have been several deaths in the United States among Viagra users. This has prompted more caution in prescribing it to patients with known cardiovascular disease and those taking commonly prescribed short- and long-acting nitrates, such as nitroglycerin.[55]

Another drug that can help prolong erection is Trazodone, an antidepressant. Several other Viagra-like drugs are being developed that will have different side effects. Another potential treatment is the internal penile pump, a soft-fluid-filled (saline) device that expands and contracts. The pump transfers saline into the penis, which causes an erection.

Orgasm Disorders

Premature ejaculation—ejaculation that occurs prior to or almost immediately following the insertion of the penis into the vagina—affects up to 50 percent of the male population at some time in their lives. Treatment for premature ejaculation involves a physical examination to rule out organic causes. If the cause of the problem is not physiological, therapy is available to help a man learn how to control the timing of his ejaculation. Fatigue, stress, performance pressure, and alcohol use all can contribute to orgasmic disorders in men.

In a woman, the inability to achieve orgasm is termed **female orgasmic disorder.** A woman with this disorder often blames herself and learns to fake orgasm to avoid embarrassment or preserve her partner's ego. Contributing to this response are the messages women have historically been given about sex as a duty rather than as a pleasurable act. As with men who experience orgasmic disorders, the first step in treatment is a physical exam to rule out organic causes.

However, the problem often is solved by simple self-exploration to learn more about what forms of stimulation are arousing enough to produce orgasm. Through masturbation, a woman can learn how her body responds sexually to various types of touch. Once she has become orgasmic through masturbation, she learns to communicate her needs to her partner.

Sexual Performance Anxiety

Both men and women can experience **sexual performance anxiety** in which they anticipate some sort of problem during the sex act. A man may become anxious and unable to maintain an erection, or he may experience premature ejaculation. A woman may be unable to achieve orgasm or to allow penetration because of the involuntary contraction of vaginal muscles. Both can overcome performance anxiety by learning to focus on immediate sensations and pleasures rather than on orgasm.

Sexual Pain Disorders

Two common sexual pain disorders are dyspareunia and vaginismus. **Dyspareunia** is pain experienced by a woman during intercourse. This pain may be caused by diseases such as endometriosis, uterine tumors, chlamydia, gonorrhea, or urinary tract infections. Damage to tissues during childbirth and insufficient lubrication during intercourse also may cause discomfort. Dyspareunia also can be psychological in origin. As with other problems, dyspareunia can be treated with good results.

Vaginismus is the involuntary contraction of vaginal muscles, which makes penile insertion painful or impossible. Most cases of vaginismus are related to fear of intercourse or to unresolved sexual conflicts. Treatment involves teaching a woman to achieve orgasm through nonvaginal stimulation.

Erectile dysfunction (impotence) Difficulty in achieving or maintaining a penile erection sufficient for intercourse.

Premature ejaculation Ejaculation that occurs prior to or almost immediately following penile penetration of the vagina.

Female orgasmic disorder The inability to achieve orgasm.

Sexual performance anxiety A condition of sexual difficulties caused by anticipating some sort of problem with the sex act.

Dyspareunia Pain experienced by women during intercourse.

Vaginismus Involuntary contraction of the vaginal muscles, which makes penile insertion painful or impossible.

Seeking Help for Sexual Dysfunction

Many theories and treatment models can help people with sexual dysfunction. A first important step is choosing a qualified sex therapist or counselor. A national organization, the American Association of Sex Educators, Counselors, and Therapists (AASECT) has been in the forefront of establishing criteria for certifying sex therapists. These criteria include appropriate degree(s) in the helping professions, specialized coursework in human sexuality, and sufficient hours of practical therapy work under the direct supervision of a certified sex therapist. Lists of certified counselors and sex therapists, as well as clinics that treat sexual dysfunctions, are available from AASECT and SIECUS.

Drugs and Sex

Because psychoactive drugs affect the entire physiology, it is only logical that they affect sexual behavior. Promises of increased pleasure make drugs tempting to those seeking greater sexual satisfaction. Too often, however, drugs become central to sexual activities and damage the relationship.

Rohypnol   A drug sometimes used in combination with alcohol to facilitate date rape by making a woman unaware of what is happening to her.

Gammahydroxybutyrate (GHB)   A drug sometimes used in combination with alcohol to facilitate date rape by making a woman unaware of what is happening to her.

Alcohol is notorious for reducing inhibitions and promoting feelings of well-being and desirability. At the same time, alcohol inhibits sexual response; thus, the mind may be willing, but the body is not.

Perhaps the greatest danger associated with use of drugs and alcohol during sex is the tendency to blame the drug for negative behavior. "I can't help what I did last night because I was drunk" is a response that demonstrates sexual immaturity. A sexually mature person carefully examines risks and benefits and makes decisions accordingly. If drugs and alcohol are necessary to increase erotic feelings, it is likely that the partners are being dishonest about their feelings for each other. Good sex should not depend on chemical substances.

Of growing concern in recent years is the increased use of date rape drugs. These have become popular among college students and often are used in combination with alcohol.[56] Both **Rohypnol** ("roofies," "rope," "forget pill") and **GHB**, or **gammahydroxybutyrate** ("Liquid X," "Grievous Bodily Harm," "Easy Lay," "Mickey Finn"), have been used to facilitate rape. The dangers of these drugs are discussed in more detail in Chapter 7.

What do you think?

Why do we find it so difficult to discuss sexual dysfunction in our society? ✳ Do you think it is more difficult for men than for women to talk about dysfunction? ✳ Have you ever used alcohol or some other drug to enhance your sexual performance? ✳ Why are date rape drugs of major concern on college campuses?

Taking Charge

Make It Happen!

Assessment: The Assess Yourself box on page 108 gave you the chance to look at how you communicate in certain situations. It is important to be able to communicate assertively and to feel that you can stand up for yourself. Now that you have considered your responses to the statements, you may want to take steps toward becoming a more assertive communicator.

Making a Change: In order to change your behavior, you need to develop a plan. Follow these steps.

1. Evaluate your behavior, and identify patterns. What can you change now? What can you change in the near future?
2. Select one pattern of behavior that you want to change.
3. Fill out a Behavior Change Contract. It should include your long-term goal for change, your short-term goals,

the rewards you'll give yourself for reaching these goals, potential obstacles along the way, and strategies for overcoming these obstacles. For each goal, list the small steps and specific actions that you will take.

4. Chart your progress in a journal. At the end of a week, consider how successful you were in following your plan. What helped you be successful? What made change more difficult? What will you do differently next week?

5. Revise your plan as needed: Are the short-term goals attainable? Are the rewards satisfying?

Example: When Stacey assessed her responses to the statements about assertiveness, she realized that she tended to say yes when someone asked her for a favor, no matter how busy or stressed out she was. Stacey decided she wanted to learn to say no when necessary. She set a goal of imagining certain situations that she had faced recently and how she would handle them more assertively. The first week, she imagined her older sister asking her to babysit her son at the last minute and her roommates asking her for car rides while she was in the middle of studying. She planned what she would say and how she would explain her reasons for saying no. The second week, when her roommates asked for a ride to the movies, Stacey calmly stated that she was busy and needed two hours more for studying before she could take a break. Her roommates decided to walk to the video store instead and rented a movie they could all watch together when Stacey was ready for a break.

Summary

✸ Intimate relationships have several different characteristics, including behavioral interdependence, need fulfillment, emotional attachment, and emotional availability. These characteristics influence how we interact with others and the types of intimate relationships we form. Family, friends, and partners or lovers provide the most common opportunities for intimacy. Each relationship may include healthy and unhealthy characteristics that may affect daily functioning.

✸ Gender differences in communication include conversation styles as well as differences in sharing feelings and disclosing personal facts and fears. These differences explain why men and women may relate differently in intimate relationships. Understanding these differences and learning how to deal with them are important aspects of healthy relationships.

✸ Barriers to intimacy often include the different emotional needs of both partners, jealousy, and emotional wounds that could result from being raised in a dysfunctional family.

✸ For most people, commitment is an important ingredient in successful relationships. The major types of committed relationships are marriage, cohabitation, and gay and lesbian partnerships.

✸ Success in committed relationships requires understanding the roles of partnering scripts, the importance of self-nurturance, and the elements of a good relationship.

✸ Life decisions such as whether to marry or whether to have children require serious consideration. Remaining single is more common than ever. Most single people lead healthy, happy, and well-adjusted lives. Those who decide to have or not to have children also can lead rewarding, productive lives as long as they have given this decision the utmost thought and weighed the pros and cons of each alternative in the context of their lifestyle. Today's family structure may look different from that of previous generations, but love, trust, and commitment to a child's welfare continue to be the cornerstones of successful childrearing.

✸ Before relationships fail, often many warning signs appear. By recognizing these signs and taking action to change behaviors, partners can save and enhance their relationships.

✸ Sexual identity is determined by a complex interaction of genetic, physiological, and environmental factors. Biological sex, gender identity, gender roles, and sexual orientation all are blended into our sexual identity.

✸ The major components of the female sexual anatomy include the mons pubis, labia minora and majora, clitoris, urethral and vaginal openings, vagina, cervix, fallopian tubes, and ovaries. The major components of the male sexual anatomy are the penis, scrotum, testes, epididymides, vasa deferentia, ejaculatory ducts, and urethra.

✸ Physiologically, males and females experience four phases of sexual response: excitement/arousal, plateau, orgasm, and resolution.

✸ Humans can express their sexual selves in a variety of ways, including celibacy, autoerotic behaviors, kissing and erotic touch, oral–genital stimulation, vaginal intercourse, and anal intercourse. Sexual orientation refers to a person's enduring emotional, romantic, sexual, or affectionate attraction to other persons. Irrational hatred or fear of homosexuality or gay and lesbian persons is termed *homophobia*.

✸ Sexual dysfunctions can be classified into disorders of sexual desire, sexual arousal, orgasm, sexual performance anxiety, and sexual pain. Drug use also can lead to sexual dysfunction.

Questions for Discussion and Reflection

1. What are the characteristics of intimate relationships? What are behavioral interdependence, need fulfillment, emotional attachment, and emotional availability, and why is each important in relationship development?
2. Why are relationships with family important? Explain how your family unit was similar to or different from the traditional family unit in early America. Who made up your family of origin? Your nuclear family?
3. How can you tell the difference between a love relationship and one that is based primarily on attraction? What characteristics do love relationships share?
4. What problems can form barriers to intimacy? What actions can you take to reduce or remove these barriers?
5. What are common elements of good relationships? What are some common warning signs of trouble? What actions can you take to improve your own interpersonal relationships?
6. Name some common misconceptions about people who choose to remain single and about couples who choose not to have children. Do you want to have children? Why or why not? What characteristics show that a couple is ready to have children?
7. How have gender roles changed over the past 20 years? Do you view the changes as positive for both men and women?
8. Discuss the cycle of changes that occurs in our bodies in response to various hormones (e.g., sexual differentiation while in the womb, development of secondary sex characteristics at puberty, menopause).
9. What is "normal" sexual behavior? What criteria should we use to determine healthful sexual practice?
10. If scientists ever establish the combination of factors that interact to produce homosexual, heterosexual, or bisexual orientation, will that put an end to antigay prejudice? Why or why not?
11. How can we remove the stigma that surrounds sexual dysfunction so that individuals feel more open to seeking help? Are men and women impacted differently by sexual dysfunction?

Accessing Your Health on the Internet

Visit the following Internet sites to explore further topics and issues related to personal health. To visit an organization's website, go to the Companion Website for *Health: The Basics, Sixth Edition* at www.aw-bc.com/donatelle, click on the book image, and select "Accessing Your Health on the Internet" from the navigation menu on the left.

1. *American Association of Sex Educators, Counselors, and Therapists (AASECT).* Professional organization providing standards of practice for treatment of sexual issues and disorders.
2. *Couples National Network.* Provides a link into a network for same-gender couples and singles, with resources about gay and lesbian issues.
3. *Go Ask Alice.* An interactive question-and-answer line from the Columbia University Health Services. "Alice" is available to answer questions each week about any health-related issues, including relationships, nutrition and diet, exercise, drugs, sex, alcohol, and stress.
4. *Mental Health Notes.* Offers user-friendly information about dysfunctional families from a licensed clinical psychologist. Includes links to related mental health articles.
5. *Relationship Growth Online.* Provides information, quizzes, games, advice, and links to more information on how to build better relationships.
6. *Sexuality Information and Education Council of the United States (SIECUS).* A source for information, guidelines, and materials for advancement of healthy and proper sex education.
7. *Teen Sexual Health.* Provides current research and other resources dealing with sexual health for high school and college-age students.
8. *University of Missouri Counseling Center Self-Help Area.* Provides a bibliography on books and other resources on issues dealing with intimacy.

Further Reading

Busby, D., and V. Loyer-Carlson. *Pathways to Marriage with RELATE Online Relationship Inventory: Premarital and Early Marital Relationships.* Boston: Allyn & Bacon, 2003.

A step-by-step approach to building better relationships.

Caron, S.L. *Sex Matters for College Students: Sex FAQ's in Human Sexuality.* Englewood Cliffs, NJ: Prentice Hall, 2002.

A brief, easy-to-read, and affordable paperback designed specifically to answer basic sexual questions in a friendly and age-appropriate way.

Firestone, R., and J. Cattlet. *Fear of Intimacy.* Washington, DC: American Psychological Association, 2001.

Two therapists provide insightful information about how we think about relationships and family and why relationships fail or thrive.

Galvin, K., and P. Cooper. *Making Connections.* Los Angeles: Roxbury Publishing, 2000.

Outstanding overview of the importance of interpersonal communication in everyday lives. Provides practical strategies to assist us at all stages of life.

Koman, A. *How to Mend a Broken Heart: Letting Go and Moving On.* Chicago: Contemporary Books, 1997.

A step-by-step program for dealing with the end of a relationship, including working through the emotional stages, strategies for coping, and gaining strength to move on.

SIECUS (Sexuality Information and Education Council of the United States) *Report.* 130 West 42nd Street, New York, NY 10036.

Highly acclaimed and readable journal. Includes timely and thought-provoking articles on human sexuality, sexuality education, and AIDS.

Wingood, G.M., and R. DiClemente, eds. *Handbook of Women's Sexual and Reproductive Health.* Boston: Plenum Publishing, 2002.

Researchers, including those in behavioral sciences and health education, summarize the epidemiology, social and behavioral factors, policies, and intervention and prevention strategies related to women's sexual and reproductive health.

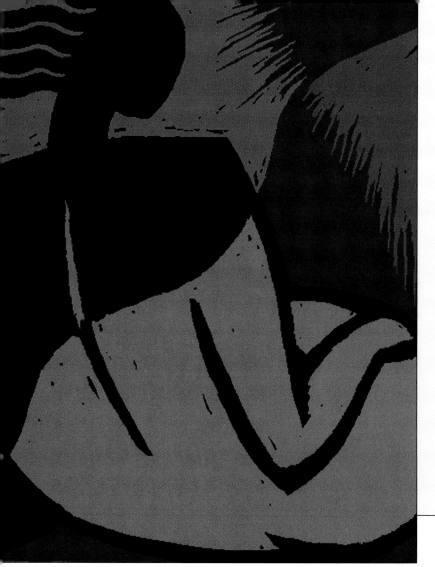

Birth Control, Pregnancy, and Childbirth

Managing Your Fertility

Objectives

❋ Discuss the different types of contraceptive methods, and compare their effectiveness in preventing pregnancy and sexually transmitted infections.

❋ Summarize the legal decisions surrounding abortion and the various types of abortion procedures used today.

❋ Discuss key issues to consider when planning a pregnancy.

❋ Explain the importance of prenatal care and the physical and emotional aspects of pregnancy.

❋ Describe the basic stages of childbirth, methods of managing childbirth, and the complications that can arise during labor and delivery.

❋ Review primary causes of and possible solutions to infertility.

A Contraceptive Clears a Hurdle to Wider Access

By Gina Kolata

GAITHERSBURG, MD In a 23-to-4 vote, two expert advisory committees to the Food and Drug Administration recommended Tuesday that a so-called morning-after pill to prevent unintended pregnancies be sold over the counter.

The FDA usually follows its committees' advice, although the final decision rests with its commissioner, Dr. Mark B. McClellan. But the overwhelming vote by the agency's outside advisers led proponents as well as opponents to expect that

Dr. McClellan would go along with the committees, making his decision within weeks to months.

The drug is an emergency contraceptive known as Plan B, to be taken when regular contraception either fails or is skipped. Consisting of two high-dose birth control pills, Plan B is meant to be used within 72 hours after unprotected sexual intercourse and may prevent up to 89 percent of unplanned pregnancies.

If approved, widespread availability of Plan B could have an impact second only to the advent of the birth control pill, advocates say.

Read the complete article online in the eThemes section of this book's website: www.aw-bc.com/donatelle.

Original article published December 17, 2003. Copyright © 2003 The New York Times. Reprinted with permission.

Today, we not only understand the intimate details of reproduction, but we also possess technologies that can control or enhance our **fertility,** our ability to reproduce. Along with information and technological advance comes choice, and choice goes hand in hand with responsibility. Choosing if and when to have children is one of our greatest responsibilities. A woman and her partner have much to consider before planning or risking a pregnancy. Children, whether planned or unplanned, change people's lives. They require a lifelong personal commitment of love and nurturing. Are you physically, emotionally, and financially prepared to care for another human being?

One measure of maturity is the ability to discuss reproduction and birth control with one's sexual partner before engaging in sexual activity. Men often assume that their partners are taking care of birth control. Women often feel that bringing up the subject implies they are "easy" or "loose." Both may feel that this discussion interferes with romance and spontaneity. You will find embarrassment-free discussion a lot easier if you understand human reproduction and contraception and honestly consider your attitudes toward these matters before you find yourself in a compromising situation.

Fertility   A person's ability to reproduce.

Conception   The fertilization of an ovum by a sperm.

Contraception   Methods of preventing conception.

Methods of Fertility Management

Conception refers to the fertilization of an ovum by a sperm. The following conditions are necessary for conception:

1. A viable egg
2. A viable sperm
3. Access to the egg by the sperm

The term **contraception** (sometimes called birth control) refers to methods of preventing conception. These methods offer varying degrees of control over when and whether pregnancies occur. However, since people first associated sexual activity with pregnancy, society has searched for a simple, infallible, and risk-free way to prevent pregnancy. We have not yet found one.

To evaluate the effectiveness of a particular contraceptive method, you must be familiar with two concepts: perfect failure rate and typical use failure rate. *Perfect failure rate* refers to the number of pregnancies that are likely to occur in a year (per 100 uses of the method during sexual intercourse) if the method is used absolutely perfectly, that is, without any error. The *typical use failure rate* refers to the number of pregnancies that are likely to occur with typical use, that is, with the normal number of errors, memory lapses, and incorrect or incomplete use. This information is much more practical for people in helping them make informed decisions about contraceptive methods. See Table 6.1 to find ratings of various contraceptive methods. We'll discuss many of them in this chapter.

Table 6.1
Contraceptive Effectiveness and STI Prevention

Number of Unintended Pregnancies per 100 Women during First Year of Use

Method	Typical Use*	Perfect Use**	Risk Reduction for Sexually Transmitted Infections (STIs)
Continuous Abstinence	0.00	0.00	Complete
Outercourse	N/A***	N/A	Some
Norplant Implant	0.05	0.05	None
Sterilization			
Men	0.15	0.1	None
Women	0.5	0.5	None
Depo-Provera Injection	0.3	0.3	None
IUD (Intrauterine Device)			
ParaGard (copper T380A)	0.8	0.6	None
Progestasert	2.0	1.5	None
Mirena	0.1	0.1	None
Lunelle Injection	N/A	0.1	None
Oral Contraceptives (The Pill)			
Combination	5.0	0.1	None
Progestin-only	5.0	0.5	None
Male Condom	14.0	3.0	Good against HIV (human immunodeficiency virus); reduces risk of others
Withdrawal	19.0	4.0	None
Diaphragm	20.0	6.0	Limited
Cervical Cap			
Women who have not given birth	20.0	9.0	Limited
Women who have given birth	40.0	30.0	Limited
Female Condom	21.0	5.0	Some
Predicting Fertility			
Periodic abstinence	20.0		None
Postovulation method		1.0	None
Symptothermal method		2.0	None
Cervical mucus (ovulation) method		3.0	None
Calendar method		9.0	None
Fertility Awareness Methods			
With male or female condom	N/A	N/A	None
With diaphragm or cap	N/A	N/A	None
With withdrawal or other methods	N/A	N/A	None
Spermicide	26.0	6.0	Limited
No Method	85.0	85.0	None

Emergency Contraception
Emergency contraception pills: Treatment initiated within 72 hours after unprotected intercourse reduces the risk of pregnancy by 75–89 percent (with no protection against STIs). Emergency IUD insertion: Treatment initiated within seven days after unprotected intercourse reduces the risk of pregnancy by more than 99 percent (with no protection against STIs).

Contraceptive effectiveness rates: R. Hatcher et al., *Contraceptive Technology, 17th ed.* (New York: Ardent Media, 1998).
Reprinted by permission of Ardent Media.
*"Typical Use" refers to failure rates for men and women whose use is not consistent or always correct.
**"Perfect Use" refers to failure rates for those whose use is consistent and always correct.
***N/A means that effectiveness rates are not available.

Many contraceptive methods also can protect, to some degree, against **sexually transmitted infections (STIs).** This is an important factor to consider in choosing a contraceptive. Table 6.1 compares the level of STI risk reduction various contraceptives offer.

Present methods of contraception fall into several categories. **Barrier methods** use a physical or chemical block to prevent the egg and sperm from joining. Hormonal methods introduce synthetic hormones into the woman's system that prevent ovulation, thicken cervical mucus, or prevent a fertilized egg from implanting. Surgical methods can prevent pregnancy permanently. Other methods of contraception may involve temporary or permanent abstinence, or planning intercourse in accordance with fertility patterns. (See the Assess Yourself box to determine which method is best for you and your partner.)

Barrier Methods

The Male Condom The **male condom** is a strong, thin sheath of latex rubber or other material designed to fit over an erect penis. The condom catches the ejaculate and thereby prevents sperm from migrating toward the egg. It is the only barrier method that effectively prevents the spread of STIs and HIV (human immunodeficiency virus). Condoms come in a wide variety of styles: colored, ribbed, lubricated, nonlubricated, and with or without reservoirs at the tip. All may be purchased with or without spermicide in pharmacies, in some supermarkets and public bathrooms, and in many health clinics. A new condom must be used for each act of intercourse, oral sex, or anal sex.

In addition to helping to prevent some STIs, including genital herpes and HIV, the use of latex condoms also may slow or reduce the development of cervical abnormalities in women that can lead to cancer. A condom must be rolled onto the penis before the penis touches the vagina, and held in place when removing the penis from the vagina after ejaculation (Figure 6.1). For greatest efficacy, condoms should be used with a spermicide containing nonoxynol-9 (N-9), the same agent found in many of the contraceptive foams and creams that women use. If necessary or desired, users can lubricate their own condoms with contraceptive foams,

---

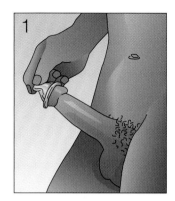
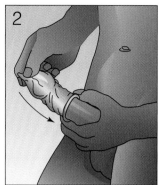
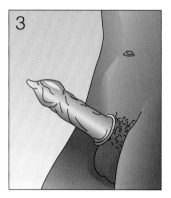
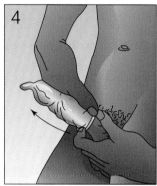

Figure 6.1

How to Use a Condom

The condom should be rolled over the erect penis before any penetration occurs. A small space (about $1/2$ inch) should be left at the end of the condom to collect the semen after ejaculation. Hold the tip of the condom, and unroll it all the way to the base of the penis. Hold the base of the condom before withdrawal to avoid spilling any semen.

---

creams, and jellies, or with other water-based lubricants, such as K-Y jelly, ForPlay Lubricants, Astroglide, or Wet or Aqua Lube, to name just a few. However, never use products such as baby oil, cold cream, petroleum jelly, vaginal yeast infection medications, or body lotion with a condom. These products contain mineral oil and will cause the latex to begin disintegrating within 60 seconds.

Condoms are less effective and more likely to break during intercourse if they are old or poorly stored. To maintain effectiveness, store them in a cool place (not in a wallet or hip pocket), and inspect them for small tears before use.

For some people, a condom ruins the spontaneity of sex because they feel that stopping to put it on breaks the mood. Others report that the condom decreases sensation. These inconveniences contribute to improper use of this barrier method of birth control. Couples who learn to put on the condom together as foreplay are generally more successful with its use.[1]

Jellies, Creams, Foams, and Suppositories Jellies, creams, foam, and suppositories, like condoms, do not require a prescription. They are referred to as **spermicides**—substances

---

Sexually transmitted infections (STIs) A variety of infections that can be acquired through sexual contact.

Barrier methods Contraceptive methods that prevent the egg and sperm from joining by means of a physical barrier (e.g., condom, diaphragm, or cervical cap), a chemical barrier (e.g., spermicide), or both.

Male condom A single-use sheath of strong, thin latex rubber or other material designed to fit over an erect penis and to catch semen upon ejaculation.

Spermicides Substances designed to kill sperm.

Contraceptive Comfort and Confidence Scale

These questions will help you assess whether the method of contraception you are using now or may consider using in the future is or will be effective for you. Answering yes to any of these questions predicts potential problems. Most individuals will have a few yes answers. If you have more than a few yes responses, however, you may want to talk to a health care provider, counselor, partner, or friend to decide whether or how to use this method so that it really will be effective. In general, the more yes answers you have, the less likely you are to use this method consistently and correctly with every act of intercourse.

Method of contraception you use now or are considering: _____

Length of time you used this method in the past: _____

Answer yes or no to the following questions:

_____ **1.** Have I ever had problems using this method?

_____ **2.** Have I ever become pregnant while using this method?

_____ **3.** Am I afraid of using this method?

_____ **4.** Would I really rather not use this method?

_____ **5.** Will I have trouble remembering to use this method?

_____ **6.** Will I have trouble using this method correctly?

_____ **7.** Do I still have unanswered questions about this method?

_____ **8.** Does this method make menstrual periods longer or more painful?

_____ **9.** Does this method cost more than I can afford?

_____ **10.** Could this method cause serious complications?

_____ **11.** Am I opposed to this method because of any religious or moral beliefs?

_____ **12.** Is my partner opposed to this method?

_____ **13.** Am I using this method without my partner's knowledge?

_____ **14.** Will using this method embarrass my partner?

_____ **15.** Will using this method embarrass me?

_____ **16.** Will I enjoy intercourse less because of this method?

_____ **17.** If this method interrupts lovemaking, will I avoid using it?

_____ **18.** Has a nurse or doctor ever told me not to use this method?

_____ **19.** Is there anything about my personality that could lead me to use this method incorrectly?

_____ **20.** Am I at risk of being exposed to HIV (the human immunodeficiency virus) or other sexually transmitted infections (STIs) if I use this method?

Total number of yes answers _____

Source: From R. A. Hatcher et al., *Contraceptive Technology, 17th ed.* (New York: Ardent Media, 1998), 238. Reprinted by permission of Ardent Media.

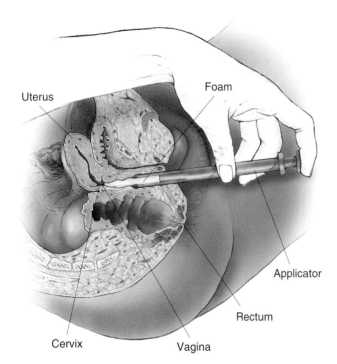

Uterus

Foam

Applicator

Rectum

Cervix

Vagina

Figure 6.2
The Proper Method of Applying Spermicide within the Vagina

designed to kill sperm. Recent studies indicate that spermicides containing N-9 are not effective in preventing certain STIs such as gonorrhea, chlamydia, and HIV. In fact, frequent use of spermicides containing N-9 has been shown to cause irritation and breaks in the mucus layer or skin of the genital tract, which creates a point of entry for viruses and bacteria that cause disease.[2] Although they are not recommended as the primary form of contraception, spermicides often are recommended for use with other forms of contraception. They are most effective when used in conjunction with a condom.

Jellies and creams are packaged in tubes, and foams are available in aerosol cans. All have tubes designed for insertion into the vagina. They must be inserted far enough to cover the cervix, thus providing both a chemical barrier that kills sperm and a physical barrier that stops sperm from continuing toward an egg (Figure 6.2).

Female condom   A single-use polyurethane sheath for internal use.

Diaphragm   A latex, saucer-shaped device designed to cover the cervix and block access to the uterus; it should always be used with spermicide.

Toxic shock syndrome (TSS)   A potentially fatal disease that occurs when specific bacterial toxins are allowed to multiply unchecked in wounds or through improper use of tampons or diaphragms.

Suppositories are waxy capsules that are inserted deep in the vagina, where they melt. They must be inserted 10 to 20 minutes before intercourse to have time to melt, but no longer than one hour prior to intercourse or they lose their effectiveness. Additional contraceptive chemicals must be applied for each subsequent act of intercourse.

The Female Condom   The **female condom** is a single-use, soft, loose-fitting polyurethane sheath meant for internal use. It is designed as one unit with two diaphragm-like rings. One ring, which lies inside the sheath, serves as an insertion mechanism and internal anchor. The other ring, which remains outside the vagina once the device is inserted, protects the labia and the base of the penis from infection. Many women like the female condom because it gives them more control over reproduction than does the male condom. When used correctly, the female condom provides protection against HIV and STIs comparable to that of a latex male condom. The condom's brand name, the Reality Condom, reflects the fact that the condom also can be used for male anal sex.

The Diaphragm with Spermicidal Jelly or Cream   Invented in the mid-nineteenth century, the **diaphragm** was the first widely used birth control method for women. The diaphragm is a soft, shallow cup made of thin latex rubber. Its flexible, rubber-coated ring is designed to fit snugly behind the pubic bone in front of the cervix and over the back of the cervix on the other side so it blocks access to the uterus. Diaphragms are manufactured in different sizes and must be fitted to the woman by a trained practitioner. The practitioner also should be certain that the user knows how to insert her diaphragm correctly before she leaves the practitioner's office.

Diaphragms must be used with spermicidal cream or jelly, which is applied to the inside of the diaphragm before insertion. The diaphragm holds the spermicide in place and creates a physical and chemical barrier against sperm. Additional spermicide must be applied before each subsequent act of intercourse; the diaphragm must be left in place for six to eight hours after intercourse to allow the chemical to kill any sperm remaining in the vagina. When used with spermicidal jelly or cream, it offers significant protection against gonorrhea and possibly chlamydia and human papilloma virus (Figure 6.3).

Using the diaphragm during the menstrual period or leaving it in place longer than 24 hours slightly increases the user's risk of **toxic shock syndrome (TSS).** This condition results from the multiplication of bacteria that spread to the bloodstream and cause sudden high fever, rash, nausea, vomiting, diarrhea, and a rapid drop in blood pressure. If not treated, TSS can be fatal. The diaphragm (as well as wounds or tampons left too long in place) creates conditions conducive to the growth of these bacteria. To reduce the risk of TSS, women should wash their hands carefully with soap and water before inserting or removing a diaphragm.

Another problem with the diaphragm is that it can put undue pressure on the urethra, which blocks urinary flow

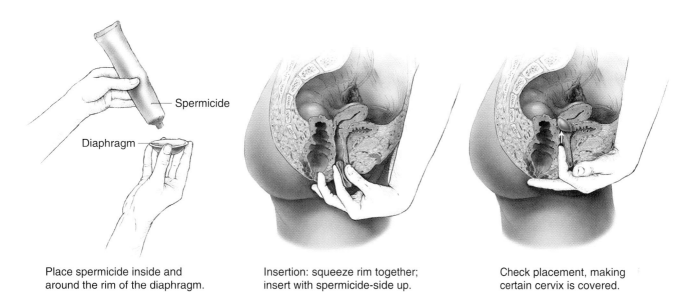

Place spermicide inside and around the rim of the diaphragm.

Insertion: squeeze rim together; insert with spermicide-side up.

Check placement, making certain cervix is covered.

Figure 6.3
The Proper Use and Placement of a Diaphragm

and predisposes the user to bladder infections. A further disadvantage is that inserting the device can be awkward, especially if the woman is rushed. When inserted incorrectly, diaphragms are much less effective.

The Cervical Cap with Spermicidal Jelly or Cream   The cervical cap is one of the oldest methods used to prevent pregnancy. Early cervical caps were made from beeswax, silver, or copper. Today's **cervical cap** is a small cup made of latex that fits snugly over the entire cervix. It must be fitted by a practitioner and is designed for use with spermicidal jelly or cream. It is somewhat more difficult to insert than a diaphragm because of its smaller size.

The cap keeps sperm out of the uterus. It is held in place by suction created during application. Insertion may take place up to two days prior to intercourse; the device must be left in place for six to eight hours after intercourse. If removed and cleaned, it can be reinserted immediately. The cervical cap may offer protection against some STIs but not HIV.

Some women report unpleasant vaginal odors after use. Because the device can become dislodged during intercourse, placement must be checked frequently. The cap cannot be used during the menstrual period or for longer than 48 hours because of the risk of TSS.

Hormonal Methods

Oral Contraceptives   **Oral contraceptive** pills were first marketed in the United States in 1960. Their convenience quickly made them the most widely used reversible method of fertility control.

Most oral contraceptives work through the combined effects of synthetic estrogen and progesterone. Because the levels of estrogen in the pill are higher than those produced by the body, the pituitary gland is never signaled to produce follicle-stimulating hormone (FSH), without which ova will not develop in the ovaries. Progesterone in the pill prevents proper growth of the uterine lining and thickens the cervical mucus, thus forming a barrier against sperm.

Pills are meant to be taken in a cycle. At the end of each three-week cycle, the user discontinues the drug or takes a placebo pill for one week. The resultant drop in hormones causes the uterine lining to disintegrate, and the user will have a menstrual period, usually within one to three days. The same cycle is repeated every 28 days. Menstrual flow is generally lighter than it is for women who don't use the pill, because the hormones in the pill prevent thick endometrial buildup.

Today's pill is different from the one introduced more than four decades ago. The original pill contained large amounts of estrogen, which caused certain risks, whereas the current pill contains the minimal amount of estrogen necessary to prevent pregnancy.

Because the chemicals in oral contraceptives change the way the body metabolizes certain nutrients, all women using the pill should check with their practitioners to see if

> **Cervical cap**   A small cup made of latex that is designed to fit snugly over the entire cervix and used with a spermicide.
>
> **Oral contraceptives**   Pills taken daily for three weeks of the menstrual cycle that prevent ovulation by regulating hormones.

dietary supplements are advisable, especially vitamin C and the B-complex vitamins—B_2, B_6, and B_{12}. A nutritious diet that includes whole grains, fresh fruits and vegetables, lean meats, fish and poultry, and nonfat dairy products is important.

Oral contraceptives can interact negatively with other drugs. For example, some antibiotics diminish the pill's effectiveness and may require an adjustment in the antibiotic dosage. Women in doubt should check with their prescribing practitioners or their pharmacists.

Return of fertility may be delayed after discontinuing the pill, but the pill is not known to cause infertility. Women who had irregular menstrual cycles before going on the pill are more likely to have problems conceiving, regardless of pill use.

The pill is convenient and does not interfere with lovemaking. It may lessen menstrual difficulties, such as cramps and premenstrual syndrome. Oral contraceptives also lower the risk of several health conditions, including endometrial and ovarian cancers, fibrocystic breast disease, ectopic pregnancies, ovarian cysts, pelvic inflammatory disease (PID), and iron deficiency anemia.[3] But possible serious health problems associated with the pill include blood clots, which can lead to strokes or heart attacks, and an increased risk for high blood pressure. The risk is low for most healthy women under 35 who do not smoke; it increases with age and especially with cigarette smoking.

Apart from these risk factors and certain side effects associated with the pill, its greatest disadvantage is that it must be taken every day. If a woman misses one pill, she should use an alternative form of contraception for the remainder of that cycle. Another drawback is that the pill does not protect against STIs. Cost also may be a problem for some women. Some teenagers report that the requirement to have a complete gynecological examination in order to get a prescription for the pill is a huge obstacle. Educating young women about what goes on in a gynecological exam certainly would help ease their anxiety.

Progestin-Only Pills   Progestin-only pills (or minipills) contain small doses of progesterone. Women who feel uncertain about using estrogen pills, who suffer from side effects related to estrogen, or who are nursing may choose these medications rather than combination pills. There is still some

question about how progestin-only pills work. Current thought is that they change the composition of the cervical mucus, thus impeding sperm travel. They also may inhibit ovulation in some women. The effectiveness rate of progestin-only pills is 96 percent, which is slightly lower than that of estrogen-containing pills. Also, their use usually leads to irregular menstrual bleeding. As with all oral contraceptives, the user has no protection against STIs.

Ortho Evra (The Patch)   A hormonal contraceptive patch, **Ortho Evra,** became available by prescription in 2002. The patch is worn for one week and replaced on the same day of the week for three consecutive weeks; the fourth week is patch-free. Ortho Evra is 99 percent effective and works by delivering continuous levels of estrogen and progestin through the skin and into the bloodstream. This patch is easy to apply, barely noticeable, and has adhesive strong enough to withstand even swimming. The patch can be worn on one of four areas of the body: buttocks, abdomen, upper torso (front and back, excluding the breasts), or upper outer arm.

Ortho Evra contains hormones similar to those in birth control pills. Some women report experiencing breast symptoms, headache, application site reaction, nausea, upper respiratory infection, menstrual cramps, and abdominal pain. However, most side effects are not serious. Serious risks, which occur infrequently but can be life threatening, include blood clots, stroke, or heart attacks; tobacco use increases these risks. The contraceptive patch does not protect against HIV or other STIs.

NuvaRing   Introduced in 2002, this effective contraceptive offers protection four weeks at a time when used as prescribed. **NuvaRing** is a soft, flexible ring about 2 inches in diameter that the user inserts into the vagina and leaves in place for three weeks. (The user then removes it for one week for her menstrual period.) Once the ring is inserted, it continuously releases a steady flow of estrogen and progestin.

Advantages to NuvaRing include protection against pregnancy for one month; no pill to take daily; no requirement to be fitted by a clinician; no requirement to use spermicide; and the quick return of the ability to become pregnant when use is stopped. Some of the side effects that women might experience include increased vaginal discharge and vaginal irritation or infection. Oil-based vaginal medicine to treat yeast infections cannot be used when the ring is in place; and a diaphragm or cervical cap cannot be used as a backup method for contraception.

Depo-Provera   Depo-Provera is a long-acting synthetic progesterone that is injected intramuscularly every three months. Researchers believe that the drug prevents ovulation. Depo-Provera encourages sexual spontaneity because the user does not have to remember to take a pill or insert a device. There are fewer health problems associated with Depo-Provera than with estrogen-containing pills. The main

---

Ortho Evra   A patch worn for three weeks at a time that releases hormones similar to those in oral contraceptives.

NuvaRing   A soft, flexible ring inserted into the vagina that releases hormones that prevent pregancy; it is left in place for three weeks and removed for one week for a menstrual period.

Depo-Provera   An injectable method of birth control that lasts for three months.

News from the World of Contraceptives Research

The introduction of a new contraceptive may take years of research and clinical trials prior to approval by the Food and Drug Administration (FDA). However, it appears that within the next few years, our contraceptive options may be expanding. Here's a look at future contraceptives.

NEW BARRIER METHODS

- Lea's Shield is a one-size-fits-all silicon rubber device that covers the cervix. The FDA has asked for more clinical studies prior to approval.
- A new vaginal sponge, Protectaid, is made of polyurethane foam and contains a combination of chemicals that serve as spermicide and microbicide to protect against sexually transmitted infections (STIs). It is available in Canada.
- FemCap is a non-latex device that covers the cervix and forms a seal against the vaginal wall. It is used with spermicide and contains a groove that traps sperm. Already in use in Europe, it was approved in 2003 by the FDA for use if fitted and prescribed by a physician. Distribution is not widespread.

CONTRACEPTIVES FOR MEN

- The often discussed "male pill" is probably about five years away.
- An injectable contraceptive that stimulates the production of antibodies to male sex hormones is in the works and will be tested more extensively within the next few years.
- A synthetic testosterone that would be delivered via a skin implant has been developed by the Population Council and is undergoing further testing to determine side effects.

IMPLANT REFINEMENTS

- The Population Council also is working on a single-rod implant delivery system that would inhibit ovulation for two years. The implant contains Nesterone, a synthetic progestin.
- Also being studied are biodegradable implants containing progestin that would be implanted under the skin of the arm or the hip. The hormone is released gradually into the body for 12 to 18 months.

INJECTIONS AND VACCINES FOR WOMEN

- Oral or injectable vaccine could stimulate the immune system to create antibodies to a crucial type of protein molecule found on the head of sperm.

UNISEX CONTRACEPTION

- A new group of drugs known as gonadotropin-releasing hormone agonists can prevent the release of FSH and LH from the pituitary gland. Blocking these hormones will temporarily suppress fertility in men and women.

Sources: J. Allen, "New Fit for U.S. Birth Control," *Los Angeles Times,* April 28, 2003; Population Council, "Biomedical Research and Products," 2003. www.popcouncil.org/biomed/biomed.html; Johns Hopkins University, "Reproductive Health Online," 2003. www.reproline.jhu.edu/

---

disadvantage is irregular bleeding, which can be troublesome at first, but within a year, most women are amenorrheic (i.e., they have no menstrual periods). Weight gain (an average of five pounds in the first year) is common. Other possible side effects include dizziness, nervousness, and headache. Unlike other methods of contraception, this method cannot be stopped immediately if problems arise. Also, women who wish to become pregnant may find that it takes up to a year after their last injection to do so.

Lunelle and Norplant Two other methods currently off the market could be reinstated in 2004. Lunelle is a monthly injection that contains the time-released synthetic hormones estrogen and progestin. It was recalled from the market due to manufacturing problems that led to pre-filled syringes containing less than the required amount of hormones.

Norplant is a set of six silicon capsules containing progestin that are surgically inserted under the skin of a woman's upper arm. The progestin works the same way that oral contraceptives do to suppress ovulation. Norplant was withdrawn from the market due to legal issues, but if they are resolved, it may become available again.

Surgical Methods

Sterilization, permanent fertility control achieved through surgical procedures, has become the leading method of contraception for women (10.7 million women), closely followed by the oral contraceptive pill (10.4 million women).[4] Although newer surgical techniques make reversal of sterilization theoretically possible, anyone considering sterilization should assume that the operation is *not* reversible. Before becoming sterilized, people should think through possibilities, such as divorce and remarriage or a future improvement in financial status, that might make a larger family realistic.

Sterilization Permanent fertility control achieved through surgical procedures.

Female Sterilization Tubal ligation is one method of sterilization for females. In this surgical procedure, the fallopian tubes are either tied shut or cut and cauterized (burned) at the edges to seal the tubes, thus blocking sperm's access to released eggs. The operation usually is done in a hospital on an outpatient basis. First, the abdomen is inflated with carbon dioxide gas through a small incision in the navel. The surgeon then inserts a *laparoscope* into another incision just above the pubic bone. This specially designed instrument has a fiberoptic light source that enables the physician to see the fallopian tubes clearly.

A tubal ligation does not affect ovarian and uterine function. The woman's menstrual cycle continues, and released eggs simply disintegrate and are absorbed by the lymphatic system. As soon as her incision heals, the woman may resume sexual intercourse with no fear of pregnancy.

As with any surgery, there are risks. Although rare, possible complications of a tubal ligation can include infection, pulmonary embolism, hemorrhage, and ectopic pregnancy.[5] Some patients are given general anesthesia, which itself presents a small risk; others receive local anesthesia. The procedure itself usually takes less than an hour, and the patient generally can return home shortly after waking up. Women considering a tubal ligation should thoroughly discuss all the risks with their physician before the operation.

The **hysterectomy,** or removal of the uterus, is a method of sterilization requiring major surgery. It usually is done only when the patient's uterus is diseased or damaged.

Male Sterilization Sterilization in men is less complicated than it is in women. A **vasectomy** is frequently done on an outpatient basis, using a local anesthetic. The surgeon (generally a urologist) makes an incision on each side of the scrotum, locates the vas deferens on each side, and removes a piece from each. The ends are usually tied or sewn shut.

In a small percentage of cases, serious complications occur, such as formation of a blood clot in the scrotum (which usually disappears without medical treatment), infection, or inflammatory reactions. Because sperm are stored in other areas of the reproductive system besides the vasa deferentia, couples must use alternative methods of birth control for at least one month after the vasectomy. The man must check with his physician (who will do a semen analysis)

to determine when unprotected intercourse can take place. The pregnancy rate in women whose partners have had vasectomies is about 15 in 10,000.

Many men are reluctant to consider sterilization, because they fear the operation will affect sexual performance. However, a vasectomy in no way affects sexual response. Because sperm constitute only a small percentage of semen, the amount of ejaculate does not change significantly. The testes continue to produce sperm, but the sperm can no longer enter the ejaculatory duct. After a time, sperm production may diminish. Any sperm that are manufactured disintegrate and are absorbed into the lymphatic system.

Although a vasectomy should be considered permanent, surgical reversal sometimes can restore fertility. Recent improvements in microsurgery techniques have resulted in annual pregnancy rates of 40 to 60 percent for women whose partners have had reversals. The two major factors influencing the success rate of reversal are the doctor's expertise and the time elapsed since the vasectomy.

What do you think?

Who do you think is responsible for deciding which method of contraception should be used in a sexual relationship? ✳ *What are some examples of good opportunities for you and your partner to have a discussion about contraceptives?* ✳ *What do you think are the biggest barriers in our society to the use of condoms?*

Other Methods of Contraception

Intrauterine Devices Women have been using **intrauterine devices (IUDs)** since 1909, but we still are not certain how they work. Although it was once thought that IUDs prevent implantation of a fertilized egg, most experts now believe that they interfere with fertilization.

Three IUDs are currently available. The first, Progestasert, is a T-shaped plastic device that slowly releases synthetic progesterone. The practitioner must remove this IUD and insert a new one every year. The second, ParaGard, is also T-shaped; it has copper wrapped around the shaft and does not contain any hormones. It can be left in place for ten years before replacement. The third and newest IUD is Mirena, a T-shaped plastic device, which is effective for five years and releases small amounts of the progestin levonorgestrel.

A physician must fit and insert an IUD. For insertion, the device is folded and placed into a long, thin plastic applicator. The practitioner measures the depth of the uterus with a special instrument and then uses these measurements to place the IUD accurately so the arms of the T open across the top of the uterus. One or two strings extend from the IUD into the vagina so the user can check that her IUD is in place. The device is removed by a practitioner when desired.

Tubal ligation Sterilization of the female that involves the cutting and tying off or cauterizing of the fallopian tubes.

Hysterectomy The removal of the uterus.

Vasectomy Sterilization of the male that involves the cutting and tying off of both vasa deferentia.

Intrauterine device (IUD) A T-shaped device that is implanted in the uterus to prevent pregnancy.

Table 6.2
Costs of Contraception

Method	Cost
Continuous abstinence	None
Outercourse (sex play without vaginal intercourse)	None
Withdrawal	None
Sterilization	
Tubal ligation: permanently blocks female's fallopian tubes where sperm join egg	$1,000–$2,500
Vasectomy: permanently blocks male's vas deferentia that carry sperm	$240–$520
Depo-Provera	$20–$40/visits to clinician; $30–$75/injection
IUD (Intrauterine device)	$175–$400/exam, insertion, and follow-up visit
Oral contraceptives	$15–$35/monthly pill-pack at drugstores, often less at clinics; $35–$125/exam
NuvaRing	$30–$35/monthly supply of rings; $35–$125/exam
Ortho Evra (patch)	$30-$35/monthly supply of patches; $35–$125/exam
Condoms/female condoms and spermicide	50¢ and up/condom—some family planning centers give them away or charge very little; $2.50/female condom; $8/applicator kit of spermicide foam and jelly ($4–$8 refills); similar prices for creams, films, and suppositories
Diaphragm or cervical cap	$13–$25/diaphragm or cap; $50–$125/examination; $4–$8/ supplies of spermicide jelly or cream
Fertility awareness methods	$5–$8 and up for temperature kits; free classes often available in health and church centers

Note: Some family planning clinics charge for services on a sliding scale according to income.
Source: Reprinted with permission from Planned Parenthood® Federation of America, Inc. © 2001 PPFA. All rights reserved.

Disadvantages of IUDs include discomfort, cost of insertion, and potential complications. The device can cause heavy menstrual flow and severe cramps. Women using IUDs have a higher risk of uterine perforation, ectopic pregnancy, PID, infertility, and tubal infections. If a pregnancy occurs while the IUD is in place, the chance of miscarriage is 25 to 50 percent, so the device should be removed as soon as possible. Doctors often offer therapeutic abortion to women who become pregnant while using an IUD because of the serious risks (including premature delivery, infection, and congenital abnormalities) associated with continuing the pregnancy.

Table 6.2 compares contraceptive costs.

Withdrawal This birth control method, which is not very effective, is used most commonly by people who have not taken the time to consider alternatives. **Withdrawal,** also called coitus interruptus, involves removing the penis from the vagina just prior to ejaculation. Because there can be up to a half-million sperm in the drop of fluid at the tip of the penis before ejaculation, this method is unreliable. Timing withdrawal is also difficult; males concentrating on accurate timing may not be able to relax and enjoy intercourse.

Emergency Contraceptive Pills There are more than 2.7 million unintended pregnancies per year in the United States, and nearly half are due to contraceptive failure. According to the Centers for Disease Control and Prevention (CDC), more than 11 million American women report using contraceptive methods associated with high failure rates, including condoms, withdrawal, periodic abstinence, and diaphragms.

Emergency contraception can be used when a condom breaks, after a sexual assault, or any time unprotected sexual intercourse occurs. **Emergency contraceptive pills (ECPs)**

Withdrawal A method of contraception that involves removing the penis from the vagina before ejaculation; also called coitus interruptus.

Emergency contraceptive pills (ECPs) Birth control pills containing estrogen and progestin taken within three days after unprotected intercourse to prevent fertilization or implantation.

are ordinary birth control pills containing estrogen and progestin. Although the therapy is commonly known as the morning-after pill, the term is misleading; ECPs can be used up to 72 hours after intercourse and can reduce the risk of pregnancy by 75 percent.

Emergency contraceptives require a prescription; the two FDA-approved products are Preven and Plan B. After a woman determines she is not already pregnant by using the pregnancy test included in the kit, she takes the first dose of two light blue emergency pills as soon as possible, within 72 hours after intercourse. She takes the second dose 12 hours later.[6] The most common side effects related to ECPs are nausea, vomiting, menstrual irregularities, breast tenderness, headache, abdominal pain and cramps, and dizziness.

Emergency minipills contain progestin only. Like ECPs, minipills can be used immediately after unprotected intercourse and up to 72 hours beyond. Emergency minipills are as effective as ECPs, but nausea and vomiting are far less common. Emergency minipills are an excellent alternative for most women who cannot use ECPs that contain estrogen.

Abstinence and "Outercourse" Strictly defined, abstinence means deliberately avoiding intercourse. This strict definition would allow one to engage in such forms of sexual intimacy as massage, kissing, and solitary masturbation. But many people today have broadened the definition of abstinence to include all forms of sexual contact, even those that do not culminate in sexual intercourse.

Couples who go a step further than massage and kissing and engage in activities such as oral–genital sex and mutual masturbation are sometimes said to be engaging in "outercourse." Like abstinence, outercourse can be 100 percent effective for birth control as long as the male does not ejaculate near the vaginal opening. Unlike abstinence, however, outercourse is not 100 percent effective against STIs.

Emergency minipills   Birth control pills containing only progestin that can be taken up to three days after unprotected intercourse.

Fertility awareness methods (FAM)   Several types of birth control that require alteration of sexual behavior rather than chemical or physical intervention into the reproductive process.

Cervical mucus method   A birth control method that relies upon observation of changes in cervical mucus to determine when the woman is fertile.

Body temperature method   A birth control method in which a woman monitors her body temperature for the rise that signals ovulation, the period during which she is fertile.

Calendar method   A birth control method in which a woman's menstrual cycle is mapped on a calendar to determine presumed fertile times.

Oral–genital contact can transmit disease, although the practice can be made safer by using a condom on the penis or a dental dam on the vaginal opening.

Fertility Awareness Methods

Methods of fertility control that rely upon the alteration of sexual behavior are called **fertility awareness methods (FAM).** These techniques include observing female fertile periods by examining cervical mucus and/or keeping track of internal temperature and then abstaining from sexual intercourse (penis–vagina contact) during these fertile times.

Two decades ago, the "rhythm method" was ridiculed because of its low effectiveness rates. However, it was the only method of birth control available to women whose religious denominations forbid the use of oral contraceptives, barrier methods, and sterilization. Our present reproductive knowledge enables women and their partners to use natural methods of birth control with less risk of pregnancy, although these methods remain far less effective than other methods.

FAMs rely upon basic physiology (Figure 6.4). A released ovum can survive up to 48 hours after ovulation. Sperm can live up to five days in the vagina. Natural methods of birth control teach women to recognize their fertile times. Changes in cervical mucus prior to and during ovulation and a rise in basal body temperature are two frequently used indicators. Another method involves charting a woman's menstrual cycle and ovulation times on a calendar. Women may use any combination of these methods to determine their fertile times more accurately.

Cervical Mucus Method The **cervical mucus method** requires women to examine the consistency and color of their normal vaginal secretions to determine when they are fertile. Prior to ovulation, vaginal mucus becomes gelatinous and stretchy, and normal vaginal secretions may increase. Sexual activity involving penis–vagina contact must be avoided while this "fertile mucus" is present and for several days following the mucus changes.

Body Temperature Method The **body temperature method** relies on the fact that the female's basal body temperature rises between 0.4 and 0.8 degree after ovulation. For this method to be effective, the woman must chart her temperature for several months to learn her body's temperature fluctuations. Abstinence from penis–vagina contact must be observed preceding the temperature rise until several days after the temperature rise is first noted.

The Calendar Method The **calendar method** requires the woman to record the exact number of days in her menstrual cycle. Because few women menstruate with complete regularity, this involves keeping a record of the menstrual cycle for 12 months, during which some other method of birth control must be used. The first day of a woman's period counts as day 1. To determine the first fertile unsafe day of the cycle, she subtracts 18 from the number of days in the

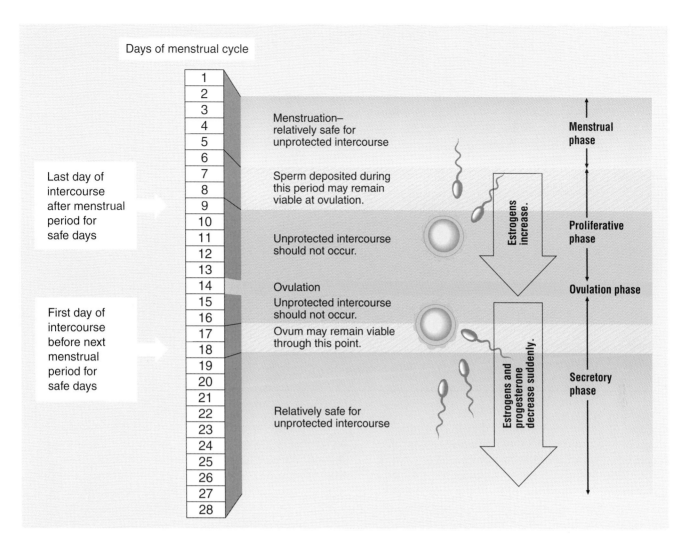

Days of menstrual cycle

| Days |
| 1 |
| 2 |
| 3 |
| 4 |
| 5 |
| 6 |
| 7 |
| 8 |
| 9 |
| 10 |
| 11 |
| 12 |
| 13 |
| 14 |
| 15 |
| 16 |
| 17 |
| 18 |
| 19 |
| 20 |
| 21 |
| 22 |
| 23 |
| 24 |
| 25 |
| 26 |
| 27 |
| 28 |

Last day of intercourse after menstrual period for safe days

First day of intercourse before next menstrual period for safe days

Menstruation–relatively safe for unprotected intercourse

Sperm deposited during this period may remain viable at ovulation.

Unprotected intercourse should not occur.

Ovulation
Unprotected intercourse should not occur.
Ovum may remain viable through this point.

Relatively safe for unprotected intercourse

Estrogens increase.

Estrogens and progesterone decrease suddenly.

Menstrual phase

Proliferative phase

Ovulation phase

Secretory phase

Figure 6.4

The Fertility Cycle

Fertility awareness methods, or FAMs, can combine the use of a calendar, the cervical mucus method, and body temperature measurements to identify the fertile period. It is important to remember that most women do not have a consistent 28-day cycle.

shortest cycle. To determine the last unsafe day of the cycle, she subtracts 11 from the number of days in the longest cycle. This method assumes that ovulation occurs during the midpoint of the cycle. The couple must abstain from penis–vagina contact during the fertile time.

Women interested in FAMs are advised to take supervised classes in their use. Women who are untrained in these techniques run a high risk of unwanted pregnancy.

Abortion

In 1973, the landmark U.S. Supreme Court decision in *Roe v. Wade* stated that the "right to privacy . . . founded on the Fourteenth Amendment's concept of personal liberty . . . is broad enough to encompass a woman's decision whether or not to terminate her pregnancy."[7] The decision maintained that during the first trimester of pregnancy, a woman and her practitioner have the right to terminate the pregnancy through **abortion** without legal restrictions. It allowed individual states to set conditions for second-trimester abortions. Third-trimester abortions were ruled illegal unless the mother's life or health was in danger.

Prior to the legalization of first- and second-trimester abortions, women wishing to terminate a pregnancy had to travel to a country where the procedure was legal, consult an illegal abortionist, or perform their own abortions. Approximately 480,000 illegal abortions were performed in the United States each year, one-third of them on married

> **Abortion** The medical means of terminating a pregnancy.

Abortion Access

The United States has had a long struggle over the issue of abortion. A review of laws and guidelines in other countries shows that different cultures have their own customs and beliefs. Here's a look at some international differences.

- Over 41% of the world's population live in countries that do not require women seeking abortion to meet specific "reason" requirements, meaning that they don't have to explain why they desire an abortion.
- Fourteen countries (including India, Great Britain, and Zimbabwe) have laws that instruct health care providers to consider a woman's economic or social situation in providing abortion services. Women who can show that carrying a baby to term would cause hardship are permitted abortions.
- Thirteen percent of the world's population (53 nations) permit abortion only when the pregnancy poses a threat to the woman's health or safety. Some countries have specific guidelines for determining threat, whereas others allow room for interpretation. For example, in Jamaica, a woman's mental health can be considered, but in Peru there must be a physical threat of permanent injury if the woman carries to term.
- The most stringent laws—those prohibiting abortion completely or allowing it only in cases where the mother's life is endangered—are in place in 74 nations (which represents 21% of the world's population), mainly in Africa and Latin America. In these nations, there can be criminal penalties for both the woman and the abortion provider.
- Fourteen countries require a husband to provide authorization before his wife can receive abortion services. These countries include Japan, Iraq, Syria, and Turkey.

Sources: From Center for Reproductive Rights, "Reproductive Rights 2000: Moving Forward." www.crlp.org/ pub_bo_rr2k.html; A. Rahman, L. Katzive, and S. Fienshaw, "A Global Review of Laws on Induced Abortion, 1985–1997," International Family Planning Perspectives (1998): 24.

---

women. These procedures sometimes led to death from hemorrhage or infection, or infertility from internal scarring.

People who oppose abortion believe that the embryo or fetus is a human being with rights that must be protected. The political debate continues as opponents of abortion pressure state and local governments to pass laws prohibiting the use of public funds for abortion and abortion counseling. In recent years, new legislation has given states the right to impose certain restrictions on abortions. In some states, abortions cannot be performed in publicly funded clinics. Other states have laws requiring parental notification before a teenager can obtain an abortion. Although *Roe v. Wade* has not been overturned, it faces many future challenges.

Although many opponents work through the courts and the political process, attacks on abortion clinics and on doctors who perform abortions are increasingly common. Nearly all clinics have faced threats or acts of violence. Recent legal changes, such as the Freedom of Access to Clinic Entrance Act, offer some relief to the harassment and violence directed at abortion clinics. However, because of such acts, the biggest threat to a woman's access to an abortion now is finding a clinic rather than legal restrictions.[8]

Vacuum aspiration An abortion technique that uses gentle suction to remove fetal tissue from the uterus.

Dilation and evacuation (D&E) An abortion technique that combines vacuum aspiration with dilation and curettage; fetal tissue is both sucked and scraped out of the uterus.

The best birth control methods can fail. Women may be raped. Pregnancies can occur despite every possible precaution. When an unwanted pregnancy does occur, the woman must decide whether to terminate, carry to term and keep the baby, or carry to term and give the baby up for adoption. This is a personal decision that each woman must make, based on her personal beliefs, values, and resources, after carefully considering all alternatives. For a discussion on how abortion is perceived in different countries, see the Health in a Diverse World box.

Methods of Abortion

The choice of abortion procedure is determined by how many weeks the woman has been pregnant. Length of pregnancy is calculated from the first day of her last menstrual period.

Surgical Abortions If performed during the first trimester of pregnancy, abortion presents a relatively low risk to the mother. The most commonly used method of first-trimester abortion is **vacuum aspiration** (Figure 6.5). The procedure is usually performed under a local anesthetic. The cervix is dilated with instruments or by placing *laminaria,* a sterile seaweed product, in the cervical canal. The laminaria is left in place for a few hours or overnight and slowly dilates the cervix. After it is removed, a long tube is inserted into the uterus through the cervix, and gentle suction removes fetal tissue from the uterine walls.

Pregnancies that progress into the second trimester can be terminated through **dilation and evacuation (D&E),**

a procedure that combines vacuum aspiration with a technique called **dilation and curettage (D&C).** Second-trimester abortions frequently are done under general anesthetic. Both procedures can be performed on an outpatient basis (usually in the physician's office), with or without pain medication. Generally, however, the woman is given a mild tranquilizer to help her relax. Both procedures may cause moderate to severe uterine cramping and blood loss.

Two other methods used in second-trimester abortions, though less common than the D&E, are prostaglandin or saline **induction abortions.** Prostaglandin hormones or saline solution are injected into the uterus, which kills the fetus and initiates labor contractions. After 24 to 48 hours, the fetus and placenta are expelled from the uterus.

A **hysterotomy** is surgical removal of the fetus from the uterus. It may be used during emergencies, when the mother's life is in danger, or when other types of abortions are deemed too dangerous.

The risks associated with abortion include infection, incomplete abortion (when parts of the placenta remain in the uterus), missed abortion (when the fetus is not actually removed), excessive bleeding, and cervical and uterine trauma. Follow-up and attention to danger signs decrease the chances of long-term problems.

The mortality rate for first-trimester abortions averages 1 death for every 530,000 at eight or fewer weeks of pregnancy. The rate for second-trimester abortions is higher than 1 per 17,000.[9] This higher rate later in the pregnancy is due to the increased risk of uterine perforation, bleeding, infection, and incomplete abortion due to the fact that the uterine wall becomes thinner as the pregnancy progresses.

One surgical method of performing abortion has been the subject of much controversy. **Intact dilation and extraction (D&X),** sometimes referred to by the nonmedical term *partial-birth abortion,* is used only in certain cases, such as when other abortion methods could injure the mother. The procedure generally involves repositioning the fetus to a breech (feet first) position before extracting most of the body except for the head. The contents of the cranium are then aspirated, which results in "vaginal delivery of a dead but otherwise intact fetus."[10] Federal legislation was passed in October 2003 banning intact dilation and extraction. However, the wording of the legislation is so general that it could be used to ban all types of abortion. For this reason, the legislation is being challenged as unconstitutional. Professional organizations such as the American College of Obstetrics and Gynecology and the American Medical Association state that physicians, acting in the best interests of their patients, should choose the safest and most appropriate method of abortion in each individual case.

Medical Abortions Unlike surgical abortions, medical abortions are performed without entering the uterus. **Mifepristone,** also known as RU-486, is a steroid hormone that induces abortion by blocking the action of progesterone, a

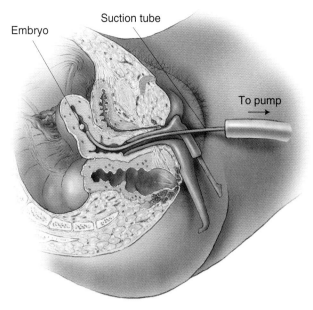

Figure 6.5
Vacuum Aspiration Abortion

hormone produced by the ovaries and placenta that maintains the lining of the uterus. Similar in structure to progesterone, mifepristone binds to cell receptor sites normally occupied by progesterone, which causes the uterine lining to break down. As a result, the uterine lining and the embryo are expelled from the uterus, which terminates the pregnancy.

Mifepristone's nickname, the abortion pill, may imply an easy process. However, this treatment actually involves more steps than a clinical abortion, which takes approximately 15 minutes followed by a physical recovery of about

---

Dilation and curettage (D&C) Abortion technique in which the cervix is dilated with laminaria for one to two days, after which the uterine walls are scraped clean.

Induction abortion Abortion technique in which chemicals are injected into the uterus through the uterine wall; labor begins, and the fetus and placenta are expelled from the uterus.

Hysterotomy The surgical removal of the fetus from the uterus.

Intact dilation and extraction (D&X) A late-term abortion procedure in which the body of the fetus is extracted up to the head and then the contents of the cranium are aspirated.

Mifepristone A steroid hormone that induces abortion by blocking the action of progesterone.

Should Student Health Insurance Cover Prescription Contraceptives?

In 2002, George Washington University (GW) changed its health insurance plan for students to add coverage of prescription contraceptives. The policy change came shortly after advocacy groups representing three female law students at the university sent a letter to school officials urging them to include birth control in the health plan or face a possible lawsuit. The letter was sent jointly by the National Women's Law Center, Trial Lawyers for Public Justice, and Planned Parenthood; it included a petition signed by more than 100 GW students. "The failure to provide coverage for prescription contraceptives is a glaring omission that causes injury to our clients and many other female students at GW, and constitutes sex discrimination," the letter said. "We strongly urge that GW take immediate action to comply with its legal obligation to its students by providing insurance coverage for all FDA-approved prescription drugs and devices, and related medical services, in the health plan it offered to its students."

The letter also cites a lawsuit, *Erickson v. Bartell Drug Co.,* in which a federal court ruled that an otherwise comprehensive health plan cannot exclude prescription contraceptives. The ruling cited Title VII of the Civil Rights Act of 1964, which prohibits employment discrimination based on race, color, religion, sex, or national origin. Although the Erickson case did not involve a university, advocacy groups argue that Title IX of the Education Amendments of 1972, a federal discrimination law, extends the same protection to college students. After receiving the letter, GW quickly complied and asked its insurance company to add birth control pills and other prescription contraceptives to its coverage.

Does your student health insurance plan provide coverage for prescription contraceptives? Do you know where to find information regarding your health insurance policy? Are you aware of your options for obtaining discounted birth control that may or may not be covered in your policy? If your school insurance does not cover prescription contraceptives, what steps can you take to change the policy? Why do you think some schools might object to adding this coverage?

Source: Jeffrey R. Young, "George Washington U. Adds Birth Control to Health Plan," *The Chronicle of Higher Education* 49, no 3 (September 13, 2002): Student Section. ©2002, The Chronicle of Higher Education. Reprinted with permission.

---

one day. With mifepristone, a first visit to the clinic involves a physical exam and a dose of three tablets, which may cause minor side effects such as nausea, headaches, weakness, and fatigue. The patient returns two days later for a dose of prostaglandins (trade name: misoprostol), which causes uterine contractions that expel the fertilized egg. The patient is required to stay under observation at the clinic for four hours.

Ninety-six percent of women who take mifepristone and prostaglandins during the first nine weeks of pregnancy will experience a complete abortion. A return visit is required 12 days later, because the pills fail to expel the fetus completely in 4 percent of cases. In such an event, a clinical abortion becomes necessary.[11]

The side effects of this treatment are similar to those reported during heavy menstruation and include cramping, minor pain, and nausea. Approximately 1 in 1,000 women requires a blood transfusion because of severe bleeding. The procedure does not require hospitalization; women may be treated on an outpatient basis.

Another drug that has been used to induce early-term medical abortions is methotrexate, although it is not approved by the FDA for this purpose. Typically a woman receives an injection from her clinician and, during an office visit three to seven days later, receives a prostaglandin dose. The pregnancy usually ends within four hours.

What do you think?

If you or your partner unexpectedly became pregnant, would you choose to terminate the pregnancy? ＊ How might an abortion affect your relationship? ＊ What factors would you consider in making your decision? ＊ Why?

Planning a Pregnancy

The many methods available to control fertility give you choices that did not exist when your parents—and even you—were born. If you are in the process of deciding whether to have children, take the time to evaluate your emotions, finances, and health.

Emotional Health

First and foremost, consider why you want to have a child: to fulfill an inner need to carry on the family? To escape loneliness? Are there any other reasons? Are you ready to make all the sacrifices necessary to bear and raise a child? Can you care for this new human being in a loving and nurturing manner?

Based on your self-evaluation, if you feel that you are ready to be a parent, the next step is preparation. You can prepare for this change in your life in several ways: read about parenthood, take classes, talk to parents of children of all ages, and join a support group. If you choose to adopt, you will find many support groups available to you as well.

Maternal Health

Before becoming pregnant, a woman should have a thorough medical examination. **Preconception care** should include assessment of potential complications that could occur during pregnancy. Medical problems such as diabetes and high blood pressure should be discussed, as well as any genetic disorders that run in the family. Additional suggestions for a healthy pregnancy include:

- Do not smoke or drink alcohol.
- Reduce or eliminate caffeine intake.
- Avoid exposure to X rays and environmental chemicals, such as lawn and garden chemicals.
- Maintain a normal weight; lose weight if necessary.
- Prior to becoming pregnant, get any dental x-ray examinations that will be needed for a checkup.[12]

Paternal Health

It is common wisdom that mothers-to-be should steer clear of toxic chemicals that can cause birth defects. Even women who are trying to conceive are cautioned to avoid toxic environments, eat a nourishing diet, stop smoking and drinking alcohol, and avoid most medications. Now, similar precautions are recommended for fathers-to-be. New research suggests that a man's exposure to chemicals influences not only his ability to father a child, but also the future health of his child.

Fathers-to-be have been overlooked in past preconception and prenatal studies for several reasons. Researchers assumed that the genetic damage leading to birth defects and other health problems occurred while a child was in the mother's womb. After all, they reasoned, that's where embryonic and fetal development take place. Conventional medical wisdom also held that defective-looking sperm (those with misshapen heads, crooked tails, or retarded swimming ability) were incapable of fertilizing an egg.

Scientists recently have discovered that how sperm look has little to do with how they act. Misshapen sperm can penetrate an egg, and they do not necessarily carry defective genetic goods. Moreover, sperm that look healthy and swim well can be true genetic culprits. DNA fluorescent markers have identified normal-looking yet genetically flawed sperm that carry too many or too few chromosomes. Fathers contribute the extra chromosome 21 in about 6 percent of children with Down syndrome, which causes mental retardation; the extra X chromosome in 50 percent of boys with **Klinefelter's syndrome,** which causes abnormal sexual development; and the shortened chromosome 15 in about 85 percent of children

with **Prader-Willi syndrome,** a disorder characterized by retardation and obesity.

Although some birth defects are caused by random errors of nature, it now appears that some genetic disorders can be traced to sperm damaged by chemicals and toxins. Many drugs and ingested chemicals can readily invade the testes from the bloodstream; others ambush sperm after they leave the testes and pass through the epididymides, where they mature and are stored. By one route or another, half of 100 chemicals studied so far (including by-products of cigarette smoke) apparently harm sperm.

Some researchers believe that vitamin C is nature's way of protecting sex cells. Bad diets, exposure to toxic chemicals, cigarette smoking, and diets low in vitamin C are implicated in sperm damage.[13]

Financial Evaluation

Finances are another important consideration. First, check your health insurance: does it provide pregnancy benefits? If not, you can expect to pay between $1,500 and $5,000 for medical care during pregnancy and birth—and substantially more if complications arise. Both partners should investigate their employers' policies concerning parental leave, including length of leave available and conditions for returning to work.

The U.S. Department of Agriculture estimates that it will cost $169,920 to raise a child born in 2001 to the age of 17. Housing costs and food are the two largest expenditures in raising children.[14] Can you afford to give your child the life you would like him or her to enjoy?

Advanced education is another consideration. If costs continue to rise by about 5 percent, the cost of a four-year education at a private college, for example, will reach almost $257,000 by the year 2019.[15]

Also consider the cost and availability of quality child care. How much family assistance can you realistically expect in helping you with a child? Is child care available if your family is not? While you may be aware of the federal tax credit available for child care, you may not realize how little assistance it actually provides: between a maximum of $480 for one child in a family with income of over $28,000 to a maximum of $720 for one child in a family having income of under $10,000. A second child doubles the credit, but no further assistance is provided for three or more children. Full-time

---

Preconception care   Medical care received prior to becoming pregnant that helps a woman assess and address potential maternal health.

Klinefelter's syndrome   A chromosome defect that causes abnormal sexual development.

Prader-Willi syndrome   A disorder characterized by mental retardation and obesity.

child care averages at least $5,000 to $10,000 a year, depending on your location (it tends to cost more in urban areas).

Contingency Planning

A final consideration is how to provide for the child should something happen to you and your partner. If both of you were to die while the child is young, do you have relatives or close friends who would raise the child? If you have more than one child, would they have to be split up, or could they be kept together? Though unpleasant to think about, this sort of contingency planning is very important. Children who lose their parents are heartbroken and confused. A prearranged plan of action will smooth their transition into new families.

> **What do you think?**
> *What factors will you consider in deciding whether or when to have children?* ✷ *Is there a certain age at which you feel you will be ready to be a parent?* ✷ *What goals do you hope to achieve first?* ✷ *What are your biggest concerns about parenthood?*

Pregnancy

Pregnancy is an important event in a woman's life. The actions taken before a pregnancy begins, as well as behaviors during pregnancy, can have a significant effect on the health of both infant and mother.

Prenatal Care

A successful pregnancy depends on a mother who takes good care of herself and the fetus. It is essential to begin regular medical checkups as soon as possible in the pregnancy (certainly within the first three months). Early detection of fetal abnormalities and identification of high-risk mothers and infants are the major purposes of prenatal care. On the first visit, the practitioner should obtain a complete medical history of the mother and her family and note any hereditary conditions that could put the woman or fetus at risk.

Regular check-ups to measure weight gain and blood pressure and to monitor the size and position of the fetus should continue throughout the pregnancy. This early care reduces infant mortality and low birth weight. The American College of Obstetricians and Gynecologists recommends

Midwives   Experienced practitioners who assist with pregnancy and delivery.

seven or eight prenatal visits for women with low-risk pregnancies. Unfortunately, prenatal care is not available to everyone. Approximately 30 percent of pregnant teenagers and unmarried women do not receive adequate prenatal attention. Babies of mothers who received no prenatal care are about 10 times more likely to die in the first month of life than babies of mothers who got prenatal care.

Additional concerns include the mother's physical condition, her level of nutrition, her confidence in her ability to give birth, her use of drugs and medications, and the availability of a skilled practitioner who can oversee the pregnancy and delivery. A woman planning a pregnancy also needs a support system (spouse or partner, family, friends, community groups) willing to give her and her child love and emotional support during and after her pregnancy.

Choosing a Practitioner   A woman should carefully choose a practitioner to attend her pregnancy and delivery and make this choice before she becomes pregnant, if possible. Recommendations from friends and from one's family physician are a good starting point.

When choosing a practitioner, parents should ask about professional credentials and experience. Besides this information, a pregnant woman must ask questions specific to her condition. Prospective parents also should inquire about the practitioner's experience in handling various complications; commitment to being at the mother's side during delivery; and beliefs and practices concerning the use of anesthesia, fetal monitoring, induced labor, and forceps delivery. What are the practitioner's attitudes toward birth control, abortion, and alternative birthing procedures? His or her approach to nutrition and medication during pregnancy should be similar to the woman's own. Finally, the parents must learn under what circumstances the practitioner would perform a cesarean section (C-section).

Two types of physicians can attend pregnancies and deliveries. The *obstetrician-gynecologist* (ob-gyn) is an M.D. who specializes in obstetrics (pregnancy and birth) and gynecology (care of women's reproductive organs). These practitioners are trained to handle all types of pregnancy-related and delivery-related emergencies. A *family practitioner* is a licensed M.D. who provides comprehensive care for people of all ages. The majority of family practitioners have obstetrical experience but will refer a patient to a specialist if necessary. Unlike the ob-gyn, the family practitioner can serve as the baby's physician after attending the birth.

Midwives are also experienced practitioners who can assist with both pregnancies and deliveries. *Certified nurse-midwives* are registered nurses that have specialized training in pregnancy and delivery. Most midwives work in private practice or in conjunction with physicians. Those who work with physicians have access to traditional medical facilities to which they can turn in an emergency. *Lay midwives* may or may not have extensive training in handling an emergency. They may be self-taught rather than trained through formal certification procedures.

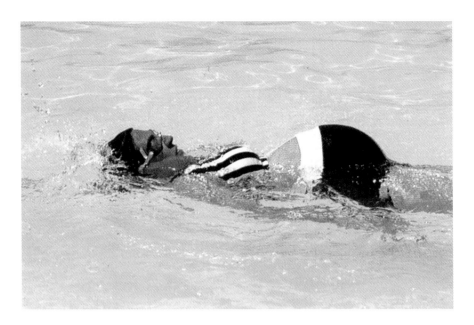

A doctor-approved exercise program during pregnancy can help control weight, make delivery easier, and have a healthy effect on the fetus.

Alcohol and Drugs A woman should avoid all types of drugs during pregnancy. Even common over-the-counter medications such as aspirin and beverages such as coffee and tea can damage a developing fetus.

During the first three months of pregnancy, the fetus is especially subject to the **teratogenic** (birth defect–causing) effects of drugs, environmental chemicals, X rays, or diseases. The fetus also can develop an addiction to or tolerance for drugs that the mother is using. Of particular concern to medical professionals is the use of tobacco and alcohol during pregnancy. The symptoms of **fetal alcohol syndrome (FAS)** include mental retardation, slowed nerve reflexes, and small head size. The exact amount of alcohol necessary to cause FAS is not known, but researchers doubt that it is safe to consume any alcohol. Therefore, they recommend total abstinence from alcohol during pregnancy.

Studies have shown a 25 to 50 percent higher rate of fetal and infant deaths among women who smoke during pregnancy compared with those who do not.[16] Women who smoke more than 10 to 15 cigarettes a day during pregnancy have higher rates of miscarriage, stillbirth, premature births, and low-birth-weight babies than do nonsmokers. Smoking restricts the blood supply to the developing fetus and thus limits oxygen and nutrition delivery and waste removal. It appears to be a significant factor in the development of cleft lip and palate, and a significant relationship has been shown between both smoking and secondhand smoke and sudden infant death syndrome.[17] Fetal research on the effects of secondhand or sidestream smoke (inhaled smoke that is produced by others) is inconclusive, but babies whose parents smoke can be twice as susceptible to pneumonia, bronchitis, and related illnesses. Recent statistics for the United States show that tobacco use among pregnant women has fallen steadily since 1989, when about 20 percent of pregnant women smoked. In 1998, that rate had declined to 12.9 percent.[18]

X rays X rays present a clear danger to the fetus. Although most diagnostic tests produce minimal amounts of radiation, even low levels may cause birth defects or other problems, particularly if several low-dose X rays are taken over a short time period. Pregnant women are advised to avoid X rays unless they are absolutely necessary.

Nutrition and Exercise Pregnant women need additional protein, calories, vitamins, and minerals, so their diets should be carefully monitored by a qualified practitioner. Special attention should be paid to getting enough folic acid (found in dark leafy greens), iron (dried fruits, meats, legumes, liver, and egg yolks), calcium (nonfat or low-fat dairy products and some canned fish), and fluids.

Vitamin supplements can correct some deficiencies, but there is no substitute for a well-balanced diet. Babies born to poorly nourished mothers run high risks of substandard mental and physical development. Folic acid, when consumed before and during early pregnancy, reduces the risk of spina bifida, a common disabling birth condition that results from failure of the spinal column to close. Manufacturers of breads, pastas, rice, and other grain products now are required to add folic acid to their products to reduce neural tube defects in newborns.

Teratogenic Causing birth defects; may refer to drugs, environmental chemicals, X rays, or diseases.

Fetal alcohol syndrome (FAS) A collection of symptoms, including mental retardation, that can appear in infants of women who drink alcohol during pregnancy.

Weight gain during pregnancy helps nourish a growing baby. For a woman of normal weight before pregnancy, the recommended weight gain during pregnancy is 25 to 35 pounds. For obese or overweight women, 15 to 25 pounds are recommended. Underweight women can gain 28 to 40 pounds, and women carrying twins should gain about 35 to 45 pounds. Gaining too much or too little weight can lead to complications. With higher weight gains, women may develop gestational diabetes, hypertension, or increased risk of delivery complications. Gaining too little weight increases the chance of a low-birth-weight baby.

Of the total number of pounds gained during pregnancy, about 6 to 8 are the baby's weight. The baby's birth weight is important, because low weight can mean health problems during labor and the baby's first few months. Pregnancy is not the time to think about losing weight—doing so may endanger the fetus.[19]

As in all other stages of life, exercise is an important factor in weight control during pregnancy and in overall maternal health. In one study, a balanced 45-minute exercise session three days per week was associated with heavier-birthweight babies, fewer surgical births, and shorter hospital stays after birth. Pregnant women should consult their physicians before starting any exercise program.

Other Factors   A pregnant woman should avoid exposure to toxic chemicals, heavy metals, pesticides, gases, and other hazardous compounds. She should not clean cat-litter boxes, because cat feces can contain organisms that cause a disease called **toxoplasmosis.** If a pregnant woman contracts this disease, her baby may be stillborn or suffer mental retardation or other birth defects.

Before becoming pregnant, a woman should be tested to determine whether she has had rubella (German measles). If not, she should be immunized for it and wait the recommended length of time before becoming pregnant. A rubella infection can kill the fetus or cause blindness or hearing disorders in the infant. If the woman has had genital herpes, she should inform her physician. The physician may want to deliver the baby by C-section, especially if the woman has active lesions. Contact with an active herpes infection during birth can be fatal to the infant.

Toxoplasmosis   A disease caused by an organism found in cat feces that, when contracted by a pregnant woman, may result in stillbirth or an infant with mental retardation or birth defects.

Down syndrome   A condition characterized by mental retardation and a variety of physical abnormalities.

Human chorionic gonadotropin (HCG)   Hormone detectable in blood or urine samples of a mother within the first few weeks of pregnancy.

A Woman's Reproductive Years

More than half of the average American woman's expected lifespan is spent between menarche (first menses) and menopause (last menses), a period of approximately 40 years. Deciding whether and when to have children, as well as how to prevent pregnancy when necessary, is a long-term concern.

Today, a woman over 35 who is pregnant has plenty of company. While births to women in their 20s are declining, the rate of first births to women between the ages of 30 and 39 has doubled in the past decade, and births to women over 39 have increased by more than 50 percent. Many women who wait until their 30s to consider motherhood find themselves wondering, "Am I too old to have a baby?" Statistically, the chances of having a baby with birth defects do rise after the age of 35. Researchers believe that there is a decline in both the quality and viability of eggs after this age.

Down syndrome, a condition characterized by mild to severe mental retardation and a variety of physical abnormalities, is the most common genetic condition. One in every 800 to 1,000 live births a year is a child with Down syndrome, which represents approximately 5,000 births per year in the United States alone. A common myth is that most children with Down syndrome have older parents. The truth is that 80 percent of children born with Down syndrome are born to women younger than 35. However, the incidence does increase with age. The incidence of Down syndrome in babies born to a mother of age 20 is 1 in 10,000 births. It rises to 1 in 400 by age 35, 1 in 110 by age 40, and 1 in 35 by age 45.[20]

Women who delay motherhood until their late 30s also worry about their physical ability to carry and deliver their babies. For them, a comprehensive exercise program will assist in maintaining good posture and promoting a successful delivery.

Despite these concerns, there are some advantages to having a baby later in life. In fact, many doctors note that older mothers tend to be more conscientious about following medical advice during pregnancy and more psychologically mature and ready to include an infant in their family than some younger women.

Pregnancy Testing

A woman may suspect she is pregnant before she has any pregnancy tests. A typical sign is a missed menstrual period, yet this is not always an accurate indicator. A woman can miss her period for a variety of reasons: stress, exercise, emotional upset. A pregnancy test scheduled in a medical office or birth control clinic will confirm the pregnancy. Women who wish to know immediately can purchase home pregnancy test kits sold over the counter in drugstores. A positive test is based on the secretion of **human chorionic gonadotropin (HCG)** found in the woman's urine (HCG is also detectable in blood). Home pregnancy test kits come

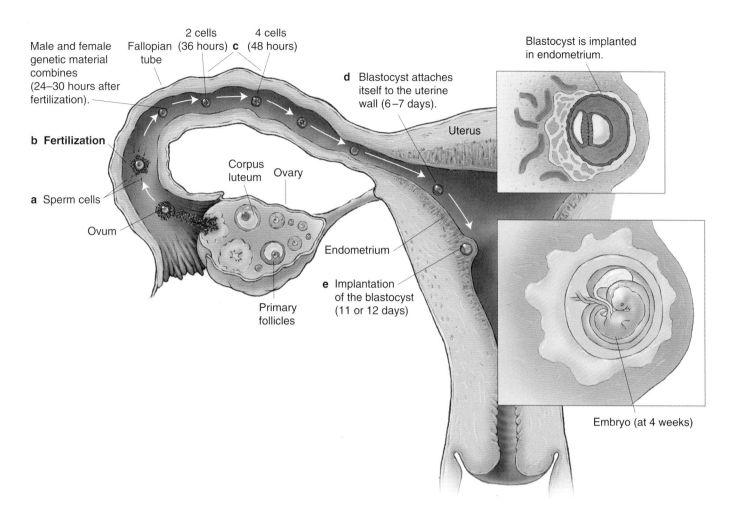

Male and female genetic material combines (24–30 hours after fertilization).

2 cells (36 hours) **c**

4 cells (48 hours)

Fallopian tube

b Fertilization

a Sperm cells

Ovum

Corpus luteum

Ovary

Primary follicles

d Blastocyst attaches itself to the uterine wall (6–7 days).

Uterus

Endometrium

e Implantation of the blastocyst (11 or 12 days)

Blastocyst is implanted in endometrium.

Embryo (at 4 weeks)

Figure 6.6

Fertilization

(**a**) The efforts of hundreds of sperm may allow one sperm to penetrate the ovum's corona radiata, an outer layer of cells, and then the zona pellucida, a thick inner membrane. (**b**) The sperm nucleus fuses with the egg nucleus at fertilization, which produces a zygote. (**c**) The zygote divides first into two cells, then four cells, etc. (**d**) The blastocyst attaches itself to the uterine wall. (**e**) The blastocyst implants itself in the endometrium.

equipped with a small sample of red blood cells coated with HCG antibodies to which the user adds a small amount of urine. If the concentration of HCG is great enough, it will clump together with the HCG antibodies, which indicates that the user is pregnant.

Home pregnancy test kits are about 85 to 95 percent reliable. If done too early in the pregnancy, they may show a false negative. Other causes of false negatives are unclean test tubes, ingestion of certain drugs, and vaginal or urinary tract infections. Accuracy also depends on the quality of the test itself and the user's ability to perform it and interpret the results. Blood tests administered and analyzed by a medical laboratory are more accurate.

The Process of Pregnancy

Pregnancy begins the moment a sperm fertilizes an ovum in the fallopian tubes (Figure 6.6). From there, the single cell multiplies and becomes a sphere-shaped cluster of cells as it travels toward the uterus, a journey that may take three to four days. Upon arrival, the embryo burrows into the thick, spongy endometrium and is nourished from this carefully prepared lining.

Early Signs of Pregnancy The first sign of pregnancy is usually a missed menstrual period (although some women "spot" in early pregnancy, which may be mistaken for a period). Other signs of pregnancy include:

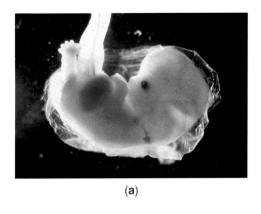
(a)

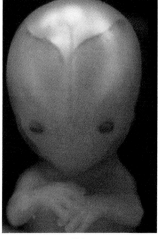
(b)

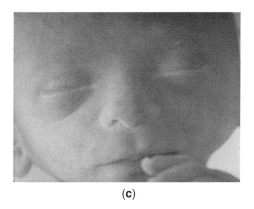
(c)

This series of fetoscopic photographs shows the development of the fetus in the first (a), second (b), and third (c) trimesters of pregnancy.

- Breast tenderness
- Emotional upset
- Extreme fatigue
- Nausea
- Sleeplessness
- Vomiting (especially in the morning)

Pregnancy typically lasts 40 weeks. The due date is calculated from the expectant mother's last menstrual period. Pregnancy is typically divided into three phases, or **trimesters,** of approximately three months each. The trimester is used to describe specific developmental changes that occur in the embryo or the fetus.

The First Trimester   During the first trimester, few noticeable changes occur in the mother's body. She may urinate more frequently and experience morning sickness, swollen breasts, or undue fatigue. But these symptoms may not be frequent or severe, so she may not even realize she is pregnant unless she has a pregnancy test.

Trimester   A three-month segment of pregnancy; used to describe specific developmental changes that occur in the embryo or the fetus.

Embryo   The fertilized egg from conception until the end of two months' development.

Fetus   The name given the developing baby from the third month of pregnancy until birth.

Placenta   The network of blood vessels connected to the umbilical cord that carries nutrients and oxygen to the developing fetus and carries fetal wastes to the mother.

During the first two months after conception, the **embryo** differentiates and develops its various organ systems, beginning with the nervous and circulatory systems. At the start of the third month, the embryo is called a **fetus,** which indicates that all organ systems are in place. For the rest of the pregnancy, growth and refinement occur in each major body system so that they can function independently, yet in coordination, at birth. The photos illustrate physical changes during fetal development.

The Second Trimester   At the beginning of the second trimester, physical changes in the mother become more visible. Her breasts swell, and her waistline thickens. During this time, the fetus makes greater demands upon the mother's body. In particular, the **placenta,** the network of blood vessels connected to the umbilical cord that carry nutrients and oxygen to the fetus and fetal waste products to the mother, becomes well established.

The Third Trimester   From the end of the sixth month through the ninth is considered the third trimester. This is the period of greatest fetal growth, when the fetus gains most of its weight. During the third trimester, the fetus must get large amounts of calcium, iron, and nitrogen from the food the mother eats. Approximately 85 percent of the calcium and iron the mother digests goes into the fetal bloodstream.

Although the fetus may live if it is born during the seventh month, it needs the layer of fat it acquires during the eighth month and time for the organs (especially the respiratory and digestive organs) to develop to their full potential. Babies born prematurely usually require intensive medical care.

Of course, the process of pregnancy involves much more than the changes in a woman's body. Many important

Table 6.3
Common Emotions Experienced throughout the Pregnancy Process

First Trimester	Second Trimester	Third Trimester	Fourth Trimester
Disbelief that one is actually pregnant	Sense that the pregnancy feels "real"	Development of emotional relationship with baby—beginning to view baby as a person as more fetal movement occurs	Sense of being overwhelmed at new responsibility—"What do we do now?"
Fear of miscarriage	Less fear of miscarriage	Fear of labor, labor complications, possible defects	Difficulty in settling limits on friend and family visits; learning to negotiate everyone's roles in baby's life
Feeling of being overwhelmed by changes	Wonder at hearing the heartbeat, feeling movement, bulging tummy	Possible tiredness of pregnancy (Pregnancy seems to take over identity—"Is that all people want to talk about?")	Exhaustion and emotional vacillation due to sleep deprivation, breast-feeding
Tendency to be more emotional, crying more easily, for example	Frustration when symptoms make fulfilling other responsibilities difficult	Impatience for due date to arrive, possible frustration with limited mobility	Surprise at how slow the physical healing process may be, impatient to get back to pre-pregnancy shape
Apprehension about upcoming decisions (screening tests, etc.)	Differing emotions about weight gain (Some enjoy it; others struggle with it.)	Interest in others' birth experiences (especially one's mother's) and parenting styles	Amazement at the birth process
Excitement about telling others about pregnancy if waiting until the end of first trimester	Excitement and anxiety in making plans for future	Excitement in making final preparations for baby, baby showers, which makes the event seem more real	Excitement about future; apprehension about post-maternity leave transition, if applicable— "How will I balance everything?"
Anxiety about being a parent	Anxiety about being a parent	Anxiety about being a parent	Anxiety about being a parent

Source: Information for second through fourth trimesters adapted from C. M. Peterson and N. L. Stotland, "Physical and Emotional Changes," *Lamaze Parents Magazine,* 2000 spring/summer issue. Reprinted by permission of Lamaze, Inc.

emotional changes occur from the time a woman learns she is pregnant through the **"fourth trimester"** (the first six weeks of an infant's life outside the womb). Table 6.3 outlines common emotions and emotional challenges that may arise over the course of a pregnancy.

Prenatal Testing and Screening

Modern technology enables medical practitioners to detect health defects in a fetus as early as the fourteenth to eighteenth weeks of pregnancy. One common testing procedure, **amniocentesis,** is strongly recommended for women over age 35. It involves inserting a long needle through the mother's abdominal and uterine walls into the **amniotic sac,** the protective pouch surrounding the fetus (Figure 6.7). The needle draws out 3 to 4 teaspoons of fluid, which are analyzed for genetic information about the baby. This test can reveal the presence of 40 genetic abnormalities, including Down syndrome, Tay-Sachs disease (a fatal disorder of the nervous system common among Jewish people of Eastern European descent), and sickle-cell anemia (a debilitating blood disorder found primarily among African Americans).

Amniocentesis also can reveal gender, a fact many parents choose not to know until the birth. Although widely used, amniocentesis is not without risk. Chances of fetal damage and miscarriage as a result of testing are 1 in 400.

Another procedure, *ultrasound,* or *sonography,* uses high-frequency sound waves to determine the size and position of the fetus. Ultrasound also can detect fetal defects in the central nervous system and digestive system. Knowing the position of the fetus helps practitioners perform amniocentesis and deliver the infant. New three-dimensional

"Fourth trimester" The first six weeks of an infant's life outside the womb.

Amniocentesis A medical test in which a small amount of fluid is drawn from the amniotic sac to test for Down syndrome and other genetic abnormalities.

Amniotic sac The protective pouch surrounding the fetus.

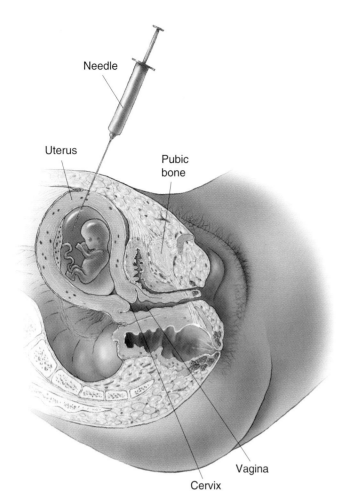

Needle

Uterus

Pubic bone

Vagina

Cervix

Figure 6.7
Amniocentesis
The process of amniocentesis can detect certain congenital problems as well as the sex of the fetus.

What do you think?

In looking at your current lifestyle, what behaviors (e.g., nutritional choices, fitness, etc.) would you cease or begin in order to promote a healthy pregnancy? ✳ *What would you look for in selecting a health care provider during your own or your partner's pregnancy?* ✳ *Would you want to know if you were carrying a child with a genetic defect or other abnormality?* ✳ *Why or why not?*

Childbirth

Prospective parents need to make a number of key decisions long before the baby is born. These include where to have the baby, whether to use drugs during labor and delivery, choice of childbirth method, and whether to breast-feed or bottle-feed. Answering these questions will ensure a smoother passage into parenthood.

Choosing Where to Have Your Baby

Today's prospective mothers have many delivery options, ranging from traditional hospital birth to home birth. Parental values are important. Many couples, for instance, feel that the modern medical establishment has dehumanized the birth process. Thus, they choose to deliver at home or at a *birthing center,* a homelike setting outside a hospital where women can give birth and receive postdelivery care by a team of professional practitioners that includes physicians and registered nurses.

However, hospitals have responded to the desire for a more relaxed, less medically oriented birthing process. Many hospitals now offer labor–delivery–postpartum birthing rooms, which allow patients with noncomplicated deliveries to spend the entire process in one room. In addition, "rooming-in," or keeping the baby in the same room with the mother at all times, is encouraged to facilitate bonding and breast-feeding. Partners are generally encouraged to room-in with mother and baby as well.

Labor and Delivery

The birth process has three stages (Figure 6.8). The exact mechanisms that initiate labor are unknown. During the few weeks preceding delivery, the baby normally shifts to a head-down position, and the cervix begins to dilate (widen). The junction of the pubic bones also loosens to permit expansion of the pelvic girdle during birth.

In the first stage of labor, the amniotic sac breaks, which causes a rush of fluid from the vagina (commonly referred to as "breaking of the waters"). Contractions in the

ultrasound techniques clarify images and improve doctors' efforts to detect and treat defects prenatally.

A third procedure, *fetoscopy,* involves making a small incision in the abdominal and uterine walls and inserting an optical viewer into the uterus to view the fetus directly. This device is used with ultrasound to determine fetal age and location of the placenta. This method is still experimental and involves some risk. It causes miscarriage in approximately 5 percent of cases.

A fourth test, *chorionic villus sampling (CVS),* involves snipping tissue from the developing fetal sac. CVS can be used at 10 to 12 weeks of pregnancy, and results are available in 12 to 48 hours. CVS is an attractive option for couples who are at high risk for having a baby with Down syndrome or a debilitating hereditary disease.

If any of these tests reveals a serious birth defect, parents are advised to undergo genetic counseling. In the case of a chromosomal abnormality such as Down syndrome, the parents usually are offered the option of a therapeutic abortion. Some parents choose this option; others research the disability and decide to go ahead with the birth.

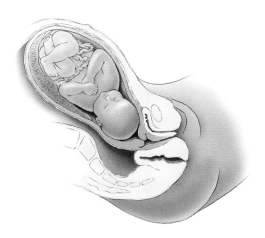

Dilation of the cervix

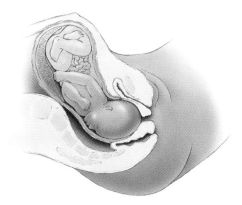

Transition ─────────── **End of Stage I**

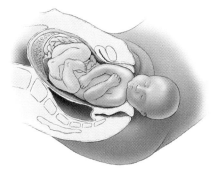

Birth of the baby (Expulsion) ───── **End of Stage II**

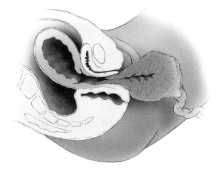

Delivery of the placenta ─────── **End of Stage III**

Figure 6.8
The Birth Process

abdomen and lower back also signal the beginning of labor. Early contractions push the baby downward, which puts pressure on the cervix and dilates it further. The first stage of labor may last from a couple of hours to more than a day for a first birth, but it is usually much shorter during subsequent births.

The end of the first stage of labor, called **transition,** is the process during which the cervix becomes fully dilated and the baby's head begins to move into the vagina, or the birth canal. Contractions usually come quickly during transition, which generally lasts 30 minutes or less.

The second stage of labor (the *expulsion stage*) follows transition when the cervix has become fully dilated. Contractions become rhythmic, strong, and more painful as the uterus pushes the baby through the birth canal. The expulsion stage lasts one to four hours and concludes when the infant is finally pushed out of the mother's body. In some cases, the attending practitioner will do an **episiotomy,** a straight incision in the mother's **perineum** (the area between the vulva and the anus), to prevent the baby's head from tearing vaginal tissues and to speed the baby's exit from the vagina. Sometimes women can avoid the need for an episiotomy by exercising and getting good nutrition throughout pregnancy, by trying different birth positions, or by having an attendant massage the perineal tissue. However, the skin's natural elasticity and the baby's size are limiting factors.

After delivery, the attending practitioner cleans the baby's mucus-filled breathing passages, and the baby takes its first breath, which is generally accompanied by a loud wail. (The traditional slap on the baby's buttocks, often romanticized in old movies, is no longer a common practice because of the trauma to the baby.) The umbilical cord is then tied and severed. The stump of cord attached to the baby's navel dries up and drops off within a few days.

In the meantime, the mother continues into the third stage of labor, during which the placenta, or **afterbirth,** is expelled from the womb. This stage is usually completed within 30 minutes after delivery.

Most mothers prefer to have their new infants next to them following the birth. Together with their spouse or partner, they feel a need to share this time of bonding with their infant.

Transition   The process during which the cervix becomes nearly fully dilated and the baby's head begins to move into the birth canal.

Episiotomy   A straight incision in the mother's perineum.

Perineum   The area between the vulva and the anus.

Afterbirth   The placenta expelled from the womb, usually within 30 minutes after delivery.

Managing Labor: Medical and Nonmedical Approaches

Because pain-killing drugs given to the mother during labor can cause sluggish responses in the newborn and other complications, many women choose drug-free labor and delivery. But it is important to keep a flexible attitude about pain relief, because each labor is different. Working in partnership with a health care provider to make the best decision for mother and baby is the best plan. Use of pain-killing medication during a delivery is not a sign of weakness. One person is not a success for delivering without medication, while another is a failure for using medical measures. Remember, pain is to be expected. In fact, many experts say that the pain of labor is the most difficult in the human experience. However, there is no one right answer in managing that pain.

Alternative Birth Methods

Expectant parents have several options beyond the traditional hospital setting for the process of their infant's birth and their participation in it. Although several of these methods have decreased in popularity, all continue to be used.

The Lamaze method is the most popular birth alternative in the United States. Prelabor classes teach the mother to control her pain through special breathing patterns, focusing exercises, and relaxation. Lamaze births usually take place in a hospital or birthing center with a physician or midwife in attendance. The partner (or labor coach) assists by giving emotional support, physical comfort (massage and ice chips), and coaching for proper breath control during contractions. Lamaze proponents discourage the use of drugs.

Other methods prospective parents can research include the Harris method, Childbirth without Fear, the Leboyer method, the Bradley Method, and water birth. These vary in their philosophies regarding painkillers, partner participation, and other issues.

Breast-Feeding and the Postpartum Period

Although the new mother's milk will not begin to flow for two or more days, her breasts secrete a thick yellow substance called *colostrum*. Because this fluid contains vital antibodies to help fight infection, the newborn baby should be allowed to suckle.

Postpartum depression   The experience of energy depletion, anxiety, mood swings, and depression that women may feel during the postpartum period four to six weeks after delivery.

The American Academy of Pediatrics strongly recommends that infants should be breast-fed for at least six months, and ideally for 12 months. Scientific findings indicate there are many advantages to breast-feeding. Breast-fed babies have fewer illnesses and a much lower hospitalization rate, because breast milk contains maternal antibodies and immunological cells that stimulate the infant's immune system. When breast-fed babies get sick, they recover more quickly. They are also less likely to be obese than babies fed on formulas, and they have fewer allergies. They may even be more intelligent: one study found that the longer a baby was breast-fed, the higher the IQ in adulthood. Researchers theorize that breast milk contains substances that enhance brain development.[21] A recent study, by Avery et al., found that women who were able to breast-feed successfully for longer periods of time generally viewed breast-feeding as more positive, had more knowledge about the process, and had higher self-efficacy in their ability to breast-feed.[22]

This does not mean that breast milk is the only way to nourish a baby. Prepared formulas can provide nourishment that allows a baby to grow and thrive.

When deciding whether to breast- or bottle-feed, mothers need to consider their own desires and preferences too. Both feeding methods can supply the physical and emotional closeness so essential to the parent–child relationship.

The *postpartum period* lasts four to six weeks after delivery. During this period, the reproductive organs revert to a nonpregnant state, and many women experience energy depletion, anxiety, mood swings, and depression. This experience, known as **postpartum depression,** appears to be a normal end-product of the birth process. For most women, the symptoms gradually disappear as their bodies return to normal. For others, the symptoms, coupled with the stresses of managing a new family, can cause more severe depression that lasts for several months.

> ### What do you think?
> *What are your thoughts on medical versus natural management of labor and delivery?* ✳ *Do you have strong preferences for how you would like to manage your own birthing process?* ✳ *If so, what are they?* ✳ *What might be the advantages and disadvantages of breast-feeding?*

Complications

Complications can occur during labor and delivery, even following a successful pregnancy. The mother should discuss these possibilities with her practitioner prior to labor so she understands the medical procedures that may be necessary for her safety and that of her child.

Cesarean Section If labor lasts too long or if a baby is presenting wrong (about to exit the uterus in any way but head first), a **cesarean section (C-section)** may be necessary. This surgical procedure involves making an incision across the mother's abdomen and through the uterus to remove the baby. This operation also is performed if labor is extremely difficult, maternal blood pressure falls rapidly, the placenta separates from the uterus too soon, the mother has diabetes, or other problems occur.

The rate of delivery by C-section in the United States has increased from 5 percent in the mid-1960s to 26.1 percent in 2002.[23] A C-section can be traumatic for the mother if she is not prepared for it. Risks to her are the same as for any major abdominal surgery; recovery from birth takes considerably longer after a C-section. Although C-sections are necessary in certain cases, some physicians and critics, including the federal government's CDC, feel that C-sections have been performed too frequently in this country. The CDC had hoped to lower the rate of C-sections in the United States to 15 per 100 births by the year 2000, a level the agency considers medically appropriate. Clearly, the goal has not been met.

However, surgical techniques allow some women who have had a C-section to deliver subsequent children vaginally. Guidelines published by the American College of Obstetricians and Gynecologists give an estimated 50 to 80 percent of women the option of a vaginal birth after cesarean. Cesarean sections still will be necessary, however, if the original incision runs from the top to the bottom of the uterus (as opposed to across); if the baby is over 9 pounds; if the birth is multiple; or if the mother has a medical condition that would make vaginal delivery difficult or dangerous, such as a very small pelvis, chronic high blood pressure, or diabetes.

Miscarriage One in ten pregnancies does not end in delivery. Loss of the fetus before it is viable is called a **miscarriage** (also referred to as spontaneous abortion). An estimated 70 to 90 percent of women who miscarry eventually become pregnant again.

Reasons for miscarriage vary. In some cases, the fertilized egg has failed to divide correctly. In others, genetic abnormalities, maternal illness, or infections are responsible. Maternal hormonal imbalance also may cause a miscarriage, as may a weak cervix or toxic chemicals in the environment. In most cases, the cause for miscarriage is not known.

A blood incompatibility between mother and father can cause **Rh factor** problems that sometimes result in miscarriage. Rh is a blood protein. Rh problems occur when the mother is Rh-negative and the fetus is Rh-positive. During a first birth, some of the baby's blood passes into the mother's bloodstream. An Rh-negative mother may manufacture antibodies to destroy the Rh-positive blood introduced into her bloodstream at the time of birth. Her first baby will be unaffected, but subsequent babies with positive Rh factor will be at risk for a severe anemia called *hemolytic disease* because the mother's Rh antibodies will attack the fetus's red blood cells.

If prenatal testing reveals Rh incompatibility, intrauterine transfusions can be given or an early delivery by C-section can be done. Prevention is preferable to treatment. All women with Rh-negative blood should be injected with a medication called RhoGAM within 72 hours of any birth, miscarriage, or abortion. This injection will prevent them from developing the Rh antibodies.

Another cause of miscarriage is **ectopic pregnancy,** or implantation of a fertilized egg outside the uterus. A fertilized egg may implant itself in the fallopian tube or, occasionally, in the pelvic cavity. Because these structures are not capable of expanding and nourishing a developing fetus, the pregnancy cannot continue and is terminated surgically. Most often, the affected fallopian tube also is removed.

Ectopic pregnancy generally is accompanied by pain in the lower abdomen or aching in the shoulders as the blood flows up toward the diaphragm. If bleeding is significant, blood pressure drops, and the woman can go into shock. If an ectopic pregnancy goes undiagnosed and untreated, the fallopian tube will rupture, which puts the woman at great risk of hemorrhage, peritonitis (infection in the abdomen), and even death.

Over the past 12 years, the incidence of ectopic pregnancy has tripled, and no one really understands why. We do know that ectopic pregnancy is a potential side effect of PID, which has become increasingly common in recent years. The scarring or blockage of the fallopian tubes that is characteristic of this disease prevents the fertilized egg from passing to the uterus. About 50 percent of women who have had an ectopic pregnancy conceive again. But women who have had one ectopic pregnancy run a higher risk of having another.

Stillbirth is one of the most traumatic events a couple can face. A stillborn baby is born dead, often for no apparent reason. The grief experienced following a stillbirth is usually devastating. Nine months of happy anticipation have been thwarted. Family, friends, and other children may be in a state of shock and need comfort but not know where to turn.

Cesarean section (C-section) A surgical procedure in which a baby is removed through an incision made in the mother's abdominal and uterine walls

Miscarriage Loss of the fetus before it is viable; also called spontaneous abortion.

Rh factor A blood protein related to the production of antibodies. If an Rh-negative mother is pregnant with an Rh-positive fetus, the mother will manufacture antibodies that can kill the fetus, which causes miscarriage.

Ectopic pregnancy Implantation of a fertilized egg outside the uterus, usually in a fallopian tube; a medical emergency that can end in the mother's death from hemorrhage or peritonitis.

Stillbirth The birth of a dead baby.

The mother's breasts produce milk, and there is no infant to be fed. A room with a crib and toys is left empty.

The grief can last for years, and both partners may blame themselves or each other. In many cases, no amount of reassurance from the attending physician, relatives, or friends can assuage the grief or guilt. Well-intended comments such as, "Oh, you'll have another baby someday," may bring no comfort.

Some communities have groups called the Compassionate Friends to help parents and other family members through this grieving process. This nonprofit organization is for parents who have lost a child of any age for any reason.

Sudden Infant Death Syndrome The unexpected death of a child under one year of age, for no apparent reason, is called **sudden infant death syndrome (SIDS).** Though SIDS is the leading cause of death for children aged one month to one year and affects about 1 in 1,000 infants in the United States each year, it is not a disease. Rather, it is ruled the cause of death after all other possibilities are ruled out. A SIDS death is sudden and silent; death occurs quickly, often during sleep, with no signs of suffering.

Because SIDS is a diagnosis of exclusion, doctors do not know what causes it. However, research done in countries including England, New Zealand, Australia, and Norway has shown that placing children on their backs or sides to sleep cuts the rate of SIDS by as much as half. The American Academy of Pediatrics advises parents to lay infants on their backs. Additional precautions against SIDS include breast-feeding, having a firm surface for the infant's bed, not allowing the child to become too warm, maintaining a smoke-free environment, having regular pediatric visits, and seeking prenatal care.

Infertility

An estimated one in six American couples experiences **infertility,** or difficulties in conceiving. Reasons include the trend toward delaying childbirth (as a woman gets older, she is less likely to conceive), endometriosis, and the rising incidence of PID.

Causes in Women

Endometriosis is the leading cause of infertility in women in the United States. With this disorder, parts of the endometrial lining of the uterus implant themselves outside the uterus—in the fallopian tubes, lungs, intestines, outer uterine walls or ovarian walls, and/or on the ligaments that support the uterus. The disorder can be treated surgically or with hormonal preparations. Success rates vary.

Another cause of infertility is **pelvic inflammatory disease (PID),** a serious infection that scars the fallopian tubes and blocks sperm migration. PID is a collective name for any extensive bacterial infection of the female pelvic organs, particularly the uterus, cervix, fallopian tubes, and ovaries. PID often results from chlamydia or gonorrheal infections that spread to the fallopian tubes or ovaries. Symptoms include severe pain, fever, and sometimes vaginal discharge.

The past 30 years have brought a tremendous increase in the annual number of PID cases, from 17,800 to about 1 million per year. During the reproductive years, one in seven women reports having been treated for PID,[24] and tens of thousands have been rendered sterile. One episode of PID causes sterility in 10 to 15 percent of women, and 50 to 75 percent become sterile after three or four infections.[25]

Causes in Men

Among men, the single largest fertility problem is **low sperm count.** Although only one viable sperm is needed for fertilization, research has shown that all the other sperm in the ejaculate aid in the fertilization process. There are normally 60 to 80 million sperm per milliliter of semen. When the count drops below 60 million, fertility declines.

Low sperm count may be attributable to environmental factors, such as exposure of the scrotum to intense heat or cold, radiation, or altitude; or even to wearing excessively tight underwear or outerwear. However, other factors, such as the mumps virus, can damage the cells that make sperm. Varicose veins above one or both testicles also can render men infertile. Male infertility problems account for around 40 percent of infertility cases.

Treatment

For the couple desperately wishing to conceive, the road to parenthood may be frustrating. Fortunately, medical treatment can identify the cause of infertility in about 90 percent of cases. The chances of becoming pregnant range from 30 to 70 percent, depending on the reason for infertility. The countless tests and the invasion of privacy that characterize some couples' efforts to conceive can put stress on an

---

Sudden infant death syndrome (SIDS) The sudden death of a child under one year of age for no apparent reason.

Infertility Difficulties in conceiving.

Endometriosis A disorder in which uterine lining tissue establishes itself outside the uterus; the leading cause of infertility in the United States.

Pelvic inflammatory disease (PID) An infection that causes infertility by scarring the fallopian tubes and consequently blocks sperm migration.

Low sperm count A sperm count below 60 million sperm per milliliter of semen; the leading cause of infertility in men.

otherwise strong, healthy relationship. Before starting fertility tests, couples should reassess their priorities. Some will choose to undergo counseling to help them clarify their feelings about the fertility process. A good physician or fertility team will take the time to ascertain the couple's level of motivation.

Fertility workups can be expensive, and the costs usually are not covered by insurance companies. Fertility workups for men include a sperm count, a test for sperm motility, and analysis of any disease processes present. Such procedures should be undertaken only by a qualified urologist. Women are thoroughly examined by an obstetrician–gynecologist for the composition of cervical mucus, extent of tubal scarring, and evidence of endometriosis.

Complete fertility workups may take four to five months and can be unsettling. The couple may be instructed to have sex "by the calendar" to increase their chances of conceiving. In some cases, surgery can correct structural problems, such as tubal scarring. In others, administering hormones can improve the health of ova and sperm. Sometimes pregnancy can be achieved by collecting the man's sperm from several ejaculations and inseminating the woman at a later time.

When all surgical and hormonal methods fail, the couple still has some options. These, too, can be very expensive. **Fertility drugs,** such as Clomid and Pergonal, contain hormones that stimulate ovulation in women who are not ovulating. Ninety percent of women who use these drugs will begin to ovulate, and half will conceive.

Fertility drugs can have many side effects, including headaches, irritability, restlessness, depression, fatigue, edema (fluid retention), abnormal uterine bleeding, breast tenderness, vasomotor flushes (hot flashes), and visual difficulties. Women using fertility drugs are also at increased risk of developing multiple ovarian cysts (fluid-filled growths) and liver damage. Sometimes the drugs trigger the release of more than one egg, so the woman has a one in ten chance of having multiple births. Most such births are twins, but triplets and even quadruplets are not uncommon.

Alternative insemination of a woman with her partner's sperm is another option. This technique has led to an estimated 250,000 births in the United States, primarily for couples in which the man is infertile. If this procedure fails, the couple may choose insemination by an anonymous donor through a sperm bank. Many men sell their sperm to such banks. The sperm are classified according to the physical characteristics of the donor (for example, blonde hair, blue eyes) and then frozen for future use. Frozen sperm can survive up to five years. The woman being inseminated usually chooses sperm from a man whose physical characteristics resemble those of her partner or match her own personal preferences.

In the last few years, concern has been expressed about the possibility of transmitting the AIDS virus through alternative insemination. As a result, donors are routinely screened for the disease.

In vitro fertilization, often referred to as test tube fertilization, involves collecting a viable ovum from the prospective mother and transferring it to a nutrient medium in a laboratory, where it is fertilized with sperm from the woman's partner or a donor. After a few days, the embryo is placed in the mother's uterus, where, it is hoped, it will implant and develop normally. Since 1984, in vitro fertilization has been responsible for 26,000 births in the United States alone.

Intracytoplasmic sperm injection (ICSI) was first performed successfully in 1992. Basically, a sperm cell is injected into an egg. This complex procedure required researchers to learn how to manipulate both egg and sperm without damaging them. This technique can help men with low sperm counts or motility, and even those who cannot ejaculate or have no live sperm in their semen as a result of vasectomy, chemotherapy, or a medical disorder. However, recent studies have found that infants conceived with the use of ICSI or in vitro fertilization have twice the risk of a major birth defect as those conceived naturally.[26]

In **gamete intrafallopian transfer (GIFT),** the egg is harvested from the woman's ovary and placed in the fallopian tube with the man's sperm. Less expensive and time consuming than in vitro fertilization, GIFT mimics nature by allowing the egg to be fertilized in the fallopian tube and migrate to the uterus according to the normal timetable.

In **nonsurgical embryo transfer,** a donor egg is fertilized by the man's sperm and implanted in the woman's uterus. This procedure also may be used to transfer an already fertilized ovum into the uterus of another woman.

Fertility drugs   Hormones that stimulate ovulation in women who are not ovulating; often responsible for multiple births.

Alternative insemination   Fertilization accomplished by depositing a partner's or a donor's semen into a woman's vagina via a thin tube.

In vitro fertilization   Fertilization of an egg in a nutrient medium and subsequent transfer back to the mother's body.

Intracytoplasmic sperm injection (ICSI)   Fertilization accomplished by injecting a sperm cell directly into an egg.

Gamete intrafallopian transfer (GIFT)   Procedure in which an egg harvested from the woman's ovary is placed with her partner's sperm in her fallopian tube, where it is fertilized and then migrates to the uterus for implantation.

Nonsurgical embryo transfer   In vitro fertilization of a donor egg by the male partner's (or donor's) sperm and subsequent transfer to the female partner's or another woman's uterus.

In **embryo transfer,** an ovum from a donor's body is artificially inseminated by the male partner's sperm. This inseminated ovum is allowed to stay in the donor's body for a time, and is then transplanted into the female partner's body.

Some laboratories are experimenting with **embryo freezing,** in which a fertilized embryo is suspended in a solution of liquid nitrogen. When desired, it is gradually thawed and implanted into the prospective mother. The first U.S. birth of a frozen embryo was reported in 1986. In the future, this technique may make it possible for young couples to produce an embryo and save it for later implantation when they are ready to have a child, thus reducing the risks of fertilizing older eggs.

Infertile couples have another alternative—**embryo adoption programs.** The embryos are originally collected from couples who want children via in vitro fertilization. These couples often donate and freeze extra embryos in case the procedure fails or they want to have more children at a later time. These couples can now donate their unneeded embryos to others. The adopting couple can enjoy the experience of pregnancy and control prenatal care. The cost is approximately $4,000 for the embryos to be thawed and transferred to an infertile woman's uterus or fallopian tubes.

The ethical and moral questions surrounding experimental infertility treatments are staggering. Before moving forward with any of these treatments, individuals need to ask themselves a few important questions. Has infertility been absolutely confirmed? Are reputable infertility counseling services accessible? Have they explored all possible alternatives and considered potential risks? Have all affected parties examined their attitudes, values, and beliefs about conceiving a child in this manner? Finally, they need to consider what and how they will tell the child about their method of conception.

Surrogate Motherhood

Between 60 and 70 percent of infertile couples are able to conceive after treatment. The rest decide to live without children, to adopt, or to attempt surrogate motherhood. In this option, the couple hires a woman to be alternatively inseminated by the husband. The surrogate then carries the baby to term and surrenders it upon birth to the couple. Surrogate mothers are reportedly paid about $10,000 for their services and are reimbursed for medical expenses. Legal and medical expenses can run as high as $30,000 for the infertile couple.

Couples considering surrogate motherhood are advised to consult a lawyer regarding contracts. Most of these legal documents stipulate that the surrogate mother must undergo amniocentesis and that if the fetus is defective, she must consent to an abortion. In that case, or if the surrogate miscarries, she is reimbursed for her time and expenses. The prospective parents also must agree to take the baby if it is carried to term, even if it is unhealthy or has physical abnormalities.

Adoption

For couples who have decided that biological childbirth is not an option, adoption provides an alternative. About 50,000 children are available for adoption in the United States every year. This is far fewer than the number of couples seeking adoptions. By some estimates, only 1 in 30 couples receives the child they want. On average, couples spend two years on the adoption process.

Because the number of American children available for adoption is limited, women who consider placing their child for adoption have gained new leverage. Increasingly, couples wishing to adopt have turned to independent adoptions arranged by a lawyer, or they may directly negotiate with the birth mother. Independent adoptions now surpass those arranged by social service agencies.

Increasingly, couples are choosing to adopt children from other countries. In 2000, U.S. families adopted 18,477 foreign children. The cost of intercountry adoption varies from approximately $7,000 to $25,000, including agency fees, dossier and immigration processing fees, and court costs. However, it may be a good solution for many couples, especially those who want to adopt an infant.

Embryo transfer   Artificial insemination of a donor with male partner's sperm; after a time, the embryo is transferred from the donor to the female partner's body.

Embryo freezing   The freezing of an embryo for later implantation.

Embryo adoption programs   A procedure whereby an infertile couple is able to purchase frozen embryos donated by another couple.

What do you think?

If you or your partner had infertility problems, how much time and money would you be willing to invest in treatment? ✳ *Do you think that single women and lesbians should have equal access to alternative methods of insemination?* ✳ *Why or why not?* ✳ *Do you think single women, single men, gay males, and lesbians should have equal opportunities to adopt?* ✳ *How do you think society views these types of adoptions?*

Make It Happen!

Assessment: The Assess Yourself box on page 143 gave you the chance to assess your comfort and confidence with a contraceptive method you are using now or may use in the future. Depending on the results of the assessment, you may consider making a change in your birth control method.

Making a Change: In order to change your behavior, you need to develop a plan. Follow these steps:

1. Evaluate your behavior, and identify patterns. What can you change now? What can you change in the near future?
2. Select one pattern of behavior that you want to change.
3. Fill out a Behavior Change Contract. It should include your long-term goal for change, your short-term goals, the rewards you'll give your-

self for reaching these goals, potential obstacles along the way, and strategies for overcoming these obstacles. For each goal, list the small steps and specific actions that you will take.

4. Chart your progress in a journal. At the end of a week, consider how successful you were in following your plan. What helped you be successful? What made change more difficult? What will you do differently next week?
5. Revise your plan as needed: Are the short-term goals attainable? Are the rewards satisfying?

Example: Marissa had been using a diaphragm as her form of birth control. When she completed the self-assessment, she discovered that there were several aspects of it that made her uncomfortable. The questions to which she answered "yes" showed that she sometimes forgot to bring her

diaphragm when she planned to see her boyfriend Ben, and she disliked using it because it interrupted her sexual activity. She also was embarrassed to use it because she didn't like inserting it in front of Ben. She decided she should investigate other birth control options and discuss them with her boyfriend. Her first step was to visit her student health center and, based on her likes and dislikes, to choose one or two alternatives to the diaphragm. Among the options suggested to her were the contraceptive patch (Ortho Evra) and the vaginal ring (NuvaRing), both of which she would not have to remember to use and would not interrupt sexual activity. Marissa's next step was to talk to her boyfriend about his likes and dislikes and then to make a final decision based on her confidence in the method, its convenience, and its cost.

Summary

* Latex condoms and the female condoms, when used correctly for oral sex or intercourse, provide the most effective protection in preventing sexually transmitted infections (STIs). Other contraceptive methods include abstinence, outercourse, oral contraceptives, foams, jellies, suppositories, creams, the diaphragm, the cervical cap, skin patches, the vaginal ring, monthly injections, intrauterine devices, withdrawal, and Depo-Provera. Fertility awareness methods rely on altering sexual practices to avoid pregnancy. Whereas all these methods of contraception are reversible, sterilization is permanent.
* Abortion is currently legal in the United States through the second trimester. Abortion methods include vacuum aspiration, dilation and evacuation (D&E), dilation and curettage (D&C), intact dilation and extraction (D&X), hysterotomy, induction abortion, mifepristone, and methotrexate.
* Parenting is a demanding job that requires careful planning. Emotional health, maternal health, paternal health, financial evaluation, and contingency planning all need to be taken into account when considering whether to become a parent.

* Prenatal care includes a complete physical exam within the first trimester and avoidance of those things that could have teratogenic effects on the fetus such as alcohol and drugs, cigarettes, X rays, and chemicals having teratogenic effects. Full-term pregnancy covers three trimesters.
* Childbirth occurs in three stages. Birth alternatives include the Lamaze method. Partners should jointly choose a labor method early in the pregnancy to be better prepared for labor when it occurs. Complications of pregnancy and childbirth include miscarriage, ectopic pregnancy, stillbirth, and the need for a C-section.
* Infertility in women may be caused by pelvic inflammatory disease (PID) or endometriosis. In men, it may be caused by low sperm count. Treatment may include alternative insemination, in vitro fertilization, gamete intrafallopian transfer (GIFT), nonsurgical embryo transfer, and embryo transfer. Surrogate motherhood involves hiring a fertile woman to be alternatively inseminated by the male partner.

Questions for Discussion and Reflection

1. List the most effective contraceptive methods. What are their drawbacks? What medical conditions would keep a person from using each one? What are the characteristics of the methods that you think would be most effective for you? Why do you consider them most effective for you personally?
2. What are the various methods of abortion? What are the two opposing viewpoints concerning abortion? What is *Roe v. Wade,* and what impact did it have on the abortion debate?
3. What are the most important considerations in deciding whether the time is right to become a parent? If you choose to have children, what factors will you consider regarding the number of children to have?
4. Discuss the growth of the fetus through the three trimesters. What medical check-ups or tests should be done during each trimester?
5. Discuss the emotional aspects of pregnancy. What types of emotional reactions are common in each trimester and the postpartum period (the "fourth trimester")?
6. If you and you partner are unable to have children, what alternative methods of conception would you consider? Is adoption an option you would consider?

Accessing Your Health on the Internet

Visit the following Internet sites to explore further topics and issues related to personal health. To visit an organization's website, go to the Companion Website for *Health: The Basics, Sixth Edition* at www.aw-bc.com/donatelle, click on the book image, and select "Accessing Your Health on the Internet" from the navigation menu on the left.

1. *Childbirth.Org.* Provides information to encourage parents to be good consumers who know their options and how to provide themselves with the best care essential to a healthy pregnancy.

2. *The National Parenting Center.* Invites parents to expand their parenting skills and strengths by sharing information in chat rooms and in an online newsletter.
3. *Safer Sex.* Provides information on safer sex issues. Discusses such issues as whether oral sex is safe, and women and safer sex. Provides links to related websites.

Further Reading

Boston Women's Health Collective. *Our Bodies, Ourselves for the New Century: A Book by and for Women.* New York: Simon and Schuster, 1998.

Like its earlier editions, this volume contains information about women's health from a decidedly feminist angle. Every aspect of health is covered, including nutrition, emotional health, fitness, relationships, reproduction, contraception, and pregnancy.

Eisenberg, A., S. Hathaway, and H. Murkoff. *What to Expect When You're Expecting, 3rd ed.* New York: Workman, 2002.

A month-by-month guide to all aspects of pregnancy. Provides information on what the mother can expect regarding physician visits, prenatal testing, physical and emotional changes, and important decisions to be made throughout pregnancy and delivery.

Hatcher, R. A., et al., *Contraceptive Technology, 17th ed.* New York: Ardent Media, 1998.

Perhaps the best primary reference concerning birth control for physicians, family planning centers, student health services, and educators. Contributors include many staff members of the CDC.

Hatcher, R. A., et. al. *A Pocket Guide to Managing Contraception, 2002–2003.* Atlanta: Bridging the Gap Foundation, 2002.

An excellent reference guide for students, health educators, and student health services. Provides accurate and current information about contraceptive methods, women's health, and primary care. Available free online at the foundation's website: www.managingcontraception.com.

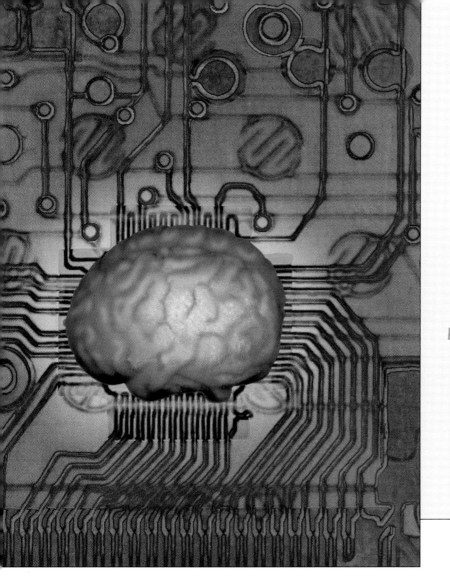

Licit and Illicit Drugs

Use, Misuse, and Abuse

7 7 7 7 7 7

Objectives

❋ Discuss the six categories of drugs and their routes of administration.

❋ Compare choices in prescription and over-the-counter drugs, and identify actions that will maximize the benefit received from these drugs.

❋ Discuss proper drug use, and explain how hazardous drug interactions occur.

❋ Discuss patterns of illicit drug use, including who uses illicit drugs and why.

❋ Describe the use and abuse of controlled substances, including cocaine, amphetamines, marijuana, opiates, hallucinogens, designer drugs, inhalants, and steroids.

❋ Profile illegal drug use in the United States, including frequency, financial impact, arrests for drug offenses, and impact on the workplace.

❋ Describe the signs of addiction.

Panel Rejects Pleas to Curb Sales of a Widely Abused Painkiller

By Gardiner Harris

A federal drug advisory panel yesterday rejected pleas from members of Congress and drug enforcement officials that sales of the widely abused painkiller OxyContin be severely restricted.

But officials from the Bush administration told the panel they were seriously considering even broader rules requiring doctors to get special training before being allowed to prescribe OxyContin or any other controlled narcotic. The changes are intended to stem a growing tide of prescription drug abuse.

OxyContin is responsible for 500 to 1,000 deaths a year, a panel member estimated yesterday. Some two million people used narcotics recreationally in 2001, the last year for which figures were available, up from 1.5 million in 1998 and 400,000 in the mid-1980s, according to data presented to the panel.

Introduced in 1995, OxyContin is a pill that gradually releases steady amounts of narcotics for 12 hours. Before OxyContin, patients were required to take pills every four hours to achieve significant pain relief.

Read the complete article online in the eThemes section of this book's website: www.aw-bc.com/donatelle.

D rug misuse and abuse are problems of staggering proportions in our society. Each year drug and alcohol abuse contributes to the deaths of more than 120,000 Americans. It also costs taxpayers more than $294 billion in preventable health care costs, extra law enforcement, auto crashes, crime, and lost productivity.[1] It's impossible to put a dollar amount on the pain, suffering, and dysfunction that drugs cause in our everyday lives.

While overall use of drugs in the United States has fallen by 50 percent in the last 20 years, the past 10 years have shown an increase in the use of certain drugs by adolescents.[2] Why so many people use drugs and the mechanisms by which drugs cause harm are topics of ongoing research. Human beings appear to have a need to alter their consciousness, or mental state. We like to feel good, to escape and feel different. Consciousness can be altered in many ways: Children spinning until they become dizzy and adults enjoying the rush of thrilling high-intensity activities are examples. To change our awareness, many of us listen to music, skydive, ski, read, daydream, meditate, pray, or have sexual relations. Others turn to drugs to alter consciousness.

Receptor sites Specialized cells to which drugs can attach themselves.

Drug Dynamics

Drugs work because they physically resemble the chemicals produced naturally within the body (Figure 7.1). Most bodily processes result from chemical reactions or from changes in electrical charge. Because drugs possess an electrical charge and a chemical structure similar to those of chemicals that occur naturally in the body, they can affect physical functions in many different ways. For example, many painkillers resemble the endorphins (the "morphine within") that are manufactured in the body.

A current explanation of how drugs work is the *receptor site theory,* which states that drugs bind to specific **receptor sites** in the body. These sites are specialized cells to which, because of their size, shape, electrical charge, and chemical properties, drugs can attach themselves. Most drugs attach to multiple receptor sites located throughout the body in places such as the heart and blood system and the lungs, liver, kidneys, brain, and gonads (testicles or ovaries).

Types of Drugs

Scientists divide drugs into six categories: prescription, over-the-counter, recreational, herbal, illicit, and commercial drugs. These classifications are based primarily on drug action, although some are based on the source of the chemical in question. Each category includes some drugs that stimulate the body, some that depress body functions, and others that produce hallucinations (auditory or visual images that

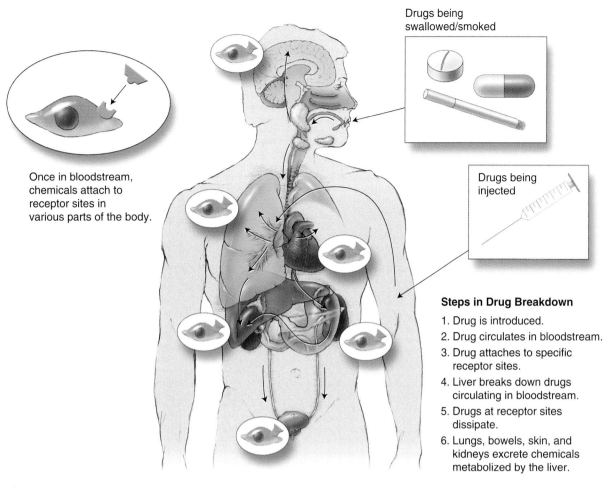

Once in bloodstream, chemicals attach to receptor sites in various parts of the body.

Drugs being swallowed/smoked

Drugs being injected

Steps in Drug Breakdown
1. Drug is introduced.
2. Drug circulates in bloodstream.
3. Drug attaches to specific receptor sites.
4. Liver breaks down drugs circulating in bloodstream.
5. Drugs at receptor sites dissipate.
6. Lungs, bowels, skin, and kidneys excrete chemicals metabolized by the liver.

Figure 7.1
How the Body Metabolizes Drugs

are perceived but are not real). Each category also includes **psychoactive drugs,** which have the potential to alter a person's mood or behavior.

- **Prescription drugs** are those substances that can be obtained only with the written prescription of a licensed physician. More than 10,000 types of prescription drugs are sold in the United States.
- **Over-the-counter (OTC) drugs** can be purchased without a prescription. Each year, Americans spend more than $14 billion on OTC products, and the market is increasing at the rate of 20 percent annually. More than 300,000 OTC products are available, and an estimated three out of four people routinely self-medicate with them.
- **Recreational drugs** belong to a somewhat vague category whose boundaries depend on how the term *recreation* is defined. Generally, these drugs contain chemicals used to help people relax or socialize. Most of them are legally sanctioned even though they are psychoactive. Alcohol, tobacco, coffee, tea, and chocolate products are usually included in this category.

- **Herbal preparations** form another vague category. Included among these approximately 750 substances are herbal teas and other products of botanical, or plant, origin that are believed to have medicinal properties.

Psychoactive drugs Drugs that have the potential to alter mood or behavior.

Prescription drugs Medications that can be obtained only with the written prescription of a licensed physician.

Over-the-counter (OTC) drugs Medications that can be purchased without a physician's prescription.

Recreational drugs Legal drugs that contain chemicals that help people relax or socialize.

Herbal preparations Substances of plant origin that are believed to have medicinal properties.

- **Illicit (illegal) drugs** are the most notorious type of drug. Although laws governing their use, possession, cultivation, manufacture, and sale differ from state to state, illicit drugs generally are recognized as harmful. All of them are psychoactive.
- **Commercial preparations** are the most universally used yet least commonly recognized chemical substances having drug action. More than 1,000 of these substances exist, including seemingly benign items such as perfumes, cosmetics, household cleansers, paints, glues, inks, dyes, gardening chemicals, pesticides, and industrial by-products.

Routes of Administration of Drugs

Route of administration refers to the way in which a given drug is taken into the body. Common routes are oral ingestion, injection, inhalation, inunction, and suppository.

Oral ingestion is the most common route of administration. Drugs that are swallowed include tablets, capsules, and liquids. Oral ingestion generally results in relatively slow absorption compared to other methods of administration because the drug must pass through the stomach, where digestive juices act upon it, and then move to the small intestine before it enters the bloodstream.

Many oral preparations are coated to keep them from being dissolved by corrosive stomach acids before they reach the intestine and to protect the stomach lining from irritating chemicals in the drugs. A stomach that contains food slows the absorption of drugs. Some drugs must not be taken with certain foods because the food will inhibit their action. Others should be ingested with food to prevent stomach irritation.

Depending on the drug and the amount of food in the stomach, drugs taken orally produce their effects within 20 to 60 minutes after ingestion. The only exception is alcohol, which takes effect sooner because some of it is absorbed directly into the bloodstream from the stomach.

Injection, another common form of drug administration, involves using a hypodermic syringe to introduce a drug into the body. **Intravenous injection,** or injection directly into a vein, puts the chemical in its most concentrated form directly into the bloodstream. Effects will be felt within three minutes, which makes this route extremely effective, particularly in medical emergencies. But injection of many substances into the bloodstream may cause serious or even fatal reactions. In addition, some serious diseases, such as hepatitis and AIDS (acquired immune deficiency syndrome), can be transferred in this way. For this reason, intravenous injection can be one of the most dangerous routes of administration.

Intramuscular injection places the hypodermic needle into muscular tissue, usually in the buttocks or the back of the upper arm. Normally used to administer antibiotics and vaccinations, this route of administration results in much slower absorption than intravenous injection does, but it ensures slow and consistent dispersion of the drug into body tissues.

Subcutaneous injection puts the drug into the layer of fat directly beneath the skin. Its common medical uses include administration of local anesthetics and insulin replacement therapy. A drug injected subcutaneously will circulate even more slowly than will an intramuscularly injected drug because it takes longer to be absorbed into the bloodstream.

Inhalation refers to administration of drugs through the nostrils or mouth. This method transfers the drug rapidly into the bloodstream through the alveoli (air sacs) in the lungs. Examples of illicit inhalation include cocaine sniffing; inhaling aerosol sprays, gases, or fumes from solvents; or smoking marijuana. Effects are frequently immediate but do not last as long as effects associated with slower routes of administration, because only small amounts of a drug can be absorbed and metabolized in the lungs.

Inunction introduces chemicals into the body through the skin. A common example is the small adhesive patch that is used to alleviate motion sickness. This patch, which contains a prescription medicine, is applied to the skin behind one ear, where it slowly releases its chemicals to provide relief for nauseated travelers. Another example is the nicotine patch.

Suppositories are drugs that are mixed with a waxy medium designed to melt at body temperature. The most common type is inserted into the anus past the rectal sphincter muscles, which hold the suppository in place. As the wax melts, the drug is released and absorbed through the rectal

---

Illicit (illegal) drugs   Drugs whose use, possession, cultivation, manufacture, and/or sale are against the law because they generally are recognized as harmful.

Commercial preparations   Commonly used chemical substances including cosmetics, household cleaning products, and industrial by-products.

Route of administration   The manner in which a drug is taken into the body.

Oral ingestion   Intake of drugs through the mouth.

Injection   The introduction of drugs into the body via a hypodermic needle.

Intravenous injection   The introduction of drugs directly into a vein.

Intramuscular injection   The introduction of drugs into muscles.

Subcutaneous injection   The introduction of drugs into the layer of fat directly beneath the skin.

Inhalation   The introduction of drugs through the nostrils or mouth.

Inunction   The introduction of drugs through the skin.

Suppositories   Mixtures of drugs and a waxy medium designed to melt at body temperature that are inserted into the anus or vagina.

walls into the bloodstream. Since this area of the anatomy contains many blood vessels, the effects usually are felt within 15 minutes. Other types of suppositories are for use in the vagina. Vaginal suppositories usually release drugs, such as antifungal agents, that treat problems in the vagina itself rather than drugs meant to travel through the bloodstream.

Using, Misusing, and Abusing Drugs

Although drug abuse usually is referred to in connection with illicit psychoactive drugs, many people abuse and misuse prescription and OTC medications. **Drug misuse** involves the use of a drug for a purpose for which it was not intended. For example, taking a friend's high-powered prescription painkiller for your headache is a misuse of that drug. This is not too far removed from **drug abuse,** or the excessive use of any drug, and may result in serious harm.

The misuse and abuse of any drug may lead to *addiction*. Both risks and benefits are involved in the use of any chemical substance. Intelligent decision making requires a clear-headed evaluation of these risks and benefits.

> ### What do you think?
> *What are some situations in which students misuse drugs?* ✷ *Other than alcohol, which drugs (prescription or OTC) do students tend to abuse while they are in college?*

Defining Addiction

Addiction is continued involvement with a substance or activity despite ongoing negative consequences. Addictive behaviors initially provide a sense of pleasure or stability that is beyond the addict's power to achieve in other ways. Eventually, the addicted person needs to be involved in the behavior in order to feel normal.

Physiological dependence is only one indicator of addiction. Psychological dynamics play an important role, which explains why behaviors not related to the use of chemicals—gambling, for example—may also be addictive. In fact, psychological and physiological dependence are so intertwined that it is not really possible to separate the two. For every psychological state, there is a corresponding physiological state. In other words, everything you feel is tied to a chemical process occurring in your body.[3] Thus, addictions once thought to be entirely psychological in nature are now understood to have physiological components.

To be addictive, a behavior must have the potential to produce a positive mood change. Chemicals are responsible for the most profound addictions, not only because they alter mood dramatically, but also because they cause cellular changes to which the body adapts so well that it eventually requires the chemical in order to function normally. Yet, other behaviors, such as gambling, spending money, working, and engaging in sex, also create changes at the cellular level along with positive mood changes. Although the mechanism is not well understood, all forms of addiction probably reflect dysfunction of certain biochemical systems in the brain.[4]

Traditionally, diagnosis of an addiction was limited to drug addiction and was based on three criteria.

1. **Withdrawal,** or the presence of an abstinence syndrome— a series of temporary physical and psychological symptoms that occurs when the addicted person abruptly stops using the drug
2. An associated pattern of pathological behavior (deterioration in work performance, relationships, and social interaction)
3. **Relapse**—the tendency to return to the addictive behavior after a period of abstinence

Until recently, health professionals were unwilling to diagnose an addiction until medical symptoms appeared in the patient. Now we know that although withdrawal, pathological behavior, relapse, and medical symptoms are valid indicators of addiction, they do not characterize all addictive behavior.

Signs of Addiction

Studies show that all animals share the same basic pleasure and reward circuits in the brain that turn on when they come into contact with addictive substances or engage in something pleasurable, such as eating or orgasm. We all engage in potentially addictive behaviors to some extent because some are essential to our survival and are highly reinforcing, such as eating, drinking, and sex. At some point along the continuum, however, some individuals are not able to engage in these behaviors moderately, and they become addicted.

Drug misuse   The use of a drug for a purpose for which it was not intended.

Drug abuse   The excessive use of a drug.

Addiction   Continued involvement with a substance or activity despite ongoing negative consequences.

Withdrawal   A series of temporary physical and biopsychosocial symptoms that occur when the addict abruptly abstains from an addictive chemical or behavior.

Relapse   The tendency to return to the addictive behavior after a period of abstinence.

All addictions are characterized by four common symptoms: (1) **compulsion,** or excessive need to perform the behavior (characterized by **obsession,** or mental preoccupation with the behavior); (2) **loss of control,** or the inability to predict reliably whether any isolated occurrence of the behavior will be healthy or damaging; (3) **negative consequences,** such as physical damage, legal trouble, financial problems, academic failure, or family dissolution, which do not occur with healthy involvement in any behavior; and (4) **denial,** the inability to perceive that the behavior is self-destructive. These four components are present in all addictions, whether chemical or behavioral.

> **What do you think?**
>
> *Have you ever seen signs of addiction in a friend or family member?* ✳ *What types of negative consequences have you witnessed?* ✳ *Can you think of any habits you have that potentially could become addictive?*

Prescription Drugs

Even though prescription drugs are administered under medical supervision, the wise consumer still takes precautions. Hazards and complications arising from the use of prescription drugs are common.

Compulsion An overwhelming need to perform a behavior or obtain an addictive object.

Obsession Excessive preoccupation with an addictive object or behavior.

Loss of control Inability to predict reliably whether a particular instance of involvement with the addictive object or behavior will be healthy or damaging.

Negative consequences Physical damage, legal trouble, financial ruin, academic failure, family dissolution, and other severe problems associated with addiction.

Denial Inability to perceive or accurately interpret the self-destructive effects of the addictive behavior.

Antibiotics Prescription drugs designed to fight bacterial infection.

Sedatives Central nervous system depressants that induce sleep and relieve anxiety.

Tranquilizers Central nervous system depressants that relax the body and calm anxiety.

Antidepressants Prescription drugs used to treat clinically diagnosed depression.

Generic drugs Medications marketed by chemical name rather than brand name.

Types of Prescription Drugs

Antibiotics are drugs used to fight bacterial infection. Bacterial infections continue to be among the most common serious diseases throughout the world, but the vast majority can be cured with antibiotics. There are close to 100 different antibiotics, which may be dispensed by intramuscular injection or in tablet or capsule form. Some, called broad-spectrum antibiotics, are designed to control disease caused by a number of bacterial species. These medications may also kill off helpful bacteria in the body, thus triggering secondary infections. For example, some vaginal infections are related to long-term use of antibiotics. The misuse of antibiotics has led to an increase in drug-resistant bacteria (see the Consumer Health box).

Sedatives are central nervous system depressants that induce sleep and relieve anxiety. Because of the high incidence of anxiety and sleep disorders in the United States, drugs that encourage relaxation and drowsiness are frequently prescribed. The potential for addiction is high. Detoxification can be life-threatening and must be supervised medically. Because doctors do not prescribe sedatives as frequently as they did in past decades, users often purchase them illegally.

Tranquilizers, another form of central nervous system depressant that relaxes the body and calms anxiety, are classified as major and minor tranquilizers. The most powerful tranquilizers are used to treat major psychiatric illnesses. When used appropriately, these strong sedatives can reduce violent aggressiveness and self-destructive impulses.

The so-called minor tranquilizers gained much notoriety in the late 1970s when consumer groups discovered that these drugs—known by their trade names Valium, Librium, and Miltown—were the most commonly prescribed medications in the United States. They often were prescribed for women who suffered from anxiety. These drugs have a high potential for addiction, and many people became physically and psychologically dependent on them. When the media reported on the widespread and casual prescribing of these drugs, physicians were forced to reevaluate the practice. Today a doctor is as likely to suggest psychotherapy or counseling for patients suffering from anxiety as he or she is likely to prescribe sedatives.

Antidepressants are medications typically used to treat major depression, although occasionally they are used for other forms of depression that resist conventional therapy. There are several groups of antidepressant medications approved for use in the United States. Prozac, Zoloft, and Paxil are among the most frequently prescribed antidepressants.

Generic Drugs

Generic drugs, medications sold under a chemical name rather than under a brand name, have gained popularity in recent years. They contain the same active ingredients as brand-name drugs but are less expensive.

Preserving the Usefulness of Antibiotics

In the 1300s, the scourge known as bubonic plague killed up to one-third of Europe's population. In modern times, we've been told that such a plague isn't possible. It would be controlled handily with antibiotic drugs such as streptomycin, gentamicin, and chloramphenicol. These drugs once were thought to be invincible—that is, until 1995, when a 16-year-old boy from Madagascar, who was infected with bubonic plague, failed to respond to the usual antibiotic treatments. This was the first documented case of antibiotic-resistant plague, which eventually did succumb to another antibiotic.

To some, this development was not all that surprising. Throughout the world, many other infectious bacteria, including those that cause pneumonia, ear infections, acne, gonorrhea, urinary tract infections, meningitis, and tuberculosis, can now outwit commonly used antibiotics and their synthetic counterparts, antimicrobials. Every time a patient takes penicillin or another antibiotic for a bacterial infection, the drug kills most of the bacteria. But a few tenacious germs may survive by mutating or acquiring resistance genes from other bacteria. These surviving genes can multiply quickly and create drug-resistant strains. The presence of these strains may mean the patient's next infection may not respond to the first-choice antibiotic therapy. Also, the resistant bacteria may be transmitted to other people in the community.

According to the Centers for Disease Control and Prevention, each year nearly 2 million people in the United States acquire an infection while in the hospital, which results in 90,000 deaths. More than 70% of the bacteria that cause these infections are resistant to at least one of the antibiotics commonly used to treat them. Although resistant bacteria have existed for a long time, the number of bacteria resistant to many different antibiotics has increased tenfold or more in the past ten years alone.

What is causing the increase in drug-resistant strains? Two factors: One has to do with the medical community, the other with patients. Experts say that doctors are sometimes too quick to prescribe antibiotics for all sorts of symptoms, despite the fact that antibiotics work only against bacteria and not against viruses or the common cold. It is estimated that more than 50–150 million antibiotic prescriptions written for patients each year outside of hospitals are unnecessary. And even when patients need the antibiotics that are prescribed, they don't always follow instructions properly. To be completely effective, antibiotics should be taken for a specific number of days. Many people, however, often stop taking the drug after symptoms have cleared or they start feeling better. Unfortunately, some of the bacteria may still be present in their bodies where they are free to attack again and able to mutate.

Organisms that have already developed defenses against antibiotic attack include the following.

- *Staphylococcus aureus.* One of the primary causes of infections in U.S. hospital patients; can infect burns, skin, and surgical wounds
- *Enterococcus.* Can cause everything from urinary tract infections to heart valve infections
- *Streptococcus pneumoniae.* Up to 30% of the strains of this bacterium, which can cause pneumonia, meningitis, and ear infections, are at least partially resistant to antibiotics in the penicillin family

Other bacteria that have grown resistant to once-reliable antibiotics are *Neisseria gonorrhoeae,* which causes the sexually transmitted infection gonorrhea; *Salmonella, Escherichia coli (E. coli),* the culprit behind food poisoning; and *Mycobacterium tuberculosis,* which causes tuberculosis.

What can you do to help curb the problem of antibiotic-resistant bacteria?

- Don't demand an antibiotic when your health care provider determines that one is not appropriate. Remember, antibiotics won't help a cold or flu.
- Finish each prescription. Even when your symptoms have disappeared, some bacteria may still survive and reproduce if you don't complete the course of treatment.
- Don't take leftover antibiotics or antibiotics prescribed for someone else.

Sources: FDA Consumer Magazine (July–August 2002); FDA Consumer Magazine (November–December 1998).

Generic drugs can help reduce health care costs because their price is often less than half that of brand-name medications. If your doctor prescribes a drug, always ask whether a generic equivalent exists and whether it would be safe and effective for you to try. Not all drugs are available as generics.

Be aware, though, that there is some controversy about the effectiveness of generic drugs because substitutions often are made in minor ingredients that can affect the way the drug is absorbed, which causes discomfort or even an allergic reaction in some users. Always note any reactions you have to medications, and tell your doctor about them.

Over-the-Counter Drugs

OTC drugs are nonprescription substances we use in the course of self-diagnosis and self-medication. More than one-third of the time, people treat their routine health problems with OTC medications. In fact, American consumers spend billions of dollars yearly on OTC preparations for relief of everything from runny noses to ingrown toenails. There are 40,000 OTC drugs and more than 300,000 brand names for them.

Most OTC drugs are manufactured from a basic group of 1,000 chemicals. The many different products available to us are produced by combining as few as two and as many as ten substances.

How Prescription Drugs Become Over-the-Counter Drugs

The Food and Drug Administration (FDA) regularly reviews prescription drugs to evaluate how suitable they would be as OTC products. For a drug to be switched from prescription to OTC status, it must meet the following criteria.

1. The drug has been marketed as a prescription medication for at least three years.
2. The use of the drug has been relatively high during the time it was available as a prescription drug.
3. Adverse drug reactions are not alarming, and the frequency of side effects has not increased during the time it was available to the public.

Since this policy has been in effect, the FDA has moved hundreds of drugs to OTC status. Some examples are ibuprofen (Advil, Nuprin), Benadryl, Bronkaid Mist, and Cortaid. Many more prescription drugs are currently being considered for OTC status.

Types of Over-the-Counter Drugs

The FDA has categorized 26 types of OTC preparations. Those most commonly used are analgesics, cold/cough/ allergy and asthma relievers, stimulants, sleeping aids, and dieting aids.

Analgesics   We spend more than $2 billion annually on **analgesics** (pain relievers), the largest sales category of OTC drugs in the United States. Although these pain relievers come in several forms, aspirin, acetaminophen (Tylenol, Pamprin, Panadol), ibuprofen (Advil, Motrin, Nuprin), and ibuprofen-like drugs such as naproxen sodium (Aleve, Anaprox) and ketoprofen (Orudis) are the most common.

Analgesics   Pain relievers.

Prostaglandin inhibitors   Drugs that inhibit the production and release of prostaglandins, hormone-like substances associated with arthritis or menstrual pain.

Generally Recognized as Safe (GRAS)   A list of drugs generally recognized as safe; they seldom cause side effects when used properly.

Most pain relievers work at receptor sites by interrupting pain signals. Some are categorized as NSAIDs (nonsteroidal anti-inflammatory drugs), also called **prostaglandin inhibitors.** Prostaglandins are chemicals that resemble hormones and are released by the body in response to pain. (Scientists believe that the additional pain caused by the release of prostaglandins signals the body to begin the healing process.) Prostaglandin inhibitors restrain the release of prostaglandins and thus reduce the pain. Common NSAIDs include ibuprofen, naproxen sodium, and aspirin.

Besides relieving pain, aspirin lowers fever by increasing the flow of blood to the skin surface, which causes sweating and cools the body. In addition, aspirin long has been used to reduce the inflammation and swelling associated with arthritis. Recently it has been discovered that aspirin's anticoagulant (interference with blood clotting) effects can reduce the risk of heart attack and stroke.

Although aspirin has been popular for nearly a century, it is not as harmless as many people think. Possible side effects—for it and many other NSAIDS—include allergic reactions, ringing in the ears, stomach bleeding, and ulcers. Combining aspirin with alcohol can compound aspirin's gastric irritant properties. As with all drugs, read the labels. Some analgesic labels caution against driving or operating heavy machinery when using the drug, and most warn that analgesics should not be taken with alcohol.

In addition, research has linked aspirin to a potentially fatal condition called *Reye's syndrome.* Children, teenagers, and young adults (up to age 25) who are treated with aspirin while recovering from the flu or chickenpox are at risk for developing this syndrome. Aspirin substitutes are recommended for people in these age groups.

Acetaminophen is an aspirin substitute found in Tylenol and related medications. Like aspirin, acetaminophen is an effective analgesic and antipyretic (fever-reducing drug). However, it does not relieve inflamed or swollen joints. The side effects associated with acetaminophen generally are minimal, though overdose can cause liver damage.

Several analgesics are available as prescription or OTC drugs. Generally, the OTC products (for example, Nuprin, Advil, and Aleve) are milder versions of the prescription varieties. Aleve's main distinction is its lasting effect: While other analgesics must be taken every 4 to 6 hours, once every 8 to 12 hours is sufficient for Aleve.

Cold, Cough, Allergy, and Asthma Relievers   The operative word in this category is *reliever.* Most of these medications are designed to alleviate the discomforting symptoms associated with maladies of the upper respiratory tract. Unfortunately, no drugs exist to cure the actual diseases. The drugs available provide only temporary relief until the sufferer's immune system prevails over the disease. Both aspirin and acetaminophen are on the government's lists of medications that are **Generally Recognized as Safe (GRAS)** and

Generally Recognized as Effective (GRAE). Basic types of OTC cold, cough, and allergy relievers include the following.

- *Expectorants.* These drugs loosen phlegm, which allows the user to cough it up and clear congested respiratory passages. GRAS and GRAE reviewers question the effectiveness of many expectorants. In addition, when combined with other medications, particularly among those used by frail or very ill individuals, safety issues may arise.
- *Antitussives.* These OTC drugs calm or curtail the cough reflex. They are most effective when the cough is dry, or does not produce phlegm. Oral codeine, dextromethorphan, and diphenhydramine are the most common antitussives that are on both the GRAE and GRAS lists.
- *Antihistamines.* These central nervous system depressants dry runny noses, clear postnasal drip, clear sinus congestion, and reduce tears.
- *Decongestants.* These remedies reduce nasal stuffiness due to colds.
- *Anticholinergics.* These substances often are added to cold preparations to reduce nasal secretions and tears. None of the preparations tested was found to be GRAE or GRAS. Some cold compounds contain alcohol in concentrations that may exceed 40 percent.

Stimulants   Nonprescription stimulants are sometimes used by college students who have neglected assignments and other obligations until the last minute. The active ingredient in OTC stimulants is caffeine, which heightens wakefulness, increases alertness, and relieves fatigue. None of the OTC stimulants has been judged GRAS or GRAE.

Sleeping Aids   Nearly 50 percent of the U.S. population experiences insomnia at least five nights each month. About 1 percent of adults routinely treat their insomnia with OTC sleep aids (such as Nytol, Sleep-Eze, and Sominex) that are advertised as providing "safe and restful" sleep.[5] These drugs often are used to induce the drowsy feelings that precede sleep. The principal ingredient in OTC sleeping aids is an antihistamine called pyrilamine maleate. Chronic reliance on sleeping aids may lead to addiction; people accustomed to using these products eventually may find it impossible to sleep without them.

Dieting Aids   In the United States, there is a $200 million market for dieting aids that are designed to help people lose weight. Some of these drugs (e.g., Acutrim, Dexatrim) are advertised as "appetite suppressants." The FDA has pulled several appetite suppressants off the market because their active ingredient was phenylpropanolamine (PPA), which has been linked to increased risk of stroke.[6]

Estimates show that when taken as recommended, even the best OTC dieting aids significantly reduce appetite in fewer than 30 percent of users, and tolerance occurs in only one to three days of use. Manufacturers of appetite suppressants often include a written 1,200-calorie diet

Drug Facts

Active ingredient (in each tablet)	Purpose
Chlorpheniramine maleate 2 mg	Antihistamine

Uses temporarily relieves these symptoms due to hay fever or other upper respiratory allergies:
■ sneezing   ■ runny nose   ■ itchy, watery eyes   ■ itchy throat

Warnings
Ask a doctor before use if you have
■ glaucoma   ■ a breathing problem such as emphysema or chronic bronchitis
■ trouble urinating due to an enlarged prostate gland

Ask a doctor or pharmacist before use if you are taking tranquilizers or sedatives

When using this product
■ You may get drowsy   ■ avoid alcoholic drinks
■ alcohol, sedatives, and tranquilizers may increase drowsiness
■ be careful when driving a motor vehicle or operating machinery
■ excitability may occur, especially in children

If pregnant or breast-feeding, ask a health professional before use.
Keep out of reach of children. In case of overdose, get medical help or contact a Poison Control Center right away.

Directions

adults and children 12 years and over	take 2 tablets every 4 to 6 hours; not more than 12 tablets in 24 hours
children 6 years to under 12 years	take 1 tablet every 4 to 6 hours; not more than 6 tablets in 24 hours
children under 6 years	ask a doctor

Other information store at 20-25° C (68-77° F)   ■ protect from excessive moisture

Inactive ingredients D&C yellow no. 10, lactose, magnesium stearate, microcrystalline cellulose, pregelatinized starch

Figure 7.2
The OTC Drug Label
The FDA requires most over-the-counter drugs to have a label that looks like this one, so the information is standardized and easy to read. Use it to compare drug ingredients and to follow dosage instructions and warnings.

to complement their drug. However, most people who limit themselves to 1,200 calories per day will lose weight—without any help from appetite suppressants. Clearly, these products have no value in treating obesity.

Some people rely on laxatives and diuretics to lose weight. Frequent use of **laxatives** disrupts the body's natural elimination patterns and may cause constipation or even obstipation (inability to have a bowel movement). The use of laxatives to produce weight loss has generally unspectacular results and can rob the body of needed fluids, salts, and minerals.

Taking **diuretics** (water pills) to lose weight is also dangerous. Not only will the user gain the weight back upon drinking fluids, but diuretic use may also contribute to dangerous chemical imbalances. The potassium and sodium eliminated by diuretics play important roles in maintaining electrolyte balance. Depletion of these vital minerals may cause weakness, dizziness, fatigue, and sometimes death.

Generally Recognized as Effective (GRAE)   A list of drugs generally recognized as effective; they work for their intended purpose when used properly.

Laxatives   Medications used to soften stool and relieve constipation.

Diuretics   Drugs that increase the excretion of urine from the body.

Rules for Proper Use of Over-the-Counter Drugs

Despite a common belief that OTC products are safe and effective, indiscriminate use and abuse can occur with these drugs as with all others. For example, people who frequently drop medication into their eyes to "get the red out" or pop antacids after every meal are likely to be addicted. Many people also experience adverse side effects because they ignore the warnings on the labels or simply do not read them.

The FDA has developed a standard label that appears on most OTC products (see Figure 7.2 on page 179). It provides directions for use, warnings, and other useful information. (Diet supplements, which are regulated as food products, have their own type of label that includes a Supplements Facts panel.)

OTC products are far more powerful than ever before, and the science behind them is stronger as well. Therefore, as with any type of medication, do your homework. Observe the following rules when taking nonprescription drugs.

1. Always know what you are taking. Identify the active ingredients in the product.
2. Know the effects, both desired and undesired, of each active ingredient.
3. Read the warnings and cautions.
4. Don't use anything for more than one or two weeks.
5. Be particularly cautious if you are also taking prescription drugs.
6. If you have questions, ask your pharmacist.
7. *If you don't need it, don't take it!*

Drug Interactions

Sharing medications, using outdated prescriptions, taking higher doses than recommended, or using medications as a substitute for dealing with personal problems may result in serious health consequences. **Polydrug use,** taking several medications or illegal drugs simultaneously, also can lead to very dangerous health problems associated with drug

---

Polydrug use The use of multiple medications or illicit drugs simultaneously.

Synergism An interaction of two or more drugs that produces more profound effects than would be expected if the drugs were taken separately.

Antagonism A type of interaction in which two or more drugs work at the same receptor site.

Inhibition A type of interaction in which the effects of one drug are eliminated or reduced by the presence of another drug at the receptor site.

Intolerance A type of interaction in which two or more drugs produce extremely uncomfortable symptoms.

Cross-tolerance The development of a tolerance to one drug that reduces the effects of another similar drug.

---

interactions. The most hazardous interactions are synergism, antagonism, inhibition, and intolerance.

Synergism, also known as potentiation, is an interaction of two or more drugs in which the effects of the individual drugs are multiplied beyond what normally would be expected if they were taken alone. Synergism can be expressed mathematically as $2 + 2 = 10$.

A synergistic interaction is most likely to occur when *central nervous system depressants* are combined. Included in this category are alcohol, opiates (OxyContin, heroin), antihistamines (cold remedies), sedative hypnotics (Quaaludes), minor tranquilizers (Valium, Librium, and Xanax), and barbiturates. The worst possible combination is alcohol and barbiturates (sleeping preparations such as Seconal and phenobarbital) because combining these depressants slows down brain centers that normally control vital functions. Respiration, heart rate, and blood pressure can drop to the point of inducing coma and even death.

Prescription and OTC medications carry labels warning the user not to combine them with certain other drugs or with alcohol. Because the dangers associated with synergism are so great, you should always verify any possible drug interactions before using a prescribed or OTC drug. Pharmacists, physicians, drug information centers, or community drug education centers can answer your questions. Even if one of the drugs in question is illegal, you still should attempt to determine the dangers involved in combining it with other drugs. Health care professionals are legally bound to maintain confidentiality even when they know that a client is using illegal substances.

Antagonism, although not usually as serious as synergism, can produce unwanted and unpleasant effects. In an antagonistic reaction, drugs work at the same receptor site so that one blocks the action of the other. The blocking drug occupies the receptor site and prevents the other substance from attaching, thus altering its absorption and action.

With **inhibition,** the effects of one drug are eliminated or reduced by the presence of another drug at the receptor site. One common inhibitory reaction occurs between antacid tablets and aspirin. The antacid inhibits the absorption of aspirin and makes it less effective as a pain reliever. Other inhibitory reactions occur between alcohol and contraceptive pills and between antibiotics and contraceptive pills. Both alcohol and antibiotics may make birth control pills less effective.

Intolerance occurs when drugs combine in the body to produce extremely uncomfortable reactions. The drug Antabuse, used to help alcoholics give up alcohol, works by producing this type of interaction. It binds liver enzymes (the chemicals the liver produces to break down alcohol), which makes it impossible for the body to metabolize alcohol. As a result, an Antabuse user who drinks alcohol experiences nausea, vomiting, and, occasionally, fever.

Cross-tolerance occurs when a person develops a physiological tolerance to one drug and shows a similar tolerance to selected other drugs as a result. Taking one drug may actually increase the body's tolerance to another substance. For example, cross-tolerance can develop between alcohol and barbiturates, two depressant drugs.

Illicit Drugs

Whereas some people become addicted to prescription drugs and painkillers, others use *illicit drugs*—those drugs that are illegal to possess, produce, or sell. The problem of illicit drug use touches us all. We may use illicit substances ourselves, watch someone we love struggle with drug abuse, or become the victim of a drug-related crime. At the very least, we are forced to pay increasing taxes for law enforcement and drug rehabilitation. An estimated 9.4 percent of full-time employees in the U.S. workforce is under the influence of illicit drugs or alcohol on any given day.[7] When our coworkers use drugs, the effectiveness of our own work is diminished. If the car we drive was assembled by drug-using workers at the plant, we are in danger. A drug-using bus driver, train engineer, or pilot jeopardizes our safety.

The good news is that the use of illicit drugs has declined significantly in recent years in most segments of society. Use of most drugs increased from the early 1970s to the late 1970s, peaked between 1979 and 1986, and declined until 1992, from which point it has not changed. In 2002, an estimated 19.5 million Americans were illicit drug users, about half the 1979 peak level of 25 million users. Among youth, however, illicit drug use, notably of marijuana, has been increasing in recent years.[8]

Who Uses Illicit Drugs?

While many of us have stereotypes in our minds of who uses illicit drugs, it is difficult to generalize about this. Illicit drug users span all age groups, ethnicities, occupations, and socio-economic groups. What can be said is that in the United States, as in many other countries, illicit drug use has a devastating effect on both users and their families.

After more than a decade of declining use on American college campuses, illicit drugs have reappeared. In 2002, the number of college students nationwide who had tried any drug stood at almost 52 percent; more than one-third had smoked pot in the past year, and 20 percent had done so in the past month. Daily use of marijuana was at its highest point since 1989.[9] Cocaine use is down sharply, but LSD use has more than doubled. These figures vary from school to school.

The reasons for using drugs vary. Age, gender, genetic background, physiology, personality, experiences, and expectations are all factors.

Patterns of drug use vary considerably by age. For example, a nationwide study of college campuses reported that approximately 35 percent of students had tried marijuana during the previous year[10] (see Table 7.1). In contrast, only 9 percent of all Americans used marijuana during that time. Approximately 4.8 percent of college students surveyed reported using cocaine in the past year, whereas only 2.2 percent of all Americans said they had used cocaine during the previous year.

Table 7.1
Annual Prevalence of Use for Various Types of Drugs, 2002: Full-Time College Students vs. Respondents 1–4 Years beyond High School

	Full-Time College (%)	Others (%)
Any illicit drug	37.0	39.6
Any illicit drug other than marijuana	16.6	23.0
Marijuana	34.7	36.3
Inhalants	2.0	2.8
Hallucinogens	6.3	7.1
LSD	2.1	3.3
Cocaine	4.8	9.6
Crack	0.4	2.6
MDMA (Ecstasy)	6.8	9.3
Heroin	0.1	0.4
Other narcotics	5.9	7.4
OxyContin	1.5	3.3
Vicodin	6.9	12.9
Amphetamines, adjusted	7.0	9.6
Ritalin	5.7	2.5
Methamphetamine	1.2	5.4
Ice	0.8	3.5
Sedatives (barbiturates)	3.7	6.7
Tranquilizers	6.7	10.8
Rohypnol	0.7	0.2
GHB	0.6	1.2
Ketamine	1.3	1.3
Alcohol	82.9	80.1
Cigarettes	38.3	47.7
Approximate weighted N =	*1,260*	*880*

Source: Monitoring the Future Study (Ann Arbor: MI: The University of Michigan, 2003).

Most anti-drug programs have not been effective because they have focused on only one aspect of drug abuse. The pressures to take drugs are often tremendous, and the reasons for using them are complex. However, since most illegal drugs produce physical and psychological dependency, it is unrealistic to think that a person can use them regularly without becoming addicted. Consider whether you are controlled by drugs or a drug user by answering the questions in the Assess Yourself box on page 182.

Recognizing a Drug Problem

ARE YOU CONTROLLED BY DRUGS?

How do you know whether you are chemically dependent? A dependent person can't stop using drugs. This abuse hurts the user and everyone around him or her. Take the following assessment. The more yes checks you make, the more likely it is that you have a problem.

Yes	No	
❏	❏	Do you use drugs to handle stress or escape from life's problems?
❏	❏	Have you unsuccessfully tried to cut down or quit using your drug?
❏	❏	Have you ever been in trouble with the law or been arrested because of your drug use?
❏	❏	Do you think a party or social gathering isn't fun unless drugs are available?
❏	❏	Do you avoid people or places that do not support your usage?
❏	❏	Do you neglect your responsibilities because you would rather use your drug?
❏	❏	Have your friends, family, or employer expressed concern about your drug use?
❏	❏	Do you do things under the influence of drugs that you would not normally do?
❏	❏	Have you seriously thought that you might have a chemical dependence problem?

ARE YOU CONTROLLED BY A DRUG USER?

Is your life controlled by a chemical abuser? Your love and care (codependence) may actually be enabling the chemical abuser to continue the abuse and hurt you and others. Try this assessment; the more yes checks you make, the more likely it is that there's a problem.

Yes	No	
❏	❏	Do you often have to lie or cover up for the chemical abuser?
❏	❏	Do you spend time counseling the person about the problem?
❏	❏	Have you taken on additional financial or family responsibilities that the chemical abuser cannot handle?
❏	❏	Do you feel that you have to control the chemical abuser's behavior?
❏	❏	At the office, have you done work or attended meetings for the abuser?
❏	❏	Do you often put your own needs and desires after the user's?
❏	❏	Do you spend time each day worrying about your situation?
❏	❏	Do you analyze your behavior to find clues to how it might affect the chemical abuser?
❏	❏	Do you feel powerless and at your wit's end about the abuser's problem?

Source: Reprinted by permission of Krames Communications, 1100 Grundy Lane, San Bruno, CA 94066-3030. www.krames.com

What do you think?

What factors do you believe influence illicit drug use in the United States? ✳ *What is the attitude toward drug use on your campus?* ✳ *Are some substances considered more acceptable than others?* ✳ *Is drug use considered more acceptable at certain times or occasions? Explain your answer.*

Controlled Substances

Drugs are classified into five "schedules," or categories, based on their potential for abuse, their medical uses, and accepted standards of safe use (Table 7.2). Schedule I drugs, those with the highest potential for abuse, are considered to have no valid medical uses. Although Schedule II, III, IV, and V drugs have known and accepted medical applications, many of them present serious threats to health when abused or misused. Penalties for illegal use are tied to the drugs' schedule level.

Table 7.2
How Drugs Are Scheduled

Schedule	Characteristics	Examples
Schedule I	High potential for abuse and addiction; no accepted medical use	Amphetamine (DMA, STP) Heroin Phencyclidine (PCP) LSD Marijuana GHB
Schedule II	High potential for abuse and addiction; restricted medical use	Cocaine Codeine* Methadone Morphine Opium OxyContin Vicodin
Schedule III	Some potential for abuse and addiction; currently accepted medical use	Anabolic steroids Nalorphine Noludar
Schedule IV	Low potential for abuse and addiction; currently accepted medical use	Rohypnol Xanax Minor tranquilizers
Schedule V	Lowest potential for abuse; accepted medical use	Robitussin AC OTC preparations

*Can also be Schedule III or Schedule IV, depending on use.
Source: National Institute on Drug Abuse, "Commonly Abused Drugs," 2003.
www.drugabuse.gov/DrugPages/DrugsofAbuse.html

Hundreds of illegal drugs exist. For general purposes, they can be divided into seven representative categories: stimulants, such as cocaine; marijuana and its derivatives; depressants, such as the opiates; hallucinogens/psychedelics; designer drugs; inhalants; and steroids.

Stimulants

Cocaine   A white crystalline powder derived from the leaves of the South American coca shrub (not related to cocoa plants), **cocaine** (coke) has been described as one of the most powerful naturally occurring stimulants.

Methods of Cocaine Use   Cocaine can be taken in several ways. The powdered form of the drug is "snorted" through the nose. When cocaine is snorted, it can damage mucous membranes in the nose and cause sinusitis. It can destroy the user's sense of smell; occasionally it even eats a hole through the septum.

Smoking (known as *freebasing*) and intravenous injections are even more dangerous means of taking cocaine. Freebasing has become more popular than injecting in recent years because of the fear of contracting diseases such as AIDS and hepatitis by sharing contaminated needles. But

freebasing involves other dangers as well. Because the volatile mixes it requires are very explosive, some people have been killed or seriously burned while freebasing. Smoking cocaine can also cause lung and liver damage.

Many cocaine users still occasionally shoot up, which introduces large amounts into the body rapidly by injection. Within seconds, a sense of euphoria sets in. This intense high lasts for 15 to 20 minutes, and then the user heads into a crash. To prevent the unpleasant effects of the crash, users must shoot up frequently, which can severely damage veins. Injecting users place themselves at risk not only for AIDS and hepatitis, but also for skin infections, inflamed arteries, and infection of the lining of the heart.

Physical Effects of Cocaine   The effects of cocaine are felt rapidly. Snorted cocaine enters the bloodstream through the lungs in less than one minute and reaches the brain in less than three minutes. When cocaine binds at its receptor sites in the central nervous system, it produces intense pleasure.

Cocaine   A powerful stimulant drug made from the leaves of the South American coca shrub.

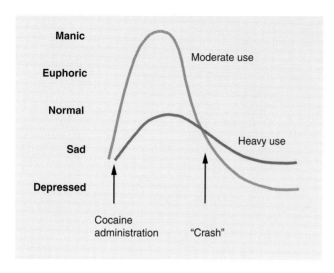

Figure 7.3
Ups and Downs of a Typical Dose of Cocaine
Source: C. Levinthal, *Drugs, Behavior, and Modern Society, 2nd ed.*
(Boston: Allyn & Bacon, 1999). © Pearson Education. Reprinted
by permission of the publisher.

The euphoria quickly abates, however, and the desire to regain the pleasurable feelings makes the user want more cocaine (see Figure 7.3).

Cocaine is both an anesthetic and a central nervous system stimulant. In tiny doses, it can slow heart rate. In larger doses, the physical effects are dramatic: increased heart rate and blood pressure, loss of appetite that can lead to dramatic weight loss, convulsions, muscle twitching, irregular heartbeat, and even eventual death due to overdose. Other effects of cocaine include temporary relief of depression, decreased fatigue, talkativeness, increased alertness, and heightened self-confidence. However, as the dose increases, users become irritable and apprehensive, and their behavior may turn paranoid or violent.

Cocaine-Affected Babies   Because cocaine rapidly crosses the placenta (as virtually all drugs do), the fetus is vulnerable when a pregnant woman snorts, freebases, or shoots up. It is estimated that 2.4 to 3.5 percent of pregnant women between the ages of 12 and 34 abuse cocaine. It is difficult to gauge how many newborns have been exposed to cocaine, because pregnant users are reluctant to discuss their drug habit with health care providers for fear of prosecution. The most threatening problem for a cocaine user during pregnancy is the increased risk of a miscarriage.

Fetuses exposed to cocaine or crack (the drug in chip form) in the womb are more likely to suffer a small head, premature delivery, reduced birthweight, increased irritabil-

Freebase   The most powerful distillate of cocaine.

Crack   A distillate of powdered cocaine that comes in small, hard chips or rocks.

ity, and subtle learning and cognitive deficits. Recent research suggests that a significant number of these children develop problems with learning and language skills that require remedial attention.[11] It is critical to identify these children early so they can receive immediate intervention. For both financial and humane reasons, prenatal care and education programs for mothers at risk should be a priority for state and local government.[12]

Freebase Cocaine   Freebase is a form of cocaine that is more powerful and costly than powder or crack. Street cocaine (cocaine hydrochloride) is converted to pure base by removing the hydrochloride salt and many of the cutting agents. The end product, freebase, is smoked through a water pipe. Because freebase cocaine reaches the brain within seconds, it is more dangerous than is snorted cocaine. It produces a quick, intense high that disappears quickly and leaves an intense craving for more. Freebasers typically increase the amount and frequency of the dose. They often become severely addicted and experience serious health problems.

Side effects of freebasing cocaine include weight loss, increased heart rate and blood pressure, depression, paranoia, and hallucinations. Freebase is an extremely dangerous drug and is responsible for a large number of cocaine-related hospital emergency room visits and deaths.

Crack   The street name **crack** is given to freebase cocaine processed from cocaine hydrochloride by using ammonia or sodium bicarbonate (baking soda), water, and heat to remove the hydrochloride. (Crack also can be processed with ether, but this is much riskier because ether is flammable.) The mixture (90 percent pure cocaine) is then dried. The soapy-looking substance that results can be broken into rocks and smoked. These rocks are approximately five times as strong as cocaine. Crack gets its name from the popping noises it makes when burned. Sometimes crack is called rock, an alias that should not be confused with rock cocaine. Rock cocaine is a cocaine hydrochloride substance that is primarily sold in California. White in color, it is about the shape of a pencil eraser and is typically snorted.

Because crack is such a pure drug, it takes much less time to achieve the desired high. One puff of a pebble-size rock produces an intense high that lasts for approximately 20 minutes. The user can usually get three or four hits off a rock before it is used up. Crack is typically sold in small vials, folding papers, or heavy tinfoil containing two or three rocks that cost between $10 and $20.

A crack user can become addicted quickly. Addiction is accelerated by the speed at which crack is absorbed through the lungs (it hits the brain within seconds) and by the intensity of the high. It is not uncommon for crack addicts to spend more than $1,000 a day on the habit.

Cocaine Addiction and Society   Cocaine addicts often suffer both physiological damage and serious disruption in lifestyle, including loss of employment and self-esteem. It is estimated that the annual cost of cocaine addiction in the

Table 7.3
Effects of Amphetamines on the Body and Mind

	Body	Mind
Low Dose	Increased heartbeat	Decreased fatigue
	Increased blood pressure	Increased confidence
	Decreased appetite	Increased feeling of alertness
	Increased breathing rate	Restlessness, talkativeness
	Inability to sleep	Increased irritability
	Sweating	Fearfulness, apprehension
	Dry mouth	Distrust of people
	Muscle twitching	Repetitive behaviors
	Convulsions	Hallucinations
	Fever	Psychosis
	Chest pain	
	Irregular heartbeat	
High Dose	Death due to overdose	

Source: G. Hanson and P. Venturelli, *Drugs and Society* (Sudbury, MA: Jones and Bartlett 1998), 229. © Jones and Bartlett, www.jbpub.com. Reprinted with permission.

United States exceeds $3.8 billion. However, there is no way to measure the cost in wasted lives. An estimated 5 million Americans from all socioeconomic groups are addicted, and 5,000 new users try cocaine or crack every day. Federal agencies estimate that 3 million to 4 million people had used the drug at least once in the past year. Experts suggest that 10 percent of recreational users will go on to heavy use.[13]

To date, we have not found a successful weapon to combat cocaine and crack use in the United States. Cocaine has been called unpredictable by drug experts, deadly by coroners, dangerous by former users, and disastrous by the media. Apparently, the risks do not override users' desire to experience the euphoria it produces.

Because cocaine is illegal, a complex underground network has developed to manufacture and sell the drug. Buyers may not get the product they think they are purchasing. Cocaine marketed for snorting may be only 60 percent pure. Usually, it is mixed, or cut, with other white powdery substances such as mannitol or sugar; occasionally it is cut with arsenic or other cocaine-like powders that may themselves be highly dangerous.

What do you think?

Have all segments of society been affected by crack use? ✳ If not, which segments of the U.S. population experience the greatest impact from crack use? ✳ Why might this be the case? ✳ Is there a difference in the profile of a person who uses crack rather than cocaine? Explain your answer.

Amphetamines The **amphetamines** include a large and varied group of synthetic agents that stimulate the central nervous system. Small doses of amphetamines improve alertness, lessen fatigue, and generally elevate mood. With repeated use, however, physical and psychological dependency develops. Sleep patterns are affected (insomnia); heart rate, breathing rate, and blood pressure increase; restlessness, anxiety, appetite suppression, and vision problems are common. High doses over long time periods can produce hallucinations, delusions, and disorganized behavior. Abusers become paranoid, fearing everything and everyone. Some become aggressive or antisocial (see Table 7.3).

Amphetamines for recreational use are sold under a variety of names: Bennies (amphetamine/Benzedrine), dex (dextroamphetamine/Dexedrine), and meth or speed (methamphetamine/Methedrine). Other street terms for amphetamines are cross tops, uppers, wake-ups, lid poppers, cartwheels, and blackies. Amphetamines do have therapeutic uses in the treatment of attention deficit/hyperactivity disorder in children (Ritalin, Cylert) and of obesity (Pondimin).

Newer-Generation Stimulants Methamphetamine, a form of amphetamine, is a powerfully addictive drug that strongly

Amphetamines A large and varied group of synthetic agents that stimulate the central nervous system.

Methamphetamine A powerfully addictive drug that strongly activates certain areas of the brain and affects the central nervous system.

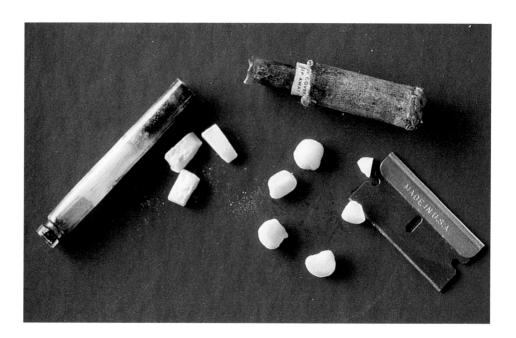

Although new drugs of choice often make the news, the availability of crack cocaine continues to be a major problem.

activates certain areas of the brain and affects the central nervous system in general. Methamphetamine is closely related chemically to amphetamine, but its central nervous system effects are greater.

Methamphetamine is relatively easy to make. People nicknamed cookers produce methamphetamine batches using cookbook-style recipes that often include common OTC ingredients such as ephedrine and pseudoephedrine. Laws have strengthened the penalties associated with manufacturing methamphetamine.

The effects of methamphetamine last six to eight hours, considerably longer than those produced by crack and cocaine. The immediate effects can include irritability and anxiety; increased body temperature, heart rate, and blood pressure; and possible death. The high state of irritability and agitation has been associated with violent behavior among some users.

Ice is a potent methamphetamine that is imported primarily from Asia, particularly from South Korea and Taiwan. It is purer and more crystalline than the version manufactured in many U.S. cities. Because it is odorless, public use of ice often goes unnoticed.

Ice   A potent, inexpensive methamphetamine that has long-lasting effects.

Marijuana   Chopped leaves and flowers of the *Cannabis indica* or *Cannabis sativa* plant (hemp); a psychoactive stimulant that intensifies reactions to environmental stimuli.

Tetrahydrocannabinol (THC)   The chemical name for the active ingredient in marijuana.

Typically, ice quickly becomes addictive. Some users have reported severe cravings after using it only once. The effects of ice are long lasting. They include wakefulness, mood elevation, and excitability, all of which appeal to work-addicted young adults, particularly those who must put in long hours in high-stress jobs. Because the drug is inexpensive and produces such an intense high that lasts from 4 to 14 hours, it has become popular among young people looking for a quick high. However, as is true of other methamphetamines, the down side of this drug is devastating. Prolonged use can cause fatal lung and kidney damage as well as long-lasting psychological damage. In some instances, major psychological dysfunction has lasted as long as two and one-half years after last use.

Marijuana

Although archaeological evidence documents the use of **marijuana** (grass, weed, pot) as far back as 6,000 years, the drug did not become popular in the United States until the 1960s. Marijuana receives less media attention today than it did then, but it is still the illicit drug used most frequently. Nearly one of every three Americans over the age of 12 has tried marijuana at least once. Some 12 million Americans have used it; more than 1 million cannot control their use of it.

Physical Effects of Marijuana   Marijuana is derived from either the *Cannabis sativa* or *Cannabis indica* (hemp) plants. Current American-grown marijuana is a turbocharged version of the hippie weed of the late 1960s. Developed using cross-breeding, genetic engineering, and American farming ingenuity, top-grade cannabis packs a punch very similar to that of hashish. **Tetrahydrocannabinol (THC)** is the psychoactive substance in marijuana and the key to determining how powerful a high it will produce. Whereas marijuana from three decades ago had a potency of 1 to 2 percent THC, a current crop averages 4 to 6 percent. Thus the modern-day marijuana user may be exposed to doses of THC many times greater than were users in the 1960s and 1970s.[14]

Hashish, a potent cannabis preparation derived mainly from the thick, sticky resin of the plant, contains high concentrations of THC. Hash oil, a substance produced by percolating a solvent such as ether through dried marijuana to extract the THC, is a tar-like liquid that may contain up to 300 milligrams (mg) of THC in a dose.

Most of the time, marijuana is rolled into cigarettes (joints) or smoked in a pipe or water pipe (bong). Effects generally are felt within 10 to 30 minutes and usually wear off within three hours.

The most noticeable effect of THC is the dilation of the eyes' blood vessels, which produces the characteristic blood-shot eyes. Smokers of the drug also exhibit coughing, dry mouth and throat (cotton mouth), increased thirst and appetite, lowered blood pressure, and mild muscular weakness primarily exhibited in drooping eyelids. Users also can experience severe anxiety, panic, paranoia, and psychosis, as well as intensified reactions to various stimuli. Colors and sounds, as well as the speed at which things move, may seem magnified. High doses of hashish may produce vivid visual hallucinations.

Effects of Chronic Marijuana Use

Because marijuana is illegal in most parts of the United States and has been used widely only since the 1960s, long-term studies of its effects have been difficult to conduct. Also, studies conducted in the 1960s involved marijuana with THC levels constituting only a fraction of today's plant levels, so their results may not apply to the stronger forms available today. Most current information about chronic marijuana use comes from countries such as Jamaica and Costa Rica, where the drug is not illegal. These studies of long-term users (ten or more years) indicate that it causes lung damage comparable to that caused by tobacco smoking. Indeed, smoking a single joint may be as bad for the lungs as smoking three tobacco cigarettes. The chemicals themselves do not injure the heart, but inhaling burning material does. Inhalation of marijuana transfers carbon monoxide to the bloodstream. Because the blood has a greater affinity for carbon monoxide than it does for oxygen, this diminishes the oxygen-carrying capacity of the blood. The heart must work harder to pump the vital element to oxygen-starved tissues. As well, the tar from cannabis contains higher levels of carcinogens than does tobacco smoke. Smoking marijuana results in three times more tar inhalation and retention in the respiratory tract than does tobacco use.

Other risks associated with marijuana include suppression of the immune system, blood pressure changes, and impaired memory function. Recent studies suggest that pregnant women who smoke marijuana are at a higher risk for stillbirth or miscarriage and for delivering low birth-weight babies and babies with abnormalities of the nervous system. Babies born to marijuana smokers are five times more likely to have features similar to those exhibited by children with fetal alcohol syndrome.

Debates concerning the effects of marijuana on the reproductive system have yet to be resolved. Studies conducted in the mid-1970s suggested that marijuana inhibited testosterone (and thus sperm) production in males and caused chromosomal breakage in both ova and sperm. Subsequent research in these areas is inconclusive. The question of whether the high-level THC plants currently available will increase the risks associated with this drug is, as yet, unanswered.

Marijuana and Medicine

Although recognized as a dangerous drug by the U.S. government, marijuana has several medical purposes. It helps control the side effects such as severe nausea and vomiting produced by chemotherapy, the chemical treatment for cancer. It improves appetite and forestalls the loss of lean muscle mass associated with AIDS-related wasting syndrome. Marijuana reduces the muscle pain and spasticity caused by diseases such as multiple sclerosis. It also temporarily relieves the eye pressure of glaucoma, although it is unclear whether it is more effective than legal glaucoma drugs.[15] Marijuana's legal status for medicinal purposes continues to be hotly debated (see the New Horizons in Health box on page 188).

Marijuana and Driving

Marijuana use presents clear hazards for drivers of motor vehicles as well as others on the road. The drug substantially reduces a driver's ability to react and to make quick decisions. Studies reveal that 60 to 80 percent of marijuana users sometimes drive while high.[16] Studies of automobile accident victims show that 6 to 12 percent of nonfatally injured drivers and 4 to 16 percent of fatally injured drivers had THC in their bloodstreams. Perceptual and other performance deficits resulting from marijuana use may persist for some time after the high subsides. Users who attempt to drive, fly, or operate heavy machinery often fail to recognize their impairment.

> **What do you think?**
> *Why do you think that marijuana is the most popular illicit drug on college campuses?* * *How widespread is marijuana use at your school?*

Hashish The sticky resin of the cannabis plant, which is high in THC.

Medicinal Use of Marijuana: Legal Challenges Continue

For years, marijuana's legal status for medicinal purposes has been hotly debated. So far, 30 states and the District of Columbia have laws that recognize marijuana's medical value. Nevertheless, 12 states with Therapeutic Research Program laws are unable to give patients legal access to medical marijuana because of federal laws. Ten states and the District of Columbia have symbolic laws that recognize marijuana's medical value but fail to provide patients with protection from arrest for possession of an illegal drug. Voters in Alaska, California, Colorado, Hawaii, Maine, Nevada, Oregon, and Washington state have chosen to legalize marijuana for medicinal uses (see the accompanying figures). These new state laws, however, conflict with federal laws against the possession of marijuana and have led to new, as yet unresolved, battles in court.

Source: R. Schmitz and C. Thomas, "State-by-State Medical Marijuana Laws: How to Remove the Threat of Arrest," 2001. Copyright Marijuana Policy Project; used by permission. http://mpp.org/statelaw/index.html

States with effective medical marijuana laws

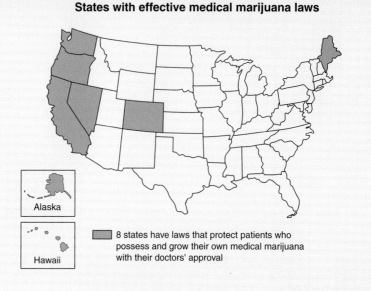

8 states have laws that protect patients who possess and grow their own medical marijuana with their doctors' approval

States with other medical marijuana laws

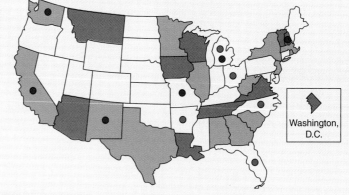

These states have laws to allow therapeutic research programs, provided that the federal government cooperates (California and Washington also have effective laws)

These states and the District of Columbia have symbolic medical marijuana laws

● States that used to have favorable laws, which have expired or been repealed

● States where legislatures have passed favorable non-binding resolutions

---

Narcotics Drugs that induce sleep and relieve pain; primarily the opiates.

Opium The parent drug of the opiates; made from the seedpod resin of the opium poppy.

Morphine A derivative of opium; sometimes used by medical practitioners to relieve pain.

Codeine A drug derived from morphine; used in cough syrups and certain painkillers.

Opiates

Opiates cause drowsiness, relieve pain, and induce euphoria. Also called **narcotics,** they are derived from the parent drug **opium,** a dark, resinous substance made from the milky juice of the opium poppy. Other opiates include morphine, codeine, heroin, and black tar heroin.

The word *narcotic* comes from the Greek word for "stupor" and generally is used to describe sleep-inducing substances. For many years, opiates were used widely by the medical community. More powerful than opium, **morphine** (named after Morpheus, the Greek god of sleep) was used widely as a painkiller during the Civil War. **Codeine,** a less powerful analgesic derived from morphine, also became popular. As opiates became more common, physicians noted that patients tended to become dependent on them. Contrary to earlier belief, all of the opiates are highly addictive. Growing concern about addiction led to government controls of narcotic use. The Harrison Act of 1914 prohibited the production, dispensation, and sale of opiate products unless prescribed by a physician. Subsequent legislation required physicians prescribing opiates to keep careful records. Physicians are still subject to audits of their prescriptions.

Some opiates still are used today for medical purposes. Doctors sometimes prescribe morphine for severe pain. Codeine is found in prescription cough syrups and other painkillers. Several prescription drugs, including Percodan, Demerol, and Dilaudid, contain synthetic opiates. Although all opiate use is strictly regulated, illicit use of OxyContin, another powerful opiate, has increased dramatically in recent years (see the Reality Check box on page 190).

Physical Effects of Opiates   Opiates are powerful depressants of the central nervous system. In addition to relieving pain, these drugs lower heart rate, respiration, and blood pressure. Side effects include weakness, dizziness, nausea, vomiting, euphoria, decreased sex drive, visual disturbances, and lack of coordination. Of all the opiates, heroin has the greatest notoriety as an addictive drug. The following section discusses the progression of heroin addiction; addiction to any opiate follows a similar path.

Heroin Addiction   Heroin is a white powder derived from morphine. **Black tar heroin** is a sticky, dark brown, foul-smelling form of heroin that is relatively pure and inexpensive. It is estimated that 600,000 Americans are addicted to heroin, with men outnumbering women addicts by three to one.[17] Authorities believe that the United States is at the beginning of a new heroin epidemic. There is concern that this epidemic will be worse than previous ones because the drug is now two to three times more available than ever before. The contemporary version of heroin is so potent that users can get high by snorting or smoking the drug rather than by injecting it and putting themselves at risk for AIDS, although many addicts continue to inject the drug. Once an inner-city drug, heroin use now is becoming more widespread among middle-class people who tend to try whatever is new and trendy.

Once considered a cure for morphine dependency, heroin was later discovered to be even more addictive and potent than is morphine. Today, heroin has no medical use.

Heroin is a depressant that produces drowsiness and a dreamy, mentally slow feeling. It can cause drastic mood swings, with euphoric highs followed by depressive lows. Heroin also slows respiration and urinary output and constricts the pupils of the eyes. In fact, pupil constriction is a classic sign of narcotic intoxication; hence, the stereotype of the drug user hiding behind a pair of dark sunglasses.

Symptoms of tolerance and withdrawal can appear within three weeks of first use.

The most common route of administration for heroin addicts is mainlining—intravenous injection of powdered heroin mixed in a solution. Many users describe the rush they feel when injecting themselves as intensely pleasurable, but others report unpredictable and unpleasant side effects. The temporary nature of the rush contributes to the drug's high potential for addiction—many addicts shoot up four or five times a day. Mainlining can cause veins to scar and eventually collapse. Once a vein has collapsed, it can no longer be used to introduce heroin into the bloodstream. Addicts become expert at locating new veins to use: in the feet, the legs, even in the temples. When they do not want their needle tracks (scars) to show, they inject themselves under the tongue or in the groin.

The physiology of the human body could be said to encourage opiate addiction. Opiate-like substances called **endorphins** are manufactured in the body and have multiple receptor sites, particularly in the central nervous system. When endorphins attach themselves at these points, they create feelings of painless well-being. Medical researchers refer to them as "the body's own opiates." When endorphin levels are high, people feel euphoric. The same euphoria occurs when opiates or related chemicals are active at the endorphin receptor sites.

Treatment for Heroin Addiction   Programs to help heroin addicts kick the habit have not been very successful. Some addicts resume drug use even after years of drug-free living because the craving for the injection rush is very strong. It takes a great deal of discipline to seek alternative, nondrug highs.

Heroin addicts experience a distinct pattern of withdrawal. They begin to crave another dose four to six hours after their last dose. Symptoms of withdrawal include intense desire for the drug, yawning, a runny nose, sweating, and crying. About 12 hours after the last dose, addicts experience sleep disturbance, dilated pupils, loss of appetite, irritability, goose bumps, and muscle tremors. The most difficult time in the withdrawal process occurs 24 to 72 hours following last use. All of the preceding symptoms continue, along with nausea, abdominal cramps, restlessness, insomnia, vomiting, diarrhea, extreme anxiety, hot and cold flashes, elevated blood pressure, and rapid heartbeat and

---

Heroin   An illegally manufactured derivative of morphine, usually injected into the bloodstream.

Black tar heroin   A dark brown, sticky form of heroin.

Endorphins   Opiate-like hormones that are manufactured in the human body and contribute to natural feelings of well-being.

OxyContin: A New and Dangerous Opiate Threat

OxyContin, a prescription central nervous system depressant in the opiate drug family, has catapulted to the top of the drug abuse scene in America. Since its 1995 approval by the FDA as a painkiller, it has become a major contributor to young adult drug abuse, which has caused the diversion of pills and theft of prescriptions in many regions of the country. According to a National Drug and Intelligence Center drug threat survey and Drug Enforcement Administration reporting in 2002, OxyContin has become the drug of choice in many Eastern states and has now hit Midwestern and Western states at an epidemic pace. Some 4% of all high school seniors reported using OxyContin without a prescription in 2002. In fall 2003, political commentator Rush Limbaugh was treated for OxyContin addiction.

Why the popularity? OxyContin is the brand name for *oxycodone hydrochloride*, one of a large group of pain relief products commonly prescribed for people suffering chronic pain. Other drugs in this category include Percocet, Percodan, Vicodan, and other high-strength painkillers; most are highly addictive if taken for prolonged periods of time. Most of these drugs contain only 2.5–5 mg of oxycodone. In contrast, OxyContin is marketed in doses of 10, 20, 40, 80 and even 160 mg tablets. The strength, duration, and known dosage of OxyContin make it a powerful painkiller, but also make it extremely attractive to abusers. OxyContin has become a substitute for heroin for some addicts who find pharmaceutical drugs to be purer and cheaper than street drugs.

Due to OxyContin's widespread availability, the crimes, addictions, and fatal overdoses associated with it have skyrocketed—many people have no idea of the risks they take when abusing the drug. Although exact numbers of deaths are unavailable, it is likely that there are hundreds every year among unsuspecting young adults. Formulated as a 12-hour time release pill, OxyContin has a low addiction rate among those who take it as prescribed for the most acute pain of cancer or injury. However, abusers disable the time release structure of the pill by chewing it, crushing it, or dissolving it into liquid form and then eating, snorting, or injecting the solution. When taken orally or injected in this form, the user experiences a rush similar to heroin. The mind and body easily become obsessed with this pleasurable rush, and a physical craving can develop causing addiction. Chronic use results in increasing tolerance so that more of the drug is needed to feel the same effects that smaller doses once provided. Often the user is unaware this is happening and goes from using two pills a day, to two pills an hour, to two pills every 15 minutes as drug tolerance builds rapidly. Self-control in using the drug is lost as the brain becomes dependent.

Because many OxyContin abusers do not know of its dangers, they may make the situation even more risky by drinking alcohol or taking sleeping pills and OTC pain medications with it. These drug interactions have caused many serious side effects, even coma and death.

The good news is that complete recovery from addiction is possible, but addicted users cannot do it on their own. Medical supervision and appropriate therapeutic techniques must be utilized to ensure recovery.

Sources: L. D. Johnston, P. M. O'Malley, and J. G. Bachman, *Monitoring the Future National Survey Results on Drug Use, 1975–2002. Volume I: Secondary School Students* (NIH Publication No. 03-5375) (Bethesda, MD: National Institute on Drug Abuse, 2003); Drug Enforcement Administration, "OxyContin: Pharmaceutical Diversion," 2002. www.dea.gov; Center for Drug Evaluation and Research. "OxyContin: Questions and Answers," 2002. www.fda.gov/cder/drug/infopage/oxycontin/oxycontin-qa.htm

respiration. Once the peak of withdrawal has passed, all these symptoms begin to subside. Still, the recovering addict has many hurdles to jump.

Methadone maintenance is one treatment available for people addicted to heroin or other opiates. Methadone is a synthetic narcotic that blocks the effects of opiate withdrawal. It is chemically similar enough to the opiates to control the tremors, chills, vomiting, diarrhea, and severe abdominal pains of withdrawal. Methadone dosage is decreased over a period of time until the addict is weaned off the drug.

Methadone maintenance is controversial because of the drug's own potential for addiction. Critics contend that the program merely substitutes one addiction for another. Proponents argue that people on methadone maintenance are less likely to engage in criminal activities to support their habits than heroin addicts are. For this reason, many methadone maintenance programs are financed by state or federal government and are available to clients free of charge or at reduced costs.

A number of new drug therapies for opiate dependence are emerging. Naltrexone (Trexan), an opiate antagonist, has been approved as a treatment. While on Naltrexone,

> **Methadone maintenance** A treatment for people addicted to opiates that substitutes methadone, a synthetic narcotic, for the opiate of addiction.

recovering addicts do not have the compulsion to use heroin. If they do use it, they don't get high, so there is no point in using the drug. More recently, researchers have reported promising results with Temgesic (buprenorphine), a mild, nonaddicting synthetic opiate. Like heroin and methadone, Temgesic bonds to certain receptors in the brain, blocks pain messages, and persuades the brain that its cravings for heroin have been satisfied. Addicts report that they do not crave heroin while they are taking buprenorphine.

Hallucinogens (Psychedelics)

Hallucinogens are substances that are capable of creating auditory or visual hallucinations. These drugs are also known as **psychedelics,** a term adapted from the Greek phrase meaning "mind manifesting." Hallucinogens are a group of drugs whose primary pharmacological effect is to alter feelings, perceptions, and thoughts in a user. The major receptor sites for most of these drugs are in the part of the brain that is responsible for interpreting outside stimuli before allowing these signals to travel to other parts of the brain. This area, the **reticular formation,** is located in the brain stem at the upper end of the spinal cord (see Figure 7.4). When a hallucinogen is present at a reticular formation site, messages become scrambled, and the user may see wavy walls instead of straight ones or may smell colors and hear tastes. This mixing of sensory messages is known as **synesthesia.**

In addition to synesthetic effects, users may become less inhibited or recall events long buried in the subconscious mind. The most widely recognized hallucinogenics are LSD, mescaline, psilocybin, psilocin, and PCP. All are illegal and carry severe penalties for manufacture, possession, transportation, or sale.

LSD Of all the psychedelics, **lysergic acid diethylamide (LSD)** is the most notorious. First synthesized in the 1930s by Swiss chemist Albert Hoffman, LSD resulted from experiments to derive medically useful drugs from the ergot fungus found on rye and other cereal grains. Because LSD seemed capable of unlocking the secrets of the mind, psychiatrists initially felt it could be beneficial to patients unable to remember suppressed traumas. From 1950 through 1968, the drug was used for such purposes.

Media attention focused on LSD in the 1960s. Young people used the drug to "turn on" and "tune out" the world that gave them the war in Vietnam, race riots, and political assassinations. In 1970, federal authorities, under intense pressure from the public, placed LSD on the list of controlled substances (Schedule I). LSD's popularity peaked in 1972, then tapered off, primarily because of users' inability to control dosages accurately.

Because of the recent wave of nostalgia for the 1960s, this dangerous psychedelic drug has been making a comeback. Known on the street as acid, LSD is now available in virtually every state. More than 11 million Americans, most of them under age 35, have tried LSD at least once. LSD

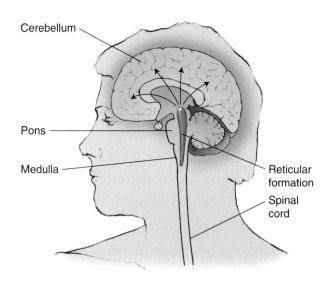

Figure 7.4
Reticular Formation

especially attracts younger users. Approximately 10 percent of high school seniors report having tried it at least once. A national survey of college students showed that 2 percent had used the drug.[18]

An odorless, tasteless, white crystalline powder, LSD most frequently is dissolved in water to make a solution that can be used to manufacture the street forms of the drug: tablets, blotter acid, and windowpane. What the LSD consumer usually buys is blotter acid—small squares of blotter-like paper that have been impregnated with the liquid. The blotter is swallowed or chewed briefly. LSD also comes in tiny thin squares of gelatin called windowpane and in tablets called microdots, which are less than an eighth of an inch across (it would take ten or more to add up to the size of an aspirin tablet). Microdots and windowpane are just a sideshow; blotter is the medium of choice. As with any illegal drug, purchasers run the risk of buying an impure product.

Hallucinogens   Substances capable of creating hallucinations.

Psychedelics   Drugs that distort the processing of sensory information in the brain.

Reticular formation   An area in the brain stem that is responsible for relaying messages to other areas in the brain.

Synesthesia   A (usually) drug-created effect in which sensory messages are incorrectly assigned—for example, hearing a taste or smelling a sound.

Lysergic acid diethylamide (LSD)   Psychedelic drug causing sensory disruptions; also called acid.

One of the most powerful drugs known to science, LSD can produce strong effects in doses as low as 20 micrograms. (To give you an idea of how small a dose this is, the average postage stamp weighs approximately 60,000 micrograms.) The potency of the typical dose currently ranges from 20 to 80 micrograms, compared to 150 to 300 micrograms commonly used in the 1960s.

Despite its reputation for being primarily a psychedelic, LSD produces a number of physical effects, including increased heart rate, elevated blood pressure and temperature, goose flesh (roughened skin), increased reflex speeds, muscle tremors and twitches, perspiration, increased salivation, chills, headaches, and mild nausea. Since the drug also stimulates uterine muscle contractions, it can lead to premature labor and miscarriage in pregnant women. Research into long-term effects has been inconclusive.

The psychological effects of LSD vary. Euphoria is the common psychological state produced by the drug, but *dysphoria* (a sense of evil and foreboding) also may occur. The drug also shortens attention span, which causes the mind to wander. Thoughts may be interposed and juxtaposed, so the user experiences several different thoughts simultaneously. Synesthesia occurs occasionally. Users become introspective, and suppressed memories may surface that often take on bizarre symbolism. Many more effects are possible, including decreased aggressiveness and enhanced sensory experiences.

Although LSD rarely produces hallucinations, it can create illusions. These distortions of ordinary perceptions may include movement of stationary objects. Bad trips, the most publicized risk of LSD, are commonly related to the user's mood. The person, for example, may interpret increased heart rate as a heart attack (a bad body trip). Often bad trips result when a user confronts a suppressed emotional experience or memory (a bad head trip).

While there is no evidence that LSD creates physical dependency, it may create psychological dependency. Many LSD users become depressed for one or two days following a trip and turn to the drug to relieve this depression. The result is a cycle of LSD use to relieve post-LSD depression, which often leads to psychological addiction.

Mescaline   A hallucinogenic drug derived from the peyote cactus.

Peyote   A cactus with small "buttons" that, when ingested, produce hallucinogenic effects.

Psilocybin   The active chemical found in psilocybe mushrooms; it produces hallucinations.

Phencyclidine (PCP)   A hallucinogen commonly called angel dust.

What do you think?

Are people today using LSD for the same reasons they did in the 1960s? ☀ *What are the perceived attractions and the real dangers of LSD?*

Mescaline   Mescaline is one of hundreds of chemicals derived from the **peyote** cactus, a small, buttonlike cactus that grows in the southwestern United States and parts of Latin America. Natives of these regions have long used the dried peyote buttons for religious purposes. In fact, members of the Native American Church (a religion practiced by thousands of North American Indians) have been granted special permission to use the drug during religious ceremonies in some states.

Users typically swallow 10 to 12 dried peyote buttons. These buttons taste bitter and generally induce immediate nausea or vomiting. Long-time users claim that the nausea becomes less noticeable with frequent use.

Those who are able to keep the drug down begin to feel the effects within 30 to 90 minutes, when mescaline reaches maximum concentration in the brain. (It may persist for up to nine or ten hours.) Unlike LSD, mescaline is a powerful hallucinogen. It is also a central nervous system stimulant.

Products sold on the street as mescaline are likely to be synthetic chemical relatives of the true drug. Street names of these products include DOM, STP, TMA, and MMDA. Any of these can be toxic in small quantities.

Psilocybin   Psilocybin and *psilocin* are the active chemicals in a group of mushrooms sometimes called magic mushrooms. Psilocybe mushrooms, which grow throughout the world, can be cultivated from spores or harvested wild. Because many mushrooms resemble the psilocybe variety, people who harvest wild mushrooms for any purpose should be certain of what they are doing. Mushroom varieties can be easily misidentified, and mistakes can be fatal. Psilocybin is similar to LSD in its physical effects, which generally wear off in four to six hours.

PCP   Phencyclidine, or **PCP,** is a synthetic substance that became a black-market drug in the early 1970s. PCP was originally developed as a dissociative anesthetic, which means that patients administered this drug could keep their eyes open and apparently remain conscious but feel no pain during a medical procedure. Afterward, patients would experience amnesia for the time the drug was in their system. Such a drug had obvious advantages as an anesthetic, but its unpredictability and drastic effects (postoperative delirium, confusion, and agitation) made doctors abandon it, and it was withdrawn from the legal market.

On the illegal market, PCP is a white, crystalline powder that users often sprinkle onto marijuana cigarettes. It is dangerous and unpredictable regardless of the method of administration. Common street names for PCP are angel dust for the crystalline powdered form and peace pill and horse tranquilizer for the tablet form.

The effects of PCP depend on the dosage. A dose as small as 5 mg will produce effects similar to those of strong central nervous system depressants—slurred speech, impaired coordination, reduced sensitivity to pain, and reduced heart and respiratory rate. Doses between 5 and 10 mg cause fever, salivation, nausea, vomiting, and total loss of sensitivity to pain. Doses greater than 10 mg result in a drastic drop in blood pressure, coma, muscular rigidity, violent outbursts, and possible convulsions and death.

Psychologically, PCP may produce either euphoria or dysphoria. It also is known to produce hallucinations as well as delusions and overall delirium. Some users experience a prolonged state of nothingness. The long-term effects of PCP use are unknown.

Designer Drugs (Club Drugs)

Designer drugs are synthetic drugs that produce effects similar to existing illegal drugs. They are manufactured in chemical laboratories and in homes, and sold illegally. These drugs are easy to produce from available raw materials. The drugs themselves were once technically legal because the law had to specify the exact chemical structure of an illicit substance. However, a law is now in place that bans all chemical cousins of illegal drugs.

Collectively known as *club drugs,* these dangerous substances include Ecstasy, GHB, Special K, and Rohypnol. Although users may think them harmless, research has shown that club drugs can produce a range of unwanted effects, including hallucinations, paranoia, amnesia, and in some cases, death. Some club drugs work on the same brain mechanisms as alcohol does and can boost the effects of both substances dangerously. Since the drugs are odorless and tasteless, people can easily slip them into drinks. Some of them have been associated with sexual assaults; for this reason they are referred to as date rape drugs.

Ecstasy (methylenedioxymethylamphetamine, or *MDMA*), once dubbed the "LSD of the 80s," has had a resurgence of popularity. Almost one of every four students at some universities report having used it. Ecstasy creates feelings of openness and warmth, combined with the mind-expanding characteristics of hallucinogens. Effects begin within 30 minutes and can last for four to six hours. Young people may use Ecstasy initially to improve mood or get energized so they can keep dancing; it also increases heart rate and blood pressure and may raise body temperature to the point of kidney and/or cardiovascular failure. Chronic use appears to damage the brain's ability to think and regulate emotion, memory, sleep, and pain. Combined with alcohol, Ecstasy can be extremely dangerous and sometimes fatal. Recent studies indicate that Ecstasy may cause long-lasting neurotoxic effects by damaging brain cells that produce serotonin; it is unknown whether these brain cells will regenerate.[19]

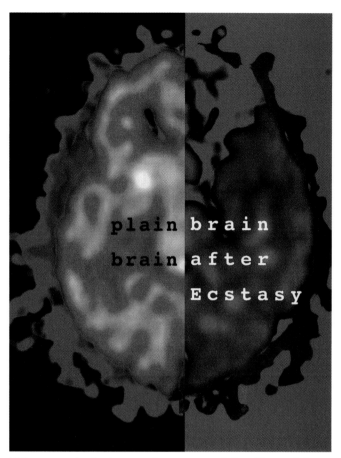

This composite brain scan shows some of the effects of the drug Ecstasy. The left side shows healthy serotonin sites. The dark sections on the right are serotonin sites no longer present even after three weeks without Ecstasy. Serotonin helps regulate mood, learning, and sleep.

Inhalants

Inhalants are chemicals that produce vapors that, when inhaled, can cause hallucinations and create intoxicating and euphoric effects. Not commonly recognized as drugs, inhalants are legal to purchase and universally available, but dangerous when used incorrectly. They generally appeal to young people who can't afford or obtain illicit substances.

Some of these agents are organic solvents representing the chemical by-products of the distillation of petroleum products. Rubber cement, model glue, paint thinner, lighter fluid, varnish, wax, spot removers, and gasoline belong to this group. Most of these substances are sniffed by users in search of a quick, cheap high.

> **Designer drug**   A synthetic analog (a drug that produces similar effects) of an existing illicit drug.
>
> **Inhalants**   Products that are sniffed or inhaled in order to produce highs.

Because they are inhaled, the volatile chemicals in these products reach the bloodstream within seconds. An inhaled substance is not diluted or buffered by stomach acids or other body fluids and thus is more potent than it would be if swallowed. This characteristic, along with the fact that dosages are extremely difficult to control because everyone has unique lung and breathing capacities, makes inhalants particularly dangerous.

The effects of inhalants usually last fewer than 15 minutes. Users may experience dizziness, disorientation, impaired coordination, reduced judgment, and slowed reaction times. Signs of inhalant use include an unjustifiable collection of glues, paints, lacquer thinner, cleaning fluid, and ether; sniffles similar to those produced by a cold; and a smell on the breath similar to the inhalable substance. The effects of inhalants resemble those of central nervous system depressants, and combining inhalants with alcohol produces a synergistic effect. In addition, combining these substances can cause severe liver damage that can be fatal.

An overdose of fumes from inhalants can cause unconsciousness. If the user's oxygen intake is reduced during the inhaling process, death can result within five minutes. Whether a user is a first-time or chronic user, sudden sniffing death syndrome can be a fatal consequence. This syndrome can occur if a user inhales deeply and then participates in physical activity or is startled.

Amyl Nitrite   Sometimes called poppers or rush, **amyl nitrite** is packaged in small, cloth-covered glass capsules that can be crushed to release the active chemical. The drug often is prescribed to alleviate chest pain in heart patients, because it dilates small blood vessels and reduces blood pressure. Dilation of blood vessels in the genital area is thought to enhance sensations or perceptions of orgasm. It also produces fainting, dizziness, warmth, and skin flushing.

Nitrous Oxide   **Nitrous oxide** is sometimes used as an adjunct to dental anesthesia or minor surgical anesthesia. It is also a propellant chemical in aerosol products such as whipped toppings. Users experience a state of euphoria, floating sensations, and illusions. Effects also include pain relief and a silly feeling demonstrated by laughing and giggling (hence its nickname laughing gas). Regulating dosages

---

Amyl nitrite   A drug that dilates blood vessels and is properly used to relieve chest pain.

Nitrous oxide   The chemical name for laughing gas, a substance properly used for surgical or dental anesthesia.

Anabolic steroids   Artificial forms of the hormone testosterone that promote muscle growth and strength.

Ergogenic drugs   Substances that enhance athletic performance.

---

of this drug can be difficult. Sustained inhalation can lead to unconsciousness, coma, and death.

Steroids

Public awareness of **anabolic steroids** recently has been heightened by media stories about their use by amateur and professional athletes, including Arnold Schwarzenegger during his competitive bodybuilding days. Anabolic steroids are artificial forms of the male hormone testosterone that promote muscle growth and strength. These **ergogenic drugs** are used primarily by young men who believe the drugs will increase their strength, power, bulk (weight), speed, and athletic performance.

Most steroids are obtained through the black market. It once was estimated that approximately 17 to 20 percent of college athletes used them. Now that stricter drug-testing policies have been instituted by the National College Athletic Association (NCAA), reported use of anabolic steroids among intercollegiate athletics has dropped to 1.1 percent. However, a recent survey among high school students found a significant increase in the use of anabolic steroids since 1991. Few data exist on the extent of steroid abuse by adults. It has been estimated that hundreds of thousands of people age 18 and older abuse anabolic steroids at least once a year. Among both adolescents and adults, steroid abuse is higher among males than among females. However, steroid abuse is growing most rapidly among young women.[20]

Steroids are available in two forms: injectable solution and pills. Anabolic steroids produce a state of euphoria, diminished fatigue, and increased bulk and power in both sexes. These qualities give steroids an addictive quality. When users stop, they can experience psychological withdrawal and sometimes severe depression that in some cases leads to suicide attempts. If untreated, such depression associated with steroid withdrawal has been known to last for a year or more after steroid use stops.

Adverse effects occur in both men and women who use steroids. These drugs cause mood swings (aggression and violence) sometimes known as "roid rage," acne, liver tumors, elevated cholesterol levels, hypertension, kidney disease, and immune system disturbances. There is also a danger of transmitting AIDS through shared needles. In women, large doses of anabolic steroids may trigger the development of masculine attributes such as lowered voice, increased facial and body hair, and male pattern baldness; they also may result in an enlarged clitoris, smaller breasts, and changes in or absence of menstruation. When taken by healthy males, anabolic steroids shut down the body's production of testosterone, which causes men's breasts to grow and testicles to atrophy.

To combat the growing problem of steroid use, Congress passed the Anabolic Steroids Control Act of 1990. This law makes it a crime to possess, prescribe, or distribute anabolic steroids for any use other than the treatment of specific diseases. Anabolic steroids are now classified as a Schedule III drug. Penalties for their illegal use include up to five years'

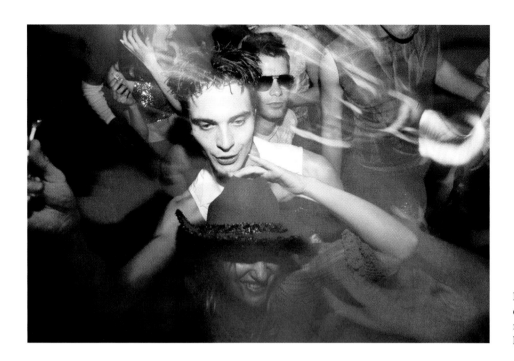

Beware of claims that the latest club drugs are "totally harmless" or "all natural." Such substances can be hazardous.

imprisonment and a $250,000 fine for the first offense, and up to ten years' imprisonment and a $500,000 fine for subsequent offenses.

A new and alarming trend is the use of other drugs to achieve the supposed performance-enhancing effects of steroids. The two most common steroid alternatives are gamma hydroxybutyrate (GHB) and clenbuterol. GHB is a deadly, illegal drug that is a primary ingredient in many performance-enhancing formulas. GHB does not produce a high. However, it does cause headaches, nausea, vomiting, diarrhea, seizures and other central nervous system disorders, and possibly death. Clenbuterol is used in some countries for veterinary treatments, but it is not approved for any use—in animals or humans—in the United States.

New attention was drawn to the issue of steroids and related substances when St. Louis Cardinals slugger Mark McGwire admitted to using a supplement containing androstenedione (andro), an adrenal hormone that is produced naturally in both men and women. Andro raises levels of the male hormone testosterone, which helps build lean muscle mass and promotes quicker recovery after injury. McGwire had done nothing illegal, since the supplement can be purchased OTC (with estimated sales of up to $800 million a year). Also, its use is legal in baseball, although it is banned by the National Football League, the NCAA, and the International Olympic Committee. A recent study found that when men take 100 mg of andro three times daily, it increases estrogen levels up to 80 percent, enlarges the prostate gland, and increases heart disease risk by 10 to 15 percent. This finding may or may not affect its use in major league baseball—no decision has yet been made.

Although andro has been banned by many sports organizations, visits to the locker rooms of many teams belonging to these organizations would disclose large containers of other alleged muscle-building supplements, such as creatine. Although they are legal, questions remain whether enough research has been done concerning the safety of these supplements. Some people worry that they may bring consequences similar to those of steroids, such as liver damage and heart problems.

What do you think?

Do you think androstenedione should be declared illegal? ✳ Would you consider using supplements for the sole purpose of increasing your body build and potentially your athletic performance? ✳ Are steroid users stigmatized in our society in the same way as users of other illicit drugs? ✳ Do you think they should be? ✳ Why or why not?

Illegal Drug Use in the United States

Stories of people who have tried illegal drugs, enjoyed them, and suffered no consequences may tempt you to try them yourself. You may tell yourself it's "just this once," convincing yourself that one-time use is harmless. Given the dangers surrounding these substances, however, you should think twice. The risks associated with drug use extend beyond the personal. The decision to try any illicit substance encourages illicit drug manufacture and transport and thus contributes to the national drug problem. The financial burden of illegal drug use on the U.S. economy is staggering, with an estimated economic cost of around $160 billion.[21] This estimate includes costs associated with substance abuse treatment and prevention, health care, reduced job productivity and lost earnings, and social consequences such as crime and social welfare.

In addition, roughly one-half of all expenditures to combat crime are related to illegal drugs. The burden of these costs is absorbed primarily by the government (46 percent), followed by those who abuse drugs and members of their households (44 percent). One study found that Americans spend $64 billion on illicit drugs annually. The major categories are as follows: $35 billion on cocaine, $10 billion each on marijuana and heroin, and $5 billion on methamphetamines. This is eight times what the federal government spends on research for HIV/AIDS, cancer, and heart disease put together.[22]

Drugs in the Workplace

The National Institute on Drug Abuse (NIDA) estimates that 8.5 percent of all U.S. workers use dangerous drugs on the job at some time. With approximately 70 to 75 percent of drug users in the United States employed to some degree, the cost to American businesses soars into the billions of dollars annually.[23] These costs reflect reduced work performance and efficiency, lost productivity, absenteeism and turnover, increased use of health benefits, accidents, and indirect losses stemming from impaired judgment.

The highest rates of illicit drug use among workers exist among people in the construction, food preparation, restaurant, transportation, and material-moving industries. Workers who require a considerable amount of public trust, such as police officers, teachers, and child-care workers, report the lowest use. In addition, younger employees (18 to 24 years old) are more likely to report drug use than are employees aged 25 and older. Drug users are 1.6 times more likely than are nonusers to quit their jobs or be fired, and 1.5 times more likely to be disciplined by their supervisor.[24]

Many companies have instituted drug testing for their employees. Mandatory drug urinalysis is controversial. Critics argue that such testing violates Fourth Amendment rights of protection from unreasonable search and seizure. Proponents believe the personal inconvenience entailed in testing pales in comparison to the problems caused by drug use in the workplace. Several court decisions have affirmed the right of employers to test their employees for drug use. They contend that Fourth Amendment rights pertain only to employees of government agencies, not to those of private businesses. Most Americans apparently support drug testing for certain types of jobs.

Drug testing is expensive; costs run as high as $100 per individual test. Moreover, some critics question the accuracy and reliability of the results. Both false positives and false negatives can occur. As drug testing becomes more common in the work environment, it is gaining greater acceptance by employees, who see testing as a step to improving safety and productivity.

What do you think?

*What do you believe are the moral and ethical issues surrounding drug testing? * Are you in favor of drug testing? * Should all employees be subjected to drug tests or just those in high-risk jobs? * Is it the employer's right to conduct drug testing at the worksite? Explain your answer.*

Solutions to the Problem

For many years, the most popular antidrug strategies were total prohibition and scare tactics. Both approaches proved ineffective. Prohibition of alcohol during the 1920s created more problems than it solved, as did prohibition of opiates in 1914. Outlawing other illicit drugs has neither eliminated them nor curtailed their traffic across U.S. borders.

In general, researchers in the field of drug education agree that a multimodal approach is best. Students should be taught the difference between drug use and abuse. Factual information that is free of scare tactics must be presented; lecturing and moralizing do not work. Emphasis should be placed on things that are important to young people. Telling adolescent males that girls will find them disgusting if their breath stinks of cigarettes or pot will get their attention. Likewise, lecturing on the negative effects of drug use is a much less effective deterrent than teaching young people how to negotiate the social scene. Drug Abuse Resistance Education, commonly called DARE, is one program intended to educate students, but it has been largely ineffective. Education efforts need to focus on achieving better outcomes for preventing drug use.

We must study at-risk groups so we can better understand the circumstances that make them susceptible to drug use. Time, money, and effort by educators, parents, and policy makers are needed to ensure that today's youth receive the love and security essential for building productive and meaningful lives.

Among the strategies suggested for combating drug abuse are stricter border surveillance to reduce drug trafficking, longer prison sentences for drug pushers, increased government spending on preventing and enforcing antidrug laws, and greater cooperation between government agencies and the private sector. All of these approaches will help up to a point, but neither alone nor in combination do they offer a total solution. Drug abuse has been a part of human behavior for thousands of years, and it is not likely to disappear in the near future. Therefore, it is necessary to educate ourselves and to develop the self-discipline necessary to avoid dangerous drug dependence.

What do you think?

*Do you feel the public has a social responsibility to fight drug abuse? * What is the cost society pays for drug use? * Have you personally known someone who has suffered because of addiction to drugs? * How did you respond?*

Make It Happen!

Assessment: The Assess Yourself box on page 182 describes signs of being controlled by drugs or by a drug user. Depending on your results, you may need to take steps toward changing certain behaviors that may be detrimental to your health.

Making a Change: In order to change your behavior, you need to develop a plan. Follow these steps.

1. Evaluate your behavior and identify patterns and specific things you are doing. What can you change now? What can you change in the near future?
2. Select one pattern of behavior that you want to change.
3. Fill out a Behavior Change Contract. It should include your long-term goal for change, your short-term goals, the rewards you'll give yourself for reaching these goals, potential obstacles along the way, and

strategies for overcoming these obstacles. For each goal, list the small steps and specific actions that you will take.
4. Chart your progress in a journal. At the end of a week, consider how successful you were in following your plan. What helped you be successful? What made change more difficult? What will you do differently next week?
5. Revise your plan as needed. Are the short-term goals attainable? Are the rewards satisfying?

Example: Tranh was surprised to find he had several yes answers to the self-assessment section about being controlled by a drug user. He realized that his girlfriend Kim's drug use was hurting their relationship and negatively affecting his well-being. Kim smoked marijuana almost every day and took club drugs at least twice a month. Tranh often had to lie to Kim's employer if she was too incapacitated to go to work. Recently, she had been

in a car accident after smoking pot for several hours, which damaged Tranh's car and increased his insurance rate. And he worried whenever she went out for an evening that she was taking Ecstasy and would find herself in a compromising situation.

These worries, financial consequences, and pressure to lie all made Tranh resolve to take steps to make a change in his responses to Kim's behavior. His first step was to plan what he wanted to say to Kim about her drug use and how it affected both of them. He also started investigating drug counseling resources at school and in the community, both for Kim and for himself to help him cope with the issues raised by Kim's drug use. Finally, he began talking to Kim's friends who, it turned out, also were concerned by her behavior. They worked together to develop strategies to help Kim and provide alternatives to her drug use; Tranh also felt less alone and more supported as soon as he started reaching out to his peers.

Summary

※ The six categories of drugs are prescription drugs, over-the-counter (OTC) drugs, recreational drugs, herbal preparations, illicit drugs, and commercial preparations. Routes of administration include oral ingestion, injection (intravenous, intramuscular, and subcutaneous), inhalation, inunction, and suppositories.

※ Prescription drugs are administered under medical supervision. There are dozens of categories, including antibiotics, sedatives, tranquilizers, and antidepressants. Generic drugs often can be substituted for more expensive brand-name products.

※ OTC drug categories include analgesics; cold, cough, allergy, and asthma relievers; stimulants; sleeping aids and relaxants; and dieting aids. Exercise personal responsibility by reading directions for OTC drugs and asking your pharmacist or doctor if any special precautions are advised when taking these substances.

※ Addiction is the continued involvement with a substance or activity despite ongoing negative consequences.

※ People from all walks of life use illicit drugs, although college students report higher usage rates than does the general population. Drug use has declined since the mid-1980s.

※ Controlled substances include cocaine and its derivatives, amphetamines, newer-generation stimulants, marijuana, opiates, hallucinogens, designer drugs, inhalants, and steroids. Users tend to become addicted quickly to such drugs.

※ The drug problem reaches everyone through crime and elevated health care costs. Drugs are a major problem in the workplace; workplace drug testing is one proposed solution to this problem.

Questions for Discussion and Reflection

1. What is the current theory that explains how drugs work in the body? Explain how this theory works.
2. Explain the terms *synergism, antagonism,* and *inhibition.*
3. What are the advantages and disadvantages associated with use of generic drugs?
4. Do you think there is such a thing as responsible use of illicit drugs? Would you change any of the current laws governing drugs? How would you determine what is legitimate use and illegitimate use?
5. Why do you think many people today feel that marijuana use is not dangerous? What are the arguments in favor of legalizing marijuana? What are the arguments against legalization? How common is the use of marijuana on your campus?
6. How do you and your peers feel about illicit drug use? Has your opinion changed in recent years? If so, how and why?
7. Debate the issue of workplace drug testing. Would you apply for a job that had drug testing as an interview requirement? As a continuing requirement?
8. What could you do to help a friend who is fighting a substance abuse problem? What resources on your campus could help you?
9. What types of programs do you think would be effective in preventing drug abuse among high school and college students? How would programs for high school students differ from those for college students?
10. Discuss how addiction affects family and friends. What role do family and friends play in helping the addict get help and maintain recovery?

Accessing Your Health on the Internet

Visit the following Internet sites to explore further topics and issues related to personal health. To visit an organization's website, go to the Companion Website for *Health: The Basics, Sixth Edition* at www.aw-bc.com/donatelle, click on the book image, and select "Accessing Your Health on the Internet" from the navigation menu on the left.

1. *Club Drugs.* A website that disseminates science-based information about club drugs.
2. *Food and Drug Administration (FDA).* The federal agency responsible for approving prescription and over-the-counter drugs, with information on product approvals, recalls, and more.
3. *Join Together.* An excellent site for the most current information related to substance abuse. Also includes information on gun violence and provides advice on organizing and taking political action.
4. *National Institute on Drug Abuse (NIDA).* The home page of this U.S. government agency has information on the latest statistics and findings in drug research.
5. *Substance Abuse and Mental Health Services Administration (SAMHSA).* Outstanding resource for information about national surveys, ongoing research, and national drug interventions.

Further Reading

Elster, J., ed. *Addiction: Entries and Exits.* New York: Russell Sage Foundation, 2000.

> Addresses current addiction controversies from an international perspective, with authors from the United States and Norway. Topics include whether addicts have a choice in their behavior and current addiction theories.

Goldstein, Avram. *Addiction: From Biology to Drug Policy.* New York: Oxford University Press, 2001.

> Discusses how drugs impact the brain, how each drug causes addiction, and how addictive drugs impact society. The author explains what we know about drug addiction, how we know what we know, and what we can and cannot do about the drug problem.

Greenburg, S. *2003 Physician's Desk Reference for Nonprescription Drugs and Dietary Supplements.* Montvale, NJ: Thomson Medical Economics, 2003.

> Outlines proper uses, possible dangers, and effective ingredients of nonprescription medications.

Griffith, W. H., and S. Moore. *Complete Guide to Prescription and Nonprescription Drugs 2003.* New York: Perigee, 2002.

> This essential guide answers every conceivable question about prescription and nonprescription drugs and contains information about dosages, side effects, precautions, interactions, and more. More than 5,000 brand-name and 800 generic drugs are profiled in an easy-to-use format.

West, J. W. *The Betty Ford Center Book of Answers: Help for Those Struggling with Substance Abuse and the People Who Love Them.* New York: Pocket Books, 1997.

> Written by the former director of the Betty Ford Center, one of the leading alcohol and drug treatment centers in the United States. Provides answers to the most frequently asked questions about treatment and recovery; includes comprehensive coverage of drug abuse issues for addicts and their families.

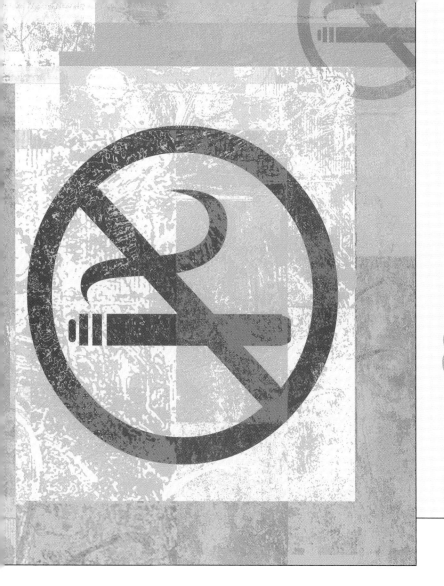

Alcohol, Tobacco, and Caffeine

Daily Pleasures, Daily Challenges

8 8 8 8 8 8

Objectives

* Discuss the alcohol use patterns of college students and overall trends in consumption.

* Explain the physiological and behavioral effects of alcohol, including blood alcohol concentration, absorption, metabolism, and immediate and long-term effects of alcohol consumption.

* Explain the symptoms and causes of alcoholism, its cost to society, and its effects on the family.

* Explain the treatment of alcoholism, including the family's role, varied treatment methods, and whether alcoholics can be cured.

* Discuss the social and political issues involved in tobacco use.

* Discuss how the chemicals in tobacco products affect a smoker's body.

* Review the health effects of smoking and smokeless tobacco.

* Evaluate the risks that environmental tobacco smoke may pose to nonsmokers.

* Summarize the benefits, risks, and long-term health consequences associated with caffeine use.

A Smoke-Free England? Expert Says It's Essential

By Warren Hoge

LONDON Smoking should be banned in all public places to reduce the threat of illness caused by secondhand inhalation, England's chief medical officer, Sir Liam Donaldson, said today.

Sir Liam called on the government to legislate a wide-ranging prohibition that would cover restaurants, shopping centers, clubs and the country's famously smoky pubs.

One in four adults in England smokes, though many workplaces have banned the practice. Smokers standing on balconies, outside doorways or on the fire escape stairways of downtown office buildings have become a common sight.

Sir Liam's report said an estimated three million people are exposed to secondhand smoke at work. He warned that smoke was a direct threat to the health of nonsmokers who are exposed to it; people who live with smokers have up to a 30 percent higher risk of developing cancer and a 25 percent higher risk of heart disease.

Sir Liam noted that smoking kills 120,000 people each year across Britain, and he cited a British Medical Association estimate that at least 1,000 people a year die as a result of exposure to other people's smoke.

Read the complete article online in the eThemes section of this book's website: www.aw-bc.com/donatelle.

Usually the word *drug* conjures up images of people abusing illegal substances. We use the term to describe dangerous chemicals such as heroin or cocaine without recognizing that socially accepted substances can be drugs, too—for example, alcohol, tobacco, and caffeine.

Alcohol: An Overview

Moderate use of alcohol can enhance celebrations and special times. Research shows that very low levels of use may actually decrease some health risks. However, always remember that alcohol is a chemical substance that affects your physical and mental behavior.

An estimated 65 percent of Americans consume alcoholic beverages regularly, though consumption patterns are unevenly distributed throughout the drinking population. Ten percent are heavy drinkers, and they account for half of all the alcohol consumed. The remaining 90 percent of the drinking population are infrequent, light, or moderate drinkers.

Alcohol and College Students

Alcohol is the most widely used (and abused) recreational drug in our society. It is also the most popular drug on college campuses, where approximately 84 percent of students consume alcoholic beverages.[1] About one-third of college students are classified as heavy drinkers, meaning that they consume large amounts of alcohol per drinking occasion. Therefore, students who might drink only once a week are considered heavy drinkers if they consume a great deal of alcohol. In a new trend on college campuses, women's consumption of alcohol is close to equaling men's. Exactly how much does a typical college student consume? Colleges and universities have been described as among the "alcohol-drenched institutions" (see the Reality Check box). Every year, America's 12 million undergraduates drink 4 billion cans of beer, which averages 55 six-packs per person, and spend $446 per person on alcoholic beverages—more than they spend on soft drinks and textbooks combined.[2]

Despite these figures, fewer students are drinking alcohol than in the past. In 1980, 9.5 percent of students nationwide said they abstained from alcohol; in 2001, 19 percent were abstainers.[3] According to the University of Michigan's Institute for Social Research, the percentage of students who report drinking daily also has declined, from 6.5 percent in 1980 to 5 percent in 2002.[4]

College is a critical time to become aware of and responsible for drinking. There is little doubt that drinking is a part of campus culture and tradition. Students are away from home, often for the first time, and many are excited by their newfound independence. For some students, this independence and the rite of passage into the college culture are symbolized by the use of alcohol. It provides the answer to one of the most commonly heard statements on any college campus: "There is nothing to do." Additionally, many students say they drink to have fun. Having fun, which often means drinking simply to get drunk, may really be a way of coping with stress, boredom, anxiety, or pressures created by academic and social demands.

The Facts about College Students and Drinking

Perhaps you've heard conflicting reports in the media about the prevalence and effects of drinking on campus. What are the real facts? The following statistics reveal the scope of the problem.

- Alcohol kills more people below age 21 than cocaine, marijuana, and heroin combined.
- One night of heavy drinking can impair the ability to think abstractly for up to 30 days. This limits a student's ability to relate textbook reading to a professor's lecture or to think through a football play.
- College administrators estimate that alcohol is involved in 29% of dropouts, 38% of academic failures, 64% of violent behaviors, and 6% of unsafe sexual practices.
- All-women colleges saw a 135% increase in frequent binge drinking between 1993 and 2001.
- An estimated 259,000 students think that wine coolers or beer cannot get a person drunk.
- There has been a threefold increase since 1993 in the number of college women who reported having been drunk on ten or more occasions in the previous month.
- The National Bureau of Economic Research found that areas of a college campus offering cheap beer prices had more violent and nonviolent crime, including trouble between students and police or other campus authorities, arguments, physical fighting, property damage, false fire alarms, and sexual misconduct.
- Alcohol is involved in more than two-thirds of the suicides among college students, one-third of all emotional and academic problems, 90% of campus rapes and sexual assaults, and 95% of violent crime on campus.
- Close to 40% of students surveyed reported binge drinking in high school.
- Women who drink heavily are 40% more likely to experience unwanted sexual advances than are those who drink less.
- In cases of acquaintance rape, 75% of male students and 55% of female students had been drinking or using drugs at the time.
- College binge drinking occurs more frequently among male students, students who reside on campus, intercollegiate athletes, and members of fraternities and sororities.
- Approximately 40% of fraternity and sorority members report being frequent binge drinkers.
- College students under the age of 21 are more prone to binge drinking and pay less for their alcohol than their older classmates do, according to researchers at the Harvard University School of Public Health.
- Though underage students are likely to drink less often, they consume more per occasion than students age 21 and older who are allowed to drink legally.
- College students who have serious alcohol problems and engage in dangerous behaviors are more likely than other students to have guns with them at school.

Sources: Data were compiled from the numerous studies cited throughout this chapter and from: Center for Science in the Public Interest, "Booze News" (2002). http://cspi.net.org/booze; L. D. Johnston, P. M. O'Malley, and J. G. Bachman, *Monitoring the Future National Survey Results on Drug Use 1975–2002 Volume II: College Students and Adults Ages 19–40,* NIH Publication No. 03-5376 (Bethesda, MD: National Institute on Drug Abuse, 2003); H. Wechsler et al., "College Binge Drinking in the 1990s: A Continuing Problem," *Journal of American College Health* 48 (2000); A. Cohen, "Battle of the Binge," *Time,* September 8, 1997.

Statistics about college students' drinking may not always reflect actual consumption. Students consistently report that their friends drink much more than they do and that average drinking within their own social living group is higher than actual self-reports. Such misinformation may promote or be used to excuse excessive drinking practices. In a survey of students at a large Midwestern university, 42 percent reported not having a hangover in the past six months. Yet, that same group of surveyed students believed that only 3 percent of their peers had not had a hangover in the past month.

Many colleges are working to change misperceptions of normal drinking behavior. An example of such a social norms campaign is Oregon State University's "Just the Facts" program, which publicizes the fact that the majority of the university's students are responsible and moderate drinkers. Students are often surprised to learn that 87 percent of their peers have never driven a car while under the influence of alcohol, and almost 90 percent have never performed poorly on a test or important project due to their alcohol use. Almost 75 percent have zero to four drinks per week, and 60 percent consumed four or fewer drinks the last time they went to a party. Clearly there are many students who use alcohol responsibly and in moderation.

Binge Drinking and College Students

Binge drinking is defined as five drinks in a row by men and four in a row by women on a single occasion. The stakes

---

Binge drinking Drinking for the express purpose of becoming intoxicated; five drinks in a single sitting for men and four drinks in a sitting for women.

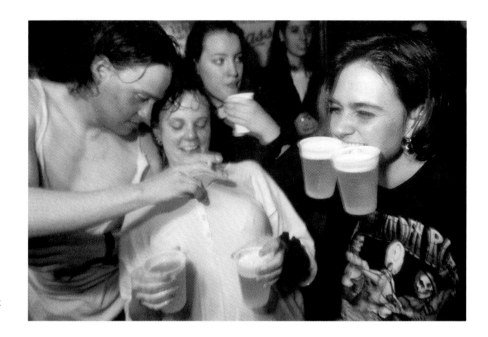

Deciding when to drink, and how much, is no small matter. Irresponsible consumption of alcohol can easily result in disaster.

of binge drinking are high because of the increased risk for alcohol-related injuries or death. An estimated 50 students die annually from alcohol poisoning.

A 2001 study by the Harvard School of Public Health found that almost 45 percent of students were binge drinkers. Of those, 22.8 percent were frequent bingers—people who binge drink three times or more in a two-week period[5] (see Table 8.1). Compared with nonbingers, frequent binge drinkers are 16 times more likely to miss class, 8 times more likely to get behind in their school work, and more apt to get into trouble with campus or local police.[6]

Although everyone is at some risk for alcohol-related problems, college students seem to be particularly vulnerable for the following reasons.

- Alcohol exacerbates their already high risk for suicide, automobile crashes, and falls.
- Many university customs and traditions encourage dangerous practices of alcohol use.
- University campuses are heavily targeted by advertising and promotions from the alcoholic beverage industry.
- It is more common for college students than for their noncollegiate peers to drink recklessly and to engage in drinking games and other dangerous drinking practices.
- College students are particularly vulnerable to peer influence and have a strong need to be accepted by their peers.
- There is institutional denial by college administrators that alcohol problems exist on their campuses.

A recent study shows that 6 percent of college students meet the criteria for a diagnosis of alcohol dependence (also

referred to as alcoholism), and 31 percent meet the criteria for alcohol abuse. Students who attend colleges with heavy drinking environments are more likely to be diagnosed with abuse or dependence. Those students at most risk are the frequent bingers; male students are generally at greater risk than are females. Despite the prevalence of alcohol disorders on campus, very few students seek treatment.[7]

To prevent alcohol abuse, many colleges and universities are instituting strong policies against drinking. University presidents have formed a leadership group to help curb the problem of alcohol abuse. Many fraternities have elected to have dry houses. At the same time, colleges and universities are making more help available to students with drinking problems. Today, both individual counseling and group counseling are offered on most campuses, and more attention is being directed toward preventing alcohol abuse. Student organizations such as BACCHUS (Boost Alcohol Consciousness Concerning the Health of University Students) promote responsible drinking and party hosting.

What do you think?

Why do college students drink excessive amounts of alcohol? ✳ *Are there particular traditions or norms related to when and why students drink on your campus?* ✳ *Have you ever had your sleep or studies interrupted because of drinking?* ✳ *Have you had to baby-sit a friend because of his or her drinking? Did you say anything about it to your friend? How did the person respond?*

Table 8.1
College Students' Patterns of Alcohol Use, 2001

Category	Total (%)	Men (%)	Women (%)
Abstainer (past year)	19.3	20.1	18.7
Non-binge drinker	36.3	31.3	40.4
Occasional binge drinker	21.6	23.4	20.0
Frequent binge drinker	22.8	25.2	20.9

Source: H. Wechsler et al., "Trends in College Binge Drinking during a Period of Increased Prevention Efforts: Findings from Four Harvard School of Public Health College Study Surveys: 1993–2001," *Journal of American College Health* 50, no. 5 (2002): 207. Reprinted with permission of Helen Dwight Reid Educational Foundation.

Physiological and Behavioral Effects of Alcohol

The Chemical Makeup of Alcohol

The intoxicating substance found in beer, wine, liquor, and liqueurs is **ethyl alcohol,** or **ethanol.** It is produced during a process called **fermentation** in which yeast organisms break down plant sugars, yielding ethanol and carbon dioxide. Fermentation continues until the solution of plant sugars (called mash) reaches a concentration of 14 percent alcohol. At this point, the alcohol kills the yeast and halts the chemical reactions that produce it.

For beers and ales, which are fermented from malt barley, the process stops when the alcohol concentration is 14 percent. Manufacturers then add other ingredients that dilute the alcohol content of the beverage. Other alcoholic beverages are produced through further processing called **distillation,** during which alcohol vapors are released from the mash at high temperatures. The vapors are then condensed and mixed with water to make the final product.

The **proof** of an alcoholic drink is a measure of the percentage of alcohol in the beverage. The term *proof* comes from the term *gunpowder proof,* a reference to the gunpowder test in which potential buyers would test the distiller's product by pouring it on gunpowder and attempting to light it. If the alcohol content was at least 50 percent, the gunpowder would burn; otherwise the water in the product would put out the flame. Thus, alcohol percentage is 50 percent of the given proof. For example, 80 proof whiskey or scotch is 40 percent alcohol by volume, and 100 proof vodka is 50 percent alcohol by volume. The proof of a beverage indicates its strength. Lower-proof drinks will produce fewer alcohol effects than the same amount of higher-proof drinks will produce.

Most wines are between 12 and 15 percent alcohol, and ales are between 6 and 8 percent. The alcoholic content of beers is between 2 and 6 percent, which varies according to state laws and type of beer.

Behavioral Effects

Blood alcohol concentration (BAC) is the ratio of alcohol to total blood volume. It is the factor used to measure the physiological and behavioral effects of alcohol. Despite individual differences, alcohol produces some general behavioral effects, depending on BAC (see Table 8.2 on page 204). At a BAC of 0.02, a person feels slightly relaxed and in a good mood. At 0.05, relaxation increases, there is some motor impairment, and a willingness to talk becomes apparent. At 0.08, the person feels euphoric and experiences further motor impairment. At 0.10, the depressant effects of alcohol become apparent, drowsiness sets in, and motor skills are further impaired, followed by a loss of judgment. Thus, a driver may not be able to estimate distances or speed, and some drinkers lose their ability to make value-related decisions and may do things they would not do when sober. As BAC increases, the drinker suffers increased physiological and psychological effects. All these changes are negative. Alcohol ingestion does not enhance any physical skills or mental functions.

People can acquire physical and psychological tolerance to the effects of alcohol through regular use. The nervous system adapts over time, so greater amounts of alcohol are required to produce the same physiological and psychological effects. Some people can learn to modify their behavior so that they appear to be sober even when their BAC is quite high. This ability is called **learned behavioral tolerance.**

Absorption and Metabolism

Unlike the molecules found in most foods and drugs, alcohol molecules are sufficiently small and fat-soluble to be absorbed throughout the entire gastrointestinal system. A negligible amount of alcohol is absorbed through the lining of the mouth. Approximately 20 percent of ingested alcohol

---

Ethyl alcohol (ethanol) An addictive drug produced by fermentation and found in many beverages.

Fermentation The process whereby yeast organisms break down plant sugars to yield ethanol and carbon dioxide.

Distillation The process whereby mash is subjected to high temperatures to release alcohol vapors, which are then condensed and mixed with water to make the final product.

Proof A measure of the percentage of alcohol in a beverage.

Blood alcohol concentration (BAC) The ratio of alcohol to total blood volume; the factor used to measure the physiological and behavioral effects of alcohol.

Learned behavioral tolerance The ability of heavy drinkers to modify behavior so that they appear to be sober even when they have high BAC levels.

Table 8.2
Psychological and Physical Effects of Various Blood-Alcohol Concentration Levels*

Number of Drinks†	Blood Alcohol Concentration (%)	Psychological and Physical Effects
1	0.02–0.03	No overt effects, slight mood elevation
2	0.05–0.06	Feeling of relaxation, warmth; slight decrease in reaction time and in fine-muscle coordination
3	0.08–0.09	Balance, speech, vision, and hearing slightly impaired; feelings of euphoria, increased confidence; loss of motor coordination
	0.10	Legal intoxication in most states; some have lower limits
4	0.11–0.12	Coordination and balance becoming difficult; distinct impairment of mental faculties, judgment
5	0.14–0.15	Major impairment of mental and physical control; slurred speech, blurred vision, lack of motor skills
7	0.20	Loss of motor control—must have assistance in moving about; mental confusion
10	0.30	Severe intoxication; minimal conscious control of mind and body
14	0.40	Unconsciousness, threshold of coma
17	0.50	Deep coma
20	0.60	Death from respiratory failure

*For each hour elapsed since the last drink, subtract 0.015 percent blood alcohol concentration, or approximately one drink.
†One drink = one beer (4 percent alcohol, 12 ounces), one highball (1 ounce whiskey), or one glass table wine (5 ounces).
Source: Modified from data given in Ohio State Police Driver Information Seminars and the National Clearinghouse for Alcohol and Alcoholism Information, Rockville, MD.

diffuses through the stomach lining into the bloodstream, and nearly 80 percent passes through the linings of the upper third of the small intestine. Absorption into the bloodstream is rapid and complete.

Several factors influence how quickly your body will absorb alcohol: the alcohol concentration in your drink, the amount of alcohol you consume, the amount of food in your stomach, pylorospasm (spasm of the pyloric valve in the digestive system), and your mood. The higher the concentration of alcohol in your drink, the more rapidly it will be absorbed in your digestive tract. As a rule, wine and beer are absorbed more slowly than distilled beverages. Carbonated alcoholic beverages, such as champagne and sparkling wines, are absorbed more rapidly than those containing no sparkling additives, or fizz. Carbonated beverages and drinks served with mixers cause the pyloric valve—the opening from the stomach into the small intestine—to relax, thereby emptying the contents of the stomach more rapidly into the small intestine. Because the small intestine is the site of the greatest absorption of alcohol, carbonated beverages increase the rate of absorption. In contrast, if your stomach is full, absorption slows because the surface area exposed to alcohol is smaller. A full stomach also retards the emptying of alcoholic beverages into the small intestine.

In addition, the more alcohol you consume, the longer absorption takes. Alcohol can irritate the digestive system, which causes a spasm in the pyloric valve (pylorospasm).

When the pyloric valve is closed, nothing can move from the stomach to the upper third of the small intestine, which slows absorption. If the irritation continues, it can cause vomiting.

Mood is another factor, because emotions affect how long it takes for the contents of the stomach to empty into the intestine. Powerful moods, such as stress and tension, are likely to cause the stomach to dump its contents into the small intestine. That is why alcohol is absorbed much more rapidly when people are tense than when they are relaxed.

Alcohol is metabolized in the liver, where it is converted by the enzyme alcohol dehydrogenase to acetaldehyde. It is then rapidly oxidized to acetate, converted to carbon dioxide and water, and eventually excreted from the body. Acetaldehyde is a toxic chemical that can cause immediate symptoms, such as nausea and vomiting, as well as long-term effects, such as liver damage. A very small portion of alcohol is excreted unchanged by the kidneys, lungs, and skin.

Like food, alcohol contains calories. Proteins and carbohydrates (starches and sugars) each contain 4 kilocalories (kcal) per gram. Fat contains 9 kcal per gram. Alcohol, although similar in structure to carbohydrates, contains 7 kcal per gram. The body uses the calories in alcohol in the same manner it uses those found in carbohydrates: for immediate energy or for storage as fat if not immediately needed.

When compared to the variable breakdown rates of foods and other beverages, the breakdown of alcohol occurs at a fairly constant rate of 0.5 ounce per hour. This amount of alcohol is equivalent to 12 ounces of 5 percent beer, 5 ounces of 12 percent wine, or 1.5 ounces of 40 percent (80 proof) liquor. Legal limits of BAC for operating motor vehicles vary from state to state. Most states set the legal limit at 0.08 to 0.10 percent. A driver whose BAC exceeds the state's legal limit is considered legally intoxicated.

A drinker's BAC depends on weight and body fat, the water content in body tissues, the concentration of alcohol in the beverage consumed, the rate of consumption, and the volume of alcohol consumed. Heavier people have larger body surfaces through which to diffuse alcohol; therefore, they have lower concentrations of alcohol in their blood than do thin people after drinking the same amount. Because alcohol does not diffuse as rapidly into body fat as into water, alcohol concentration is higher in a person with more body fat. Because a woman is likely to have more body fat and less water in her body tissues than a man of the same weight, she will be more intoxicated than a man will be after drinking the same amount of alcohol.

Alcohol Poisoning   Alcohol poisoning occurs much more frequently than people realize, and all too often it can be fatal. Drinking large amounts of alcohol in a short period of time can cause the blood alcohol level to reach the lethal range relatively quickly. Alcohol, either used alone or in combination with other drugs, is probably responsible for more toxic overdose deaths than any other substance.

Death from alcohol poisoning can be caused by either central nervous system (CNS) and respiratory depression or the inhalation of vomit or fluid into the lungs. The amount of alcohol it takes for a person to become unconscious is dangerously close to the lethal dose. Signs of alcohol poisoning include inability to be roused; a weak, rapid pulse; an unusual or irregular breathing pattern; and cool (possibly damp), pale, or bluish skin. If you are with someone who has been drinking heavily and who exhibits these conditions, or if you are unsure about the person's condition, call 911 for emergency help right away.

Women and Alcohol   Body fat is not the only contributor to the differences in alcohol's effects on men and women. Compared to men, women have half as much alcohol hydrogenase, the enzyme that breaks down alcohol in the stomach before it has a chance to reach the bloodstream and the brain. Therefore, if a man and a woman drink the same amount of alcohol, the woman's BAC will be approximately 30 percent higher than the man's BAC, leaving her more vulnerable to slurred speech, careless driving, and other drinking-related impairments.

> **What do you think?**
> *Have you noticed that some types of alcoholic beverages affect people more quickly than others?* * *What factors affect BAC levels?* * *Are these factors different for men and women? If so, how?*

Breathalyzer and Other Tests   The Breathalyzer tests used by law enforcement officers determine BAC based on the amount of alcohol exhaled in the breath. Urinalysis also can yield a BAC based on the concentration of unmetabolized alcohol in the urine. Both breath analysis and urinalysis are used to determine whether a driver is legally intoxicated, but blood tests are more accurate measures. An increasing number of states are requiring blood tests for people suspected of driving under the influence of alcohol. In some states, refusal to take the breath or urine test results in immediate revocation of the person's driver's license.

Immediate Effects

The most dramatic effects produced by ethanol occur within the CNS. The primary action of the drug is to reduce the frequency of nerve transmissions and impulses at synaptic junctions. This depresses CNS functions, which results in decreased respiratory rate, pulse rate, and blood pressure. As CNS depression deepens, vital functions become noticeably depressed. In extreme cases, coma and death can result.

Alcohol is a diuretic that causes increased urinary output. Although this effect might be expected to lead to automatic **dehydration** (loss of water), the body actually retains water, most of it in the muscles or in the cerebral tissues. The reason is that water is usually pulled out of the **cerebrospinal fluid** (fluid within the brain and spinal cord), leading to what is known as mitochondrial dehydration at the cellular level within the nervous system. Mitochondria are miniature organs within cells that are responsible for specific functions, and they rely heavily upon fluid balance. When mitochondrial dehydration occurs from drinking, the mitochondria cannot carry out their normal functions. This results in symptoms that include the "morning-after" headaches some drinkers suffer.

Alcohol irritates the gastrointestinal system and may cause indigestion and heartburn if taken on an empty stomach. Long-term use of alcohol causes repeated irritation that has been linked to cancers of the esophagus and stomach. In addition, people who engage in brief drinking sprees during which they consume unusually high amounts of alcohol put themselves at risk for irregular heartbeat or even total loss of heart rhythm, which can disrupt blood flow and damage the heart muscle.

A **hangover** is often experienced the morning after a drinking spree. The symptoms of a hangover are familiar to

> **Dehydration**   Loss of water from body tissues.
> **Cerebrospinal fluid**   Fluid within and surrounding the brain and spinal cord tissues.
> **Hangover**   The physiological reaction to excessive drinking, including symptoms such as headache, muscle aches, upset stomach, anxiety, depression, diarrhea, and thirst.

Table 8.3
Drugs and Alcohol: Actions and Interactions

Drug Class/Trade Name(s)	Effects with Alcohol
Antialcohol: Antabuse	Severe reactions to even small amounts; headache, nausea, blurred vision, convulsions, coma, possible death.
Antibiotics: Penicillin, Cyantin	Reduced therapeutic effectiveness.
Antidepressants: Elavil, Sinequan, Tofranil,	Increased central nervous system (CNS) depression, blood pressure changes.
Nardil, Prozac, Zoloft	Combined use of alcohol and MAO inhibitors, SSRIs, specific types of antidepressant can trigger massive increases in blood pressure, even brain hemorrhage and death.
Antihistamines: Allerest, Dristan	Drowsiness and CNS depression. Driving ability impaired.
Aspirin: Anacin, Excedrin, Bayer	Irritates stomach lining. May cause gastrointestinal pain, bleeding.
Depressants: Valium, Ativan, Placidyl	Dangerous CNS depression, loss of coordination, coma. High risk of overdose and death.
Narcotics: heroin, codeine, Darvon	Serious CNS depression. Possible respiratory arrest and death.
Stimulants: caffeine, cocaine	Masks depressant action of alcohol. May increase blood pressure, physical tension.

Source: Reprinted by permission from *Drugs and Alcohol: Simple Facts about Alcohol and Drug Combinations* (Phoenix: DIN Publications, 1988), no. 121.

most people who drink: headache, muscle aches, upset stomach, anxiety, depression, diarrhea, and thirst. **Congeners** are thought to play a role in the development of a hangover. Congeners are forms of alcohol that are metabolized more slowly than ethanol and are more toxic. The body metabolizes the congeners after the ethanol is gone from the system, and their toxic by-products may contribute to the hangover. In addition, alcohol upsets the water balance in the body, which results in excess urination and thirst the next day. Increased production of hydrochloric acid can irritate the stomach lining and cause nausea. It usually takes 12 hours to recover from a hangover. Bed rest, solid food, and aspirin may help relieve its discomforts, but unfortunately, nothing cures it but time.

When you use any drug (and alcohol is a drug), you need to be aware of its possible interactions with any other drugs, whether prescription or over-the-counter. Table 8.3 summarizes possible interactions. Note that alcohol may cause a negative interaction even with aspirin.

Long-Term Effects

Alcohol is distributed throughout most of the body and may affect many organs and tissues. Problems associated with long-term, habitual use of alcohol include diseases of the nervous system, cardiovascular system, and liver, as well as some cancers.

Congeners   Forms of alcohol that are metabolized more slowly than ethanol and produce toxic by-products.

Effects on the Nervous System   The nervous system is especially sensitive to alcohol. Even people who drink moderately experience shrinkage in brain size and weight and a loss of some degree of intellectual ability. The damage that results from alcohol use is localized primarily in the left side of the brain, which is responsible for written and spoken language, logic, and mathematical skills. The degree of shrinkage appears to be directly related to the amount of alcohol consumed. In terms of memory loss, the evidence suggests that having one drink every day is better than saving up for a binge and consuming seven or eight drinks in a night. The amount of alcohol consumed at one time is critical. Alcohol-related brain damage can be partially reversed with good nutrition and staying sober.

Cardiovascular Effects   Alcohol affects the cardiovascular system in a number of ways. Numerous studies have associated light to moderate alcohol consumption (no more than two drinks a day) with a reduced risk of coronary artery disease. Several mechanisms have been proposed to explain how this might happen. The strongest evidence favors an increase in high-density lipoprotein (HDL) cholesterol, which is known as the "good" cholesterol. Studies have shown that drinkers have higher levels of HDL. Another factor that might help is an *antithrombotic* effect. Alcohol consumption is associated with a decrease in clotting factors that contribute to the development of atherosclerosis.

However, this does not mean that alcohol consumption is recommended as a preventive measure against heart disease—it causes many more cardiovascular health hazards than benefits. Alcohol contributes to high blood pressure and slightly increased heart rate and cardiac output. Those who report drinking three to five drinks a day, regardless of race or sex, have higher blood pressure than those who drink less.

Liver Disease   One of the most common diseases related to alcohol abuse is **cirrhosis** of the liver. It is among the top ten causes of death in the United States. One result of heavy drinking is that the liver begins to store fat—a condition known as fatty liver. If there is insufficient time between drinking episodes, this fat cannot be transported to storage sites, and the fat-filled liver cells stop functioning. Continued drinking can cause a further stage of liver deterioration called fibrosis, in which the damaged area of the liver develops fibrous scar tissue. Cell function can be partially restored at this stage with proper nutrition and abstinence from alcohol. If the person continues to drink, however, cirrhosis results. At this point, the liver cells die, and the damage becomes permanent.

Alcoholic hepatitis is a serious condition resulting from prolonged use of alcohol. A chronic inflammation of the liver develops, which may be fatal in itself or progress to cirrhosis.

Cancer   The repeated irritation caused by long-term use of alcohol has been linked to cancers of the esophagus, stomach, mouth, tongue, and liver. Research has also shown a link between breast cancer and moderate levels of alcohol consumption in women. One compelling report has demonstrated that "drinkers of three or more glasses of alcoholic beverages per day appear to be at greater risk for breast cancer."[8]

Other Effects   An irritant to the gastrointestinal system, alcohol may cause indigestion and heartburn if ingested on an empty stomach. It also damages the mucous membranes and can cause inflammation of the esophagus, chronic stomach irritation, problems with intestinal absorption, and chronic diarrhea.

Alcohol abuse is a major cause of chronic inflammation of the pancreas, the organ that produces digestive enzymes and insulin. Chronic abuse of alcohol inhibits enzyme production, which further inhibits the absorption of nutrients. Drinking alcohol can block the absorption of calcium, a nutrient that strengthens bones. This should be of particular concern to women because as they age, their risk for osteoporosis (bone thinning and calcium loss) increases. Heavy consumption of alcohol worsens this condition.

Evidence also suggests that alcohol impairs the body's ability to recognize and fight foreign bodies such as bacteria and viruses. The relationship between alcohol and acquired immune deficiency syndrome (AIDS) is unclear, especially since some of the populations at risk for AIDS are also at risk for alcohol abuse. But any stressor like alcohol, with a known effect on the immune system, would probably contribute to the development of the disease.

Alcohol and Pregnancy

Of the 30 known **teratogens** in the environment, alcohol is one of the most dangerous and common. Alcohol can harm fetal development.

More than 10 percent of all children have been exposed to high levels of alcohol in utero. All will suffer varying degrees of effects, ranging from mild learning disabilities to major physical, mental, and intellectual impairment. It takes very little alcohol to cause serious damage. Research has shown that even a single exposure to high levels of alcohol can cause significant brain damage in the infant.[9] A disorder called **fetal alcohol syndrome (FAS)** is associated with alcohol consumption during pregnancy. Alcohol consumed during the first trimester poses the greatest threat to organ development; exposure during the last trimester, when the brain is developing rapidly, is most likely to affect CNS development. FAS is the third most common birth defect and the second leading cause of mental retardation in the United States. The incidence of FAS is estimated to be 1 to 2 of every 1,000 live births. It is the most common preventable cause of mental impairment in the Western world.

FAS occurs when alcohol ingested by the mother passes through the placenta into the infant's bloodstream. Because the fetus is so small, its BAC will be much higher than that of the mother. Among the symptoms of FAS are mental retardation; small head; tremors; and abnormalities of the face, limbs, heart, and brain.

Children with a history of prenatal alcohol exposure but with fewer than the full physical or behavioral symptoms of FAS may be categorized as having **fetal alcohol effects (FAE)**. FAE is estimated to occur three to four times as

---

Cirrhosis   The last stage of liver disease associated with chronic heavy use of alcohol during which liver cells die and damage becomes permanent.

Alcoholic hepatitis   Condition resulting from prolonged use of alcohol in which the liver is inflamed. It can result in death.

Teratogens   Certain chemicals, some therapeutic and illicit drugs, radiation, and intrauterine viral infections that cause fetal malformations.

Fetal alcohol syndrome (FAS)   A disorder that may affect the fetus when the mother consumes alcohol during pregnancy. Among its effects are mental retardation; small head; tremors; and abnormalities of the face, limbs, heart, and brain.

Fetal alcohol effects (FAE)   A syndrome describing children with a history of prenatal alcohol exposure but without all the physical or behavioral symptoms of FAS. Among its symptoms are low birth weight, irritability, and possible permanent mental impairment.

often as FAS, although it is much less recognized. The signs of FAE in newborns are low birth weight and irritability, and there may be permanent mental impairment. Infants whose mothers habitually consumed more than 3 ounces of alcohol (approximately six drinks) in a short time period when pregnant are at high risk for FAE. Risk levels for babies whose mothers consume smaller amounts are uncertain.

Alcohol also can be passed to a nursing baby through breast milk. For this reason, most doctors advise nursing mothers not to drink for at least four hours before nursing their babies and preferably to abstain altogether.

> **What do you think?**
>
> *Why do we hear so little about FAS in this country when it is the third most common birth defect and second leading cause of mental retardation?*
> *✳ Is this a reflection of our society's denial of alcohol as a dangerous drug?*

Drinking and Driving

The leading cause of death for all age groups from 5 to 45 years (including college students) is traffic accidents. Approximately 41 percent of all traffic fatalities in 2002 were alcohol related.[10] Unfortunately, college students are over-represented in alcohol-related crashes. The College Alcohol Study findings indicated that 20 percent of non-binge drinkers, 43 percent of occasional bingers, and 59 percent of frequent bingers reported driving while intoxicated.[11] Furthermore, it is estimated that three out of every ten Americans will be involved in an alcohol-related accident at some time in their lives.[12] Studies show that those involved in car crashes who had been drinking have a 40 to 50 percent higher chance of dying than do nondrinkers involved in car crashes.

In 2002, there were 17,419 alcohol-related traffic fatalities (ARTFs), a 5 percent reduction from the ARTF data reported in 1982. This number represents an average of one alcohol-related fatality every 30 minutes.[13] The highest intoxication rates in fatal crashes in 2002 were recorded for drivers ages 21 to 24 (33 percent), followed by ages 25 to 34 (28 percent) and 35 to 44 (26 percent). In the most current data reported, approximately 1.4 million drivers were arrested in 2001 for driving under the influence of alcohol or drugs. This is an arrest rate of 1 for every 137 licensed drivers in the United States.[14]

Several factors probably contributed to these reductions in ARTFs: laws that raised the drinking age to 21; stricter law enforcement; increased emphasis on zero tolerance (laws prohibiting those under 21 from driving with *any* detectable BAC); and educational programs designed to discourage drinking and driving. Most states have set 0.10 percent as the

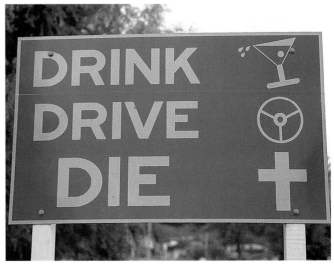

All too often, drinking and driving can be a deadly combination. Approximately 40 percent of U.S. traffic fatalities are alcohol related.

BAC at which drivers are considered to be legally drunk (refer to Table 8.2). However, several states have lowered the standard to 0.08 percent, and others are likely to follow.

Laboratory and test track research shows that the vast majority of drivers, even experienced drinkers, are impaired at a BAC of 0.08 percent with regard to critical driving tasks. Braking, steering, lane changing, judgment, and divided attention, among other measures, are all affected significantly at 0.08 BAC. National groups such as MADD (Mothers Against Drunk Driving), started by a mother whose child was killed by a drunk driver, go as far as tracking drunk driving cases through the court systems to ensure that drunk drivers are punished. Members of the high school group SADD (Students Against Drunk Driving) educate their peers about the dangers of drinking and driving.

Despite all these measures, the risk of being involved in an alcohol-related automobile crash remains substantial. Researchers have shown a direct relationship between the amount of alcohol in a driver's bloodstream and the likelihood of a crash. A driver with a BAC level of 0.10 percent is approximately ten times more likely to be involved in a car accident than a driver who has not been drinking. At a BAC of 0.15 on weekend nights, the likelihood of dying in a single-vehicle crash is more than 380 times higher than for nondrinkers. Alcohol involvement is highest during nighttime (9:00 P.M. to 6:00 A.M.) single-vehicle crashes. In these crashes in 2002, 52 percent of fatally injured drivers had BACs at or over 0.08 percent. Only 27 percent of fatally injured drivers involved in nighttime single-vehicle crashes had no alcohol in their blood.[15]

Not only does the time of day increase the risk of being involved in an alcohol-related crash, but it also makes a difference whether it is a weekday or weekend. In 2002, 31 percent of all fatal crashes during the week were alcohol-related, compared with 54 percent on weekends.[16]

What do you think?

What do you think the legal BAC for drivers should be? ✳ *Why do you think that many states have not lowered the legal limit to 0.08?* ✳ *What should the penalty be for people arrested for driving under the influence of alcohol (DUI) for the first offense? The second offense? The third offense?*

Alcohol Abuse and Alcoholism

Alcohol use becomes **alcohol abuse** when it interferes with work, school, or social and family relationships, or when it entails any violation of the law, including driving under the influence (DUI). **Alcoholism** results when personal and health problems related to alcohol use are severe, and stopping alcohol use results in withdrawal symptoms. Some 6 million Americans can be described as alcoholics.

Identifying a Problem Drinker

As in other drug addictions, tolerance, psychological dependence, and withdrawal symptoms must be present to qualify a drinker as an addict. Addiction results from chronic use over a period of time that varies from person to person. Irresponsible or problem drinkers, such as people who get into fights or embarrass themselves or others when they drink, are not necessarily alcoholics. The stereotype of the alcoholic on skid row applies to only 5 percent of the alcoholic population. The remaining 95 percent live in some type of extended family unit. Alcoholics can be found at all socioeconomic levels and in all professions, ethnic groups, geographical locations, religions, and races.

Studies suggest that the lifetime risk of alcoholism in the United States is about 10 percent for men and 3 percent for women. Moreover, almost 25 percent of the American population (50 million people) is affected by the alcoholism of a friend or family member. The 2001 National Household Survey on Drug Abuse found that 5.7 percent of Americans were heavy drinkers, and 20.7 percent were binge drinkers.

Recognizing and admitting the existence of an alcohol problem can be difficult. Alcoholics themselves deny their problem, often making statements such as, "I can stop any time I want to. I just don't want to right now." Their families also tend to deny the existence of a problem, saying things such as, "He really has been under a lot of stress lately. Besides, he only drinks beer." The fear of being labeled a "problem drinker" often prevents people from seeking help.

Women are the fastest-growing population of alcohol abusers. They tend to become alcoholic at a later age and after fewer years of heavy drinking than do male alcoholics. Women at highest risk for alcohol-related problems are those who are unmarried but living with a partner, in their 20s or early 30s, or have a husband or partner who drinks heavily.

The Causes of Alcohol Abuse and Alcoholism

We know that alcoholism is a disease with biological and social/environmental components. But we do not know what role each component plays in the disease.

Biological and Family Factors Research into the hereditary and environmental causes of alcoholism has found higher rates of alcoholism among family members of alcoholics. In fact, alcoholism is four to five times more common among children of alcoholics than in the general population.

Male alcoholics are more likely than nonalcoholics to have alcoholic parents and siblings. Two distinct subtypes of alcoholism provide important information about the inheritance of alcoholism. *Type 1 alcoholics* are drinkers who had at least one parent of either sex who was a problem drinker and who grew up in an environment that encouraged heavy drinking. Their drinking is reinforced by environmental events during which there is heavy drinking. Type 1 alcohol abusers share certain personality characteristics. They avoid novelty and harmful situations and are concerned about the thoughts and feelings of others. *Type 2 alcoholism* is seen in males only. These alcoholics are typically the biological sons of alcoholic fathers who have a history of both violence and drug use. Type 2 alcoholics display the opposite characteristics of Type 1 alcoholics. They do not seek social approval, they lack inhibition, and they are prone to novelty-seeking behavior.[17]

One study found a strong relationship between alcoholism and alcoholic patterns within the family.[18] Children with one alcoholic parent had a 52 percent chance of becoming alcoholics themselves. With two alcoholic parents, the chances of becoming alcoholic jumped to 71 percent.

Social and Cultural Factors Although a family history of alcoholism may predispose a person to problems, numerous other factors may mitigate or exacerbate that tendency. Social and cultural factors may trigger the affliction for many people who are not genetically predisposed to alcoholism.

> **Alcohol abuse** Use of alcohol that interferes with work, school, or personal relationships or that entails violations of the law.
>
> **Alcoholism** Condition when personal and health problems related to alcohol use are severe, and stopping alcohol use results in withdrawal symptoms

Alcohol Abuse and Alcoholism: Common Questions

Although many people think that they have a clear understanding of the disease alcoholism, there is much that remains in question. Answering the following questions will indicate your own level of knowledge about the disease. For further information, particularly as it relates to alcohol use on college campuses, check out the National Institute of Alcohol Abuse and Alcoholism (www.niaaa.nih.gov).

1. Alcoholism is a disease characterized by what four symptoms?
   a.
   b.
   c.
   d.

2. Is alcoholism an inherited trait?   Yes   Probably   No
3. Do you have to be an alcoholic to experience alcohol-related problems?   Yes   No
4. What groups of individuals tend to have the most problems with alcoholism?

ANSWERS

1. The four symptoms of alcoholism include:
   a. Craving (a strong need or urge to drink alcohol)
   b. Loss of control (not being able to stop drinking once drinking begins)
   c. Physical dependence (withdrawal symptoms, such as nausea, sweating, shakiness, and anxiety after stopping drinking)
   d. Tolerance: (the need to drink greater amounts of alcohol to get high) (See also the *Diagnostic Statistical Manual IV* published by the American Psychological Association for more information.)

2. Probably yes. The risk for developing alcoholism does indeed run in families. While part of this may be explained by genetics, lifestyle is a major factor. Currently, researchers are trying to locate the actual genes that put you at risk. Your friends, the amount of stress in your life, and the ready availability alcohol are also factors that increase risk. Remember that risk is not destiny. A child of an alcoholic won't automatically become an alcoholic. Others develop alcoholism even though no one in their family is an alcoholic. If you know you are at risk, you can take steps to protect yourself.

3. No. Alcoholism is only one type of alcohol problem. Alcohol abuse can be just as harmful. A person can abuse alcohol without being an alcoholic—that is, he or she may drink too much, too often and still not be dependent on alcohol. Some of the problems of alcohol abuse include not being able to meet work, school, or family responsibilities; drunk driving arrests and car crashes; and drinking-related medical conditions. Under some circumstances, even social or moderate drinking is dangerous—for example, when driving, during pregnancy, or when taking certain medications.

4. Alcohol abuse and alcoholism cut across gender, race, and nationality. Nearly one in three adults abuse alcohol in the United States today. In general, more men than women are alcohol dependent or have alcohol problems. Alcohol problems are highest among young adults, ages 18–29, and lowest among adults ages 65 and older. We also know that the younger you start, the more likely that you will have a problem.

Source: National Institute on Alcohol Abuse and Alcoholism, "College Drinking: FAQs on Alcohol Abuse and Alcoholism," 2002. www.collegedrinkingprevention.gov/facts/faq.aspx.

Some people begin drinking as a way to dull the pain of an acute loss or an emotional or social problem. For example, college students may drink to escape the stress of college life; disappointment over unfulfilled expectations; difficulties in forming relationships; or loss of the security of home, loved ones, and close friends. Involvement in a painful relationship, death of a family member, and other problems may trigger a search for an anesthetic. Unfortunately, the emotional discomfort that causes many people to turn to alcohol also ultimately causes them to become even more uncomfortable as the depressant effect of the drug begins to take its toll. Thus, the person who is already depressed may become even more depressed, antagonizing friends and other social supports. Eventually, the drinker becomes physically dependent on the drug.

Family attitudes toward alcohol also seem to influence whether a person will develop a drinking problem. It has been clearly demonstrated that people who are raised in cultures in which drinking is a part of religious or ceremonial activities or in which alcohol is a traditional part of the family meal are less prone to alcohol dependence. In contrast, in societies in which alcohol purchase is carefully controlled and drinking is regarded as a rite of passage to adulthood, the tendency for abuse appears to be greater.

Certain social factors have been linked with alcoholism as well. These include urbanization, increased mobility, the weakening of links to the extended family and a general loosening of kinship ties, and changing religious and philosophical values. Apparently, then, some combination of heredity and environment plays a decisive role in the development of alcoholism. Some ethnic and racial groups also have special alcohol abuse problems.

> **What do you think?**
> *How was alcohol used in your family when you were growing up?* ✳ *Was alcohol used only on special occasions or not at all?* ✳ *How much do you think your family's attitudes and behaviors toward alcohol have shaped your behavior?*

Effects of Alcoholism on the Family

Only recently have people begun to recognize that it is not only the alcoholic that suffers, but also the alcoholic's entire family. Although most research focuses on family effects during the late stages of alcoholism, the family unit actually begins to react early on as the person starts to show symptoms of the disease.

An estimated 76 million Americans (about 43 percent of the U.S. adult population) have been exposed to alcoholism in the family.[19] Twenty-two million members of alcoholic families are age 18 or older, and many have carried childhood emotional scars into adulthood. Approximately one in four children under age 18 lives in an atmosphere of anxiety, tension, confusion, and denial.[20]

In dysfunctional families, children learn certain rules from a very early age: don't talk, don't trust, and don't feel. These unspoken rules allow the family to avoid dealing with real problems and real issues. Family members unconsciously adapt to the alcoholic by adjusting their own behavior. Unfortunately, these behaviors actually help keep the alcoholic drinking. Children in such dysfunctional families generally assume at least one of the following roles.

- *Family hero.* Tries to divert attention from the problem by being too good to be true.
- *Scapegoat.* Draws attention away from the family's primary problem through delinquency or misbehavior.
- *Lost child.* Becomes passive and quietly withdraws from upsetting situations.
- *Mascot.* Disrupts tense situations by providing comic relief.

For children in alcoholic homes, life is a struggle. They have to deal with constant stress, anxiety, and embarrassment.

Because the alcoholic is the center of attention, the children's wants and needs often are ignored. It is not uncommon for these children to be victims of violence, abuse, neglect, or incest. As we have seen, when such children grow up, they are much more prone to alcoholic behaviors themselves than are children from nonalcoholic families.

In the past decade, we have come to recognize the unique problems of adult children of alcoholics whose difficulties in life stem from a lack of parental nurturing during childhood. Among these problems are difficulty in developing social attachments, a need to be in control of all emotions and situations, low self-esteem, and depression. Fortunately, not all individuals who have grown up in alcoholic families are doomed to lifelong problems. As many of these people mature, they develop a resilience in response to their families' problems. They thus enter adulthood armed with positive strengths and valuable career-oriented skills, such as the ability to assume responsibility, strong organizational skills, and realistic expectations of their jobs and others.

Costs to Society

The entire society suffers the consequences of individuals' alcohol abuse. Close to half of all traffic fatalities are attributable to alcohol. According to the National Institute on Alcohol Abuse and Alcoholism, in 1998, alcohol-related costs to society were at least $184.6 billion, after factoring in health insurance, criminal justice, treatment costs, and lost productivity. Reportedly, alcoholism is directly and indirectly responsible for more than 25 percent of the nation's medical expenses and lost earnings. More than 50 percent of all child abuse cases are the result of alcohol-related problems. Finally, the costs in emotional health are impossible to measure.[21]

Women and Alcoholism

In the past, women have consumed less alcohol and have had fewer alcohol-related problems than have men. But now, greater percentages of women, especially college-age women, are choosing to drink and are drinking more heavily.

Studies indicate that there are now almost as many female as male alcoholics. Risk factors for drinking problems among *all women* include:

- A family history of drinking problems
- Pressure to drink from a peer or spouse
- Depression
- Stress

Risk factors among *young women* include:

- College attendance: Women in college drink more, and more frequently, than they do after they graduate
- Nontraditional, low-status, and part-time jobs; unemployment
- Being single, divorced, or separated

Risk factors among *middle-aged women* include:

- Loss of social roles (e.g., through divorce, children growing up and leaving the home)
- Abuse of prescription drugs
- Heavy drinking by spouse
- Presence of other disorders, such as depression

Risk factors among *older women* include:

- Heavy- or problem-drinking spouse
- Retirement, with a loss of social networks centered on the workplace

Drinking patterns among *different age groups* also differ in these ways.

- Younger women drink more overall, drink more often, and experience more alcohol-related problems, such as drinking and driving, assaults, suicide attempts, and difficulties at work.
- Middle-aged women are more likely to develop drinking problems in response to a traumatic or life-changing event, such as divorce, surgery, or death of a significant other.
- Older women are more likely than are older men to have developed drinking problems within the past ten years.[22]

It is estimated that only 14 percent of women who need treatment get it. In one study, women cite potential loss of income, not wanting others to know they may have a problem, inability to pay for treatment, and fear that treatment would not be confidential as reasons for not seeking treatment.[23] Another major obstacle is child care. Most residential treatment centers do not allow women to bring their children with them.

> ### What do you think?
> *Why do women appear to be drinking more heavily today than they did in the past?* ✳ *Does society look at men's and women's drinking habits in the same way?* ✳ *Can you think of ways to increase support for women in their recovery process?*

Recovery

Most problem drinkers who seek help have experienced a turning point: a spouse walks out, taking children and

---

Intervention   A planned confrontation with an alcoholic in which family members and friends plus professional counselors express their concern about the alcoholic's drinking.

Delirium tremens (DTs)   A state of confusion brought on by withdrawal from alcohol. Symptoms include hallucinations, anxiety, and trembling.

---

possessions; the boss issues an ultimatum to dry out or ship out. Devoid of hope, physically depleted, and spiritually despairing, the alcoholic finally recognizes that alcohol controls his or her life. The first steps on the road to recovery are to regain that control and to assume responsibility for personal actions.

The Family's Role

Members of an alcoholic's family sometimes take action before the alcoholic does. They may go to an organization or a treatment facility to seek help for themselves and their relative. An effective method of helping an alcoholic to confront the disease is a process called **intervention.** Essentially, an intervention is a planned confrontation with the alcoholic that involves several family members and friends plus professional counselors. Family members express their love and concern, telling the alcoholic that they will no longer refrain from acknowledging the problem and affirming their support for appropriate treatment. A family intervention is the turning point for a growing number of alcoholics.

Treatment Programs

The alcoholic who is ready for help has several avenues of treatment: psychologists and psychiatrists specializing in the treatment of alcoholism, private treatment centers, hospitals specifically designed to treat alcoholics, community mental health facilities, and support groups such as Alcoholics Anonymous.

Private Treatment Facilities   Private treatment facilities have been making concerted efforts to attract patients through advertising. On admission to the treatment facility, the patient receives a complete physical exam to determine whether underlying medical problems will interfere with treatment. Alcoholics who decide to quit drinking will experience withdrawal symptoms, such as:

- Hyperexcitability
- Confusion
- Sleep disorders
- Convulsions
- Agitation
- Tremors of the hands
- Brief hallucinations
- Depression
- Headache
- Seizures

For a small percentage of people, alcohol withdrawal results in a severe syndrome known as **delirium tremens (DTs).** The DT syndrome is characterized by confusion, delusions, agitated behavior, and hallucinations.

For any long-term addict, medical supervision is usually necessary. *Detoxification,* the process by which addicts end their dependence on a drug, is commonly carried out in a medical facility, where patients can be monitored to prevent fatal reactions. Withdrawal takes 7 to 21 days. Shortly after detoxification, alcoholics begin their treatment for psychological addiction. Most treatment facilities keep their patients three to six weeks. Treatment at private treatment centers costs several thousand dollars, but some insurance programs or employers will assume most of this expense.

Family Therapy, Individual Therapy, and Group Therapy

In family therapy, the person and family members gradually examine the psychological reasons underlying the addiction. In individual and group therapy with fellow addicts, alcoholics learn positive coping skills for situations that have regularly caused them to turn to alcohol. On some college campuses, the problems associated with alcohol abuse are so great that student health centers are opening their own treatment programs.

Other Types of Treatment

Two other treatments are drug and aversion therapy. Disulfiram (trade name: Antabuse) is the drug of choice for treating alcoholics. If alcohol is consumed, the drug causes unpleasant effects—headache, nausea, vomiting, drowsiness, and hangover—that discourage the alcoholic from drinking. Aversion therapy, based on conditioning therapy, works on the premise that the sight, smell, and taste of alcohol will acquire aversive properties if repeatedly paired with a noxious stimulus. For ten days, the alcoholic takes drugs that induce vomiting when combined with several drinks. These treatments work best in conjunction with some type of counseling.

Alcoholics Anonymous (AA) is a private, nonprofit, self-help organization founded in 1935. The organization, which relies upon group support to help people stop drinking, currently has more than 1 million members and branches all over the world. At meetings, last names are never used, and no one is forced to speak. Members are taught to believe that their alcoholism is a lifetime problem and they may never use alcohol again. They share their struggles with each other and talk about the devastating effects alcoholism has had on their personal and professional lives. All members are asked to place their faith and control of the habit into the hands of a "higher power." The road to recovery is taken one step at a time. AA offers specialized meetings for gays, atheists, people who have the human immunodeficiency virus (HIV), and a variety of other people with alcohol problems.

Alcoholics Anonymous also has auxiliary groups to help spouses or partners, friends, and children of alcoholics. *Al-Anon* is the group dedicated to helping adult relatives and friends of alcoholics understand the disease and how they can contribute to the recovery process. Spouses and other adult loved ones often play an unwitting role in perpetuating the alcoholic's problems. For example, they may call the alcoholic's boss and lie about why the alcoholic missed work. At Al-Anon, these people examine their roles in their loved one's alcoholism and explore alternative behaviors.

Alateen, another AA-related organization, helps adolescents live with alcoholic parents. They learn that they are not at fault for their parents' problems. They develop their self-esteem to overcome guilt and function better socially.

Other self-help groups include Women for Sobriety and Secular Organizations for Sobriety (SOS). Women for Sobriety addresses the differing needs of female alcoholics, who often have more severe problems than do males. Unlike AA meetings, where attendance can be quite large, each group has no more than ten members. SOS was founded to help people who are uncomfortable with AA's spiritual emphasis.

Relapse

Success in recovery from alcoholism varies with the individual. A return to alcoholic habits often follows what appears to be a successful recovery. Some alcoholics never recover. Some partially recover and improve other parts of their lives but remain dependent on alcohol. Many alcoholics refer to themselves as "recovering" throughout their lifetime; they never use the word *cured*.

Roughly 60 percent of alcoholics relapse (resume drinking) within the first three months of treatment. Why is the relapse rate so high? Treating an addiction requires more than getting the addict to stop using a substance; it also requires getting the person to break a pattern of behavior that has dominated his or her life.

People who are seeking to regain a healthy lifestyle must not only confront their addiction, but also must guard against the tendency to relapse. Drinkers with compulsive personalities need to learn to understand themselves and take control. Others need to view treatment as a long-term process that takes a lot of effort beyond attending a weekly self-help group meeting. In order to work, a recovery program must offer the alcoholic ways to increase self-esteem and resume personal growth. Alcoholics most likely to recover completely are those who developed their dependence after age 20, those with intact and supportive families, and those who have reached a high level of personal disgust coupled with strong motivation to recover.

Our Smoking Society

Tobacco use is the single most preventable cause of death in the United States.[24] Every year more than 440,000 Americans die of tobacco-related diseases (Figure 8.1).[25] This is 50 times as many as will die from all illegal drugs combined.

> **Alcoholics Anonymous (AA)** An organization whose goal is to help alcoholics stop drinking; includes auxiliary branches such as Al-Anon and Alateen.

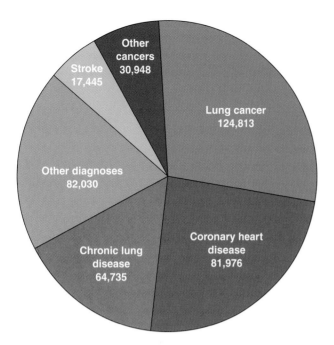

Figure 8.1

Annual Deaths Attributable to Smoking in the United States

Source: Centers for Disease Control, "Annual Smoking-Attributable Mortality, Years of Potential Life Lost, and Economic Costs," *Morbidity and Mortality Weekly Report* 51, no. 14 (2002): 300–303.

In addition, 10 million will suffer from diseases caused by tobacco. To date, tobacco is known to be the probable cause of about 25 diseases, and one in every five deaths in the United States is smoking related. About half of all regular smokers die of smoking-related diseases.

In 1991, the Youth Risk Assessment Survey, which includes only middle school and high school students, indicated that 27.5 percent of teenagers smoke; by 2001, 28.5 percent were current smokers. The most recent survey of adolescent smokers has shown a downward trend from the earlier survey. Currently, the percentage of teenage males and females who smoke is equal at approximately 28.5 percent.[26] The number of teenagers who become daily smokers before the age of 18 is estimated to be more than 3,000 per day. Every day another 6,000 teens under the age of 18 smoke their first cigarette. The increase in cigarette use is attributed in part to the ready availability of tobacco products through vending machines and the aggressive drive by tobacco companies to entice young people to smoke.

Tobacco and Social Issues

The production and distribution of tobacco products in the United States and abroad involve many political and economic issues. Tobacco-growing states derive substantial income from tobacco production, and federal, state, and local governments benefit enormously from cigarette taxes. More recently, nationwide health awareness has led to a decrease in the use of tobacco products among U.S. adults.

Advertising The tobacco industry spends $18 million per day on advertising and promotional materials. With the number of smokers declining by about 1 million each year, the industry must actively recruit new smokers. Campaigns are directed at all age, social, and ethnic groups. But because children and teenagers constitute 90 percent of all new smokers, much of the advertising has been directed toward them. Evidence of product recognition with underage smokers is clear: 86 percent of underage smokers prefer one of the three most heavily advertised brands—Marlboro, Newport, or Camel.

Advertisements in women's magazines imply that smoking is the key to financial success, independence, and social acceptance. Many brands also have thin spokeswomen pushing "slim" and "light" cigarettes to cash in on women's fear of gaining weight. These ads have apparently been working. From the mid-1970s through the early 2000s, cigarette sales to women increased dramatically. Not coincidentally, by 1987 cigarette-induced lung cancer had surpassed breast cancer as the leading cancer killer among women.

Women are not the only targets of gender-based cigarette advertisements. Males are depicted changing clothes in a locker room, charging over rugged terrain in off-road vehicles, or riding bay stallions into the sunset in blatant appeals to a need to feel and appear masculine. In addition, minorities often are targeted.

Clearly, 18- to 24-year-olds have become the new target for tobacco advertisers. The tobacco industry has set up aggressive marketing promotions at bars, music festivals, and similar places where young people congregate, specifically targeted to this age group. Additionally, modeling and peer influence have an impact on smoking initiation. This potential impact is heightened by the fact that although over half of campuses are considered smoke-free, they do permit smoking in residence hall rooms, student centers, and cafeterias, and many sell tobacco products in campus stores and student lounges.

Financial Costs to Society The use of tobacco products is costly to all of us in terms of lost productivity and lost lives. Estimates show that tobacco use caused more than $150 billion in annual health-related economic losses from 1995 to 1999. Its economic burden totaled more than $75.5 billion in medical expenditures (these include hospital, physician, and nursing home costs; prescription drugs; and home health care costs) and $89.1 billion in indirect costs, such as absenteeism, added cost of fire insurance, training costs to replace employees who die prematurely, and disability payments. The economic costs of smoking are estimated to be about $3,391 per smoker per year. In effect, each pack of cigarettes sold in the U.S. costs the nation $7.18 in medical costs and lost productivity.[27]

College Students and Smoking

College students are especially vulnerable when placed in a new, often stressful social and academic environment. For

Table 8.4
What's in Cigarette Smoke?

Cigarette smoke contains more than 4,000 chemicals, including these:

Cancer-Causing Agents	Metals	Other Chemicals	
Benzo(a)pyrene	Aluminum	Acetic acid (vinegar)	Hydrogen cyanide (gas chamber poison)
B-Napthylamine	Copper	Acetone (nail polish remover)	Methane (swamp gas)
Cadmium	Gold	Ammonia (floor/toilet cleaner)	Methanol (rocket fuel)
Crysenes	Lead	Arsenic (poison)	Napthalene (mothballs)
Diberiz acidine	Magnesium	Butane (cigarette lighter fluid)	Nicotine (insecticide/addictive drug)
Nickel	Mercury	Cadmium (rechargeable batteries)	Nitrobenzene (gasoline additive)
Nitrosamines	Silicon	Carbon monoxide (car exhaust fumes)	Nitrous oxide phenols (disinfectant)
N. nitrosonornicotine	Silver	DDT/dieldrin (insecticides)	Stearic acid (candle wax)
P.A.H.'s	Titanium	Ethanol (alcohol)	Toluene (industrial solvent)
Polonium 210	Zinc	Formaldehyde (preserver of body tissue and fabric)	Vinyl chloride (makes PVC)
Toluidine			
		Hexamine (barbecue lighter)	

many, the college years are their initial taste of freedom from parental supervision. Smoking may begin earlier, but most college students are a part of the significant age group in which people initiate smoking and become hooked.

A recent study found that cigarette smoking among U.S. college students increased by 32 percent between 1991 and 1999. In 1999, researchers surveyed more than 14,000 students from 119 U.S. colleges. This poll took into account all types of tobacco use, including cigars, smokeless tobacco, and pipe smoking as well as cigarettes. Researchers found that more than 60 percent of college students had tried some tobacco product. One-third of all students had used tobacco in the month before the study, and just under half had used tobacco in the past year, although they did not consider themselves "smokers." Among current smokers, the survey found a wide range of smoking behaviors. For example, 32 percent smoked less than a cigarette a day, while 13 percent smoked a pack or more per day. Furthermore, the study found students who used tobacco products were more likely to smoke marijuana, binge drink, have multiple sex partners, earn lower grades, rate parties as more important than academic activities, and spend more time socializing with friends.[28]

A common perception is that students are not interested in smoking cessation efforts. However, a recent study reported that 70 percent of cigarette smokers had tried to quit smoking. Unfortunately, three out of four were still smokers.[29] It is important for colleges and universities to engage in antismoking efforts, strictly control tobacco advertising, provide smoke-free residence halls, and offer greater access to smoking cessation programs.

What do you think?

Have you noticed an increase in the number of your friends who have become regular smokers or occasional smokers? ✳ *How many of them smoked prior to coming to college, and how many picked up the habit at college?* ✳ *What are their reasons for smoking?* ✳ *What barriers keep your friends from quitting?*

Tobacco and Its Effects

The chemical stimulant **nicotine** is the major psychoactive substance in all tobacco products. In its natural form, nicotine is a colorless liquid that turns brown upon oxidation (exposure to oxygen). When tobacco leaves are burned in a cigarette, pipe, or cigar, nicotine is released and inhaled into the lungs. Sucking or chewing a quid (a pinch of snuff typically tucked between the gum and lower lip) of tobacco releases nicotine into the saliva, and the nicotine is then absorbed through the mucous membranes in the mouth.

Smoking is the most common form of tobacco use. Smoking delivers a strong dose of nicotine to the user, along with an additional 4,000 chemical substances (Table 8.4). Among these chemicals are various gases and vapors that carry

Nicotine The stimulant chemical in tobacco products.

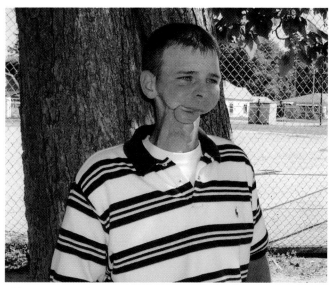

This 25-year-old cancer survivor has undergone almost 30 disfiguring surgeries. One operation removed half his neck muscles, lymph nodes, and tongue. He first tried smokeless tobacco at age 13; by age 17, he was diagnosed with squamous cell carcinoma. He now speaks out about the dangers of smokeless tobacco.

particulate matter in concentrations that are 500,000 times greater than those of the most air-polluted cities in the world.[30]

Particulate matter condenses in the lungs to form a thick, brownish sludge called **tar.** Tar contains various carcinogenic (cancer-causing) agents such as benzo(a)pyrene and chemical irritants such as phenol. Phenol has the potential to combine with other chemicals to contribute to the development of lung cancer.

In healthy lungs, millions of tiny hairlike tissues called cilia sweep away foreign matter, to be expelled from the lungs by coughing. Nicotine impairs the cleansing function of the cilia by paralyzing them for up to one hour following the smoking of a single cigarette. This allows tars and other solids in tobacco smoke to accumulate and irritate sensitive lung tissue.

Tar and nicotine are not the only harmful chemicals in cigarettes. In fact, tars account for only 8 percent of tobacco smoke. The remaining 92 percent consists of various gases, the most dangerous of which is **carbon monoxide.** In tobacco smoke, the concentration of carbon monoxide is 800 times higher than the level considered safe by the U.S. Environmental Protection Agency (EPA). In the human body, carbon monoxide reduces the oxygen-carrying capacity of the red blood cells by binding with the receptor sites for oxygen. This causes oxygen deprivation in many body tissues.

Tar   A thick, brownish substance condensed from particulate matter in smoked tobacco.

Carbon monoxide   A gas found in cigarette smoke that binds at oxygen receptor sites in the blood.

The heat from tobacco smoke, which can reach 1,616 degrees Fahrenheit, is also harmful. Inhaling hot gases exposes sensitive mucous membranes to irritating chemicals that weaken the tissues and contribute to cancers of the mouth, larynx, and throat.

Tobacco Products

Tobacco comes in several forms. Cigarettes, cigars, pipes, and bidis are used for burning and inhaling tobacco. Smokeless tobacco is inhaled or placed in the mouth.

Filtered cigarettes designed to reduce levels of gases such as hydrogen cyanide and hydrocarbons may actually deliver more hazardous carbon monoxide to the user than do nonfiltered brands. Some smokers use low-tar and low-nicotine products as an excuse to smoke more cigarettes. This practice is self-defeating because they wind up exposing themselves to more harmful substances than they would with regular-strength cigarettes.

Clove cigarettes contain about 40 percent ground cloves (a spice) and about 60 percent tobacco. Many users mistakenly believe that these products are made entirely of ground cloves and that smoking them eliminates the risks associated with tobacco. In fact, clove cigarettes contain higher levels of tar, nicotine, and carbon monoxide than do regular cigarettes. In addition, the numbing effect of eugenol, the active ingredient in cloves, allows smokers to inhale the smoke more deeply.

Cigars   Those big stogies that we see celebrities and government figures puffing on these days are nothing more than tobacco fillers wrapped in more tobacco. Since 1991, cigar sales in the United States have increased 250 percent. This growing fad is especially popular among young men and women, fueled in part by the willingness of celebrities to be photographed puffing on a cigar. Among some women, cigar smoking symbolizes an impulse to be slightly outrageous and liberated. Many people believe that cigars are safer than cigarettes, when in fact nothing could be further from the truth.[31] Cigar smoke contains 23 poisons and 43 carcinogens.

Smoking as little as one cigar per day can increase the risk of several cancers, including cancer of the oral cavity (lip, tongue, mouth, and throat), esophagus, larynx, and lungs. Daily cigar smoking, especially for people who inhale, also increases the risk of heart disease (cigar smokers double their risk of heart attack and stroke) and a type of lung disease known as chronic obstructive pulmonary disease. Smoking one or two cigars doubles the risk for oral cancers and esophageal cancer, compared with risk for someone who has never smoked. The risks increase with the number of cigars smoked per day.

A common question asked is whether cigars are addictive. Most cigars have as much nicotine as several cigarettes do, and nicotine is highly addictive. When cigar smokers inhale, nicotine is absorbed as rapidly as it is with cigarettes. For those who don't inhale, nicotine is still absorbed through the mucous membranes in the mouth.

Bidis Gaining in popularity, **bidis** are small, hand-rolled, flavored cigarettes generally made in India or Southeast Asia. They come in a variety of flavors, such as vanilla, chocolate, and cherry. Bidis resemble a marijuana joint or a clove cigarette and have become increasingly popular with college students, who view them as safer, cheaper, and easier to obtain than cigarettes. However, they are far more toxic than cigarettes. A study by the Massachusetts Department of Health found that bidis produced three times more carbon monoxide and nicotine and five times more tar than cigarettes during an identical testing process. The tendu leaf wrappers are nonporous, which means that smokers have to pull harder to inhale and inhale more to keep the bidi lit. During testing, it took an average of 28 puffs to smoke a bidi, compared to only 9 puffs for a regular cigarette. This results in much more exposure to the higher amounts of tar, nicotine, and carbon monoxide, and bidis lack any sort of filter to lower these levels. Bidi smokers are at the same, if not higher, risk for coronary heart disease and cancer due to smoking.[32]

Smokeless Tobacco Approximately 5 million U.S. adults use smokeless tobacco. Most of them are teenage (20 percent of male high school students) and young adult males, who are often emulating a professional sports figure or family member. There are two types of smokeless tobacco: chewing tobacco and snuff.

Chewing tobacco is placed between the gums and teeth for sucking or chewing. It comes in three forms: loose leaf, plug, or twist. Chewing tobacco contains tobacco leaves treated with molasses and other flavorings. The user places a quid of tobacco in the mouth between the teeth and gums and then sucks or chews the quid to release the nicotine. Once the quid becomes ineffective, the user spits it out and inserts another. **Dipping** is another method of using chewing tobacco. The dipper places a small amount of tobacco between the lower lip and teeth to stimulate the flow of saliva and release the nicotine. Dipping rapidly releases nicotine into the bloodstream.

Snuff is a finely ground form of tobacco that can be inhaled, chewed, or placed against the gums. It comes in dry or moist powdered form or sachets (tea bag–like pouches). Usually snuff is placed inside the cheek. Inhaling dry snuff is more common in Europe than in the United States.[33]

Smokeless tobacco is just as addictive as cigarettes because of its nicotine content. There is nicotine in all tobacco products, but smokeless tobacco contains even more than cigarettes. Holding an average-sized dip or chew in the mouth for 30 minutes delivers as much nicotine as smoking four cigarettes. A two-can-a-week snuff dipper gets as much nicotine as a one-and-a-half-pack-a-day smoker.

Smokeless tobacco contains 10 times the amount of cancer-producing substances found in cigarettes and 100 times more than the Food and Drug Administration (FDA) allows in foods and other substances used by the public. A major risk of chewing tobacco is leukoplakia, a condition characterized by leathery white patches inside the mouth produced by contact with irritants in tobacco juice. Between 3 and 17 percent of diagnosed leukoplakia cases develop into oral cancer.

It is estimated that 75 percent of the 28,900 oral cancer cases in 2002 resulted from either smokeless tobacco or cigarettes.[34] Users of smokeless tobacco are 50 times more likely to develop oral cancers than are nonusers. Warning signs of oral cancers include lumps in the jaw or neck; color changes or lumps inside the lips; white, smooth, or scaly patches in the mouth or on the neck, lips, or tongue; a red spot or sore on the lips or gums or inside the mouth that does not heal in two weeks; repeated bleeding in the mouth; and difficulty or abnormality in speaking or swallowing.

The lag time between first use and contracting cancer is shorter for smokeless tobacco users than for smokers because absorption through the gums is the most efficient route of nicotine administration. A growing body of evidence suggests that long-term use of smokeless tobacco also increases the risk of cancer of the larynx, esophagus, nasal cavity, pancreas, kidney, and bladder. Moreover, many smokeless tobacco users eventually "graduate" to cigarettes.

The stimulant effects of nicotine may create the same circulatory and respiratory problems for chewers as for smokers. Chronic smokeless tobacco use also results in delayed wound healing and peptic ulcer disease.

Like smoked tobacco, smokeless tobacco impairs the senses of taste and smell. This causes the user to add salt and sugar to food, which may contribute to high blood pressure and obesity. Some smokeless tobacco products contain high levels of sodium (salt), which also contributes to high blood pressure. In addition, dental problems are common among smokeless tobacco users. Contact with tobacco juice causes receding gums, tooth decay, bad breath, and discolored teeth. Damage to both the teeth and jawbone can contribute to early loss of teeth. Users of any tobacco products may not be able to absorb the vitamins and other nutrients in food effectively. The Health in a Diverse World box on page 220 describes a new form of smokeless tobacco.

What do you think?

Should smokeless tobacco be banned in all venues that also ban smoking? ✳ *What is attractive about the use of smokeless tobacco?* ✳ *Why is it popular with athletes and males, in general?*

Bidis Hand-rolled flavored cigarettes.

Chewing tobacco A stringy type of tobacco that is placed in the mouth and then sucked or chewed.

Dipping Placing a small amount of chewing tobacco between the front lip and teeth for rapid nicotine absorption.

Snuff A powdered form of tobacco that is sniffed and absorbed through the mucous membranes in the nose or placed inside the cheek and sucked.

Physiological Effects of Nicotine

Nicotine is a powerful CNS stimulant that produces a variety of physiological effects. Its stimulant action in the cerebral cortex produces an aroused, alert mental state. Nicotine also stimulates the adrenal glands, which increases the production of adrenaline. The physical effects of nicotine stimulation include increased heart and respiratory rate, constricted blood vessels, and subsequent increased blood pressure because the heart must work harder to pump blood through the narrowed vessels.

Nicotine decreases blood sugar levels and the stomach contractions that signal hunger. These factors, along with decreased sensation in the taste buds, reduce appetite. For this reason, many smokers eat less than nonsmokers do and weigh, on average, seven pounds less than nonsmokers.

Beginning smokers usually feel the effects of nicotine with their first puff. These symptoms, called **nicotine poisoning,** include dizziness, lightheadedness, rapid and erratic pulse, clammy skin, nausea, vomiting, and diarrhea. The effects of nicotine poisoning cease as tolerance to the chemical develops. Tolerance develops almost immediately in new users, perhaps after the second or third cigarette. In contrast, tolerance to most other drugs, such as alcohol, develops over a period of months or years. Regular smokers often do not experience the "buzz" of smoking. They continue to smoke simply because stopping is too difficult.

Health Hazards of Smoking

Cigarette smoking adversely affects the health of every person who smokes. Each day cigarettes contribute to more than 1,000 deaths from cancer, cardiovascular disease, and respiratory disorders.

Cancer

The American Cancer Society estimates that tobacco smoking causes 85 to 90 percent of all cases of lung cancer; fewer than 10 percent of cases occur among nonsmokers. Lung cancer is the leading cause of cancer deaths in the United States. There were an estimated 171,900 *new* cases of lung cancer in the United States in 2003 alone, and an estimated 157,200 Americans died of the disease in 2003.[35] Figure 8.2 illustrates how tobacco smoke damages the lungs.

Nicotine poisoning   Symptoms often experienced by beginning smokers, including dizziness, diarrhea, lightheadedness, rapid and erratic pulse, clammy skin, nausea, and vomiting.

Platelet adhesiveness   Stickiness of red blood cells associated with blood clots.

Lung cancer can take 10 to 30 years to develop, and the outlook for its victims is poor. Most lung cancer is not diagnosed until it is fairly widespread in the body; at that point, the five-year survival rate is only 13 percent. When a malignancy is diagnosed and recognized while still localized, the five-year survival rate rises to 47 percent.

If you are a smoker, your risk of developing lung cancer depends on several factors. First, the number of cigarettes you smoke per day is important. Someone who smokes two packs a day is 15 to 25 times more likely to develop lung cancer than a nonsmoker will. If you started smoking in your teens, you have a greater chance of developing lung cancer than do people who started later. If you inhale deeply when you smoke, you also increase your chances. Occupational or domestic exposure to other irritants, such as asbestos and radon, will also increase your likelihood of developing lung cancer.[36]

Tobacco is linked to other cancers as well. Cigarette smoking increases the risk of pancreatic cancer by 70 percent. Smokers can reduce those odds by 30 percent if they quit for 11 years or more.[37] Cancers of the lip, tongue, salivary glands, and esophagus are five times more likely to occur among smokers than among nonsmokers. Smokers are also more likely to develop kidney, bladder, and larynx cancers.

Cardiovascular Disease

Half of all tobacco-related deaths occur from some form of heart disease.[38] Smokers have a 70 percent higher death rate from heart disease than nonsmokers do, and heavy smokers have a 200 percent higher death rate than moderate smokers do. In fact, smoking cigarettes poses as great a risk for developing heart disease as high blood pressure and high cholesterol levels do.

Smoking contributes to heart disease by adding the equivalent of ten years of aging to the arteries.[39] One explanation is that smoking encourages atherosclerosis, the buildup of fatty deposits in the heart and major blood vessels. For unknown reasons, smoking decreases blood levels of HDLs, which help protect against heart attacks. Smoking also contributes to **platelet adhesiveness,** the sticking together of red blood cells that is associated with blood clots. The oxygen deprivation associated with smoking decreases the oxygen supply to the heart and can weaken tissues. Smoking also contributes to irregular heart rhythms, which can trigger a heart attack. Both carbon monoxide and nicotine in cigarette smoke can precipitate angina attacks (pain spasms in the chest when the heart muscle does not get the blood supply it needs).

The number of years a person has smoked does not seem to bear much relation to cardiovascular risk. If a person quits smoking, the risk of dying from a heart attack is reduced by half after only one year without smoking and declines gradually thereafter. After about 15 years without smoking, the ex-smoker's risk of cardiovascular disease is similar to that of people who have never smoked.

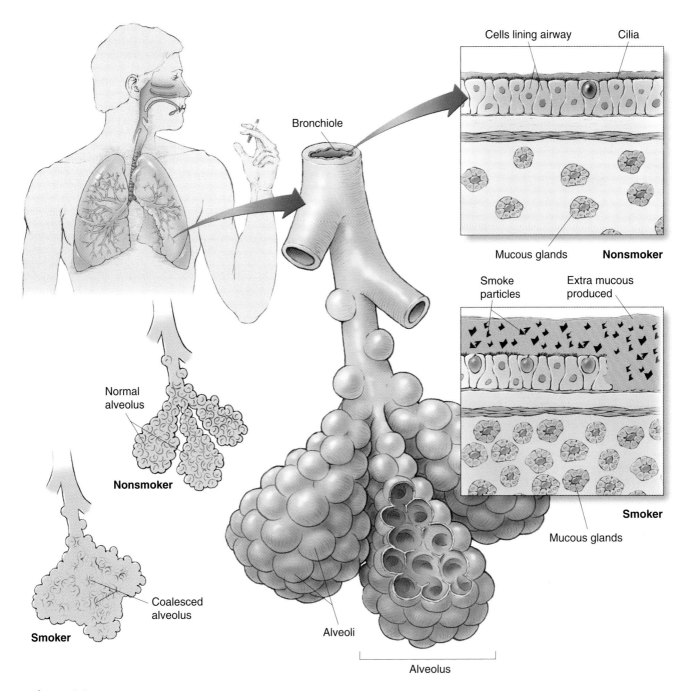

Figure 8.2

How Cigarette Smoking Damages the Lungs

Smoke particles irritate the lung pathways, which causes excess mucous production. They also indirectly destroy the walls of the lungs' alveoli, which coalesce. Both factors reduce lung efficiency. In addition, tar in tobacco smoke has a direct cancer-causing action.

Stroke Smokers are twice as likely to suffer strokes as non-smokers are. A stroke occurs when a small blood vessel in the brain bursts or is blocked by a blood clot, which denies oxygen and nourishment to vital portions of the brain. Depending on the area of the brain affected, stroke can result in paralysis, loss of mental functioning, or death. Smoking contributes to strokes by raising blood pressure, which thereby increases the stress on vessel walls. Platelet adhesiveness contributes to clotting. Five to 15 years after they stop smoking, ex-smokers face the same risk of stroke as do people who have never smoked.

A Sweet but Deadly Addiction in India

Promoted by a slick advertising campaign, *gutka,* an indigenous form of smokeless tobacco, has become a fixture in the mouths of millions of Indians over the last two decades. It has spread through the subcontinent and even to South Asians in England. But what prompts particular concern is the popularity that gutka—as portable as chewing gum and sometimes as sweet as candy—has gained during the last ten years with Indian children.

Young people have become gutka consumers in large numbers, and they have become an alarming avant-garde in what doctors say is an oral cancer epidemic. That, among other factors, has prompted the state of Maharashtra, which includes Bombay, to take an unusual step. It enacted a five-year ban, the longest permitted by law, on the production, sale, transport and possession of gutka, a $30 million business in the state. The ban started in 2002. Several other states have undertaken similar bans, although some have been stayed by the courts.

On the streets of Bombay it is easy to find young men like Raga Vendra, now 19, a railway worker who began taking gutka at age 11. It is also easy to find gutka sellers like Ahmed Maqsood who say they have had customers as young as 6.

Dr. Surendra Shastri, the head of preventive oncology at Tata Memorial Hospital, noticed about five years ago that his patients were getting younger by about eight to ten years. "High school and college students were coming in with precancerous lesions," he says. "Usage was starting much earlier."

India has 75,000 to 80,000 new cases of oral cancer a year—the world's highest incidence. About 2,000 deaths a day are tobacco related.

A 1998 survey of 1,800 boys ages 13 to 15 from a wide range of socioeconomic groups found that up to 20% were already using three to five packets of gutka daily. The price is low: sometimes less than two cents a packet. The contents, a mixture of ingredients including tobacco, are usually placed in the cheek lining, savored, then expelled.

Gutka was the product of a packaging revolution that made an Indian tradition portable and cheap. Many Indians have long chewed paan, a betel leaf wrapped around a mixture of lime paste, spices, areca nut, and often tobacco. But obtaining paan required a visit to a paanwallah— it was too messy to be transported.

All of that changed with gutka, a dried version of the concoction minus the betel leaf, preserved and perfumed with chemicals, and sealed in a plastic or foil pack. Gutka could be used at will, at work or at home or at school, and it was used in very large quantities. Sales of gutka and its tobaccoless counterpart, paan masala, are now more than $1 billion a year, having quintupled during the 1990s.

"What caused this boom of oral cancers was this packaging of tobacco," says Dr. A. K. D'Cruz, the lead head-and-neck surgeon at Tata Memorial Hospital. "Convenience got them hooked."

Many consumers say they welcome the ban, because they see no other way to curb their addiction. Even some vendors like Mr. Maqsood have embraced the ban, saying they felt they were trading in toxins. "The chemicals used in gutka were poisonous," he says. "I have seen some customers who can't open their mouth."

Doctors view gutka as particularly insidious because it is inexpensive and contains many unhealthful additives such as magnesium carbonate. For children and teenagers, smoking cigarettes remains taboo. Gutka has no social stigma among peers, and it is easy to hide from parents.

Padmini Samini, who started an antitobacco advocacy group after her father developed oral cancer, knows of gutkamakers who give free samples to children after school. Sometimes it is sweetened to mask the harsh tobacco taste, until the children consider it candy.

About 30% of the cancers in India are located in the head and neck, compared with 4.5% in the West. Furthermore, Dr. D'Cruz adds, "Most of our cancers come a decade earlier than the West." They occur in the cheek and jaw, often preceded by submucosal fibrosis, a hardening of the palate that can make it almost impossible to open the mouth.

Source: A. Waldman, "Sweet but Deadly Addiction Is Seizing the Young in India," *The New York Times,* August 13, 2002. © The New York Times Company. Reprinted with permission.

Respiratory Disorders

Smoking quickly impairs the respiratory system. Smokers can feel its impact in a relatively short period of time—they are more prone to breathlessness, chronic cough, and excess phlegm production than are nonsmokers their age. Smokers tend to miss work one-third more often than nonsmokers do, primarily because of respiratory problems, and they are up to 18 times more likely to die of lung disease.

Chronic bronchitis is the presence of a productive cough that persists or recurs frequently. It may develop in smokers because their inflamed lungs produce more mucus and constantly try to rid themselves of this mucus and foreign particles. The effort to do so results in "smoker's hack," the persistent cough most smokers experience. Smokers are more prone than are nonsmokers to respiratory ailments such as influenza, pneumonia, and colds.

Emphysema is a chronic disease in which the alveoli (the tiny air sacs in the lungs) are destroyed, which impairs the lungs' ability to obtain oxygen and remove carbon dioxide. As a result, breathing becomes difficult. Whereas healthy people expend only about 5 percent of their energy in breathing, people with advanced emphysema spend nearly 80 percent of their energy. A simple movement such as rising from a seated position becomes painful and difficult for the emphysema patient. Because the heart has to work harder to do even the simplest tasks, it may become enlarged, and the person may die from heart damage. There is no known cure for emphysema. Approximately 80 percent of all cases are related to cigarette smoking.

Sexual Dysfunction

Despite attempts by tobacco advertisers to make smoking appear sexy, research shows just the opposite: It can cause impotence in men. A number of recent studies have found that male smokers are about two times more likely than are nonsmokers to suffer from some form of impotence. Toxins in cigarette smoke damage blood vessels, which reduces blood flow to the penis and leads to an inadequate erection. It is thought that impotence could indicate oncoming cardiovascular disease.

Other Health Effects of Smoking

Gum disease is three times more common among smokers than among nonsmokers, and smokers lose significantly more teeth.[40] Smokers are also likely to use more medications. Nicotine and the other ingredients in cigarettes interfere with the metabolism of drugs. Nicotine speeds up the process by which the body uses and eliminates drugs, so that medications become less effective. The smoker may therefore have to take a larger dose of a drug or take it more frequently.

> **What do you think?**
>
> *Most people are very aware of the long-term hazards associated with tobacco use, yet despite prevention efforts, people continue to smoke.*
> ✳ *Why do you think this is so?* ✳ *What strategies might be effective at reducing the number of people who begin smoking?*

Environmental Tobacco Smoke

Although fewer than 30 percent of Americans smoke, air pollution from smoking in public places continues to be a problem. **Environmental tobacco smoke (ETS)** is divided into two categories: mainstream and sidestream smoke (also called secondhand smoke). **Mainstream smoke** refers to smoke drawn through tobacco while inhaling; **sidestream smoke** refers to smoke from the burning end of a cigarette or smoke exhaled by a smoker. People who breathe smoke from someone else's smoking product are said to be *involuntary* or *passive* smokers. Nearly nine out of ten nonsmoking Americans are exposed to environmental tobacco smoke. In fact, measurable levels of nicotine were found in the blood of 88 percent of all nontobacco users.

Risks from Environmental Tobacco Smoke

Although involuntary smokers breathe less tobacco than active smokers do, they still face risks from exposure to tobacco smoke. Sidestream smoke actually contains more carcinogenic substances than the smoke that a smoker inhales. According to the American Lung Association, sidestream smoke has about 2 times more tar and nicotine, 5 times more carbon monoxide, and 50 times more ammonia than does mainstream smoke. Every year, ETS is responsible for approximately 3,000 lung cancer deaths, 37,000 cardiovascular disease deaths, and 13,000 deaths from other cancers.[41] The EPA has designated secondhand tobacco smoke a *group A cancer-causing agent* that is even worse than other group A threats, such as benzene, arsenic, and radon. There is also evidence that sidestream smoke poses an even greater risk for death due to heart disease than for death due to lung cancer.[42]

Sidestream smoke is estimated to cause more deaths per year than does any other environmental pollutant. The risk of dying because of exposure to passive smoking is 100 times greater than the risk that requires the EPA to label a pollutant as carcinogenic and 10,000 times greater than the risk that requires the labeling of a food as carcinogenic.[43]

Lung cancer and heart disease are not the only dangers involuntary smokers face. Children's exposure to ETS increases their risk of infections of the lower respiratory tract. An estimated 300,000 children are at greater risk of pneumonia and bronchitis as a result.[44] Children exposed to sidestream smoke have a greater chance of developing other respiratory problems, such as cough, wheezing, asthma, and chest colds,

---

Emphysema   A chronic lung disease in which the tiny air sacs in the lungs are destroyed, which makes breathing difficult.

Environmental tobacco smoke (ETS)   Smoke from tobacco products, including sidestream and mainstream smoke.

Mainstream smoke   Smoke that is drawn through tobacco while inhaling.

Sidestream smoke   The cigarette, pipe, or cigar smoke nonsmokers breathe; also called secondhand smoke.

Tobacco Companies and Social Responsibility

Philip Morris is the world's largest producer and marketer of consumer packaged goods and the largest food company in the nation. It is also the world's largest and most profitable tobacco corporation. To many Americans, Philip Morris, which owns Kraft Foods, is firmly linked to the more than 400,000 people in the United States and the 3.4 million worldwide who die each year from smoking-related illnesses. This company has also led the way, in the United States and internationally, in spreading the tobacco epidemic, in particular to girls and women in regions where they traditionally have not smoked. In addition, Philip Morris and other tobacco companies have been charged with lying and deliberately deceiving the public regarding the safety of tobacco and creating and marketing a chemical addiction for profit.

However, a visit to the Philip Morris headquarters in New York paints a different picture. The company aggressively promotes its charitable work, in particular its youth smoking-prevention program. It houses the Whitney Museum exhibit of an Indian artist and sponsors the "Thurgood Marshall Scholars." Furthermore, Philip Morris employees are involved in efforts to fight hunger and combat domestic violence. The company donates $60 million a year to charity and spends another $100 million in advertising to inform the public about its good deeds. The advertising campaign is a concerted strategy to improve Philip Morris's corporate image and build credibility. In addition to the advertising campaign, the company has established a speakers' bureau in which top company executives go on the road to address PTA meetings and other groups about the company's charitable work.

Is there an ethical dilemma associated with this corporation? Does a tobacco company have an ethical obligation to society, and if so what is it? Do you think Philip Morris is attempting to do the right thing, or are these initiatives a public relations effort? Since smokers choose to start smoking, is it fair to blame Philip Morris if they develop tobacco-related health problems?

along with a decrease in lung function. The greatest effects of sidestream smoke are seen in children under the age of five. Children exposed to sidestream smoke daily in the home miss 33 percent more school days and have 10 percent more colds and acute respiratory infections than those not exposed. A recent study found that 31.2 percent of children are exposed to cigarette smoke daily in the home. This study found wide regional, income, and education differences: Children of high-income, high-education-level parents in California are exposed far less than are children of low-income, low-education-level parents in the Midwest.[45]

Cigarette, cigar, and pipe smoke in enclosed areas presents other hazards. Ten to 15 percent of nonsmokers are extremely sensitive (hypersensitive) to cigarette smoke. These people suffer itchy eyes, difficulty in breathing, painful headaches, nausea, and dizziness in response to minute amounts of smoke. The level of carbon monoxide in cigarette smoke contained in enclosed places is 4,000 times higher than the clean air standard recommended by the EPA.

Efforts to reduce the hazards associated with passive smoking have been gaining momentum in recent years. Groups such as GASP (Group Against Smokers' Pollution) and ASH (Action on Smoking and Health) have been working since the early 1970s to reduce smoking in public places. In response to their efforts, some 44 states have enacted laws restricting smoking in public places such as restaurants, theaters, and airports. The federal government has restricted smoking in all government buildings. Hotels and motels now set aside rooms for nonsmokers, and car rental agencies designate certain vehicles for nonsmokers. Since 1990, smoking has been banned on all domestic airline flights.

What do you think?

What rights, if any, should smokers have with regard to smoking in public places? ✳ *Does your campus allow smoking in residence halls?* ✳ *Does your community have nonsmoking restaurants, or does it only have nonsmoking sections?* ✳ *Do you think your community would support nonsmoking restaurants and bars? Why or why not?*

Tobacco and Politics

It has been nearly 40 years since the government began warning that tobacco use is hazardous. Today the tobacco industry is under fire—46 states have sued to recover health care costs related to treating smokers. In 1998, the tobacco industry reached a Master's Settlement Agreement with these states. Key provisions include the following.[46]

- The tobacco payments will total approximately $206 billion to be paid over 25 years nationwide.
- The industry will pay $1.5 billion over ten years to support antismoking measures, including education and advertising. An additional $250 million will fund research to determine the most effective ways to stop kids from smoking.

- The industry is barred from billboard advertising, including advertisements on transit systems. In-store ads are still permitted but will be limited in size.
- All outdoor advertising is banned, including billboards, signs, and placards larger than a poster in arenas, stadiums, shopping malls, and video arcades.
- The agreement bans youth access to free samples, proof-of-purchase gifts, and sale and distribution of "branded" merchandise, such as t-shirts, hats, and other items bearing tobacco brand names or logos.
- There is a ban on the use of cartoon characters in advertising. (Such advertising is considered particularly appealing to young children.)
- Tobacco company sponsorship of concerts, athletic events, or any event in which a significant portion of the audience consists of young people is forbidden.
- The industry agreed not to market cigarettes to children and not to misrepresent the health effects of cigarettes.

Other states and communities are advocating for stricter tobacco control. A number of states have imposed extra taxes on cigarette sales in an effort to discourage use. The monies are then used for various purposes, including prevention and cessation programs and school health programs. Two community-based programs, ASSIST (American Stop Smoking Intervention Study) and IMPACT (Initiatives to Mobilize for the Prevention and Control of Tobacco Use), are tobacco control initiatives focused on creating legislation to help prohibit the sale of tobacco to minors and assist with enforcement.

Quitting

Quitting smoking isn't easy. Smokers must break both the physical addiction to nicotine and the habit of lighting up at certain times of day.

From what we know about successful quitters, quitting is often a lengthy process involving several unsuccessful attempts before success is finally achieved. Even successful quitters suffer occasional slips, which emphasizes the fact that stopping smoking is a dynamic process that occurs over time.

Approximately one-third of all smokers attempt to quit each year. Unfortunately, 90 percent or more of those attempts fail. The person who wishes to quit smoking has several options. Most try to quit "cold turkey"—that is, they decide simply not to smoke again. Others resort to short-term quitting programs, such as those offered by the American Cancer Society, which are based on behavior modification and a system of self-rewards. Still others turn to treatment centers that are part of large franchises or part of a local medical clinic's community outreach plan. Finally, some people work privately with their physicians to reach their goal.

Prospective quitters must decide which method or combination of methods will work best for them. Programs that combine several approaches have shown the most promise. Financial considerations, personality characteristics, and level of addiction are all factors to consider.

Breaking the Nicotine Addiction

Nicotine addiction may be one of the toughest addictions to overcome. Symptoms of **nicotine withdrawal** include irritability, restlessness, nausea, vomiting, and intense cravings for tobacco.

Nicotine Replacement Products
Nontobacco products that replace depleted levels of nicotine in the bloodstream have helped some people stop using tobacco. The two most common are nicotine chewing gum and the nicotine patch, both of which are available over the counter. The FDA also has approved a nicotine nasal spray, a nicotine inhaler, and a nicotine pill.

Some patients use Nicorette, a chewing gum containing nicotine, to reduce nicotine consumption over time. Under the guidance of a physician, the user chews between 12 and 24 pieces of gum per day for up to six months. Nicorette delivers about as much nicotine as a cigarette does. But because it is absorbed through the mucous membrane of the mouth, it doesn't produce the same rush. Users experience no withdrawal symptoms and fewer cravings for nicotine as the dosage is reduced until they are completely weaned.

Some controversy surrounds the use of nicotine gum. Opponents believe that it substitutes one addiction for another. Successful users counter that it is a valid way to help break a deadly habit without suffering the unpleasant cravings that often lead to relapse.

The nicotine patch, first marketed in 1991, is generally used in conjunction with a comprehensive smoking-behavior cessation program. A small, thin, 24-hour patch placed on the smoker's upper body delivers a continuous flow of nicotine through the skin, which helps to relieve cravings. The patch is worn for 8 to 12 weeks under the guidance of a physician. The dose of nicotine is gradually reduced until the smoker is fully weaned from the drug. Occasional side effects include mild skin irritation, insomnia, dry mouth, and nervousness. The patch costs the equivalent of two packs of cigarettes a day—about $4—and some insurance plans will pay for it.

How effective is the nicotine patch? According to an analysis of 17 studies involving 5,098 people, the nicotine patch was at least twice as effective as placebo (fake) patches. At the end of treatment periods lasting at least four weeks, 27 percent of nicotine patch wearers were free of cigarettes versus 13 percent of placebo patch users. Six months later, 22 percent of the nicotine patch users were abstinent compared with only 9 percent of the placebo users. The study also showed that the patch was effective with or without intensive counseling.[47]

> **Nicotine withdrawal** Symptoms, including nausea, headaches, and irritability, suffered by smokers who cease using tobacco.

The nasal spray, which requires a prescription, is much more powerful and delivers nicotine to the bloodstream faster than gum or the patch. Patients are warned to be careful not to overdose; as little as 40 milligrams of nicotine taken at once could be lethal. The spray is somewhat unpleasant to use. The FDA has advised that it should be used for no more than three months and never for more than six months, so that smokers don't find themselves as dependent on nicotine in spray form as they were on cigarettes. The FDA also advises that no one who experiences nasal or sinus problems, allergies, or asthma should use it.

The nicotine inhaler, which also requires a prescription, consists of a mouthpiece and cartridge. By puffing on the mouthpiece, the smoker inhales air saturated with nicotine, which is absorbed through the lining of the mouth, not the lungs. This nicotine enters the body much more slowly than the nicotine in cigarettes does. Using the inhaler mimics the hand-to-mouth actions used in smoking and causes the back of the throat to feel as it would when inhaling tobacco smoke. Each cartridge lasts for 80 long puffs and is designed for 20 minutes of use.

Approved in 1997 by the FDA, Zyban, the smoking cessation pill, offers new hope to many who thought they could never quit. Zyban is thought to work on dopamine and norepinephrine receptors in the brain to decrease craving and withdrawal symptoms. Because of the way this prescription medication works, it is important to start the pills 10 to 14 days before the targeted quit date; it requires planning ahead.

Breaking the Habit

For many smokers, the road to quitting includes antismoking therapy. Among the more common techniques are aversion therapy, operant conditioning, and self-control therapy.

Aversion Therapy   Aversion techniques attempt to reduce smoking by pairing the act of smoking with a noxious stimulus so that smoking itself is perceived as unpleasant. For example, the technique of rapid smoking instructs patients to smoke rapidly and continuously until they exceed their tolerance for cigarette smoke, which produces unpleasant sensations. Short-term rates of success are high, but many patients relapse over time.

Operant Strategies   Pairing the act of smoking with an external stimulus is a typical example of this method. For example, one technique requires smokers to carry a timer that

---

Caffeine   A stimulant found in coffee, tea, chocolate, and some soft drinks.

Xanthines   The chemical family of stimulants to which caffeine belongs.

---

sounds a buzzer at different intervals. When the buzzer sounds, the patient is required to smoke a cigarette. Once the smoker is conditioned to associate the buzzer with smoking, the buzzer is eliminated, and, one hopes, so is the smoking.

Self-Control   Self-control strategies view smoking as a learned habit associated with specific situations. Therapy is aimed at identifying these situations and teaching smokers the skills necessary to resist smoking.

Benefits of Quitting

According to the American Cancer Society, many tissues damaged by smoking can repair themselves. As soon as smokers stop, the body begins the repair process (Figure 8.3). Within eight hours, carbon monoxide and oxygen levels return to normal, and "smoker's breath" disappears. Often, within a month of quitting, the mucus that clogs airways is broken up and eliminated. Circulation and the senses of taste and smell improve within weeks. Many ex-smokers say they have more energy, sleep better, and feel more alert. By the end of one year, the risk for lung cancer and stroke decreases. In addition, ex-smokers reduce considerably their risks of developing cancers of the mouth, throat, esophagus, larynx, pancreas, bladder, and cervix. They also cut their risk of peripheral artery disease, chronic obstructive lung disease, coronary heart disease, and ulcers. Women are less likely to bear babies with low birth weight. Within two years, the risk for heart attack drops to near normal. At the end of ten smoke-free years, the ex-smoker can expect to live out his or her normal life span.

What do you think?

Do you know people who have tried to quit smoking? ✴ *What was this experience like for them?* ✴ *Were they successful? If not, what factors contributed to relapse?*

Caffeine

Caffeine is the most popular and widely consumed drug in the United States. Almost half of all Americans drink coffee every day, and many others consume caffeine in some other form, mainly for its well-known "wake-up" effect. Drinking coffee is legal, even socially encouraged. Many people believe caffeine is not a drug and not really addictive. Coffee and other caffeine-containing products seem harmless; with no cream or sugar added, they are calorie-free and therefore a good way to fill up if you are dieting. If you share these attitudes, you should think again because research in the past decade has linked caffeine to certain health problems.

Caffeine is a drug derived from the chemical family called **xanthines.** Two related chemicals, *theophylline* and

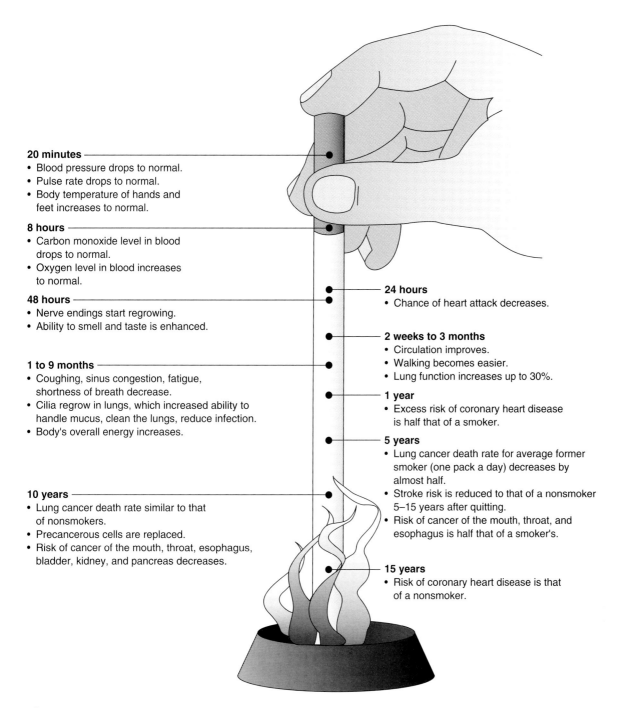

20 minutes
- Blood pressure drops to normal.
- Pulse rate drops to normal.
- Body temperature of hands and feet increases to normal.

8 hours
- Carbon monoxide level in blood drops to normal.
- Oxygen level in blood increases to normal.

48 hours
- Nerve endings start regrowing.
- Ability to smell and taste is enhanced.

1 to 9 months
- Coughing, sinus congestion, fatigue, shortness of breath decrease.
- Cilia regrow in lungs, which increased ability to handle mucus, clean the lungs, reduce infection.
- Body's overall energy increases.

10 years
- Lung cancer death rate similar to that of nonsmokers.
- Precancerous cells are replaced.
- Risk of cancer of the mouth, throat, esophagus, bladder, kidney, and pancreas decreases.

24 hours
- Chance of heart attack decreases.

2 weeks to 3 months
- Circulation improves.
- Walking becomes easier.
- Lung function increases up to 30%.

1 year
- Excess risk of coronary heart disease is half that of a smoker.

5 years
- Lung cancer death rate for average former smoker (one pack a day) decreases by almost half.
- Stroke risk is reduced to that of a nonsmoker 5–15 years after quitting.
- Risk of cancer of the mouth, throat, and esophagus is half that of a smoker's.

15 years
- Risk of coronary heart disease is that of a nonsmoker.

Figure 8.3

When Smokers Quit

Within 20 minutes of smoking that last cigarette, the body begins a series of changes that continues for years. However, by smoking just one cigarette a day, the smoker loses all these benefits, according to the American Cancer Society.

Source: G. Hanson and P. Venturelli, *Drugs and Society, 5th ed.* (Sudbury, MA: Jones and Bartlett, 1998), 320. © Jones and Bartlett, www.jbpub.com. Reprinted with permission.

Table 8.5
Caffeine Content of Various Products

Product	Caffeine Content (Average mg per Serving)
Coffee (5-oz. cup)	
Regular brewed	65–115
Decaffeinated brewed	3
Decaffeinated instant	2
Tea (6-oz. cup)	
Hot steeped	36
Iced	31
Bottled (12 oz.)	15
Soft Drinks (12-oz. servings)	
Jolt Cola	100
Dr. Pepper	61
Mountain Dew	54
Coca-Cola	46
Pepsi Cola	36–38
Chocolate	
1 oz. baking chocolate	25
1 oz. chocolate candy bar	15
½ cup chocolate pudding	4–12
Over-the-Counter Drugs	
No Doz (2 tablets)	200
Excedrin (2 tablets)	130
Midol (2 tablets)	65
Anacin (2 tablets)	64

Source: Office of Department of Health and Welfare, October 2001.

theobromine, are found in tea and chocolate, respectively. The xanthines are mild CNS stimulants that enhance mental alertness and reduce feelings of fatigue. Other stimulant effects include increases in heart muscle contractions, oxygen consumption, metabolism, and urinary output. These effects are felt within 15 to 45 minutes of ingesting a product that contains caffeine.

Side effects of the xanthines include wakefulness, insomnia, irregular heartbeat, dizziness, nausea, indigestion, and sometimes mild delirium. Some people also experience heartburn. As with some other drugs, the user's psychological outlook and expectations will influence the effects.

Different products contain different concentrations of caffeine. A five-ounce cup of coffee contains 65 to 115 milligrams. Caffeine concentrations vary with the brand of the beverage and the strength of the brew. Small chocolate bars

Caffeinism   Caffeine intoxication brought on by excessive caffeine use; symptoms include chronic insomnia, irritability, anxiety, muscle twitches, and headaches.

contain up to 15 milligrams of caffeine and theobromine. Table 8.5 compares various caffeine-containing products.

Caffeine Addiction

As the effects of caffeine wear off, users may feel let down—mentally or physically depressed, exhausted, and weak. To counteract this, people commonly choose to drink another cup of coffee. Habitually engaging in this practice leads to tolerance and psychological dependency. Until the mid-1970s, caffeine was not medically recognized as addictive. Chronic caffeine use and its attendant behaviors were called "coffee nerves." This syndrome is now recognized as *caffeine intoxication,* or **caffeinism.**

Symptoms of caffeinism include chronic insomnia, jitters, irritability, nervousness, anxiety, and involuntary muscle twitches. Withdrawing the caffeine may compound the effects and produce severe headaches. (Some physicians ask their patients to take a simple test for caffeine addiction: Don't consume anything containing caffeine, and if you get a severe headache within four hours, you are addicted.) Because caffeine meets the requirements for addiction—tolerance, psychological dependency, and withdrawal symptoms—it can be classified as addictive.

Although you would have to drink 67 to 100 cups of coffee in a day to produce a fatal overdose of caffeine, you may experience sensory disturbances after consuming only 10 cups of coffee within a 24-hour period. These symptoms include tinnitus (ringing in the ears), spots before the eyes, numbness in arms and legs, poor circulation, and visual hallucinations. Because 10 cups of coffee is not an extraordinary amount to drink in one day, caffeine use clearly poses health threats.

The Health Consequences of Long-Term Caffeine Use

Long-term caffeine use has been suspected of being linked to a number of serious health problems, ranging from heart disease and cancer to mental dysfunction and birth defects. However, no strong evidence exists to suggest that moderate caffeine use (less than 500 milligrams daily, approximately five cups of coffee) produces harmful effects in healthy, nonpregnant people.

It appears that caffeine does not cause long-term high blood pressure and has not been linked to strokes. Nor is there any evidence of a relationship between coffee and heart disease.[48] However, people who suffer from irregular heartbeat are cautioned against caffeine because the resultant increase in heart rate might be life-threatening. Both decaffeinated and caffeinated coffee products contain ingredients that can irritate the stomach lining and be harmful to people with stomach ulcers.

For years, caffeine consumption was linked with fibrocystic breast disease, a condition characterized by painful, noncancerous lumps in the breast. Reports claim that caffeine promotes cyst formation in female breasts. Although these conclusions have been challenged, many clinicians advise patients with mammillary cysts to avoid caffeine. In addition, some reports indicate that very high doses of caffeine given to pregnant laboratory animals can cause stillbirths or offspring with low birth weight or limb deformations. Studies have found that moderate consumption of caffeine (less than 300 milligrams per day) did not significantly affect human fetal development.[49] Mothers usually are advised to avoid or at least reduce caffeine use during pregnancy.

> **What do you think?**
> *How much caffeine do you consume, and why?* ✳ *What is your pattern of caffeine consumption for the day?* ✳ *Have you ever experienced any ill effects after going without caffeine for a period of time?*

Taking Charge

Make It Happen!

Assessment: The Assess Yourself box on page 210 gave you the chance to test your knowledge about alcoholism. If you couldn't answer some of the questions, or if you were surprised by some of the answers, you may want to take steps to learn more or to change your behavior.

Making a Change: In order to change your behavior, you need to develop a plan. Follow these steps.

1. Evaluate your behavior, and identify patterns and specific things you are doing. What can you change now? What can you change in the near future?
2. Select one pattern of behavior that you want to change.
3. Fill out a Behavior Change Contract. It should include your long-term goal for change, your short-term goals, the rewards you'll give yourself for reaching these goals, potential obstacles along the way, and strategies for overcoming these obstacles. For each goal, list the small steps and specific actions that you will take.

4. Chart your progress in a journal. At the end of a week, consider how successful you were in following your plan. What helped you be successful? What made change more difficult? What will you do differently next week?
5. Revise your plan as needed. Are the short-term goals attainable? Are the rewards satisfying?

Example: After completing the Assess Yourself box, Mark was surprised to discover that he had held several misperceptions about alcohol abuse and alcoholism. In particular, his answers showed that he exhibited one of the symptoms that characterize alcoholism. Mark realized that in his three years in college he had developed a tolerance to alcohol that caused him to drink greater amounts of it to achieve the same effect. He decided to address his concerns about his alcohol use in several steps.

First, Mark kept a log of his alcohol consumption over two weeks. He saw that he was drinking almost every night of the week. Mark decided he wanted to reduce his drinking and set

two goals: taking a break from drinking altogether for three weeks and after that, drinking only on Friday and Saturday nights for the rest of the semester. Mark explained to his friends that he was taking a break and invited them to go with him on hikes, to the movies, and to other alcohol-free environments.

After successfully taking this break, Mark decided to set some goals and limits for himself on the alcohol he would consume in the future. He went to a fraternity party on a Friday night and drank two beers, his predetermined limit. He was happy to notice when he woke up the next morning that he felt refreshed, not hungover. When he went out for dinner with his friends Saturday night, they wanted to go barhopping afterward. He volunteered to be the designated driver, and the bar gave him free sodas for the night. The next weekend, Mark found he had extra money that he had not spent on beer during the week and bought himself a new DVD.

Summary

* Alcohol is a central nervous system (CNS) depressant used by 70 percent of all Americans and 83 percent of all college students; 44 percent of college students are binge drinkers. While consumption trends are slowly creeping downward, college students are under extreme pressure to consume alcohol.

* Alcohol's effect on the body is measured by the blood alcohol concentration (BAC), the ratio of alcohol to total blood volume. The higher the BAC, the greater the impaired judgment and coordination and drowsiness. Some negative consequences associated with alcohol use and college students are lower grade point averages, academic problems, traffic accidents, dropping out of school, unplanned sex, hangovers, and injury. Long-term alcohol overuse includes damage to the nervous system, cardiovascular damage, liver disease, and increased risk for cancer. Use during pregnancy can cause fetal alcohol effects (FAE) or fetal alcohol syndrome (FAS). Alcohol is also a causative factor in traffic accidents.

* Alcohol use becomes abuse or even alcoholism when it interferes with school, work, or social and family relationships, or entails violations of the law. Causes of alcoholism include biological, family, social, and cultural factors. Alcoholism has far-reaching effects on families, especially on children.

* Treatment options for alcoholism include detoxification at private medical facilities, therapy (family, individual, or group), and programs such as Alcoholics Anonymous.

* The use of tobacco involves many social and political issues, including advertising targeted at youth and women, the largest growing populations of smokers. Health care and lost productivity resulting from smoking cost the nation as much as $150 billion per year.

* Tobacco is available in smoking and smokeless forms, both containing addictive nicotine (a psychoactive substance). Smoking also delivers 4,000 other chemicals to the lungs of smokers.

* Health hazards of smoking include markedly higher rates of cancer, heart and circulatory disorders, respiratory diseases, and gum diseases. Smoking while pregnant presents risks for the fetus, including miscarriage and low birth weight.

* Smokeless tobacco contains more nicotine than do cigarettes and dramatically increases risks for oral cancer and other oral problems.

* Environmental tobacco smoke (sidestream smoke) puts nonsmokers at risk for cancer and heart disease.

* Nicotine replacement products (gum and the patch) can help wean smokers off nicotine. Several therapy methods can help smokers break the habit.

* Caffeine is a widely used CNS stimulant. No long-term ill-health effects have been proven, although chronic users who try to quit may experience withdrawal.

Questions for Discussion and Reflection

1. When it comes to drinking alcohol, how much is too much? How can you avoid drinking amounts that will affect your judgment? When you see a friend having too many drinks at a party, what actions do you normally take? What actions could you take?

2. What are some of the most common negative consequences college students experience as a result of drinking? What are secondhand effects of binge drinking? Why do students tolerate negative behaviors of students who have been drinking?

3. Determine what your BAC would be if you drank four beers in two hours (assume they are spaced at equal intervals). What physiological effects will you feel after each drink? Would a person of similar weight show greater effects after having four gin and tonics instead of beer? Why or why not? At what point in your life should you start worrying about the long-term effects of alcohol abuse?

4. Describe the difference between a problem drinker and an alcoholic. What factors can cause someone to slide from responsibly consuming alcohol to becoming an alcoholic? What effect does alcoholism have on an alcoholic's family?

5. Does anyone ever recover from alcoholism? Why or why not? Do you think society's views on drinking have changed over the years? Explain your answer.

6. New research suggests that genetic factors might be more influential than environmental factors in smoking initiation and nicotine dependence. How might this information change current prevention efforts? How would you design smoking prevention strategies targeted at adolescents?

7. Discuss short-term and long-term health hazards associated with tobacco. How will increased tobacco use among adolescents and college students impact the medical system in the future? Who should be responsible for the medical expenses of smokers? Insurance companies? Smokers themselves?

8. Restrictions on smoking are increasing in our society. Do you think these restrictions are fair? Do they infringe on people's rights? Are the restrictions too strict or not strict enough?

9. Describe the pros and cons of each method of tobacco cessation. Which would be most effective for you? Explain why.

10. Discuss problems related to the ingestion of caffeine. How much caffeine do you consume? Why?

Accessing Your Health on the Internet

Visit the following Internet sites to explore further topics and issues related to personal health. To visit an organization's website, go to the Companion Website for *Health: The Basics, Sixth Edition* at www.aw.-bc.com/donatelle, click on the book image, and select "Accessing Your Health on the Internet" from the navigation menu on the left.

1. *American Lung Association.* This site offers a wealth of information regarding smoking trends, environmental smoke, and advice on smoking cessation.
2. *ASH (Action on Smoking and Health).* The nation's oldest and largest antismoking organization, ASH regularly takes hard-hitting legal actions and does other work to fight smoking and protect the rights of nonsmokers. ASH provides nonsmokers with legal forms and valuable information about protecting their rights and about the problems and costs of smoking to nonsmokers. ASH's actions have helped prohibit cigarette commercials; ban smoking on planes, buses, and in many public places; and lower insurance premiums for nonsmokers.
3. *College Drinking: Changing the Culture.* This online resource center is based on a series of reports published by the Task Force of the National Advisory Council on Alcohol Abuse and Alcoholism. It targets three audiences: the student population as a whole, the college and its surrounding environment, and the individual at-risk or alcohol-dependent drinker.
4. *Had Enough.* This entertaining site is designed for college students who have suffered the secondhand effects (baby-sitting a roommate who has been drinking, having sleep interrupted, etc.) of other students' drinking. It offers suggestions for taking action and being proactive about policy issues on your campus.
5. *Higher Education Center for Alcohol and Other Drug Prevention.* This site is funded through the U.S. Department of Education and provides information relevant to colleges and universities. A specific site exists for students who are seeking information regarding alcohol.
6. *TIPS (Tobacco Information and Prevention Source).* This site provides access to a variety of information regarding tobacco use in the United States, with specific information for and about young people.

Further Reading

Glantz, S. A., and E. D. Balbach. *The Tobacco War: Inside the California Battles.* Berkeley: University of California Press, 2000.

Charts the dramatic and complex history of tobacco politics in California over the past quarter century. Shows how the accomplishments of tobacco-control advocates have changed how people view the tobacco industry and its behavior.

Jersild, Devon. *Happy Hours: Alcohol in a Woman's Life.* New York: HarperCollins, 2001.

This book, a combination of cutting-edge research and personal stories of women who have struggled with alcohol problems, examines the role that alcohol plays in women's lives.

Kluger, R. *Ashes to Ashes: America's Hundred-Year Cigarette War, the Public Health, and the Unabashed Triumph of Philip Morris.* New York: Vintage Books, 1997.

A definitive history of America's controversial tobacco industry, focusing on Philip Morris. Traces the development of the cigarette, revelations of its toxicity, and the impact of political and corporate shenanigans on the battle over smoking.

National Institute on Alcohol Abuse and Alcoholism (NIAAA). *Research Monographs.* Washington, DC: U.S. Department of Health and Human Services.

A series of monographs containing the results of a number of studies conducted by research scientists under the auspices of NIAAA through 2002. They address issues such as alcohol use among the elderly, occupational alcoholism, social drinking, and the relationship between heredity and alcoholism.

Nuwer, H. *Wrongs of Passage: Fraternities, Sororities, Hazing, and Binge Drinking.* Bloomington: Indiana University Press, 1999.

A comprehensive exposé on the continuing crisis of death and injury among fraternity and sorority pledges. The book provides an overview of Greek customs and demands that encouraged hazing as well as the recent deaths of students at some of the nation's most prestigious universities. The author argues that we need to control the Greek system as well as other organizations that employ similar, sometimes deadly, hazing practices.

Whelan, E. *Cigarettes: What the Warning Label Doesn't Tell You—The First Comprehensive Guide to the Health Consequences of Smoking.* New York: Prometheus Books, 1997.

From impotence to diabetes, cataracts to psoriasis, the proven dangers of smoking go well beyond heart and lung disease. This book details all the known health threats of smoking. Twenty-one experts explain how smoking can affect the body.

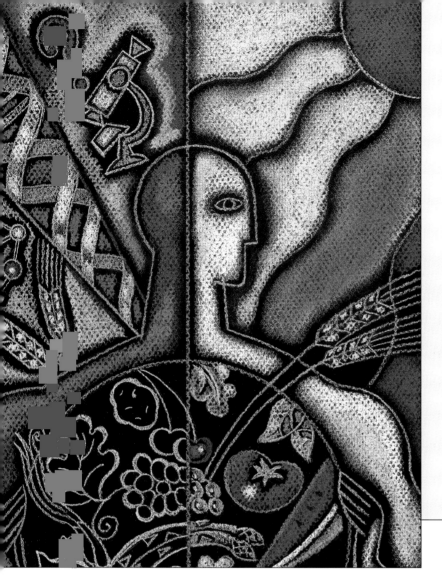

Nutrition

Eating for Optimum Health

Objectives

❋ Examine the factors that influence dietary choices.

❋ Discuss how to change old eating habits, including using the Food Guide Pyramid appropriately, eating nutrient-dense foods, and improving other behaviors that enhance health.

❋ Summarize the major essential nutrients and indicate what purpose they serve in maintaining overall health. Explain any controversies related to these substances.

❋ Discuss food as a form of medicine and the facts related to new trends in nutrition, food supplements, and their roles in health and well-being.

❋ Distinguish among the various forms of vegetarianism and discuss possible health benefits and risks from these dietary alternatives.

❋ Discuss issues surrounding gender and nutrition, food safety, and the unique dietary issues facing college students.

❋ Discuss the unique problems that college students face when trying to eat healthy foods and the actions they can take to comply with the Food Guide Pyramid.

❋ Explain some of the food safety concerns facing Americans and people from other regions of the world.

U.S. Diet Proposals Reflect Nation's Lack of Fitness

By Marian Burros

The Department of Agriculture is proposing dietary advice that for the first time recognizes that a majority of Americans, 64 percent, are overweight and sedentary and need to eat less.

Until now, that dietary advice, reflected in the department's Food Guide Pyramid, has been geared to the nation's healthy population. Under the proposals, recommendations for these more active people would continue to be available but would no longer serve as the cornerstone of government nutrition information.

The new recommendations call for most women from 35 to 70 years old, for instance, to eat 1,600 to 1,800 calories a day, and for most men in that age group to eat 2,000 to 2,200 calories. Previously, the recommendation for most such people, then assumed to be active, was about 600 calories more.

"Over all, the message is that people have to eat a lot less than they are currently eating," said Dr. Marion Nestle, chairwoman of the department of nutrition and food studies at New York University. "People will be shocked at how little it is."

Read the complete article online in the eThemes section of this book's website: www.aw-bc.com/donatelle.

Original article published September 10, 2003. Copyright © 2003 The New York Times. Reprinted with permission.

D o you ever get frustrated by conflicting information about diet and nutritional supplements? If so, you are like millions of other Americans. In fact, three out of four Americans say that there is far too much contradictory information about nutrition, and they feel overwhelmed by the daunting task of trying to distinguish fact from fiction.[1] Just when we think we know the answers, a new research study tells us that what we thought was true probably isn't.

Today, we face dietary choices and nutritional challenges that our grandparents never dreamed of such as exotic foreign foods; dietary supplements; artificial sweeteners; no-fat, low-fat, and artificial-fat alternatives; and cholesterol-free, high-protein, low-carbohydrate, and low-calorie products. Thousands of alternatives bombard us daily. Caught in the crossfire of advertised claims by the food industry and advice provided by health and nutrition experts, most of us find it difficult to make wise dietary decisions. The good news is that, according to the American Dietetic Association, more Americans are seeking out information on food and nutrition and taking action to improve their habits than ever before.[2]

When you are living away from home for the first time, suddenly having to make your own choices about food may seem a formidable task. A study of more than 2,000 college students indicated that students often face considerable difficulty planning healthy menus and having the resources to prepare balanced meals.[3] On the other hand, a subsequent study showed that college students and graduates tend to practice more healthful habits and make healthier food choices than do nonstudents.[4] Many students' eating behaviors appear to mirror eating patterns that they learned in their homes.

Assessing Eating Behaviors

Although we have all undoubtedly experienced **hunger** before mealtime, few Americans have experienced the type of hunger that continues for days and threatens survival. Most of us do not eat to sustain physical survival. Instead, we eat because we experience **appetite**—the desire to eat—or because some inner signal tells us that it's time to eat. Appetite may cause a person to eat even when the person is quite full.

Many factors influence when we eat, what we eat, and how much. Sensory stimulation, such as smelling, seeing, and tasting food, can stimulate appetite even if we're not hungry. Finding the right balance between eating to maintain body function (eating to live) and eating to satisfy appetite (living to eat) is a constant struggle for many of us. The following are among the most powerful influences that make us who we are nutritionally.[5]

- *Personal preferences.* We all choose certain foods because we like the taste.
- *Habit.* Many of us select foods because they are familiar and provide comfort.

Hunger The feeling associated with the physiological need to eat.

Appetite The desire to eat; normally accompanies hunger but is more psychological than physiological.

- *Ethnic heritage or tradition.* People eat the foods they grew up eating.
- *Social interactions.* For many of us, eating and socializing go hand in hand.
- *Availability, convenience, and economy.* Those with lower incomes find some foods too expensive, whereas others with higher incomes have more choice. Most of us eat foods that are readily available, quick and easy to prepare, and friendly to our budgets.
- *Emotional comfort.* We learn from birth that eating is a pleasant experience associated with warmth, pleasure, and sensory delights.
- *Values.* Food choices often reflect one's religious or spiritual beliefs, political views, or environmental concerns.
- *Body image.* Many people select certain foods because they believe the foods will enhance appearance, improve health, or act as a preventive agent.
- *Nutrition.* Many people make nutrition choices based purely on health concerns.

Nutrition is the science that investigates the relationship between physiological function and the essential elements of the foods we eat. With our country's overabundance of food and vast array of choices, media that prime us to want the tasty morsels shown on advertisements, and easy access to almost every type of **nutrient** (proteins, carbohydrates, fats, vitamins, minerals, and water), Americans should have few nutritional problems. However, these "diets of affluence" contribute to several major diseases, including obesity-related problems with heart disease, certain cancers, diabetes, hypertension (high blood pressure), cirrhosis of the liver, sleep apnea, varicose veins, gout, gallbladder disease, respiratory problems, abdominal hernias, flat feet, complications in pregnancy and surgery, and even higher accident rates, to name but a few.[6] Diabetes, in particular, has reached epidemic proportions in the United States and is largely a product of poor diet, excess weight, and lack of exercise. A weight gain of 11 to 18 pounds increases a person's risk of developing diabetes to twice that of individuals who have not gained weight.[7]

Eating for Health

Americans consume more calories per person than any other group of people in the world. Not coincidentally, we also have the highest rates of obesity. A **calorie** is a unit of measure that indicates the amount of energy we obtain from a particular food. We consume calories in the form of *proteins, fats,* and *carbohydrates,* three of the basic nutrients necessary for life. Three other nutrients, *vitamins, minerals,* and *water,* are necessary for bodily function but do not contribute any calories to our diet.

Excess calorie consumption is a major factor in our tendency to be overweight. However, it is not so much the quantity of food we eat that is likely to cause weight problems and resultant diseases as it is the relative proportion of

nutrients and lack of physical activity. Americans typically get approximately 38 percent of their calories from fat, 15 percent from proteins, 22 percent from complex carbohydrates, and 24 percent from simple sugars.[8] Nutritionists recommend increasing complex carbohydrates to make up 48 percent of our total calories and reducing proteins to 12 percent, simple sugars to 10 percent, and fats to no more than 30 percent of our total diet.

It is the high concentration of fats in the American diet, particularly saturated fats (largely animal fats), that appears to increase risk for heart disease. Although excessive consumption of sugar has been implicated in the development of many diseases, much of this information is inaccurate. Contrary to popular opinion, American consumption of sugar has not changed dramatically in recent years. In addition, the only disease associated with long-term excessive sugar intake is dental cavities. Most diet-related diseases result from excess calories and increased consumption of fat. Over the years, several federal agencies have worked to modify the average American's diet through a series of dietary goals and guidelines. How healthy are your eating habits? Find out by completing the quiz in the Assess Yourself box on pages 238 and 239.

The Food Guide Pyramid

The Food Guide Pyramid, promoted by the United States Department of Agriculture (USDA) since 1993, illustrates graphically the importance of grains, cereals, vegetables, and fruits compared to meat, fish, poultry, dairy products, and other foods. Figure 9.1 on page 234 shows the Food Guide Pyramid with recommended servings and examples of servings from each group.

A Call for a New Pyramid

Researchers have begun a collective movement to significantly up-end the current pyramid. They favor a pyramid that downplays meat and dairy products and moves whole-grain foods and plant oils to the top of the list of foods that should make up your daily intake. Several experts have proposed a pyramid that looks much like the guidelines in Figure 9.2 on page 235 and will be the topic of much debate in the coming years. The USDA plans to release a revised pyramid, along with revised Dietary Guidelines, in 2005.

Nutrition The science that investigates the relationship between physiological function and the essential elements of foods eaten.

Nutrients The constituents of food that sustain us physiologically: proteins, carbohydrates, fats, vitamins, minerals, and water.

Calorie A unit of measure that indicates the amount of energy obtained from a particular food.

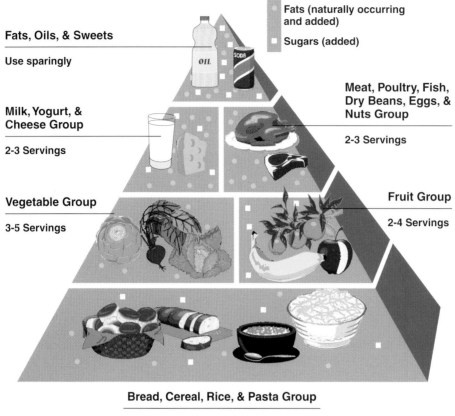

Fats, Oils, & Sweets

Use sparingly

■ Fats (naturally occurring and added)

□ Sugars (added)

Milk, Yogurt, & Cheese Group

2-3 Servings

Meat, Poultry, Fish, Dry Beans, Eggs, & Nuts Group

2-3 Servings

Vegetable Group

3-5 Servings

Fruit Group

2-4 Servings

Bread, Cereal, Rice, & Pasta Group

6-11 Servings

Figure 9.1

Food Guide Pyramid: A Guide to Daily Food Choices

Source: U.S. Department of Agriculture, Center for Nutrition Policy and Promotion, "The Food Guide Pyramid," *Home and Garden Bulletin,* no. 252. (1996).

Making the Pyramid Work for You

Many people are overwhelmed by their first glance at the pyramid. However, take a look at what the USDA considers a serving: 1 ounce of ready-to-eat cereal, for example. A normal bowl of cereal contains 3 to 4 ounces of cereal. When was the last time you ate a quarter bowl of cereal? When you consider breakfast, lunch, dinner, and snacks, it is really quite easy to get all the servings in this group that you need.

Understanding Serving Sizes How much is a *serving*? Is it different from a *portion*? While these two terms often are used interchangeably, they actually mean different things. A serving is the amount of food recommended in materials such as the Food Guide Pyramid, while a portion is the amount of food you choose to eat at any one time and that may be more or less than a serving. Most people have trouble judging what a serving looks like and eat 2 to 3 servings when they think they are only having 1. In a national survey, more than half of Americans overestimated the serving size of cooked pasta and rice, and took at least 2 times the amount that they should have.[9]

The amount of food that counts as 1 serving in the various food groups is listed below. If you eat a larger portion, count it as more than 1 serving. Be sure to eat at least the lowest number of servings from the major food groups; you need them for the nutrients they provide. (Some people need more servings from the milk, yogurt, and cheese group; teens and breast-feeding or pregnant women should get 3 servings, and pregnant or breast-feeding teens should get 4.) No specific serving size is given for fats, oils, and sweets because they should be used sparingly.

Breads, Cereal, Rice, and Pasta Group
- 1 slice of bread or medium dinner roll
- 1/2 cup cooked rice, pasta, or other grains
- 1 ounce ready-to-eat cereal
- 3 cups popped popcorn

Fruit Group
- Whole fruit such as 1 medium apple, banana, or orange
- 1/2 cup of raw, cooked, or canned fruit
- 3/4 cup of fruit juice
- 1/2 cup canned fruit
- 1/4 cup dried fruit

Vegetable Group
- 1 cup leafy raw vegetables
- $\frac{1}{2}$ cup chopped fresh, frozen, or canned vegetables

Meat, Poultry, Fish, Dry Beans, Eggs, and Nuts Group
- 2–3 ounces lean, trimmed, and baked or roasted meat, fish, or poultry. The following can substitute for 1 ounce of meat:
  - 2 tablespoons peanut butter or other nut or seed butter
  - $\frac{1}{4}$ cup nuts
  - $\frac{1}{2}$ cup cooked legumes
  - 3 ounces tofu
  - 1 egg

Milk, Yogurt, and Cheese Group
- 1 cup milk or yogurt
- $1\frac{1}{2}$ ounces natural cheese
- 2 ounces processed cheese
- $\frac{1}{2}$ cup cottage cheese
- $1\frac{1}{2}$ cups ice cream, ice milk, or frozen yogurt

What do you think?

Which food groups from the Food Guide Pyramid are you most likely to eat enough of during a typical day? ✳ *Which ones, if any, are you most likely to skimp on?* ✳ *What are some simple changes that you could make right now in your diet to help you comply with pyramid recommendations?*

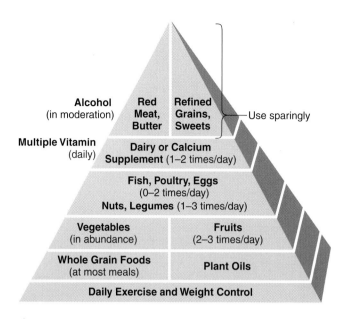

Figure 9.2

Proposed New Food Guide Pyramid

Source: W. C. Willett, *Eat, Drink, and Be Healthy* (New York: Simon and Schuster, 2001). Copyright © 2001 by President and Fellows of Harvard College.

Today's Dietary Guidelines

For several decades, the USDA and leading health and nutrition professional groups have worked together to develop guidelines to help insure optimal dietary health for Americans. A comparison of how these guidelines have changed in response to national goals and objectives is reflected in Table 9.1 on page 236. Changes include the growing recognition of physical activity as part of a healthy lifestyle, a more sophisticated understanding of differences among fats, and the increase in concerns over food safety. The most recent guidelines, published in 2000, respond in particular to our growing epidemics of obesity and diabetes; the Dietary Guidelines for 2005 will be available soon. Current guidelines are based on the ABCs for good health.

- **A**iming for Fitness— Recommendations include aiming for a healthy weight and being physically active each day. Strive to be physically active for at least 30 minutes daily, preferably with moderate activity levels on most days. (Moderate activity is any activity that requires about as much energy as walking two miles in 30 minutes.)
- **B**uilding A Healthy Base—Recommendations include using the Food Guide Pyramid to guide your choices, with plant foods (whole grains, fruits, and vegetables) serving as a foundation of your daily intake. This guideline also

includes taking care of the unique nutrient needs of special age groups or circumstances, checking food labels, exercising moderation with fats and sweets, aiming for variety, and making sure foods are safe and properly prepared and stored.

- **C**hoosing Sensibly—Recommendations include choosing a diet that is low in saturated fat and cholesterol and moderate in total fat, knowing the differences between fats, choosing beverages and foods that limit intake of sugar, consuming less salt, and drinking alcohol in moderation, if at all.

See the Skills for Behavior Change box on page 237 for some ideas on incorporating these guidelines into your daily diet.

Eating Nutrient-Dense Foods

Although eating the proper number of servings from the food pyramid is important, it is also important to recognize that there are large caloric, fat, and energy differences between food categories within pyramid groups. For example, you might get the same number of calories from a glass of beer as you would from a glass of milk, but you would get many more nutrients from the milk. Likewise, fish and hot dogs provide vastly different fat and energy levels per ounce, with fish providing better energy and calorie value per serving. Nutrient density is even more important for someone who is ill and unable to keep food down. That is why nutrient supplements such as *Ensure* and others often are provided for cancer patients who need a nutrient "hit" in a small package.

Table 9.1
Dietary Guidelines for Americans, 1980–2000

1980 7 Guidelines	1985 7 Guidelines	1990 7 Guidelines	1995 7 Guidelines	2000 10 Guidelines
Eat a variety of foods	Eat a variety of foods	Eat a variety of foods	Eat a variety of foods	**Aim for Fitness** Aim for a healthy weight
Maintain ideal weight	Maintain desirable weight	Maintain healthy weight	Balance the food you eat with physical activity—maintain or improve your weight	Be physically active each day
				Build a Healthy Base Let the Pyramid guide your food choices
Avoid too much fat, saturated fat, and cholesterol	Avoid too much fat, saturated fat, and cholesterol	Choose a diet low in fat, saturated fat and cholesterol		
Eat foods with adequate starch and fiber	Eat foods with adequate starch and fiber	Choose a diet with plenty of vegetables, fruits, and grain products	Choose a diet with plenty of grain products, vegetables, and fruits	Choose a variety of grains daily, especially whole grains
				Choose a variety of fruits and vegetables daily
				Keep food safe to eat
				Choose Sensibly
			Choose a diet low in fat, saturated fat and cholesterol	Choose a diet low in saturated fat and cholesterol and moderate in total fat
Avoid too much sugar	Avoid too much sugar	Use sugars only in moderation	Choose a diet moderate in sugars	Choose beverages and foods to moderate your intake of sugars
Avoid too much sodium	Avoid too much sodium	Use salt and sodium only in moderation	Choose a diet moderate in salt and sodium	Choose and prepare foods with less salt
If you drink alcohol, do so in moderation	If you drink alcohol, do so in moderation	If you drink alcohol, do so in moderation	If you drink alcohol, do so in moderation	If you drink alcohol, do so in moderation

Shading highlights how the order in which the guidelines are presented has changed over time.

The Digestive Process

Food provides the chemicals we need for energy and body maintenance. Because our bodies cannot synthesize or produce certain essential nutrients, we must obtain them from the foods we eat. Even though we may take in adequate amounts of foods and nutrients, if our body systems are not functioning properly, much of the nutrient value in our food may be lost. Before foods can be utilized properly, the digestive system must break down the larger food particles into smaller, more usable forms. The sequence of functions by which the body breaks down foods and either absorbs or excretes them is known as the **digestive process.**

Even before you take your first bite of pizza, your body has already begun a series of complex digestive responses. Your mouth prepares for the food by increasing production of **saliva.** Saliva contains mostly water, which aids in chewing and swallowing, but it also contains important enzymes that begin the process of food breakdown, including amylase, which breaks down carbohydrates. *Enzymes* are protein compounds that facilitate chemical reactions but are not altered in the process. From the mouth, the food passes down the

Digestive process The sequence of functions by which the body breaks down foods and either absorbs or excretes them.

Saliva Fluid secreted by the salivary glands; enzymes in the fluid aid in the breakdown of certain foods for digestion.

Making Healthy Choices

Knowing what the healthy choices for a balanced diet are is one thing, actually making those choices is another matter. Here are some ideas for changing your diet in three key areas: whole grain consumption, fruit and vegetable choices, and salt intake.

INCREASING YOUR INTAKE OF WHOLE GRAIN FOODS

Choose foods that name one of the following ingredients *first* on the label's ingredient list:

- brown rice
- bulgher
- cracked wheat
- graham flour
- oatmeal
- popcorn
- whole barley
- whole cornmeal
- whole oats
- whole rye
- whole wheat

Look for whole wheat bread, low-fat whole wheat crackers, oatmeal, corn tortillas, whole wheat pasta, whole barley in soup, and tabouli salad.

CHOOSING THE MOST NUTRITIOUS FRUITS AND VEGETABLES

All fruits and vegetables contribute to a healthy diet. These choices are especially good because they are high in important vitamins and minerals.

- Sources of vitamin A (carotenoids):
  - Bright orange vegetables (carrots, sweet potatoes, pumpkin)
  - Dark-green leafy vegetables (spinach, collards, turnip greens)
  - Bright orange fruits (mango, cantaloupe, apricots)

- Sources of vitamin C:
  - Citrus fruits and juices, kiwi, strawberries, cantaloupe
  - Broccoli, peppers, tomatoes, cabbage, potatoes
  - Leafy greens (romaine, turnip greens, spinach)

- Sources of folate:
  - Cooked dried beans and peas
  - Oranges, orange juice
  - Deep green leaves (spinach, mustard greens)

- Sources of potassium:
  - Baked white or sweet potatoes, cooked greens, winter (orange) squash
  - Bananas, plantains, many dried fruits, orange juice

DECREASING YOUR SALT INTAKE

- At the grocery store, fresh, plain, frozen, and canned vegetables without added salt are the lowest in salt.
- Fresh or frozen fish, shellfish, poultry, and meat are lower in salt than most canned and processed forms.
- Use the Nutrition Facts label to compare the amount of sodium in processed foods such as soups and cereals; the amount in different types and brands often varies widely.
- Learn to season with herbs and spices instead of salt.
- Be aware that condiments such as soy sauce, ketchup, mustard, pickles, and olives can be high in salt.
- Choose grilled or roasted entrees, baked potatoes, and salad with oil and vinegar dressing. Batter-fried foods and combination dishes such as stews tend to be high in salt.

Source: Dietary Guidelines Advisory Committee, USDA Agricultural Research Service, "Dietary Guidelines for Americans," 2000. www.ars.usda.gov/dgac/2kdiet.pdf

---

esophagus, a 9- to 10-inch tube that connects the mouth and stomach. A series of contractions and relaxations by the muscles lining the esophagus gently move food to the next digestive organ, the **stomach.** Here food mixes with enzymes and stomach acids. Hydrochloric acid begins to work in combination with pepsin, an enzyme, to break down proteins. In most people, the stomach secretes enough mucus to protect the stomach lining from these harsh digestive juices.

Further digestive activity takes place in the **small intestine,** a 20-foot coiled tube containing three sections: the *duodenum, jejunum,* and *ileum.* Each section secretes digestive enzymes that, when combined with enzymes from the liver and the pancreas, further contribute to the breakdown of proteins, fats, and carbohydrates. These nutrients are absorbed into the bloodstream to supply body cells with energy. The liver is the major organ that determines whether nutrients are stored, sent to cells or organs, or excreted. Solid wastes consisting of fiber, water, and salts are dumped into the large intestine, where most of the water and salts are reabsorbed into the system and the fiber is passed out through the anus. The entire digestive process takes approximately 24 hours.

Esophagus   Tube that transports food from the mouth to the stomach.

Stomach   Large muscular organ that temporarily stores, mixes, and digests foods.

Small intestine   Muscular, coiled digestive organ; consists of the duodenum, jejunum, and ileum.

What's Your EQ (Eating Quotient)?

Keeping up with the latest on what to eat—or not to eat—isn't easy. If you think a few facts might have slipped past you, this quiz should help. There's only one correct answer for each question.

1. Which of these foods is most likely to help prevent the most common form of blindness in older Americans?
   a. carrots
   b. oranges
   c. spinach
   d. tomato juice
   e. zucchini

2. Which claim is backed by the best research?
   a. Hot dogs increase the risk of childhood leukemia.
   b. Carnitine helps you lose weight.
   c. Cranberry juice can help treat urinary tract infections.
   d. Garlic strengthens your immune system.
   e. Coenzyme Q10 helps prevent heart disease.

3. Breast cancer kills more women than any other disease.
   a. true
   b. false

4. If you're in your 50s or 60s and your blood pressure is normal, it will stay that way.
   a. true
   b. false

5. Four of these strategies have been clearly shown to keep blood pressure from rising. Which has not?
   a. cutting salt
   b. losing excess weight
   c. eating potassium-rich foods
   d. getting enough vitamin C
   e. exercising regularly

6. Which has not been linked to a high-salt diet?
   a. stroke
   b. stomach cancer
   c. osteoporosis
   d. diabetes

7. There's evidence that the B vitamin folic acid cuts the risk of all but
   a. birth defects, such as spina bifida.
   b. stroke.
   c. colon cancer.
   d. heart disease.
   e. prostate cancer.

8. Which of the following foods is not a good source of folic acid?
   a. tuna fish
   b. corn flakes
   c. asparagus
   d. lentils
   e. orange juice

9. Which of the following does not appear to be dangerous in high doses?
   a. vitamin B_6
   b. vitamin B_{12}
   c. niacin
   d. vitamin D

10. Most multivitamin supplements contain far less than a day's worth of
    a. zinc.
    b. vitamin A.
    c. iron.
    d. calcium.
    e. vitamin D.

11. Which food poisoning symptoms warrant calling the doctor?
    a. bloody diarrhea
    b. a stiff neck, severe headache, and fever
    c. excessive vomiting
    d. any of the above

Obtaining Essential Nutrients

Water: A Crucial Nutrient

If you were to go on a survival trip, which would you take with you—food or water? You may be surprised to learn that you could survive much longer without food than you could without water. Even in severe conditions, the average person can go for weeks without certain vitamins and minerals before experiencing serious deficiency symptoms. **Dehydration,** however, which is abnormal depletion of body fluids, can cause serious problems within a matter of hours. After a few days without water, death is likely.

Fifty to 60 percent of our total body weight is water. The water in our system bathes cells, aids in fluid and electrolyte balance, maintains pH balance, and transports molecules and cells throughout the body. Water is the major component of our blood, which carries oxygen and nutrients to the tissues and is responsible for maintaining cells in working order.

Dehydration Abnormal depletion of body fluids; a result of lack of water.

12. Which is least likely to cause food poisoning?
   a. undercooked chicken
   b. Caesar salad dressing
   c. raw oysters
   d. rare hamburger
   e. mayonnaise

13. Which is least likely to have contaminants?
   a. flounder
   b. swordfish
   c. raw clams
   d. bluefish
   e. lake trout

14. What poisons the most children under the age of six?
   a. eating moldy food
   b. drinking household cleaners
   c. taking an overdose of iron pills
   d. chewing poisonous houseplant leaves

ANSWERS

1. c. Two carotenoids found in spinach—lutein and zeaxanthin—appear to protect eyes more than beta-carotene and other carotenoids do. Other good sources: red bell pepper, okra, and leafy greens, such as kale, collard greens, and romaine lettuce.

2. c. In a recent study from Harvard Medical School, women who drank a little more than a cup of cranberry juice cocktail a day were twice as likely to be cured of their urinary tract infections as women who drank a look-alike, taste-alike beverage with no cranberry juice.

3. b. When women of all ages are combined, heart disease kills 4 times as many women as breast cancer.

4. b. In the United States, blood pressure rises with age for most people.

5. d. There's convincing evidence for all but the vitamin C. Limiting alcohol to no more than two drinks a day should also keep your blood pressure from rising.

6. d. A high-salt diet is most clearly linked to the risk of stroke. But the more salt you eat, the more calcium your body excretes, which can lead to osteoporosis, or brittle bones. While stomach cancer is deadly, the kind that's linked to salty foods is on the decline in the United States.

7. e.

8. a. The best places to get folic acid are fruits, vegetables, beans, fortified cereals, and vitamin supplements.

9. b. A high dose of B_{12} (500 micrograms a day) can prevent B_{12} deficiency. And it's safe. A high dose of B_6 (possibly as little as 200 mg a day), on the other hand, can cause (reversible) nerve damage. Niacin (about 500 mg a day or more) is considered a drug. While it lowers cholesterol, it can cause side effects, such as flushing and liver damage. Vitamin D may cause side effects at levels as low as 1,200 IU a day.

10. d. If you want to get close to 100 percent of the U.S. Recommended Daily Allowance (USRDA) from a supplement, you'll need to take calcium separately.

11. d. You should also see a physician if any milder food poisoning symptom lasts for more than three days.

12. e. Despite its reputation for spoiling easily, mayonnaise is not as risky as undercooked poultry, rare hamburger, the raw egg in Caesar salad dressing, or raw shellfish.

13. a. Other low-fat seafood, such as cod, haddock, Pacific halibut, ocean perch, pollock, sole, and cooked shellfish, are also likely to be safe. Ditto for salmon and canned tuna.

14. c. Since 1986, more than 110,000 children have been poisoned by taking an overdose of their parents' (often brightly colored) iron supplements or iron-containing multivitamins, some after swallowing as few as five pills.

Individual needs for water vary drastically according to dietary factors, age, size, overall health, environmental temperature and humidity levels, and exercise. Certain diseases, such as diabetes or cystic fibrosis, cause people to lose fluids at a rate necessitating a higher volume of fluid intake.

Is bottled water healthier than tap water? In most instances, expensive "spring" water and bottled water are no healthier than are chlorinated and fluoridated city water. In fact, if you look closely at the labels, you'll find that most expensive little bottles don't contain pristine water from natural springs but rather, purified city water that has been subjected to reverse osmosis. Is it worth the extra cost? Most experts think not. If you are concerned about your current water source, have it tested. Otherwise, don't spend your money needlessly. In addition, if you buy water a few times and then refill the plastic bottles, you may cause yourself problems. Bacteria flourish in a warm, moist environment, and the bacteria from your saliva may make your "pure" water into a teeming soup of disease-causing liquid.

Proteins

Next to water, **proteins** are the most abundant substances in the human body. Proteins are major components of nearly every cell and have been called the "body builders" because of their role in developing and repairing bone, muscle, skin, and blood cells. Proteins are also the key elements of the antibodies that protect us from disease, of enzymes that control chemical activities in the body, and of hormones that regulate body functions. Moreover, proteins aid in the transport of iron, oxygen, and nutrients to all body cells and supply another source of energy to cells when fats and carbohydrates are not readily available. In short, adequate amounts of protein in the diet are vital to many body functions and ultimately to survival.

Whenever you consume proteins, your body breaks them down into smaller molecules known as **amino acids,** the building blocks of protein, which link together like beads in a necklace to form 20 different combinations. Nine of these combinations are termed **essential amino acids,** which means the body must obtain them from the diet; the other 11 are produced by the body.

Dietary protein that supplies all of the essential amino acids is called **complete (high-quality) protein.** Typically, protein from animal products is complete. When we consume foods that are deficient in some of the essential amino acids, the total amount of protein that can be synthesized from the other amino acids is decreased. For proteins to be complete, they also must be present in digestible form and in amounts proportional to body requirements.

What about plant sources of protein? Proteins from plant sources are often **incomplete proteins** in that they are missing one or two of the essential amino acids. Nevertheless, it is relatively easy for the non–meat-eater to combine plant foods effectively and eat complementary sources of plant protein. An excellent example of this mutual supplementation process is eating peanut butter on whole grain bread.

Although each of these foods lacks certain essential amino acids, eating them together provides high-quality protein.

Plant sources of protein fall into three general categories: *legumes* (beans, peas, peanuts, and soy products), *grains* (whole grains, corn, and pasta products), and *nuts and seeds.* Certain vegetables, such as leafy green vegetables and broccoli, also contribute valuable plant proteins. Mixing two or more foods from each of these categories during the same meal will provide all of the essential amino acids necessary to ensure adequate protein absorption. People who are not interested in obtaining all of their protein from plants can combine incomplete plant proteins with complete low-fat animal proteins, such as chicken, fish, turkey, and lean red meat. Low-fat or nonfat cottage cheese, skim milk, egg whites, and nonfat dry milk all provide high-quality proteins and have few calories and little dietary fat.

You need to eat enough protein, but don't consume too much. Eating too much protein, particularly animal protein, can place added stress on the liver and kidneys. It also may increase calcium excretion in urine, which can elevate the risk of osteoporosis and bone fractures.[10]

Recently, several low-calorie diets that practically eliminate carbohydrates and focus on eating large quantities of protein have reemerged in the popular press. Diets that deviate from a balanced nutritional approach are almost certainly flawed. In particular, people who have kidney or liver problems or who suffer from fluid imbalances or problems should avoid high-protein diets. For more information, see the following section on carbohydrates and Chapter 10 on weight management.

A person might need to eat extra protein if he or she is fighting off a serious infection, recovering from surgery or blood loss, or recovering from burns. In these instances, proteins that are lost to cellular repair need to be replaced. There is considerable controversy over whether someone in high-level physical training needs additional protein to build and repair muscle fibers or whether normal daily requirements should suffice.

Although protein deficiency continues to pose a threat to the global population, few Americans suffer from protein deficiencies. In fact, the average American consumes more than 100 grams of protein daily, and about 70 percent of this comes from high-fat animal flesh and dairy products.[11] The recommended protein intake for the average man is only 63 grams and 50 grams for the average woman. The typical recommendation is that in a 2,000-calorie diet, about 10 percent of calories should come from protein, 60 percent from carbohydrates, and less than 30 percent from fat. The excess is stored as extra calories that lead to extra fat.

Carbohydrates

Although the importance of proteins in the body should not be underestimated, it is **carbohydrates** that supply us with the energy needed to sustain normal daily activity. Carbohydrates actually can be metabolized more quickly and efficiently than proteins can. They are a quick source of energy

---

Proteins   The essential constituents of nearly all body cells; necessary for the development and repair of bone, muscle, skin, and blood; the key elements of antibodies, enzymes, and hormones.

Amino acids   The building blocks of protein.

Essential amino acids   Nine of the basic nitrogen-containing building blocks of protein that must be obtained from foods to ensure health.

Complete (high-quality) proteins   Proteins that contain all of the nine essential amino acids.

Incomplete proteins   Proteins that are lacking in one or more of the essential amino acids.

Carbohydrates   Basic nutrients that supply the body with the energy needed to sustain normal activity.

for the body because they are easily converted to glucose, the fuel for the body's cells. These foods also play an important role in the functioning of internal organs, the nervous system, and the muscles. They are the best fuel for endurance athletics because they provide both an immediate and a time-released energy source since they are digested easily and then consistently metabolized in the bloodstream.

For many people, a plate of pasta represents an attractive, healthy alternative to a fatty steak. However, carbohydrates also have been painted as villains recently in several popular diets promising quick weight loss. Although some studies seem to support the low carbohydrate, high protein and fat approach to weight loss, previous decades of research have consistently disagreed with these claims. See Chapter 10 for more information about these diets.

One issue that proponents of many of these diets overlook is that not all carbohydrates are the same. There are two major types of carbohydrates: **simple sugars,** which provide short-term energy, are found primarily in fruits. **Complex carbohydrates,** which provide sustained energy, are found in grains, cereals, dark green leafy vegetables, yellow fruits and vegetables (carrots, yams), *cruciferous* vegetables (such as broccoli, cabbage, and cauliflower), and certain root vegetables, such as potatoes. Most of us do not get enough complex carbohydrates in our daily diets.

A typical American diet contains large amounts of simple sugars. The most common form is *glucose.* Eventually, the human body converts all types of simple sugars to glucose to provide energy to cells. In its natural form, glucose is sweet and is obtained from substances such as corn syrup, honey, molasses, vegetables, and fruits. *Fructose* is another simple sugar found in fruits and berries. Glucose and fructose are **monosaccharides** that contain only one molecule of sugar.

Disaccharides are combinations of two monosaccharides. Perhaps the best-known example is common granulated table sugar (known as sucrose), which consists of a molecule of fructose chemically bonded to a molecule of glucose. Lactose, found in milk and milk products, is another form of disaccharide formed by the combination of glucose and galactose (another simple sugar). Disaccharides must be broken down into simple sugars before the body can use them.

Controlling the amount of sugar in your diet can be difficult because sugar, like sodium, is often present in food products that you might not expect to contain it. Such diverse items as ketchup, Russian dressing, Coffee-Mate, and Shake 'n' Bake derive 30 to 65 percent of their calories from sugar. Read food labels carefully before purchasing.

Polysaccharides are complex carbohydrates formed by long chains of saccharides. Like disaccharides, they must be broken down into simple sugars before the body can utilize them. There are two major forms of complex carbohydrates: *starches* and *fiber,* or **cellulose.**

Starches make up the majority of the complex carbohydrate group. Starches in our diets come from flours, breads, pasta, potatoes, and related foods. They are stored in body muscles and the liver in a polysaccharide form called

glycogen. When the body requires a sudden burst of energy, it breaks down glycogen into glucose.

Carbohydrates and Athletic Performance In the past decade, carbohydrates have become the health foods of many athletes. Some fitness enthusiasts consume concentrated sugary foods or drinks before or during athletic activity because they think that the sugars will provide extra energy. This may actually be counterproductive.

One possible problem involves the gastrointestinal tract. If your intestines react to activity (or the nervousness before competition) by moving material through the small intestine more rapidly than usual, undigested disaccharides and/or unabsorbed monosaccharides will reach the colon, which can result in a very inopportune bout of diarrhea.

Consuming large amounts of sugar during exercise also can have a negative effect on hydration. Concentrations exceeding 24 grams of sugar per 8 ounces of fluid can delay stomach emptying and hence absorption of water. Some fruit juices, fruit drinks, and other sugar-sweetened beverages have more than this amount of sugar. If you use these products, dilute them with ice cubes or water.

Marathon runners and other people who require reserves of energy for demanding tasks often attempt to increase stores of glycogen in the body by *carbohydrate loading.* This process involves modifying the nature of both workouts and diet, usually during the week or so before competition. The athletes train very hard early in the week while eating small amounts of carbohydrates. Right before competition, they dramatically increase their intake of carbohydrates to force the body to store more glycogen to be used during endurance activities (such as the last miles of a marathon).

The Myth of Sugar and Hyperactivity Contrary to early media reports, extensive research in recent years indicates that sugars do *not* cause hyperactivity.[12] In well-controlled dietary

---

Simple sugar   A major type of carbohydrate, which provides short-term energy.

Complex carbohydrates   A major type of carbohydrate, which provides sustained energy.

Monosaccharide   A simple sugar that contains only one molecule of sugar.

Disaccharide   A combination of two monosaccharides.

Polysaccharide   A complex carbohydrate formed by the combination of long chains of saccharides.

Cellulose   Fiber; a major form of complex carbohydrates.

Glycogen   The polysaccharide form in which glucose is stored in the liver.

challenge studies, consumption of sugar has not been shown to have negative effects on motor activity, spontaneous behavior, performance in psychological tests, learning, memory, attention span, or problem-solving ability. In addition, sugar intake is not related to violence or criminal activity.

Is Sugar Addictive?   Another sugar-related controversy is whether sugar can be addictive. A recent report on this topic summarizes the accumulated research and concludes that the evidence supporting an addiction is scant. It might be more appropriate to say that your sweet tooth is a preference.[13]

According to the report, scientists agree that babies are born with a preference for sweet and salty tastes and a dislike for sour and bitter tastes. In addition, some people are "supertasters," which means that they have more taste buds on the tip of the tongue (up to 1,100 taste buds per square centimeter) than medium, low, or non-tasters (low tasters have around 40 taste buds in the same area). Low and non-tasters require more sugar for taste and thus may have a stronger sweet tooth.

Preference for sweets is also a part of our cultural heritage, with indications that we develop a taste for sugar based on learned eating patterns rather than because of an addiction. Culture, genetics, and other factors appear to be reasons for why some of us love sugar far too much. The keys are to monitor sugar intake and eat sweet foods in moderation.

Carbohydrates and Carcinogens   The World Health Organization recently labeled *acrylamide,* a compound found in plastics, as a "probable human carcinogen" because it has been shown to cause cancer, as well as genetic, neurological, and reproductive damage in animals. While some of the concern arises from our use of plastics to cover food in microwaves, the larger issue arose because acrylamide is formed when starchy foods are cooked at high temperatures. University of Stockholm researchers found the highest concentrations of acrylamide in potato chips and crispbreads that were baked or fried, like French fries, crackers, and cereals.[14] Acrylamide was not found in raw foods, meats, or starchy foods that were boiled, such as rice or pasta. Critics of the study say that too few samples were used and that the amounts of acrylamide found were a thousandfold less than levels shown to cause cancer in mice. Follow-up research by the Center for Science in the Public Interest showed that a large order of French fries contained 39 to 82 micrograms of acrylamide, roughly 300 times what the U.S. Environmental Protection Agency allows in a glass of water.[15] At this writing, the U.S. Food and Drug Administration (FDA) and other agencies are still deciding on a course of action or whether one is justified.

Fiber   The indigestible portion of plant foods that moves food through the digestive system and absorbs water.

Fiber

Fiber, often referred to as "bulk" or "roughage," is the indigestible portion of plant foods that helps move foods through the digestive system and softens stools by absorbing water. Fiber also helps to control weight by creating a feeling of fullness without adding extra calories. Although nutritionists have been very vocal in advocating increased fiber intake, the average American consumes only about 12 grams of fiber a day, about half the recommended daily amount of 25 grams.[16]

Insoluble fiber, which is found in bran, whole grain breads and cereals, and most fruits and vegetables, is associated with these gastrointestinal benefits and also has been found to reduce the risk for several forms of cancer. *Soluble fiber* appears to be a factor in lowering blood cholesterol levels, which thereby reduces risk for cardiovascular disease. Major sources of soluble fiber in the diet include oat bran, dried beans (such as kidney, garbanzo, pinto, and navy beans), and some fruits and vegetables.

The best way to increase intake of dietary fiber is to eat more complex carbohydrates, such as whole grains, fruits, vegetables, dried peas and beans, nuts, and seeds. As with most nutritional advice, however, too much of a good thing can pose problems. Sudden increases in dietary fiber may cause flatulence (intestinal gas), cramping, or a bloated feeling. Consuming plenty of water or other liquids may reduce such side effects.

A few years ago, fiber was thought by some to be the remedy for just about everything. Much of this hope was exaggerated. However, current research does support many benefits of fiber, which include the following.[17]

- *Protection against colon and rectal cancer.* One of the leading causes of cancer deaths in the United States, colorectal cancer is much rarer in countries having diets high in fiber and low in animal fat. Several studies contributed to the theory that fiber-rich diets, particularly those including insoluble fiber, prevent the development of precancerous growths. Whether this was because more fiber helps to move foods through the colon faster, which thereby reduces the colon's contact time with cancer-causing substances, or because insoluble fiber reduces bile acids and certain bacterial enzymes that may promote cancer, remained in question. However, more recent findings indicate that fiber may not be as protective against colon cancer as once believed.[18] Earlier studies failed to adequately control for other factors that may have caused an apparent protective effect. While fiber is still promoted for its possible benefits, more research is necessary.
- *Protection against breast cancer.* Research into the effects of fiber on breast cancer risks is inconclusive. However, some studies have indicated that wheat bran (rich in insoluble fiber) reduces blood estrogen levels, which may affect the risk for breast cancer. Another theory is that people who eat more fiber have proportionally less fat in their diets, and this is what reduces overall risk.

- *Protection against constipation.* Insoluble fiber, consumed with adequate fluids, is the safest, most effective way to prevent or treat constipation. The fiber acts like a sponge, absorbing moisture and producing softer, bulkier stools that are easily passed. Fiber also helps produce gas, which in turn may initiate a bowel movement.
- *Protection against diverticulosis.* About one American in ten over the age of 40 and at least one in three over the age of 50 suffers from *diverticulosis,* a condition in which tiny bulges or pouches form on the large intestinal wall. These bulges become irritated and cause chronic pain if under strain from constipation. Insoluble fiber helps to reduce constipation and discomfort.
- *Protection against heart disease.* Many studies have indicated that soluble fiber (found in oat bran, barley, and fruit pectin) helps reduce blood cholesterol, primarily by lowering low density lipoprotein (LDL), or "bad" cholesterol. Whether this reduction is a direct effect or occurs instead through the displacement of fat calories by fiber calories or through intake of other nutrients, such as iron, remains in question.
- *Protection against diabetes.* Some studies suggest that soluble fiber improves control of blood sugar and can reduce the need for insulin or medication in people with diabetes. Exactly why isn't clear, but soluble fiber seems to delay the emptying of the stomach and slow the absorption of glucose by the intestine. The significance of this effect has been downgraded in recent years, however.[19]
- *Protection against obesity.* Because most high-fiber foods are high in carbohydrates and low in fat, they help control caloric intake. Many take longer to chew, which slows you down at the table and makes you feel full sooner.

Most experts believe that Americans should double their current consumption of dietary fiber to 20 to 30 grams per day for most people and perhaps to 40 to 50 grams for others. Here are some tips for increasing your fiber intake.

1. Eat a variety of foods. Aim for at least 5 servings of fruits and vegetables and 3 to 6 servings of whole grain breads, cereals, and legumes per day throughout the day.
2. Consume less processed food.
3. Eat the skins of fruits and vegetables.
4. Get your fiber from foods rather than from pills or powders. Pills and powders do not supply enough essential nutrients.
5. Spread out your fiber intake.
6. Drink plenty of liquids—at least 64 ounces of water daily.

Fats

Fats (or *lipids*), another group of basic nutrients, are perhaps the most misunderstood of the body's required energy sources. Fats play a vital role in maintaining healthy skin and hair, insulating body organs against shock, maintaining body

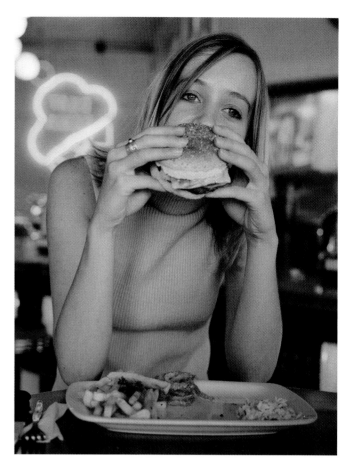

It takes information and planning to make smart menu choices, whether you are eating out, in your dining hall, or preparing a meal at home.

temperature, and promoting healthy cell function. Fats make foods taste better and carry the fat-soluble vitamins A, D, E, and K to the cells. They also provide a concentrated form of energy in the absence of sufficient amounts of carbohydrates. If fats perform all these functions, why are we constantly urged to cut back on them?

Although moderate consumption of fats is essential to health, overconsumption can be dangerous. **Triglycerides,** which make up about 95 percent of total body fat, are the most common form of fat circulating in the blood. When we consume too many calories, the liver converts the excess into triglycerides, which are stored throughout our bodies.

Fats Basic nutrients composed of carbon and hydrogen atoms; needed for the proper functioning of cells, insulation of body organs against shock, maintenance of body temperature, and healthy skin and hair.

Triglycerides The most common form of fat in the body; excess calories consumed are converted into triglycerides and stored as body fat.

The remaining 5 percent of body fat is composed of substances such as **cholesterol,** which can accumulate on the inner walls of arteries and narrow the channel through which blood flows. This buildup, called **plaque,** is a major cause of *atherosclerosis* (hardening of the arteries). At one time, the amount of circulating cholesterol in the blood was thought to be crucial. Current thinking is that the actual amount of circulating cholesterol itself is not as important as is the ratio of total cholesterol to a group of compounds called **high-density lipoproteins (HDLs).** Lipoproteins are the transport facilitators for cholesterol in the blood. High-density lipoproteins are capable of transporting more cholesterol than are **low-density lipoproteins (LDLs).** Whereas LDLs transport cholesterol to the body's cells, HDLs apparently transport circulating cholesterol to the liver for metabolism and elimination from the body. People with a high percentage of HDLs therefore appear to be at lower risk for developing cholesterol-clogged arteries. Regular vigorous exercise plays a part in reducing cholesterol by increasing HDLs.

MUFAs and PUFAs: Unsaturated "Good Guys"

Fat cells consist of chains of carbon and hydrogen atoms. Those that are unable to hold any more hydrogen in their chemical structure are labeled **saturated fats.** They generally come from animal sources, such as meats and dairy products, and are solid at room temperature. **Unsaturated fats,** which come from plants and include most vegetable oils, are generally liquid at room temperature and have room for additional hydrogen atoms in their chemical structure. The

---

Cholesterol   A form of fat circulating in the blood that can accumulate on the inner walls of arteries.

Plaque   Cholesterol buildup on the inner walls of arteries, which causes a narrowing of the channel through which blood flows; a major cause of atherosclerosis.

High-density lipoproteins (HDLs)   Compounds that facilitate the transport of cholesterol in the blood to the liver for metabolism and elimination from the body.

Low-density lipoproteins (LDLs)   Compounds that facilitate the transport of cholesterol in the blood to the body's cells.

Saturated fats   Fats that are unable to hold anymore hydrogen in their chemical structure; derived mostly from animal sources; solid at room temperature.

Unsaturated fats   Fats that do have room for more hydrogen in their chemical structure; derived mostly from plants; liquid at room temperature.

Trans-fatty acids   Fatty acids that are produced when polyunsaturated oils are hydrogenated to make them more solid.

---

terms *monounsaturated fat* (MUFA) and *polyunsaturated fat* (PUFA) refer to the relative number of hydrogen atoms that are missing. Peanut and olive oils are high in monounsaturated fats, whereas corn, sunflower, and safflower oils are high in polyunsaturated fats.

There is currently a great deal of controversy about which type of unsaturated fat is most beneficial. Although nutritional researchers in the 1980s favored PUFAs, today many believe that they may decrease beneficial HDL levels while reducing LDL levels. PUFAs come in two forms: omega-3 fatty acids and omega-6 fatty acids. MUFAs, such as olive oil, seem to lower LDL levels and increase HDL levels and thus are currently the preferred, or least harmful, fats. Nevertheless, a tablespoon of olive oil gives you a hefty 10 grams of MUFAs.

Reducing Fat in Your Diet   Want to cut the fat? These guidelines offer a good place to start.

- *Know what you are putting in your mouth.* Read food labels. Remember that no more than 10 percent of your total calories should come from saturated fat, and no more than 30 percent should come from all forms of fat.
- *Choose fat-free or low-fat versions of cakes, cookies, crackers, or chips.* Remember, though, that calories still count. Don't eat *more* chips just because they're lower in fat.
- *Use olive oil for baking and sautéing.* Animal studies have shown that it doesn't raise cholesterol or promote the growth of tumors.
- *Whenever possible, use liquid, diet, or whipped margarine.* These products have far less trans-fatty acid than solid fat.
- *Choose lean meats, fish, or poultry.* Remove skin. Broil or bake whenever possible. In general, the more well-done the meat, the fewer the calories. Drain off fat after cooking.
- *Choose fewer cold cuts, bacon, sausages, hot dogs, and organ meats.* Be careful of those products claiming to be "95 percent fat-free," because they may still have high levels of fat.
- *Select nonfat dairy products whenever possible.* Part-skim-milk cheeses, such as mozzarella, farmer's, lappi, and ricotta, are good choices.
- *When cooking, use substitutes for butter, margarine, oils, sour cream, mayonnaise, and salad dressings.* Chicken broths, wine, vinegar, and low-calorie dressings provide flavor with less fat.
- *Think of your food intake as an average over a day or a couple of days.* If you have a high-fat breakfast or lunch, balance it with a low-fat dinner.

Trans-Fatty Acids: Still Bad?   Since 1961, Americans have decreased their intake of butter by more than 43 percent. Instead, they have substituted margarine, which became known as the "better butter" after reports labeled unsaturated fats the "heart-healthy" alternative. But a widely publicized landmark study in 1990 questioned the benefits of margarine; it indicated that margarine contains fats that raise blood cholesterol at least as much as the saturated fat in butter does.[20] The culprits? **Trans-fatty acids,** fatty acids that have unusual shapes, are produced when polyunsaturated oils are *hydrogenated,* a process in which hydrogen is added to unsaturated fats to make them more solid and resistant to chemical change.[21] Besides raising cholesterol levels, trans-fatty acids have been implicated in certain types of cancer.[22]

A more recent study found that the trans-fatty acids found in margarine may in fact pose an even greater risk for heart disease than does the saturated fat in butter and lard.[23] But before you dash out and fill your refrigerator with butter, be aware that this research is controversial.

Keep in mind that trans-fatty acids, even monounsaturated acids, alter blood cholesterol the same way as some saturated fats do; they raise LDL and lower HDL cholesterol.[24] The American Heart Association has steadfastly stated that because butter is rich in both saturated fat and cholesterol, whereas margarine is made from vegetable fat with no dietary cholesterol, margarine is still preferable to butter.[25] Others disagree, claiming that the occasional use of butter is preferable to margarine.[26] The majority of experts claims that the whole area of trans-fatty acids needs much more research. As a result, they advise that moderation in all fat intake is probably the best rule of thumb.[27] Whenever possible, opt for condiments other than butter or margarine on your bread; use jams, fat-free cream cheese, garlic, or other toppings. Some experts advocate using low-fat salad dressings as toppings for bread and pasta, or using olive oil in moderation to add a bit of flavor.

New Fat Advice: Is More Fat Ever Better?   Although most of this chapter has promoted the age-old recommendation to reduce saturated fat, avoid trans-fatty acids, and eat more monounsaturated fats, some experts worry that we have gone too far. In fact, according to these researchers, our zeal to eat no fat or low-fat foods may be one of the greatest causes of obesity in America today. According to the American Heart Association, eating fewer than 15 percent of our calories as fat (less than 34 grams a day on a 2,000 calorie diet) can actually increase blood triglycerides to levels that promote heart disease, while lowering levels of protective HDLs ("good" cholesterol). There is also a concern that very low-fat diets may lead to shortages of essential fatty acid (EFA) in the diet.[28]

Not all fat is bad. In addition to the benefits already mentioned, dietary fat supplies the two EFAs that we must receive from our diets, *linoleic acid* and *alpha-linolenic acid.* These two fats are needed to make hormone-like compounds that control immune function, pain perception, and inflammation, to name a few key benefits.[29]

Although linoleic acid and alpha-linolenic acid are both polyunsaturated fats, they are actually quite different in what they do. Linoleic acid, a member of the *omega-6* family of fats (found in soybeans, peanuts, corn, and sunflower seeds), reduces blood levels of total cholesterol and LDL ("bad" cholesterol) when consumed in reasonable amounts. Alpha-linolenic acid is part of the *omega-3* fats, and is found in flax, canola oil, sardines, spinach, kale, green leafy vegetables, walnuts, and wheat germ. Alpha-linolenic acid is converted

to two other beneficial omega-3 fats in the body, but you get a much bigger dose of those nutrients by eating cold water fish such as salmon and tuna that have abundant supplies of omega-3. Today, Americans eat 17 times more omega-6 fats than omega 3s, and most experts agree that we need a more balanced approach.[30]

While both of these essential fats are important, too much linoleic acid may promote blood clots and constrict arteries, which leads to inflammation and damaged blood vessels. Recent research indicates that a form of linoleic acid known as conjugated linoleic acid (CLA) seems to be effective in inhibiting breast cancer and, in fact, may moderate the negative effects of high-fat diets. CLA is found in minute quantities in meat and dairy products, so eating small portions of these foods as part of a mostly plant-based diet may provide the health benefits of CLA without the risks of consuming too much fat.[31] Consuming more alpha-linolenic acid reduces risks for blood clots and abnormal heart rhythms and may improve immune function. The best rule of thumb is to balance, following these recommendations.[32]

- Eat fatty fish (bluefish, herring, mackerel, salmon, sardines, or tuna) at least twice weekly.
- Substitute soy and canola oils for corn, safflower, and sunflower oils. Keep using olive oil.
- Add healthy doses of green, leafy vegetables, walnuts, walnut oil, and ground flaxseed to your diet to increase intake of alpha-linolenic acid
- Limit processed and convenience foods, since they often contain harmful saturated and trans-fats.
- Pick the MUFA or PUFA with the fewest calories and most nutrients.

Vitamins

Vitamins are potent and essential organic compounds that promote growth and help maintain life and health. Every minute of every day, vitamins help maintain nerves and skin, produce blood cells, build bones and teeth, heal wounds, and convert food energy to body energy. And they do all of this without adding any calories to your diet.

Age, heat, and other environmental conditions can destroy vitamins in food. Vitamins can be classified as either *fat soluble,* which means they are absorbed through the intestinal tract with the help of fats, or *water soluble,* which means they are dissolved easily in water. Vitamins A, D, E, and K are fat soluble; B complex vitamins and vitamin C are water soluble. Fat-soluble vitamins tend to be stored in the body, and toxic accumulations in the liver may cause cirrhosis-like symptoms. Water-soluble vitamins generally are excreted and cause few toxicity problems (Table 9.2).

(text continues on page 249)

> **Vitamins**   Essential organic compounds that promote growth and reproduction and help maintain life and health.

Table 9.2
A Guide to Vitamins

Vitamin	Best Sources	Chief Functions in the Body
Water-Soluble Vitamins		
Thiamin 1.5 mg (RDA + RDI)	Meat, pork, liver, fish, poultry, whole grain and enriched breads, cereals, pasta, nuts, legumes, wheat germ, oats	Helps enzymes release energy from carbohydrate; supports normal appetite and nervous system function
Riboflavin 1.7 mg (RDA + RDI)	Milk, dark green vegetables, yogurt, cottage cheese, liver, meat, whole grain or enriched breads and cereals	Helps enzymes release energy from carbohydrate, fat, and protein; promotes healthy skin and normal vision
Niacin 20 mg NE (RDA + RDI)	Meat, eggs, poultry, fish, milk, whole grain and enriched breads and cereals, nuts, legumes, peanuts, nutritional yeast, all protein foods	Helps enzymes release energy from energy nutrients; promotes health of skin, nerves, and digestive system
Vitamin B_6 2.0 mg (RDA + RDI)	Meat, poultry, fish, shellfish, legumes, whole grain products, green, leafy vegetables, bananas	Protein and fat metabolism, formation of antibodies and red blood cells; helps convert tryptophan to niacin
Folate 400 μg (DFE + RDA)	Green, leafy vegetables, liver, legumes, seeds	Red blood cell formation; protein metabolism; new cell division; prevents neural tube defects
Vitamin B_{12} 2.4 mg (RDA)	Meat, fish, poultry, shellfish, milk, cheese, eggs, nutritional yeast	Helps maintain nerve cells; red blood cell formation; synthesis of genetic material
Pantothenic acid 5–7 mg (AI)	Widespread in foods	Coenzyme in energy metabolism
Biotin 30 μg (AI)	Widespread in foods	Coenzyme in energy metabolism; fat synthesis; glycogen formation
Vitamin C (ascorbic acid) (RDI + RDA) 60 mg	Citrus fruits, cabbage-type vegetables, tomatoes, potatoes, dark green vegetables, peppers, lettuce, cantaloupe, strawberries, mangos, papayas	Synthesis of collagen (helps heal wounds, maintains bone and teeth, strengthens blood vessels); antioxidant; strengthens resistance to infection; helps body's absorption of iron
Fat-Soluble Vitamins		
Vitamin A 5,000 I.U.	Retinal: fortified milk and margarine, cream, cheese, butter, eggs, liver. Carotene: spinach and other dark leafy greens, broccoli, deep orange fruits (apricots, peaches, cantaloupe) and vegetables (squash, carrots, sweet potatoes, pumpkin)	Vision; growth and repair of body tissues; reproduction; bone and tooth formation; immunity; cancer protection; hormone synthesis
Vitamin D 400–600 I.U. (RDA + RDI)	Self-synthesis with sunlight, fortified milk, fortified margarine, eggs, liver, fish	Calcium and phosphorus metabolism (bone and tooth formation); aids body's absorption of calcium
Vitamin E 30 I.U. (RDA + RDI)	Vegetable oils, green leafy vegetables, wheat germ, whole-grain products, butter, liver, egg yolk, milk fat, nuts, seeds	Protects red blood cells; antioxidant; stabilization of cell membranes
Vitamin K 70–140 μg	Liver; green, leafy, and cabbage-type vegetables; milk	Bacterial synthesis in digestive tract. Synthesis of blood-clotting proteins and a blood protein that regulates blood calcium

Table 9.2
A Guide to Vitamins

Deficiency Symptoms	Toxicity Symptoms
Beriberi, edema, heart irregularity, mental confusion, muscle weakness, low morale, impaired growth	Rapid pulse, weakness, headaches, insomnia, irritability
Eye problems, skin disorders around nose and mouth	None reported, but an excess of any of the B vitamins can cause a deficiency of the others
Pellagra: skin rash on parts exposed to sun, loss of appetite, dizziness, weakness, irritability, fatigue, mental confusion, indigestion	Flushing, nausea, headaches, cramps, ulcer irritation, heartburn, abnormal liver function, low blood pressure
Nervous disorders, skin rash, muscle weakness, anemia, convulsions, kidney stones	Depression, fatigue, irritability, headaches, numbness, damage to nerves, difficulty walking
Anemia, heartburn, diarrhea, smooth tongue depression, poor growth	Diarrhea, insomnia, irritability, may mask a vitamin B_{12} deficiency
Anemia, smooth tongue, fatigue, nerve degeneration progressing to paralysis	None reported
Rare; sleep disturbances, nausea, fatigue	Occasional diarrhea
Loss of appetite, nausea, depression, muscle pain, weakness, fatigue, rash	None reported
Scurvy, anemia, atherosclerotic plaques, depression, frequent infections, bleeding gums, loosened teeth, pinpoint hemorrhages, muscle degeneration, rough skin, bone fragility, poor wound healing, hysteria	Nausea, abdominal cramps, diarrhea, breakdown of red blood cells in persons with certain genetic disorders, deficiency symptoms may appear at first on withdrawal of high doses
Night blindness, rough skin, susceptibility to infection, impaired bone growth, abnormal tooth and jaw alignment, eye problems leading to blindness, impaired growth	Red blood cell breakage, nosebleeds, abdominal cramps, nausea, diarrhea, weight loss, blurred vision, irritability, loss of appetite, bone pain, dry skin, rashes, hair loss, cessation of menstruation, growth retardation
Rickets in children; osteomalacia in adults; abnormal growth, joint pain, soft bones	Raised blood calcium, constipation, weight loss, irritability, weakness, nausea, kidney stones, mental and physical retardation
Muscle wasting, weakness, red blood cell breakage, anemia, hemorrhaging, fibrocystic breast disease	Interference with anticlotting medication, general discomfort
Hemorrhaging	Interference with anticlotting medication; may cause jaundice

Note: Values increase among women who are pregnant or lactating.
Sources: From *Personal Nutrition,* 2nd ed., by Marie Boyle and Gail Zyla. Reprinted with permission of Wadsworth, a division of Thomson Learning; National Academy Press, "Reading Room." www.Nap.edu

News from the World of Nutrition Research

Nutritional experts from the international community meet bi-annually for the Linus Pauling Institute International Conference on Diet and Optimum Health, sponsored by Oregon State University. Below is a synopsis of research from the last decade and summary opinion conclusions from large clinical trials or longitudinal dietary studies, based on reports presented at these conferences.

- When considered together, genetics, sedentary lifestyle, and consumption of too much dietary fat are probably not as responsible for our steep increases in obesity in the United States as the recommendation to eat less saturated fat and to eat more carbohydrates. When these recommendations hit the public media, Americans shifted to nonfat or low-fat diets and consumed more refined carbohydrates. One need only look at the ingredients of many nonfat or low-fat foods to see the hefty doses of sugars and refined starches that tempt our palates. Experts believe that in our attempts to reduce saturated fats, we may have actually increased prevalence of cardiovascular disease (CVD) and obesity.
- There is little support for the theory that increasing your consumption of dietary fat will increase your risk of breast or colon cancer. In fact, the highest rates of these cancers appear to be among those with the lowest overall fat intake. Experts are focusing on the type of fat we consume—not the total amount consumed—and are recommending higher rates of consumption of monounsaturated, vegetable-based fats, such as olive and canola oil. As a result of

these studies, the American Heart Association is likely to move away from recommending nonfat/low-fat products, because they may actually cause people to eat more. Instead, they will focus on encouraging more olive oil and vegetable-based fats in the diet.
- Diets focusing on the glycemic index (a measure of rate of carbohydrate absorption after a meal) seem to be the most effective. Low-glycemic-index foods (which contain more complex carbohydrates, normal levels of monounsaturated fats, and reasonable amounts of proteins) suppress appetite longer, raise high-density lipoprotein (HDL) cholesterol levels, and seem to protect against disease (hence the call for more olive oil indicated above). The new U.S. Dietary Guidelines are likely to be modified to reflect this body of work. Bad news: Potatoes don't fare well on this index. Good news: Pasta remains on the positive side of the index.
- There is dramatic new evidence that eating olive oil and other monounsaturated fats found in certain salad dressings may be protective for CVD and cancer. But if you want super protection, eating olive oil and similar fats with green, leafy vegetables (which contain nutrients that are abundant in chlorophyll) may reduce risk sevenfold.
- Increases in obesity, CVD risks, and certain cancers and diabetes may in fact be attributable in large part to displacing monounsaturated fats (e.g., olive and canola oils) with refined carbohydrates and processed sugars, as well as hydrogenated fat versions found in low-fat and nonfat foods. (Check your labels when purchasing low-fat and nonfat items at the store.)
- White tea is the hottest new food/beverage surfacing as a possible protective mechanism for cancer, particularly

colon cancer. Preliminary research is indicating a sevenfold reduction in colon cancer risks and other cancers from 2 to 3 servings of white tea per day.
- Lipoic acid and acetyl carnitine (natural, not synthetic forms) have shown amazing results in mice and pig studies. (Natural forms of acetyl carnitine are currently available in health food stores, but natural forms of lipoic acid are not yet available.) When these substances are combined and given in modest doses to older animals, their brain function reverts to that of younger animals within five to six weeks. The combination of these two seems to have significant effects on the wear-and-tear of aging. Animals fed these substances regenerate brain cells and repair damaged ones. Human trials will begin soon. Doses for effectiveness are not known.
- There seems to be little evidence that supplementing with chromium or selenium is of any benefit.
- Are you using vitamin E as a health aid? You may want to rethink this practice. According to antioxidant experts, newer research implicates vitamin E supplementation with reducing HDL levels and a variety of other potential risks rather than benefits.
- Folic acid has shown promising results in reducing CVD and cancer risks. Deficiencies in folate also lead to chromosome damage.
- Researchers are gaining new information on the importance of iron. Too much or too little iron can cause damage to mitochondria and oxidative stress damage to cells.

Source: Linus Pauling Institute, Public Sessions, International Conference on Diet and Optimum Health, May 2001 and May 2003, Portland, Oregon.

Despite many media suggestions to the contrary, few Americans suffer from true vitamin deficiencies if they eat a diet containing all of the food groups at least part of the time. Nevertheless, Americans continue to purchase large quantities of vitamin supplements. For the most part, vitamin supplements are unnecessary and, in certain instances, may even be harmful. Overusing them can even lead to a toxic condition known as **hypervitaminosis.**

Minerals

Minerals are the inorganic, indestructible elements that aid physiological processes within the body. Without minerals, vitamins could not be absorbed. Minerals are readily excreted and are usually not toxic. **Macrominerals** are those minerals that the body needs in fairly large amounts: sodium, calcium, phosphorus, magnesium, potassium, sulfur, and chloride. **Trace minerals** include iron, zinc, manganese, copper, iodine, and cobalt. Only very small amounts of these minerals are needed, and serious problems may result if excesses or deficiencies occur (Table 9.3 on pages 250 and 251).

Although minerals are necessary for body function, there are limits on the amounts we should consume. Americans tend to overuse or underuse certain minerals.

Sodium   Sodium is necessary for the regulation of blood and body fluids, transmission of nerve impulses, heart activity, and certain metabolic functions. However, we consume much more than we need. It is estimated that the average adult who does not sweat profusely needs only 500 mg of sodium (about ¼ teaspoon) per day, yet the average American consumes 6,000 to 12,000 mg. The Recommended Dietary Allowance (RDA) Subcommittee recommends restricting sodium to no more than 2,400 mg per day; less is better.

The most common form of sodium in the American diet comes from table salt. However, table salt accounts for only 15 percent of sodium intake. The remainder comes from water and from highly processed foods that are infused with sodium to enhance flavor. Pickles, salty snack foods, processed cheeses, many breads and bakery products, and smoked meats and sausages often contain several hundred mg of sodium per serving. Many fast-food entrees and convenience entrees pack 500 to 1,000 mg of sodium per serving.

Many experts believe that there is a link between excessive sodium intake and hypertension (high blood pressure). Although this theory is controversial, researchers recommend that hypertensive Americans cut back on sodium to reduce their risk for cardiovascular disorders.[33] Osteoporosis researchers are confirming that high sodium intake may increase calcium loss in urine, which increases your risk for debilitating fractures as you age.

Calcium   The issue of calcium consumption has gained national attention with the rising incidence of osteoporosis among elderly women. Although calcium plays a vital role in building strong bones and teeth, muscle contraction, blood clotting, nerve impulse transmission, regulating heartbeat, and fluid balance within cells, most Americans do not consume the 1,200 mg of calcium per day established by the RDA.

Because calcium intake is so important throughout life for maintaining strong bones, it is critical to consume the minimum required amount each day. More than half of our calcium intake usually comes from milk, one of the richest sources of dietary calcium. Calcium-fortified orange juice and soy milk provide a good way to get calcium if you do not drink dairy milk. Many green, leafy vegetables are good sources of calcium, but some contain oxalic acid, which makes their calcium harder to absorb. Spinach, chard, and beet greens are not particularly good sources of calcium, whereas broccoli, cauliflower, and many peas and beans offer good supplies (pinto beans and soybeans are among the best). Other good sources include nuts, seeds, molasses, citrus fruits, and raisins. Bone meal is not a recommended calcium source because of possible contamination.

Do you consume carbonated soft drinks? Be aware that the added phosphoric acid (phosphate) in these drinks can cause you to excrete extra calcium, which may result in calcium being pulled out of your bones. Calcium/phosphorus imbalance may lead to kidney stones and other calcification problems as well as to increased atherosclerotic plaque.

We also know that sunlight increases the manufacture of vitamin D in the body and is therefore like having an extra calcium source because vitamin D improves absorption of calcium. Stress, however, contributes to calcium depletion. It is generally best to take calcium throughout the day; consume it with foods containing protein, vitamin D, and vitamin C for optimum absorption. Experts vary on which type of supplemental calcium is absorbed most readily and efficiently, although aspartate and citrate salts of calcium often are recommended. The best way to obtain calcium, like all nutrients, is to consume it as part of a balanced diet.

Iron   Worldwide, iron deficiency is the most common nutrient deficiency; it affects more than 1 billion people. In developing countries, more than one-third of the children and women of childbearing age suffer from *iron-deficiency anemia.*[34] **Anemia** is a problem resulting from the body's inability to produce

(text continues on page 252)

Hypervitaminosis   A toxic condition caused by overuse of vitamin supplements.

Minerals   Inorganic, indestructible elements that aid physiological processes.

Macrominerals   Minerals that the body needs in fairly large amounts.

Trace minerals   Minerals that the body needs in only very small amounts.

Anemia   Iron deficiency disease that results from the body's inability to produce hemoglobin.

Table 9.3
A Guide to Minerals

Mineral	Significant Sources	Chief Functions in the Body
Calcium RDA = 800–1,200 mg+ RDI = 1,000 mg	Milk and milk products, small fish (with bones), tofu, greens, legumes	Principal mineral of bones and teeth; involved in muscle contraction and relaxation, nerve function, blood clotting, blood pressure
Phosphorus RDA = 1,000 mg	All animal tissues	Part of every cell; involved in acid-base balance
Magnesium RDA = 400 mg	Nuts, legumes, whole grains, dark green vegetables, seafood, chocolate, cocoa	Involved in bone mineralization, protein synthesis, enzyme action, normal muscular contraction, nerve transmission
Sodium RDA = 500 mg DRV = 2,400 mg	Salt, soy sauce; processed foods; cured, canned, pickled, and many boxed foods	Helps maintain normal fluid and acid-base balance
Chloride RDA = 750 mg	Salt, soy sauce; processed foods	Part of stomach acid, necessary for proper digestion, fluid balance
Potassium RDA = 2,000 mg DRV = 3,500 mg	All whole foods: meats, milk, fruits, vegetables, grains, legumes	Facilitates many reactions including protein synthesis, fluid balance, nerve transmission, and contraction of muscles
Iodine RDA = 150 μg RDI = 150 μg	Iodized salt, seafood	Part of thyroxine, which regulates metabolism
Iron RDA = 18 mg RDI = 18 mg	Beef, fish, poultry, shellfish, eggs, legumes, dried fruits	Hemoglobin formation; part of myoglobin; energy utilization
Zinc RDA = 15 mg RDI = 15 mg	Protein-containing foods: meats, fish, poultry, grains, vegetables	Part of many enzymes; present in insulin; involved in making genetic material and proteins, immunity, vitamin A transport, taste, wound healing, making sperm, normal fetal development
Copper RDA = 2 mg RDI = 2 mg	Meats, drinking water	Absorption of iron; part of several enzymes
Fluoride 1.5–4.0 mg	Drinking water (if naturally fluoride-containing or fluoridated), tea, seafood	Formation of bones and teeth; helps make teeth resistant to decay and bones resistant to mineral loss
Selenium 50–70 μg	Seafood, meats, grains	Helps protect body compounds from oxidation
Chromium 50–200 μg	Meats, unrefined foods, fats, vegetable oils	Associated with insulin and required for the release of energy from glucose
Molybdenum 75–250 μg	Legumes, cereals, organ meats	Facilitates, with enzymes, many cell processes
Manganese 2.0–5.0 mg	Widely distributed in foods	Facilitates, with enzymes, many cell processes

Table 9.3
A Guide to Minerals

Deficiency Symptoms	Toxicity Symptoms
Stunted growth in children; bone loss (osteoporosis) in adults	Excess calcium is excreted except in hormonal imbalance states
Unknown	Can create relative deficiency of calcium
Weakness, confusion, depressed pancreatic hormone secretion, growth failure, behavioral disturbances, muscle spasms	Not known
Muscle cramps, mental apathy, loss of appetite	Hypertension (in salt-sensitive persons)
Growth failure in children, muscle cramps, mental apathy, loss of appetite	Normally harmless (the gas chlorine is a poison but evaporates from water); disturbed acid-base balance; vomiting
Muscle weakness, paralysis, confusion; can cause death, accompanies dehydration	Causes muscular weakness; triggers vomiting; if given into a vein, can stop the heart
Goiter, cretinism	Very high intakes depress thyroid activity
Anemia: weakness, pallor, headaches, reduced resistance to infection, inability to concentrate	Iron overload: infections, liver injury
Growth failure in children, delayed development of sexual organs, loss of taste, poor wound healing	Fever, nausea, vomiting, diarrhea
Anemia, bone changes (rare in human beings)	Unknown except as part of a rare hereditary disease (Wilson's disease)
Susceptibility to tooth decay and bone loss	Fluorosis (discoloration of teeth)
Anemia (rare)	Digestive system disorders
Diabetes-like condition marked by inability to use glucose normally	Unknown as a nutrition disorder. Occupational exposures damage skin and kidneys.
Unknown	Enzyme inhibition
In animals: poor growth, nervous system disorders, abnormal reproduction	Poisoning, nervous system disorders

Because we have less information about minerals than about vitamins, RDA recommendations are estimates of minimum requirements.

Sources: From *Personal Nutrition,* 2d ed., by Marie Boyle and Gail Zyla and *Nutrition Concepts and Controversies,* 9th ed., by F. Sizer and E. Whitney. © 2003. Reprinted with permission of Wadsworth, a division of Thomson Learning.

hemoglobin, the bright red, oxygen-carrying component of the blood. In the United States, iron deficiency anemia is less prevalent, but it still affects 10 percent of toddlers, adolescent girls, and women of childbearing age, which makes prevention a high priority.[35] People with iron-deficiency anemia also may develop a condition known as **pica,** an appetite for ice, clay, paste, and other nonfood substances that do not actually contain iron and, in fact, may inhibit iron absorption.

How much iron do adults need? Females ages 19 to 50 need about 18 mg per day, and males ages 19 to 50 need about 10 mg.

When iron deficiency occurs, body cells receive less oxygen, and carbon dioxide wastes are removed less efficiently. As a result, the iron-deficient person feels tired and run down. While iron deficiency in the diet is a common cause of anemia, anemia also can result from blood loss, cancers, ulcers, and other conditions. Generally, women are more likely to develop iron-deficiency problems because they typically eat less than men do and their diets contain less iron. Women having heavy menstrual flow may be at greater risk.

To date, considerable research has linked iron to a host of problems. Iron deficiency may tax the immune system, which causes it to function less effectively. Research suggesting a link between cardiovascular disease and elevated iron stores is inconclusive.[36] Likewise, there appears to be a slight association between iron deficiency and cancer, but the mechanism remains inconclusive.[37]

Iron overload (known as **hemochromatosis**), or iron toxicity due to ingesting too many iron-containing supplements, remains the leading cause of accidental poisoning in small children in the United States. Symptoms of iron toxicity include nausea, vomiting, diarrhea, rapid heartbeat, weak pulse, dizziness, shock, and confusion. Overdoses of as few as five iron tablets containing as little as 200 mg of iron have killed dozens of children.

The Medicinal Value of Food

The old adage "you are what you eat" is indeed a motto to live by. Beneficial foods are termed *functional foods.* This is based on the ancient belief that eating the right foods may not only prevent disease, but also actually cure it. This perspective is gaining credibility among those in the scientific community. (It is also important to be aware of potential interactions between medications you are taking and foods you are eating; see Table 9.4 on pages 254 and 255 for more information on this.)

Two major studies, the *Dietary Approaches to Stop Hypertension Study* and the *Dietary Intervention Study (DIS)* provide compelling evidence that diet may be as effective as drugs are in bringing borderline hypertension back to the normal range. Diet may also play a role in reducing cholesterol and controlling insulin-dependent diabetes.[38] In these clinically controlled trials, subjects were assigned to two groups: treatment and control. In the treatment group, subjects had to follow recommended diets, which were low in fats and high in fiber and fruits. The control group followed typical American dietary intervention. In each study, subjects in the treatment groups showed significantly improved health indicators (blood pressure, cholesterol, and blood glucose in the DIS study), which reflected the potential benefits of diet in improving health and treating disease.

Antioxidants and Your Health

Antioxidants are substances that are believed to protect active people from *oxidative stress* and resultant tissue damage at the cellular level. This damage is believed to occur in a complex process in which *free radicals* (molecules with unpaired electrons that are produced in excess when the body is overly stressed through exposure to toxic substances or events) either damage or kill healthy cells, cell proteins, or genetic material in the cells. Antioxidants produce enzymes that destroy excess free radicals by scavenging them, slowing their formation, and/or actually repairing oxidative stress damage.

There have been many claims about the benefits of antioxidants in reducing risks of cancer and heart disease, improving vision, and slowing or reversing the aging process. Whether these claims produce scientifically validated evidence that a daily dose of antioxidants is truly beneficial remains to be seen. Initial results from numerous studies appear to support the benefits of at least some antioxidants. For example, the beneficial effects of moderate doses of vitamin C appear to be well substantiated.[39] However, a recent British study of 30 healthy men and women showed that taking a daily 500 mg supplement of vitamin C had both positive and negative effects on DNA. Similarly, a widely cited Finnish study of 29,000 men reported that for those who smoked a pack of cigarettes a day and took daily beta-carotene supplements, risk of lung cancer actually increased by 18 percent over those who took no supplement.[40]

Other antioxidants that had received initial support in the research now have begun to lose their favor in scientific circles. For example, vitamin E, which was once thought capable of preventing heart disease and cancer, has increasingly received bad reviews from critics who point out that new research doesn't point to any benefits.

Pica Iron deficiency disease characterized by craving for certain foods and substances.

Hemochromatosis Iron toxicity due to excess consumption

Antioxidants Substances believed to protect active people from oxidative stress and resultant tissue damage at the cellular level.

In addition to vitamins E and C, other nutrients, including several key minerals, are also important in the destruction of free radicals. Among them are selenium, copper, zinc, iron, and manganese.[41]

Beta-carotene is one of the many compounds classified as **carotenoids.** Carotenoids are part of the red, orange, and yellow pigments found in fruits and vegetables. They are fat soluble, transported in the blood by lipoproteins, and stored in the fatty tissues of the body. Beta-carotene, the most researched carotenoid, is a precursor of vitamin A; this means that vitamin A can be produced in the body from beta-carotene. Like vitamin A, beta-carotene has antioxidant properties.[42]

Although there are more than 600 carotenoids in nature, two that have received increasing attention recently are *lycopene* (found in tomatoes), and *lutein* (found in green, leafy vegetables such as spinach, broccoli, kale, and brussels sprouts). Both are believed to be more beneficial than beta-carotene in preventing disease.

The National Cancer Institute and the American Cancer Society have endorsed lycopene as possibly having the ability to reduce the risk of cancer. A landmark study assessing the effects of tomato-based foods on cancer reported that men who ate ten or more servings of lycopene-rich foods per week had a 45 percent reduced risk of prostate cancer.[43]

Lutein is touted most often as a means of protecting aging eyes, particularly from age-related macular degeneration (ARMD), a leading cause of blindness for people aged 65 and over. Although researchers do not know what causes ARMD, they do know that older age, light-colored eyes, smoking, and exposure to sunlight increase a person's risk of developing it. They speculate that oxidative damage may be the crux of the problem, and thus, antioxidants may be a possible means of prevention.[44] Researchers at the National Eye Institute found that those with the highest blood levels of lutein and other antioxidants found in foods were 70 percent less likely to develop ARMD than were those with the lowest levels. Researchers in the Nurses Health study found that eating spinach more than five days a week lowered risk by 47 percent and also lowered risk of cataract formation.[45]

Other research points to additional potential benefits from lutein. A recent study by Tufts University and Korean investigators revealed a dramatic 88 percent drop in breast cancer in women who had the highest blood concentration of lutein. Researchers at the University of Utah Medical School found that the highest consumers of lutein had the lowest risk of colon cancer. In animals, lutein slowed the growth of breast tumors; in test tubes, it killed cancer cells. Preliminary research also has shown a possible reduction in artery clogging among those consuming the highest amounts of lutein.[46]

According to the experts, the answer is moderation. "Antioxidants should always be taken as part of a well-balanced mixture, either as a diet or as a supplement, and not singly," says Dr. John R. Smythies, a researcher at the University of California–San Diego and author of *Every Person's*

Guide to Antioxidants.[47] Smythies, like many other experts, advocates balance in intake and advises that adults take 500 mg of vitamin C daily and 400 to 800 I.U. of vitamin E, plus 10 mg of beta-carotene. Other antioxidant researchers might go to 1,000 mg of vitamin C for the general population and more vitamin E for anyone who exercises intensely for more than an hour each day.[48] Other experts, such as Dr. Balz Frei at the Linus Pauling Institute, indicate that the "200 rule" might be the best option. This recommendation calls for fruits and vegetables in the diet and a supplement of 200 mg of vitamin C, 200 I.U. of vitamin E, and 200 micrograms of selenium, along with 400 micrograms of folate and 3 mg of vitamin B_6.[49] It is believed that these combinations will reduce the body's overproduction of free radicals, those unstable molecules that can damage healthy cells and turn low-density lipoproteins into artery-clogging compounds.[50] However, even the lowering of free radicals is controversial. Many believe that free radicals are beneficial and kill germs in the same way they kill other cells. From this standpoint, killing off free radicals may lower resistance to harmful pathogens.[51]

To find the right balance, keep in mind the following.

- Keep your daily vitamin C intake (from both food and supplements) below 2,000 mg. Higher amounts may cause diarrhea.
- The upper limit for vitamin E, based only on supplements, is 1,000 mg. That's roughly equivalent to 1,500 I.U. of "D-alpha-tocopherol," sometimes labeled *natural vitamin E.* More than these amounts could increase risk of stroke and uncontrolled bleeding.
- The maximum intake level for selenium from both food and supplements is 400 micrograms per day. Taking more could cause *selenosis,* a toxic reaction marked by hair loss and brittle nails.

Folate

In 1998, the Food and Drug Administration (FDA) began requiring *folate* fortification of all bread, cereal, rice, and macaroni products sold in the United States. This practice, which will boost folate intake by an average of about 100 micrograms daily, is expected to decrease the number of infants born with spina bifida and other neural tube defects.

Folate is a form of vitamin B believed to decrease blood levels of *homocysteine,* an amino acid that has been linked to vascular diseases, and to protect against cardiovascular disease.[52] Homocysteine results from the breakdown of

(text continues on page 256)

Carotenoids   Fat-soluble compounds with antioxidant properties.

Folate   A type of vitamin B believed to decrease levels of homocysteine, an amino acid that has been linked to vascular diseases.

Table 9.4
Common Food-Medication Interactions

Interactions are listed by drug category, followed by examples of specific medications (with generic and brand names). As always, alert your physician and pharmacist to any over-the-counter medications, herbal remedies, and supplements you are taking.

Medications	Interactions with Foods/Nutrients	What to Do
Antibiotics ciprofloxacin *(Cipro)* doxycycline *(Vibramycin)* minocycline *(Minocin)* tetracycline *(Achromycin-V, surrycin)* penicillin *(Ledercillin)*	• Calcium and iron bind with these drugs, which inhibits absorption of the drug plus the calcium and iron. Results in less antibiotic effect, which risks the possibility that the bacteria causing the infection will not be killed. • Food slows down absorption of the drug.	• Do not take within three hours of taking calcium-containing antacids, iron supplements or multivitamin/minerals. • Do not take ciprofloxacin or tetracycline with foods rich in calcium, such as milk and other dairy products. • Take an hour before or two hours after eating.
Cardiovascular Medications *ACE Inhibitors:* captopril *(Capoten)* enalapril *(Vasotec)* lisinopril *(Prinivil, Zestril)* moexipril *(Univasc)*	• Some ACE inhibitors cause hyperkalemia (elevated blood potassium). • Licorice can disrupt potassium balance. • Chili pepper worsens persistent cough side effect. • Food decreases absorption of captopril and moexipril.	• Limit potassium-rich foods and salt substitutes containing potassium. • Avoid natural licorice. • Avoid chili pepper. • Take captopril, moexipril an hour before or two hours after eating.
Blood Thinners: warfarin *(Coumadin)*	• Vitamin K reduces the effectiveness of anticoagulants. If you maintain a consistent intake of vitamin K, your doctor can adjust your medication level accordingly.	• Keep a consistent intake of vitamin K-rich foods: broccoli, spinach, kale, turnip greens, Swiss chard, cauliflower, Brussels sprouts, asparagus, beet, and chicken liver.
Calcium Channel Blockers: amlodipine *(Norvasc)* felodipine *(Plendil)* nifedipine *(Adalat, Procardia)*	• Licorice can increase potassium excretion and sodium reabsorption and raise blood pressure. • Grapefruit can increase blood levels of these drugs up to twofold, which causes blood pressure to drop dangerously low.	• Avoid natural licorice. • Avoid grapefruit, grapefruit juice, and Seville oranges.
HMG-CoA Reductase Inhibitors ("statins"): atorvastatin *(Lipitor)* lovastatin *(Mevacor)* simvastatin *(Zocor)*	• Grapefruit significantly increases blood levels of the drug, which causes more side effects or toxicity. • Soluble fiber inhibits absorption of lovastatin. • Lovastatin is best absorbed with a big meal containing fat. Works best when asleep.	• Avoid grapefruit, grapefruit juice, and Seville oranges. • Don't eat foods rich in fiber, oat bran, or pectin within several hours of taking lovastatin. • If taken once a day, take lovastatin with the evening meal.
Diuretics *Potassium-Losing Diuretics:* lurosumide *(Lasix)* hydrochlorothiazide *(HydroDIURIL)*	• Cause a loss of potassium and magnesium, which require extra potassium and magnesium in the diet or supplements. A potassium deficiency can trigger a heart attack. • Licorice can cause a loss of potassium.	• Eat plenty of potassium-rich foods; apricots, bananas, cantaloupe, dairy foods, dried beans, lentils, oranges, tomatoes. • Eat magnesium-rich foods: bananas, dried beans, lentils, nuts. • Avoid natural licorice.

oz = ounces
mg = milligrams

Table 9.4
Common Food-Medication Interactions

Medications	Interactions with Foods/Nutrients	What to Do
Potassium-Sparing Diuretics: spironolactone *(Aldactone)*	• Prevent kidneys from excreting potassium. Taking in too much potassium can cause irregular heartbeat. • Licorice can disrupt potassium balance.	• Don't overdo foods rich in potassium. • Avoid salt substitutes that contain potassium. • Avoid natural licorice.
Psychotherapeutic Medications buspirone *(Buspar)*—treats anxiety	• Grapefruit significantly increases blood levels of the drug.	• Avoid grapefruit, grapefruit juice, and Seville oranges.
Monoamine Oxidase Inhibitors (MAOIs): isocarboxazid *(Marplan)* phenelzine *(Nardil)* tranylcypromine *(Parmate)*	• Combining with too much caffeine, beer or wine (even alcohol-free) or foods rich in tyramine can lead to a dangerous increase in blood pressure.	• Avoid excessive caffeine; use with caution. • Avoid foods rich in tyramine: aged cheeses and meats, beer, fava beans, sauerkraut, soy sauce, wine. Use small amounts of beer (one or two 12-oz. bottles a day) and wine (2–4 oz. a day) with caution.
Other Medications cilostazol *(Pletal)*—treats circulatory conditions colchicine—treats gout levodopa *(Dopar, Larodopa, Sinernet)*—treats Parkinson's disease theophylline *(Slo-bid, Theobid, Elixophyllin, Theo-Dur, Uniphyl)*—treats asthma and other pulmonary disorders.	• Grapefruit significantly increases blood levels of the drug, which causes increased side effects or drug toxicity. • Grapefruit significantly increases blood levels of the drug. • Pyridoxine decreases effectiveness of the drug. Keep pyridoxine (vitamin B$_6$) intake to less than 5 mg a day. • Caffeine increases theophylline's side effects: dizziness, nausea, vomiting, convulsions, or coma. • Black pepper and chili pepper increase drug blood levels. • Amount of protein and carbohydrate in diet can alter enzyme levels that affect theophylline breakdown.	• Avoid grapefruit, grapefruit juice, and Seville oranges. • Avoid grapefruit, grapefruit juice, and Seville oranges. • Limit foods rich in pyridoxine: chicken, fish, pork, liver, and kidney. Go easy on legumes, nuts, and whole grains. • Avoid excessive caffeine (e.g. coffee, tea, cola). • Avoid excessive black pepper or chili pepper. • Keep intake of protein and carbohydrate consistent to keep drug levels consistent.

oz = ounces
mg = milligrams

Sources: Reprinted by permission of *Environmental Nutrition* magazine, from K. Neville, "Foods, Too, Can Interfere with Medications, If You're Not Careful," *Environmental Nutrition* (November 2001) 52 Riverside Drive, Suite 15A, New York: NY 10024. For subscription information, 800-829-5384. Data from *Food Medication Interactions—12th edition* (2002: available at 800-746-2324); Food & Drug Interactions (Food and Drug Administration with National Consumers League. 1998, online updated 2000; available at http://vm.cfsan.fda.gov/~lrd/fdinter.html): interviews with Zaneta Pronsky, M.S., R.D., F.A.D.A., Sr. Jeanne Crowe, Pharm D., R.Ph. and Dean Elbe, B.Sc.

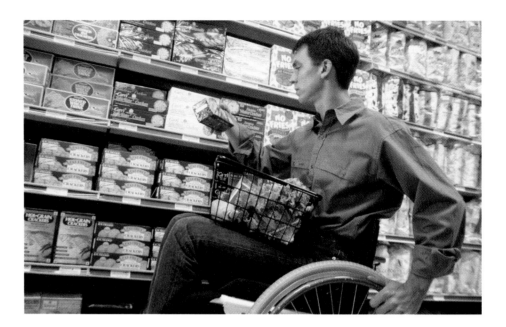

Reading food labels before you purchase products will help you make smart nutritional choices.

methionine, an amino acid found in meat and other protein-laden foods. Two B vitamins—folate and B_6—are believed to control homocysteine levels.[53] When intake of folate and B_6 is low, homocysteine levels rise in the blood. Recent studies indicate that when the level of homocysteine rises, arterial walls and blood platelets become sticky, which encourages clotting. (Note: Homocysteine levels tend to rise with age, smoking, and menopause.) When clots develop in areas already narrowed by atherosclerosis, a heart attack or stroke is likely.

Although the amount of folate needed to protect the heart has not been determined, many people have jumped on the folate bandwagon and take daily folate supplements of up to 800 micrograms. Recently, a new *dietary folate equivalent (DFE)* was established to distinguish folate in food from its synthetic counterpart, *folic acid.* As a food additive or a supplement, folic acid is absorbed about twice as efficiently as folate. The DFE for folate in women age 19 or older is approximately 400 micrograms, with higher levels for pregnant or lactating women. (See Table 9.2 for daily recommended amounts of other B vitamins.) Potential dangers of taking too much folate include a masking of B_{12} deficiencies and resulting problems, ranging from nerve damage, immuno-deficiency problems, anemia, fatigue, and headache, to constipation, diarrhea, weight loss, gastrointestinal disturbances, and a host of neurological symptoms.[54]

Gender and Nutrition

Men and women differ in body size, body composition, and overall metabolic rates. They therefore have differing needs for most nutrients throughout the life cycle (see Tables 9.2 and 9.3 on vitamin and mineral requirements) and face unique difficulties in keeping on track with their dietary goals. Some of these differences have already been discussed. However, there are some factors that need further consideration. Have you ever wondered why men can eat more than women do without gaining weight? Although there are many possible reasons, one factor is that women have a lower ratio of lean body mass to adipose (fatty) tissue at all ages and stages of life. Also, after sexual maturation, the rate of metabolism is higher in men, which means that they will burn more calories doing the same activities.

Different Cycles, Different Needs

In addition to these differences, women have many more landmark times in life when their nutritional requirements vary significantly from requirements at other times. From menarche to menopause, women undergo cyclical physiological changes that can exert dramatic effects on metabolism and nutritional needs. For example, during pregnancy and lactation, women's nutritional requirements increase substantially. Those who are unable to follow the strict dietary recommendations of their doctors may find themselves gaining much more weight during pregnancy and retaining it afterward. During the menstrual cycle, many women report significant food cravings. Later in life, with the advent of menopause, nutritional needs again change rather dramatically. With depletion of the hormone estrogen, the body's need for calcium to ward off bone deterioration becomes pronounced. Women must pay closer attention to exercise and to getting enough calcium through diet or dietary supplements, or they run the risk of osteoporosis.

Changing the "Meat-and-Potatoes" American

Since our earliest agrarian years, many Americans, especially men, have relied on a "meat-and-potatoes" diet. What's wrong with all those hot dogs, steaks, and hamburgers? Heart disease, stroke, and cancer are probably the greatest threats. Add increased risks for colon and prostate cancers, and the rationale for dietary change becomes even more compelling. Consider the following points.

- Heavy red meat eaters are more than twice as likely to get prostate cancer and nearly 5 times more likely to develop colon cancer as those who do not eat a great deal of red meat.
- For every three servings of fruits or vegetables they consume per day, men can expect a 22 percent lower risk of stroke.
- Diets high in fruit and vegetables may lower the risk of lung cancer in smokers from 20 times the risk of nonsmokers to "only" 10 times the risk. They also may protect against oral, throat, pancreatic, and bladder cancers, all of which are more common among smokers.
- The fastest-rising malignancy in the United States, particularly among white men, is cancer of the lower esophagus. Though obesity seems to be a factor, fruits and vegetables are the protectors. (The average American male eats fewer than 3 servings of them per day, although 5 to 9 servings are recommended. Women average 3 to 7 servings per day.)

Does something in meat make it inherently bad? The fat content of meat and fried potatoes and the potential carcinogenic substances produced through cooking have been implicated. Probably something more basic is also involved. By eating so much protein, a person fills up sooner and never gets around to the fruits and vegetables. Thus, the potential protective value of consuming these foods is lost.

What do you think?

*Think about the women that you know who seem to have weight problems. * How old are they? * What factors may make it more difficult for them to keep the weight off? * What factors do men have to deal with in controlling their eating and managing their weight?*

Determining Your Nutritional Needs

Determining the right amount of a given nutrient can be a challenging task. Since the early 1940s, various committees have devised several standards for nutritional needs.

Recommended Dietary Allowances–Adequate Intake The most familiar dietary guidelines are the **Recommended Dietary Allowances (RDAs),** which were originally established by the National Academy of Sciences' Food and Nutrition board in the early 1940s. First designed to prevent nutritional deficiencies, these standards have been revised periodically to reflect changes in nutrition science. In recent years, as deficiencies that lead to disease conditions have declined, the RDAs have taken on more of a prevention focus. For example, calcium requirements have been steadily increased to reflect concerns about osteoporosis. In the late 1990s, the Food and Nutrition board added these new mechanisms for assessing dietary needs.

> **Adequate Intake (AI)**—a best "guess-timate" of what nutritional needs are likely to be for most people when there hasn't been enough research conducted to fully determine an RDA for a specific nutrient.
>
> **Tolerable Upper Intake Level (UL)**—the highest amount of a nutrient that an individual can safely consume every day without risking adverse health effects.

After a careful analysis of RDAs and the new AI and UL values, Canadian and U.S. researchers developed the **Dietary Reference Intake (DRI),** a new, combined listing of more than 26 essential vitamins and minerals.[55] Although you seldom see the DRI on labels, these are the guidelines recommended for healthy adults. They are more comprehensive than RDAs alone because they indicate likely recommendations for nutrients currently being studied. Essentially, DRI should be considered the umbrella guidelines under which RDA, AI, and UL will fall.[56]

Reading Labels for Health To help consumers choose between similar types of food products, the FDA and the USDA developed the **U.S. Recommended Daily Allowances (USRDA)** as a spinoff of RDA recommendations in 1973. The

---

Recommended Dietary Allowances (RDAs) The average daily intakes of energy and nutrients considered adequate to meet the needs of most healthy people in the United States under usual conditions.

Adequate Intakes (AIs) Best estimates of nutritional needs.

Tolerable Upper Intake Level (UL) The highest amount of a nutrient that an individual can safely consume every day without risking adverse health effects.

Dietary Reference Intake (DRI) A new combined listing, developed by Canadian and U.S. researchers, of more than 26 essential vitamins and minerals.

U.S. Recommended Daily Allowances (USRDAs) Dietary guidelines developed by the FDA and the USDA.

first voluntary food labels with USRDAs were a part of this action. Eventually, in response to consumer demand, the USDA issued mandatory guidelines for food labeling in 1993.[57] These new, mandatory guidelines generally replaced USRDAs with **Reference Daily Intakes (RDIs)** and **Daily Reference Values (DRVs)**. RDIs are the recommended amounts of 19 vitamins and minerals, also known as micronutrients. DRVs are the recommended amounts for macronutrients, such as total fat, saturated fat, cholesterol, total carbohydrates, dietary fiber, sodium, potassium, and protein.

Together, RDIs and DRVs make up the **Daily Values (DV)** that you will find on food and supplement labels listed as a percentage (% DV); see Figure 9.3 for an example. When you look at a label with a % DV listing, you can tell what percentage of a nutrient is found in a serving of food. Although % DV has become widely accepted, it should be noted that it is not as up to date as RDA or DRIs. Although DVs will eventually be updated, they also do not reflect the different needs of older adults, people with conditions such as pregnancy, or differences by gender. Advocates of the DV system argue that there isn't enough room for such information on labels, and a basic, easy-to-understand system works best.

Vegetarianism: Eating for Health

For aesthetic, animal rights, economic, personal, health, cultural, or religious reasons, some people choose specialized diets. Between 5 and 15 percent of all Americans today claim to be vegetarians. Normally, vegetarianism provides a superb alternative to our high-fat, high-calorie, meat-based cuisine. But without proper information and food choices, vegetarians can also develop dietary problems.

The term **vegetarian** means different things to different people. Strict vegetarians, or *vegans,* avoid all foods of

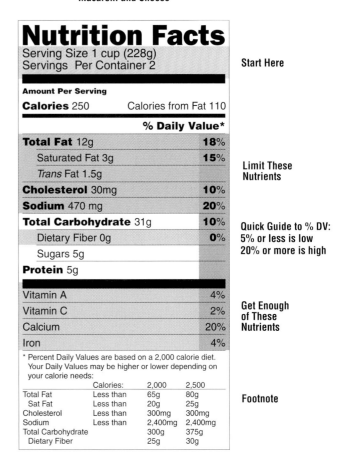

Sample Label for
Macaroni and Cheese

Figure 9.3
Reading a Food Label
Source: Center for Food Safety and Applied Nutrition, "Questions and Answers about *Trans* Fat Nutrition Labeling," 2003. www. cfsan.fda.gov/ ~ dms/qatrans2.html

---

Reference Daily Intake (RDI)   Recommended amounts of 19 vitamins and minerals, also known as micronutrients.

Daily Reference Values (DRVs)   Recommended amounts for macronutrients such as total fat, saturated fat, and cholesterol.

Daily Values (DVs)   The RDIs and DRVs together make up the Daily Values seen on food and supplement labels.

Vegetarian   A term with a variety of meanings: vegans avoid all foods of animal origin; lacto-vegetarians avoid flesh foods but eat dairy products; ovo-vegetarians avoid flesh foods but eat eggs; lacto-ovo-vegetarians avoid flesh foods but eat both dairy products and eggs; pesco-vegetarians avoid meat but eat fish, dairy products, and eggs; semi-vegetarians eat chicken, fish, dairy products, and eggs.

---

animal origin, including dairy products and eggs. Vegans must be careful to obtain all of the necessary nutrients. Far more common are *lacto-vegetarians,* who eat dairy products but avoid flesh foods. Their diet can be low in fat and cholesterol, but only if they consume skim milk and other low-fat or nonfat products. *Ovo-vegetarians* add eggs to their diet, while *lacto-ovo-vegetarians* eat both dairy products and eggs. *Pesco-vegetarians* eat fish, dairy products, and eggs, while *semivegetarians* eat chicken, fish, dairy products, and eggs. Some people in the semivegetarian category prefer to call themselves "non–red meat eaters."

Generally, people who follow a balanced vegetarian diet weigh less and have better cholesterol levels, fewer problems with irregular bowel movements (constipation and diarrhea), and a lower risk of heart disease than do nonvegetarians. Some preliminary evidence suggests that vegetarians may also have a reduced risk for colon and breast cancer.[58] Whether these lower risks are due to the vegetarian diet per se or to some combination of lifestyle variables remains unclear.

Although in the past vegetarians often suffered from vitamin deficiencies, the vegetarian of the new millennium is usually extremely adept at combining the right types of foods to ensure proper nutrient intake. People who eat dairy products and small amounts of chicken or fish are seldom nutrient-deficient; in fact, while vegans typically get 50 to 60 grams of protein per day, lacto-ovo-vegetarians normally consume between 70 and 90 grams per day, well beyond the RDA. Vegan diets may be deficient in vitamins B_2 (riboflavin), B_{12}, and D. Riboflavin is found mainly in meat, eggs, and dairy products; however, broccoli, asparagus, almonds, and fortified cereals are also good sources. Vitamins B_{12} and D are found only in dairy products and fortified products such as soy milk. Vegans are also at risk for deficiencies of calcium, iron, zinc, and other minerals, but they can obtain these nutrients from supplements. Strict vegans have to pay much more attention to what they eat than the average person does, but by eating complementary combinations of plant products, they can receive adequate amounts of essential amino acids. Examples of complementary combinations are corn and beans, and peanut butter and whole grain bread. Eating a full variety of grains, legumes, fruits, vegetables, and seeds each day will help to keep even the strictest vegetarian in excellent health. Pregnant women, the elderly, the sick, and children who are vegans need to take special care to ensure that their diets are adequate. People who take part in heavy aerobic exercise programs (over three hours per week) may need to increase their protein consumption. In all cases, seek advice from a health care professional if you have questions.

The Vegetarian Pyramid

Dr. Arlene Spark, a nutritionist at New York Medical College, has devised a food guide pyramid that conveys the essentials of a vegetarian diet. Modeled after the USDA Food Guide Pyramid discussed earlier in this chapter, the vegetarian version clarifies what people who don't eat meat need to do to stay healthy. The vegetarian pyramid defines the following categories. We include examples of single servings in each category.

Grains and Starchy Vegetables Group (6–11 servings/day)
- 1 slice bread
- 1 ounce cold cereal
- $1/2$ cup cooked cereal, rice, or pasta
- 3 cups popcorn
- $1/2$ cup corn
- 1 medium potato
- $1/2$ cup green peas

Vegetable Group (2–3 servings/day)
- $1/2$ cup cooked or chopped raw vegetables
- 1 cup raw leafy vegetables
- $3/4$ cup vegetable juice

Fruit Group (2–3 servings/day)
- 1 medium whole piece of fruit
- $1/2$ cup canned, chopped, or cooked fruit
- $3/4$ cup fruit juice

Calcium-Rich Foods (4–6 servings/day)
- $1/2$ cup milk or yogurt
- 1 ounce processed cheese

Beans and Alternatives Group (2–3 servings/day)
- $1/2$ cup cooked dry beans, peas, or lentils
- 1 egg
- $1/3$ cup bean curd or tofu
- 3–4 tablespoons seeds

Other
- 1 teaspoon flaxseed oil
- vitamins B_{12} and D supplements

What do you think?

Why are so many people today becoming vegetarians? ✳ *How easy is it to be a vegetarian on your campus?* ✳ *What concerns about vegetarianism would you be likely to have, if any?*

Improved Eating for the College Student

College students often face a challenge when trying to eat healthy foods. Some students live in dorms and do not have their own cooking or refrigeration facilities. Others live in crowded apartments where everyone forages in the refrigerator for everyone else's food. Still others eat at university food services where food choices may be limited. Most students have financial and time constraints that make buying, preparing, and eating healthy food a difficult task. What's a student to do?

Fast Foods: Eating on the Run

If your campus is like many others, you've probably noticed a distinct move toward fast-food restaurants in your student unions, so that they now resemble the food courts found in shopping malls. These new eating centers fit students' needs for a fast bite of food at a reasonable price between classes and also bring in money to your school. But many fast foods are high in fat and sodium. Are they all unhealthy?

Not all fast foods are created equal, and not all are bad for you. Even at the often-maligned burger chains, menus are healthier than ever before and offer excellent choices for the discriminating eater. The key word here is *discriminating*. It really is possible to eat healthy food if you follow these suggestions (see the Consumer Health box for even more ideas about how to eat healthily while eating out).

- Ask for nutritional analyses of items. Most fast-food chains now have them.
- Avoid mayonnaise, sauces, and other add-ons. Some places even have fat-free mayonnaise if you ask. Put a hold on extra ketchup.
- Hold the cheese. This extra contributes substantially to total fat but does not add a lot to taste.
- Order single, small burgers rather than large, high-calorie, bacon- or cheese-topped choices. Put on your own ketchup, and keep portions small.
- Order salads, and be careful how much dressing you add. Many people think they are being health-smart by eating salad, only to load it with calorie- and fat-rich dressing. Try the vinegar and oil or low-fat alternative dressings. Stay away from eggs and other high-fat add-ons such as bacon bits.
- When ordering a chicken sandwich, order the skinless broiled version rather than the deep-fried version. Many people think that a deep-fried chicken sandwich is a healthier choice when it really has more fat than a loaded double burger.
- If you must have fries, check to see what type of oil is used to cook them. Avoid lard-based or other saturated fat products.
- Order wheat bread, and ask them to hold the butter.
- Avoid fried foods in general, including hot apple pies and other crust-based fried foods.
- Opt for places where foods are broiled rather than fried.

When Funds Are Short

Maintaining a nutritious diet within the confines of student life can be challenging. However, if you take the time to plan healthy meals, you will find that you are eating better, enjoying your food more, and actually saving money. Follow these steps to ensure a healthy but affordable diet.

- Buy fruits and vegetables in season whenever possible for their lower cost, higher nutrient quality, and greater variety.
- Use coupons and specials to get price reductions.
- Shop at discount warehouse food chains; capitalize on volume discounts and no-frills products.
- Plan ahead to get the most for your dollar and avoid extra trips to the store; extra trips usually mean extra purchases. Make a list and stick to it.
- Purchase meats and other products in volume; freeze portions for future needs. Or purchase small amounts of meats and other expensive proteins and combine them with beans and plant proteins for lower cost, calories, and fat.
- Cook large meals, and freeze small portions for later use.
- Drain off extra fat after cooking. Save juices to use in soups and other dishes.
- If you find that you have no money for food, talk to staff at your county or city health department. They may know of ways for you to get assistance.

Supplements: New Research on the Daily Dose

For years, health experts touted the benefits of eating a balanced diet over popping a vitamin/mineral supplement. In fact, we were told that supplements were rarely necessary in the United States and that if we chose to pop those one-a-day pills, most of their water-soluble content would simply be replenishing the nutrient supplies of our underground sewer systems.

So eyebrows were raised in the summer of 2002 when an article in the esteemed *Journal of the American Medical Association (JAMA)* recommended that "a vitamin/mineral supplement a day just might be important in keeping the doctor away, particularly for some groups of people."[59] Essentially, the article indicated that older people, vegans, alcohol-dependent individuals, and patients with malabsorption problems may be at particular risk for deficiency of several vitamins. Although they acknowledged that there may be a risk if you overdose on fat-soluble vitamins, for the most part, inadequate amounts of nutrients such as vitamins B_6, B_{12}, D, E, and lycopene are linked to chronic diseases, including coronary heart disease, cancer, and osteoporosis. As a result of this study, *JAMA* indicated that all adults should take a basic multi-vitamin.

So should you rush out and stock up on supplements? Not so fast. According to Dr. David Bender, writing in the *British Medical Journal*,[60] the *JAMA* review article produced little convincing evidence in favor of supplements. According to Dr. Bender, if our dietary intake is adequate, supplements probably will do us little good. Surely there will be much more controversy over supplement use in the future. If you are in doubt, make sure you eat from the food groups recommended in the Food Guide Pyramid. If you are facing extreme stressors on the body from physical exercise, illness, or other nutrient-depleting events, supplements might be beneficial. In all cases, beware of overdosing. Choose inexpensive varieties, and aim to meet minimal levels.

Food Safety: A Growing Concern
Food-Borne Illnesses

Are you concerned that the chicken you are buying doesn't look pleasingly pink, or that your "fresh" fish smells a little *too* fishy? Are you *sure* that your apple juice is free of animal

What's Good on the Menu?

While some restaurants offer hints for health-conscious diners, you're on your own most of the time. To help you order wisely, here are lighter options and high-fat pitfalls. Best choices contain fewer than 30 grams of fat, a generous meal's worth for an active, medium-size woman. "Worst" choices have up to 100 grams of fat.

FAST FOOD

Best
Grilled chicken sandwich
Roast beef sandwich
Single hamburger
Salad with light vinaigrette

Worst
Bacon burger
Double cheeseburger
French fries
Onion rings

Tips
Order sandwiches without mayo or "special sauce." Avoid deep-fried items like fish fillets, chicken nuggets, and French fries.

ITALIAN

Best
Pasta with red or white clam sauce
Spaghetti with marinara or tomato-and-meat sauce

Worst
Eggplant parmigiana
Fettuccine alfredo
Fried calamari
Lasagna

Tips
Stick with plain bread instead of garlic bread made with butter or oil. Ask for the waiter's help in avoiding cream- or egg-based sauces. Try vegetarian pizza, and don't ask for extra cheese.

MEXICAN

Best
Bean burrito (no cheese)
Chicken fajitas

Worst
Beef chimichanga
Chile relleno
Quesadilla
Refried beans

Tips
Choose soft tortillas (not fried) with fresh salsa, not guacamole. Special-order grilled shrimp, fish, or chicken. Ask for beans made without lard or fat and for cheeses and sour cream provided on the side or left out altogether.

CHINESE

Best
Hot-and-sour soup
Stir-fried vegetables
Shrimp with garlic sauce
Szechuan shrimp
Wonton soup

Worst
Crispy chicken
Kung pao chicken
Moo shu pork
Sweet-and-sour pork

Tips
Share a stir-fry; help yourself to steamed rice. Ask for vegetables steamed or stir-fried with less oil. Order moo shu vegetables instead of pork. Avoid fried rice, breaded dishes, egg rolls and spring rolls, and items loaded with nuts. Avoid high-sodium sauces.

JAPANESE

Best
Steamed rice and vegetables
Tofu as a substitute for meat
Broiled or steamed chicken and fish

Worst
Fried rice dishes
Miso (very high in sodium)
Tempura

Tips
Avoid soy sauces. Use caution in eating sashimi and sushi (raw fish) dishes to avoid possible bacteria or parasites.

THAI

Best
Clear broth soups
Stir-fried chicken and vegetables
Grilled meats

Worst
Coconut milk
Peanut sauces
Deep-fried dishes

Tips
Avoid coconut-based curries. Ask for steamed, not fried, rice.

BREAKFAST

Best
Hot or cold cereal with 2% milk
Pancakes or French toast with syrup
Scrambled eggs with hash browns and plain toast

Worst
Belgian waffle with sausage
Sausage and eggs with biscuits and gravy
Ham-and-cheese omelette with hash browns and toast

Tips
Ask for whole grain cereal or shredded wheat with 1% milk or whole wheat toast without butter or margarine. Order omelettes without cheese, fried eggs without bacon or sausage.

SANDWICHES

Best
Ham and Swiss cheese
Roast beef
Turkey

Worst
Tuna salad
Reuben
Submarine

Tips
Ask for mustard; hold the mayo and cheese. See if turkey-ham is available.

SEAFOOD

Best
Broiled bass, halibut, or snapper
Grilled scallops
Steamed crab or lobster

Worst
Fried seafood platter
Blackened catfish

Tips
Order fish broiled, baked, grilled, or steamed—not pan-fried or sauteed. Ask for lemon instead of tartar sauce. Avoid creamy and buttery sauces.

Sources: American Dietetic Association, 2002. http://www.eatright.org; *Health* 10 (November/December 1996): 79.

waste? You may have good reason to be worried. In increasing numbers, Americans are becoming sick from what they eat, and many of these illnesses are life threatening. Scientists estimate, based on several studies conducted over the past ten years, that food-borne pathogens sicken more than 76 million people and cause some 9,000 deaths in the United States annually.[61] Because most of us don't go to the doctor every time we feel ill, we may not make a connection between what we eat and later symptoms.

Signs of food-borne illnesses vary tremendously and usually include one or several symptoms: diarrhea, nausea, cramping, and vomiting. Depending on the amount and virulence of the pathogen, symptoms may appear as early as 30 minutes after eating contaminated food, or as long as several days or weeks. Most of the time, symptoms occur five to eight hours after eating and last only a day or two. For certain populations, however, such as the very young, the elderly, or people with severe illnesses such as cancer, diabetes, kidney disease, or AIDS, food-borne diseases can be fatal.

Several factors may be contributing to the increase in food-borne illnesses. According to Michael T. Osterholm, Ph.D., state epidemiologist in Minneapolis,[62] the movement away from a traditional meat-and-potato American diet to heart-healthy eating—increasing consumption of fruits, vegetables, and grains—has spurred demand for fresh foods that are not in season most of the year. This means that we must import fresh fruits and vegetables, which thus puts us at risk for ingesting exotic pathogens. Depending on the season, up to 70 percent of the fruits and vegetables consumed in the United States come from Mexico alone. The upshot is that a visit to developing countries isn't necessary to be stricken with food-borne "traveler's diarrhea" because the produce does the traveling.[63] Although when we travel to developing countries we are told to "boil it, peel it, or don't eat it," we bring these foods into our kitchens and eat them often without even basic washing.[64] Food can become contaminated by being watered with contaminated water, fertilized with "organic" fertilizers (animal manure), and not subjected to the same rigorous pesticide regulations as American-raised produce is. To give you an idea of the implications, studies have shown that *E. coli* (a lethal bacterial pathogen) can survive in cow manure for up to 70 days and can multiply in foods grown with manure unless heat or additives such as salt or preservatives are used to kill the microbes.[65] There are essentially no regulations that say farmers can't use animal manure in growing their crops. Turkey manure, pig manure, and other agribusiness by-products are often sprayed on fields that ultimately grow foods for consumers. *E. coli* H7:0157 actually increases in summer months in cows awaiting slaughter in crowded, overheated pens. This increases the chances of meat coming to market already contaminated.[66]

Key factors associated with the increasing spread of food-borne diseases include the following.[67]

- *Globalization of the food supply.* Because the food supply is distributed worldwide, the possibility of exposure to pathogens native to remote regions of the world is greater. For example, a large outbreak of the bacterial disease *Shigella* occurred in Norway, Sweden, and the United Kingdom from lettuce that originated in southern Europe.

- *Inadvertent introduction of pathogens into new geographic regions.* One theory is that cholera was introduced into waters off the coast of the southern United States when a cargo ship discharged contaminated ballast as it came into harbor. Other pathogens may enter into aquatic life in a similar manner.

- *Exposure to unfamiliar food-borne hazards.* Travelers, refugees, and immigrants who move through foreign countries are exposed to food-borne hazards and bring them home with them.

- *Changes in microbial populations.* Changing microbial populations can lead to the evolution of new pathogens. As a result, old pathogens develop new virulence factors or become resistant to antibiotics, which makes diseases more difficult to treat.

- *Increased susceptibility of varying populations.* People are becoming more vulnerable to disease. The numbers of highly susceptible persons are expanding worldwide because of aging populations, HIV infection, and other underlying medical conditions, such as malnutrition and the compromised health status that results from the use of immunosuppressive drugs. High birth rates and increased longevity have increased the numbers of vulnerable populations at the margins.

- *Insufficient education about food safety.* Increased urbanization, industrialization, and travel, combined with more people eating out, raise the risk of unsafe food handling and illness.

Responsible Use: Avoiding Risks in the Home

Part of the responsibility for preventing food-borne illness lies with consumers—more than 30 percent of all such illnesses result from unsafe handling of food at home.

- When shopping, pick up packaged and canned foods first, and save frozen foods and perishables such as meat, poultry, and fish until last. Place these foods in separate plastic bags so drippings don't run onto other foods in your cart and contaminate them.
- Check for cleanliness at the salad bar and meat and fish counters.
- When shopping for fish, buy from markets that get their supplies from state-approved sources.
- Most cuts of meat, fish, and poultry should be kept in the refrigerator no more than one or two days. Check the shelf life of all products before buying.
- Eat leftovers within three days.
- Keep hot foods hot and cold foods cold.
- Use a thermometer to ensure that meats are completely cooked. Beef and lamb steaks and roasts should be

cooked to at least 145°F; ground meat, pork chops, ribs, and egg dishes to 160°F; ground poultry and hot dogs to 165°F; chicken and turkey breasts to 170°F; and chicken and turkey legs, thighs, and whole birds to 180°F.

- Fish is done when the thickest part becomes opaque and the fish flakes easily when poked with a fork.
- Never leave cooked food standing on the stove or table for more than two hours.
- Never thaw frozen foods at room temperature.
- Wash your hands and countertop with soap and water when preparing food, particularly after handling meat, fish, or poultry.
- When freezing foods like chicken, make sure juices can't spill over into ice cubes or into other areas of the refrigerator.

Food Irradiation: How Safe Is It?

Each year, thousands of people get sick from largely preventable diseases such as that caused by *E. coli* as well as other bacteria such as *Salmonella* and *Listeria*. In response to these concerns, in 2000 the USDA approved large-scale irradiation of beef, lamb, poultry, pork, and other raw animal foods.

Food irradiation is a process that involves treating foods with gamma radiation from radioactive cobalt, cesium, or other sources of X rays. When foods are irradiated, they are exposed to low doses of radiation, or ionizing energy, which breaks chemical bonds of harmful bacteria in the DNA, destroys the pathogens, and keeps them from replicating. The rays essentially pass through the food without leaving any radioactive residue.[68]

Some companies use cobalt 60, a radioactive substance, for irradiation. But others are beginning to use a new kind of irradiation that dispenses with radioactive compounds and uses electricity as the energy source instead. Thus, as foods pass along a conveyor belt, the energy used to kill bacteria comes from electron beams rather than from gamma rays.[69] Irradiation lengthens food products' shelf life and prevents the spread of deadly microorganisms, particularly in high-risk foods such as ground beef and pork. Thus, the minimal costs of irradiation should result in lower overall costs to consumers, in addition to reducing the need for toxic chemicals now used to preserve foods and prevent contamination from external pathogens.

Food irradiation has been approved for potatoes, spices, pork carcasses, and fruits and vegetables since the mid-1980s. Some environmentalists and consumer groups have raised concerns, so irradiated products are not common fare. However, the facts appear to support the use of irradiation.

Food Additives

Additives generally reduce the risk of food-borne illness (i.e., nitrates added to cured meats), prevent spoilage, and enhance the ways foods look and taste. Additives can also enhance nutrient value, especially to benefit the general public. A deficiency can be a terrible public health problem, and a solution is relatively easy to administer. Good examples include the fortification of milk with vitamin D, and of grain products with folate. Although the FDA regulates additives according to effectiveness, safety, and ability to detect them in foods, questions have been raised about those additives put into foods intentionally and those that get in unintentionally before or after processing. Whenever these substances are added, consumers should take the time to determine what they are and if there are alternatives. As a general rule, the fewer chemicals, colorants, and preservatives, the better. Also, it should be noted that certain foods and additives can interact with medications. To be a smart consumer, be aware of these potential dietary interactions. Examples of common additives include the following.

- *Antimicrobial agents.* Substances such as salt, sugar, nitrates, and others that tend to make foods less hospitable for microbes
- *Antioxidants.* Substances that preserve color and flavor by reducing loss due to exposure to oxygen. Vitamins C and E are among those antioxidants believed to play a role in reduced cancer and cardiovascular disease. The additives BHA and BHT are also antioxidant in action.
- *Artificial colors*
- *Nutrient additives*
- *Flavor enhancers such as MSG (monosodium glutamate)*
- *Sulfites.* Used to preserve vegetable color; some people have severe allergic reactions to them.
- *Substances that inadvertently get into food products from packaging and/or handling*
- *Dioxins.* Found in coffee filters, milk containers, and frozen foods
- *Methylene chloride.* Found in decaffeinated coffee
- *Hormones.* Bovine growth hormone (BGH) found in animal meat

Food Allergy or Food Intolerance?

At some point in time, a *food allergy* or *food intolerance* will affect nearly everyone. You eat something, develop gas or have an unpleasant visit to the bathroom, and assume that it is a food allergy. One out of every three people today either say they have a food allergy or avoid something in their diet because they think they are allergic to it; in fact, only 3 percent of all children and 1 percent of all adults experience genuine allergic reactions to what they eat.[70] Surprised? Most people are when they hear this.

Food irradiation Treating foods with gamma radiation from radioactive cobalt, cesium, or some other source of X rays to kill microorganisms.

A **food allergy** or hypersensitivity is an abnormal response to a food that is triggered by the immune system. Reactions range from minor rashes to severe swelling in the mouth, tongue, and throat, to violent vomiting and diarrhea and occasionally death.

In adults, the most common foods to cause true allergic reactions are shellfish (such as shrimp, crayfish, lobster, and crab); peanuts, which can cause severe anaphylaxis (a sudden drop in blood pressure that can be fatal if not treated promptly); tree nuts such as walnuts; fish; and eggs. In children, food allergens that cause the most problems are eggs, milk, and peanuts.[71]

In contrast to allergies, in cases of **food intolerance** you may have symptoms of gastric upset but they are not the result of an immune system response. Probably the best example of a food intolerance is *lactose intolerance,* a problem that affects about one in every ten adults. Lactase is an enzyme in the lining of the gut that degrades lactose, which is in dairy products. If you don't have enough lactase, lactose cannot be digested and remains in the gut to be used by bacteria. Gas is formed, and you experience bloating, abdominal pain, and sometimes diarrhea. Food intolerance also occurs in response to some food additives, such as the flavor enhancer MSG, certain dyes, sulfites, gluten, and other substances. In some cases, the food intolerance may have psychological triggers.

If you suspect that you have an actual allergic reaction to food, see an allergist to be tested. Because there are several diseases that share symptoms with food allergies (ulcers and cancers of the gastrointestinal tract can cause vomiting, bloating, diarrhea, nausea, and pain), you should have persistent symptoms checked out as soon as possible. If particular foods seem to bother you consistently, look for alternatives or modify your diet. In true allergic instances, you may not be able to consume even the smallest amount safely. For example, people have experienced severe allergic reactions to peanuts from ingesting as little as a crumb.

Is Organic for You?

Due to mounting concerns about food safety, many people refuse to buy processed foods and mass-produced agricultural products. Instead, they purchase foods that are **organically**

Food allergies   Overreaction by the body to normally harmless substances, which are perceived as allergens. In response, the body produces antibodies, triggering allergic symptoms.

Food intolerance   Adverse effects resulting when people who lack the digestive chemicals needed to break down certain substances eat those substances.

Organically grown   Foods that are grown without use of pesticides or chemicals.

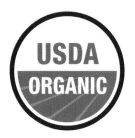

Figure 9.4
Label for Certified Organic Foods
This seal indicates that the product is at least 95 percent organic according to USDA guidelines.
Source: USDA Agriculture Marketing Program, The National Organic Program, "Organic Food Standards and Labels: The Facts," 2002. www.ams.usda.gov/nop

grown—foods reported to be pesticide- and chemical-free. Less than a decade ago, buying organic foods meant going to a specialty store and paying premium prices for produce that was likely to be wilted, wormy, and smaller than its nonorganic alternative. These products also came with no guarantee that they were really grown in organic environments. People who bought these foods did so out of a desire to eat healthier produce and avoid the chemicals that they were increasingly being told caused cancer, immune system problems, and a host of other ailments.

Enter the organics of the twenty-first century—larger, more attractive, and fresher looking, but still carrying a hefty price tag. Is buying organic really better for you? Perhaps if we could put a group of people in a pristine environment and insure that they never ate, drank, or were exposed to chemicals, we could test this hypothesis. In real life, however, it is almost impossible to assess the health impact of organic versus non-organic. Nevertheless, the market for organics has been increasing by 15 to 20 percent per year—5 times faster than food sales in general. Nearly 40 percent of U.S. consumers now reach occasionally for something labeled organic, with sales topping $11 billion per year.

As of 2002, any food sold as organic has to meet criteria set by the USDA under the National Organic Rule and can carry a new USDA seal verifying products as "certified organic" (Figure 9.4). Under this rule, something that is certified may carry one of the following terms: 100 percent Organic (100 percent compliance with organic criteria), Organic (must contain at least 95 percent organic materials), Made with Organic Ingredients (must contain at least 70 percent organic ingredients), or Some Organic Ingredients (contains less than 70 percent organic ingredients—usually listed individually). In order to use any of the above terms, the foods must be produced without hormones, antibiotics, herbicides, insecticides, chemical fertilizers, genetic modification, or germ-killing radiation.

Make It Happen!

Assessment: The Assess Yourself box on page 238 gave you the chance to test your knowledge of some of the health effects of various foods. Now that you have considered these results, you can decide whether you need to do more to keep up on what to eat and what to avoid for long-term health.

Making a Change: In order to change your behavior, you need to develop a plan. Follow these steps.

1. Evaluate your behavior, and identify patterns and specific things you are doing. What can you change now? What can you change in the near future?
2. Select one pattern of behavior that you want to change.
3. Fill out a Behavior Change Contract. It should include your long-term goal for change, your short-term goals, the rewards you'll give yourself for reaching these goals, potential obstacles along the way, and strategies for overcoming these obstacles. For each goal, list the small steps and specific actions that you will take.

4. Chart your progress in a journal. At the end of a week, consider how successful you were in following your plan. What helped you be successful? What made change more difficult? What will you do differently next week?
5. Revise your plan as needed. Are the short-term goals attainable? Are the rewards satisfying?

Example: Tara discovered that she had very little idea about what foods to eat and to avoid for long-term health. She decided to keep track of her normal diet for a week and then to evaluate it in light of some of the guidelines in this chapter. She considered her diet fairly balanced and was surprised to find that she was eating less than 2 servings of vegetables a day, instead of the recommended 3 to 5. Tara looked at her eating patterns and saw several times during the week where she snacked on foods that could be replaced with other, healthier snacks. She decided to cut carrots up into sticks that she could toss into her backpack. They stayed fresh all day and made a good snack between classes instead of a candy bar from the vending machine. She also found

that her favorite Mexican restaurant offered a vegetarian burrito full of black beans (not refried), squash, tomatoes, and other vegetables that was even tastier than her usual pork burrito. At the end of the first week, Tara and her friends decided to order pizza after a late night of studying. Instead of getting pepperoni or sausage, Tara suggested a pizza with green peppers, spinach, and onions as toppings. Tara did have a setback when she went to a baseball game and ate peanuts and hot dogs all day, but the next day she had a salad for lunch and saw that her vegetable consumption was almost at her goal.

Tara's goal for the next week is to continue to substitute healthy snacks and to look for healthy alternatives when she is eating out. When she is consistently eating the recommended servings of vegetables each week, she will start focusing on other parts of her diet that could use improvement. She is already thinking about how to replace some of the white bread and sugary breakfast cereals she eats now with more whole wheat and whole grains.

Summary

- Recognizing that we eat for more reasons than just survival is the first step toward changing our health.
- The Food Guide Pyramid provides guidelines for healthy eating.
- The major nutrients that are essential for life and health include water, proteins, carbohydrates, fiber, fats, vitamins, and minerals.
- Experts are interested in the role of food as medicine and in the benefits of functional foods. These foods may play an important role in improving certain conditions, such as hypertension.
- Men and women have differing needs for most nutrients throughout the life cycle because of different body size and composition.

- Vegetarianism can provide a healthy alternative for those wishing to cut fat from their diets or to reduce animal consumption. The vegetarian pyramid provides dietary guidelines to help vegetarians obtain needed nutrients.
- College students face unique challenges in eating healthfully. Learning to make better choices at fast-food restaurants, eat healthfully when funds are short, and eat nutritionally in the dorm are all possible when you use the information contained in this chapter.
- Food-borne illnesses, food irradiation, food allergies, and other food safety and health concerns are becoming increasingly important to health-wise consumers. Recognizing potential risks and taking steps to prevent problems are part of a sound nutritional plan.

Questions for Discussion and Reflection

1. Which factors influence the dietary patterns and behaviors of the typical college student? What factors have been the greatest influences on your eating behaviors? Why is it important to recognize influences on your diet as you think about changing eating behaviors?
2. What are the six major food groups in the Food Guide Pyramid? From which groups do you eat too few servings? What can you do to increase or decrease your intake of selected food groups? How can you remember the six groups?
3. What are the major types of nutrients that you need to obtain from the foods you eat? What happens if you fail to get enough of some of them? Are there significant differences between the sexes in particular areas of nutrition?
4. Distinguish between the different types of vegetarianism. Which types are most likely to lead to nutrient deficiencies? What can be done to ensure that even the most strict vegetarian receives enough of the major nutrients?
5. What are functional foods? What are the major functional foods discussed in this chapter? What are their reported benefits, if any?
6. What are the major problems that many college students face when trying to eat the right foods? List five actions that you and your classmates could take immediately to improve your eating.
7. What are the potential benefits and risks of food irradiation? Why is it being used? What are the major risks for food-borne illnesses, and what can you do to protect yourself? How are food illnesses and food allergies different?

Accessing Your Health on the Internet

Visit the following Internet sites to explore further topics and issues related to personal health. To visit an organization's website, go to the Companion Website for *Health: The Basics, Sixth Edition* at www.aw-bc.com/donatelle, click on the book image, and select "Accessing Your Health on the Internet" from the navigation menu on the left.

1. *American Dietetic Association (ADA).* Provides information on a full range of dietary topics, including sports nutrition, healthful cooking, and nutritional eating; also links to scientific publications and information on scholarships and public meetings.
2. *American Heart Association (AHA).* Includes information about a heart-healthy eating plan and an easy-to-follow guide to healthy eating.
3. *Food and Drug Administration (FDA).* Provides information for consumers and professionals in the areas of food safety, supplements, and medical devices. Links to other sources of information about nutrition and food.
4. *Food and Nutrition Information Center.* Offers a wide variety of information related to food and nutrition.
5. *National Institutes of Health: Office of Dietary Supplements.* Site of the International Bibliographic Database Information on Dietary Supplements (IBIDS), updated quarterly.
6. *U.S. Department of Agriculture (USDA).* Offers a full discussion of the USDA Dietary Guidelines for Americans.

Further Reading

Nutrition Action Healthletter

This newsletter, published 10 times a year, contains up-to-date information on diet and nutritional claims and current research issues. The newsletter can be obtained by writing to the Center for Science in the Public Interest, 1501 16th St. NW, Washington, DC 20036.

Nutrition Today

An excellent magazine for the interested nonspecialist. Covers controversial issues and provides a forum for conflicting opinions. Six issues per year. Order from Williams and Wilkins, 351 West Camden Street, Baltimore, MD 21201-2436.

Schlosser, E. *Fast Food Nation.* Boston: Houghton Mifflin, 2001.

Overview of the influence of the fast food industry and its effect on health and well-being in America.

Tufts University Health and Nutrition Letter.

An excellent source for quick "fixes" on current nutritional topics. Reputable sources and information. E-mail tufts@tiac.net, or phone (800) 274-7581. The Tufts Nutrition Navigator website (http://navigator.tufts.edu) rates nutrition-related websites for information and accuracy.

U.S. Department of Agriculture (USDA)

For information on the proper handling of meat and poultry and other information, call the USDA's Meat and Poultry Hot Line at (800) 535-4555 between 10:00 A.M. and 4:00 P.M. on weekdays. Write to the Meat and Poultry Hot Line, USDA-FSIS, Room 1165-S, Washington, DC, 20250 for a new booklet, A Quick Consumer's Guide to Safe Food Handling.

Whitney, E., and S. Rolfes. *Understanding Nutrition, 9th ed.* Belmont, CA: Wadsworth Publishing, 2002.

An introductory college health text that provides an outstanding overview of nutritional information in a highly accessible, easy-to-read format.

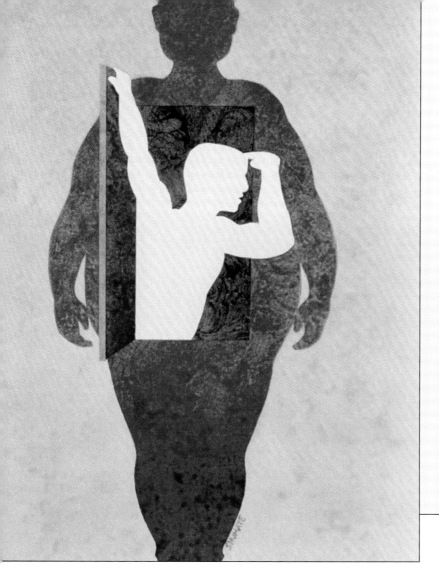

Managing Your Weight

Finding a Healthy Balance

10 10 10 10 10 10 10

Objectives

❋ Explain why so many people are obsessed with thinness and how to determine the right weight for you.

❋ Define obesity and describe the current epidemic of obesity in the United States.

❋ Discuss reliable options for determining body fat content.

❋ Describe factors that place people at risk for problems with obesity.

❋ Distinguish between risk factors that can and cannot be controlled.

❋ Discuss the roles of exercise, dieting, nutrition, lifestyle, fad diets, and other strategies of weight control.

❋ Describe the most effective methods of weight management.

❋ Describe major eating disorders, explain the health risks related to these conditions, and indicate the factors that make people susceptible to them.

Doubt Cast on Food Supplements for Weight Control

By Marian Burros and Sherri Day

For $120 a month, a dedicated dieter can buy a full month's supply of Dr. Phil's Shape Up "weight management supplement and complete multivitamin" stew.

And while Dr. Phillip C. McGraw says the products can be an important part of a weight-loss program, some experts in obesity say they know of no sound scientific evidence that supplements help anyone lose weight.

The packages of supplements make the claim, "These products contain scientifically researched levels of ingredients that can help you change your behavior to take control of your weight." A 15-day supply of each of the two kinds of supplement recommended is $60.

Dr. Jules Hirsch, a clinical researcher in nutrition and obesity and professor emeritus at Rockefeller University, said he knows of no evidence that dietary supplements help lose weight, an opinion echoed by Dr. Kelly Brownell, director of the Center for Eating and Weight Disorders at Yale University. "It sounds like gibberish," Dr. Hirsch said.

Read the complete article online in the eThemes section of this book's website: www.aw-bc.com/donatelle.

Original article published October 27, 2003. Copyright © 2003 The New York Times. Reprinted with permission.

In spite of society's messages about the need for diet and exercise, numerous studies on eating patterns suggest that Americans are doing worse with each successive decade. In fact, the most recent National Health and Nutrition Examination Survey (NHANES III), conducted by the Centers for Disease Control and Prevention, shows that 61 percent of U.S. adults are either overweight or obese—an increase of more than 5 percent over the past decade.[1]

Clearly, obesity is a major public health problem that needs to be addressed. The threats to life and overall health and happiness are staggering. In fact, officials estimate that between 300,000 and 500,000 lives are lost each year to conditions directly related to obesity, and perhaps many more deaths are indirectly related to a history of obesity throughout a person's life.[2] Associated health risks include coronary heart disease, hypertension, diabetes, gallstones, sleep apnea, osteoarthritis, and many cancers (Table 10.1). Some experts predict that the number of Americans diagnosed with diabetes will increase by a whopping 165 percent, from 11 million in 2000 to 29 million in 2050.[3] In addition, the relationship between obesity and psychosocial development, including self-esteem, is believed to be quite close.

The estimated annual health care cost due to obesity in the United States exceeds $123 billion in medical expenses and lost productivity.[4] In fact, obesity rivals smoking

as a cause of preventable death.[5] This chapter will help you understand what *underweight, normal weight, overweight,* and *obesity* really mean, and why managing your weight is essential to overall health and well-being.

Determining the Right Weight for You

What weight is right for you? This depends on a wide range of variables, including your body structure, height, weight distribution, and the ratio of fat to lean tissue. In fact, your weight can be a deceptive indicator. Many extremely muscular athletes would be considered overweight based on traditional height–weight charts. Many young women think that they are the right weight based on charts but are shocked to discover that 35 to 40 percent of their weight is body fat!

In general, weights at the lower end of the range on these charts are recommended for individuals with a low ratio of muscle and bone to fat; those at the upper end are advised for people with more muscular builds (Table 10.2 on page 270). However, since actual body composition is hard to determine, most charts give a general range.

Overweight or Obese?

Most of us cringe at the thought of being labeled as one of the "O" words. What is the distinction between the two? **Overweight** refers to increased body weight in relation to

---

Overweight Increased body weight in relation to height.

Table 10.1
Selected Health Consequences of Overweight and Obesity

Premature Death
- Obese individuals have a 50–100% increased risk of death from all causes compared with people of normal weight. Among 25- to 35-year-olds, severe obesity increases the risk of death by a factor of 12.
- At least 300,000 deaths per year may be attributable to obesity.
- The risk of death rises with increasing weight.
- Even moderate excess weight (10–20 pounds for a person of average height) increases risk of death.

Cardiovascular Disease
- High blood pressure is twice as common in obese adults as it is for those who are at healthy weights.
- Incidence of all forms of heart disease is increased among overweight and obese people.
- Obesity is associated with elevated triglycerides and decreased "good" cholesterol.

Diabetes
- A weight gain of 11–18 pounds increases a person's risk of developing type 2 diabetes to twice that of individuals who have not gained weight.
- More than 80% of people with diabetes are overweight or obese.

Cancer
- Overweight and obesity are associated with increased risk of endometrial, colon, gallbladder, prostate, kidney, and post-menopausal breast cancer.
- Women gaining more than 20 pounds between age 18 and midlife double their risk of postmenopausal breast cancer compared to women whose weight remains stable.

Additional Health Consequences
- Sleep apnea and asthma are both associated with obesity.
- For every 2-pound increase in weight, the risk of developing arthritis increases by 9–13%.
- Obesity-related complications during pregnancy include increased risk of fetal and maternal death, labor and delivery complications, and increased risk of birth defects.

Source: U.S. Department of Health and Human Services, "The Surgeon General's Call to Action to Prevent and Decrease Overweight and Obesity," 2001. www.surgeongeneral.gov/topics/obesity/calltoaction/fact_consequences.htm; D. Eberwine, "Globesity: The Crisis of Growing Proportions," *Perspectives in Health* 7, no. 3 (2003): 6–11.

height, when compared to a standard such as the height/weight charts in Table 10.2. The excess weight may come from muscle, bone, fat, and/or water. Historically, nutritionists have defined overweight as being 1 to 19 percent above one's ideal weight and obese as being above 19 percent.

Another measurement of overweight and obesity is a mathematical formula known as **Body Mass Index (BMI),** which represents weight levels associated with the lowest overall risk to health (see the next section to calculate your BMI). Desirable BMI levels may vary with age.[6] You would be classified as being overweight if you have a BMI between 25.0 and 29.9. About 35 percent of all Americans fit this category.

A person may be classified as overweight using these standards even if the weight gain is due to an increase in lean muscle mass. For example, an athlete may be very lean and muscular, with very little body fat, yet she may weigh a lot more than others of the same height who have little muscle tissue. Conversely, a person may proudly proclaim that he weighs the same that he did in high school but have a much greater proportion of body fat, particularly in the hips, buttocks or thighs, than he did at a younger age. Body weight alone may not be a good indicator of overall fitness.

Another problem with using BMI is that people who have lost muscle mass, such as older adults, people with anorexia, or those who are seriously disabled or bedridden, could be in the "healthy weight" range, even though their nutritional reserves are dangerously low. BMI is a useful guideline but by itself is not diagnostic of a person's overall health status.[7]

Obesity is defined as an excessively high amount of body fat or adipose tissue in relation to lean body mass. It is important to consider both the distribution of fat throughout the body and the size of the adipose tissue deposits. Body fat distribution can be estimated by skinfold measures; waist-to-hip circumference ratios; or techniques such as ultrasound, computed tomography or magnetic resonance imaging, or others. People 20 to 40 percent above their ideal weight are

---

Body Mass Index (BMI) A technique of weight assessment based on the relationship of weight to height.

Obesity A weight disorder generally defined as an accumulation of fat beyond that considered normal for a person based on age, sex, and body type.

Table 10.2
Healthy Weight Ranges*

Height without Shoes	Weight† without Clothes
4'10"	91–119
4'11"	94–124
5'0"	97–128
5'1"	101–132
5'2"	104–137
5'3"	107–141
5'4"	111–146
5'5"	114–150
5'6"	118–155
5'7"	121–160
5'8"	125–164
5'9"	129–169
5'10"	132–174
5'11"	136–179
6'0"	140–184
6'1"	144–189
6'2"	148–195
6'3"	152–200
6'4"	156–205
6'5"	160–211
6'6"	164–216

* Each data entry applies to both men and women.

† In pounds

Source: Center for Nutrition Policy and Promotion, "Dietary Guidelines for Americans, 2000" (2000). www.usda.gov/cnpp/Pubs/ DG2000

labeled as *mildly obese* (90 percent of the obese fall into this category). Those 41 to 99 percent above their ideal weight are described as *moderately obese* (about 7 to 8 percent of the obese fit into this category). And 2 to 3 percent are identified as fitting the *severely, morbidly, or grossly overweight* category, which means that they are 100 percent or more above their ideal weight. In the last decade, more and more people fit into the moderate and severe levels of obesity, which means increased risks at all ages and stages of their lives.[8]

The most widely used definition of obesity is based on the expert panel's report from NHANES III data. The report defined obesity as having a BMI greater than or equal to 30.0. More than 30.5 percent of Americans age 20 and over are obese; thus, the general calculation that more than 60.5 percent of all Americans are overweight or obese.

The difficulty with defining obesity lies in determining what is normal. To date, there are no universally accepted standards for the ideal body weight or *body composition* (the ratio of lean body mass to fat body mass). While sources vary slightly, men's bodies should contain between 11 and 15 percent total body fat, and women should be within the range of 18 to 22 percent body fat. At various ages and stages of life, these ranges also vary. But generally, when men exceed 20 percent body fat and women exceed 30 percent body fat, they have slipped into obesity.

Why the difference between men and women? Much of it may be attributed to the normal structure of the female body and to sex hormones. Lean body mass consists of the structural and functional elements in cells, body water, muscle, bones, and other body organs such as the heart, liver, and kidneys. Body fat is composed of two types: essential and storage fat. Essential fat is necessary for normal physiological functioning, such as nerve conduction. Essential fat makes up approximately 3 to 7 percent of total body weight in men and approximately 15 percent of total body weight in women. Storage fat, the part that many of us try to shed, makes up the remainder of our fat reserves. It accounts for only a small percentage of total body weight for very lean people and between 5 and 25 percent of body weight of most American adults. Female bodybuilders, who are among the leanest of female athletes, may have body fat percentages of 8 to 13 percent, nearly all of which is essential fat.

Too Little Fat?

A certain amount of body fat is necessary for insulating the body, cushioning parts of the body and vital organs, and maintaining body functions. In men, this lower limit is approximately 3 to 4 percent. Women generally should not go below 8 percent. Excessively low body fat in females may lead to amenorrhea, a disruption of the normal menstrual cycle. The critical level of body fat necessary to maintain normal menstrual flow is believed to be 8 to 13 percent, but there are many additional factors that affect the menstrual cycle. Under extreme circumstances, such as starvation diets and certain diseases, the body utilizes all available fat reserves and begins to break down muscle tissue as a last-ditch effort to obtain nourishment.

The fact is that too much fat and too little fat are both potentially harmful. The key is to find a healthy level at which you are comfortable with your appearance and your ability to be as active as possible. Many options are available for determining your body fat and weight.

Assessing Fat Levels

Weight-for-Height Charts

Today, most weight control authorities believe that getting on the scale to determine your weight and then looking at where you fall on some arbitrary chart may not be helpful. Height–weight charts may lead some to think they are overweight when they are not, or that they are okay when, in fact, they may be at risk. Other measures exist for calculating body content, and some provide a very precise calculation of body fat. They include body mass index, waist circumference, waist-to-hip ratio, and various measures of body fat.

Body Mass Index

A useful index of the relationship of height and weight, BMI is the measurement of choice for obesity researchers and health professionals. It is not gender specific. Although it does not directly measure percentage of body fat, it does provide a more accurate measure of overweight and obesity than weight alone.[9]

We find BMI by dividing a person's weight in kilograms by height in meters squared. The mathematical formula is:

$$\text{Weight (kg)} \div \text{height squared (m}^2)$$

To determine BMI using pounds and inches, multiply your weight in pounds by 704.5, then divide the result by your height in inches, and divide that result by your height in inches a second time. (The National Institutes of Health uses the multiplier 704.5. Other organizations, such as the American Dietetic Association, suggest multiplying by 700. The variation in outcomes between the two is insignificant, and 700 is easier for most people to remember.) You can also go to the BMI calculator at the National Heart, Lung and Blood Institute's (NHLBI) website at http://nhlbisupport.com/bmi/bmicalc.htm or see Figure 10.1 on page 272.

Healthy weights are defined as those associated with BMIs of 19 to 25, the range of lowest statistical health risk.[10] The desirable range for females falls between 21 and 23; for males, between 22 and 24.[11] A BMI greater than 25 indicates overweight and potentially significant health risks. A body mass index of 30 or more is considered obese.[12] Many experts believe that this number is too high, particularly for younger adults.

Calculating BMI is simple, quick, and inexpensive—but it does have limitations. One problem is that very muscular people may fall into the overweight category when they are actually healthy and fit. As well, certain population groups, such as Asians, tend to have higher-than-healthy body fat at normal BMI levels, while Polynesians have somewhat lower body fat than other populations at the same BMI.[13]

These standards may seem almost impossible for people who consistently exceed the target weights and who have difficulty keeping off any lost weight. Constant failure may lead them to stop trying. The secret lies in establishing a healthful weight at a young age and maintaining it—a task easier said than done. The U.S. Dietary Guidelines for Americans encourage a weight gain of no more than 10 pounds after reaching adult height and endorses small weight losses of one-half to 1 pound per week, if needed, as well as smaller weight losses of 5 to 10 percent to make a difference toward health.[14]

Waist Circumference

Waist circumference measurement is a useful tool for assessing abdominal fat and associated health risks. Research indicates that a waistline greater than 40 inches (102 cm) in men and 35 inches (88 cm) in women may indicate greater health risk. If a person has a short stature (under 5 feet tall) or a BMI of 35 or above, waist circumference standards used for the general population might not apply.[15] Measure waist circumference by wrapping a tape measure comfortably around the smallest area below the rib cage and above the belly button.

Waist-to-Hip Ratio

Another useful measure is the waist-to-hip ratio, a measure of regional fat distribution. Research has shown that excess fat in the abdominal area poses a greater health risk than does excess fat in the hips and thighs. Determine your ratio by dividing the circumference of your waist by the circumference of your hips. A waist-to-hip ratio greater than 1.0 in men and 0.8 in women indicates increased health risks.[16] Therefore, knowing where your fat is carried may be more important than knowing your total fat content.

Men and postmenopausal women tend to store fat in the upper regions of their body, particularly in the abdominal area. Premenopausal women usually store their fat in lower regions of their bodies, particularly in the hips, buttocks, and thighs.[17]

Measures of Body Fat

Hydrostatic Weighing Techniques   From a clinical perspective, **hydrostatic weighing techniques** offer the most accurate method of measuring body fat. This method measures the amount of water a person displaces when completely submerged. Because fat tissue is less dense than muscle or bone tissue, a relatively accurate indication of actual body fat can be computed by comparing underwater and out-of-water weights. Although this method may be subject to error, it is one of the most sophisticated techniques currently available.

Pinch and Skinfold Measures   Perhaps the most commonly used method of determining body fat is the **pinch test**. Numerous studies have determined that the triceps area (the

---

Hydrostatic weighing techniques   Method of determining body fat by measuring the amount of water displaced when a person is completely submerged.

Pinch test   A method of determining body fat whereby a fold of skin just behind the triceps is pinched between the thumb and index fingers to determine the relative amount of fat.

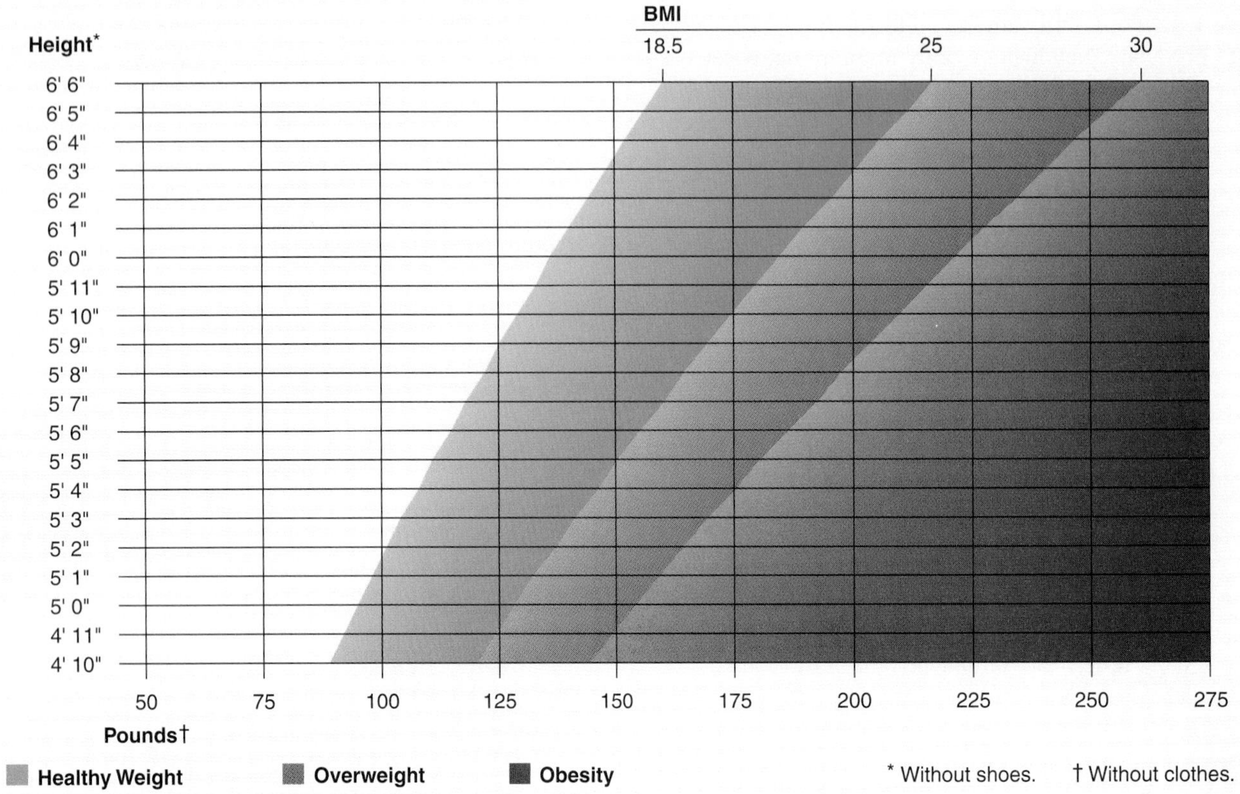
BMI
18.5
25
30
Height*
6' 6"
6' 5"
6' 4"
6' 3"
6' 2"
6' 1"
6' 0"
5' 11"
5' 10"
5' 9"
5' 8"
5' 7"
5' 6"
5' 5"
5' 4"
5' 3"
5' 2"
5' 1"
5' 0"
4' 11"
4' 10"
50
75
100
125
150
175
200
225
250
275
Pounds†
Healthy Weight
Overweight
Obesity
* Without shoes.
† Without clothes.

Directions: Find your weight on the bottom of the graph. Go straight up from that point until you come to the line that matches your height. Then look to find your weight group.

- BMI of 25 defines the upper boundary of healthy weight
- BMI of higher than 25 to 30 defines overweight
- BMI of higher than 30 defines obesity

Figure 10.1
Body Mass Index: Are You at a Healthy Weight?
Source: Dietary Guidelines Advisory Committee, USDA Agricultural Research Service. "Dietary Guidelines for Americans," 2000. www.ars.usda.gov/dgac/2kdiet.pdf

back of the upper arm) is one of the most reliable regions of the body for assessing the amount of fat in the subcutaneous (just under the surface) layer of the skin. In making this assessment, a person pinches a fold of skin just behind the triceps with the thumb and index finger and assesses the distance between thumb and finger. It is important to pinch only the fat layer and not the triceps muscle. If the size of the pinch is thicker than 1 inch, the person is generally considered overfat.

Skinfold caliper test A method of determining body fat whereby folds of skin and fat at various points on the body are grasped between thumb and forefinger and measured with calipers.

The **skinfold caliper test** resembles the pinch test but is much more accurate. This procedure involves pinching folds of skin at various points on the body with the thumb and index finger. A specially calibrated instrument called a *skinfold caliper* is used to measure the fat layer. Besides the triceps, the areas most often measured are the biceps (front of the arm), the subscapular (upper back), and the iliac crest (hip). Special formulas are employed to arrive at a combined prediction of total body fat.

Girth and Circumference Measures Girth and circumference measures involve using a measuring tape to take girth, or circumference, measurements at various body sites. These measurements are then converted into constants, and a formula is used to determine relative percentages of body fat. Although this technique is inexpensive, easy to use, and commonly performed, it is not as accurate as many of the other techniques listed here.

Soft-Tissue Roentgenogram A relatively new technique for determining body fat, the **soft-tissue roentgenogram** involves injecting a radioactive substance into the body and allowing this substance to penetrate muscle (lean) tissue, so that fat and lean tissue can be distinguished by means of imaging.

Bioelectrical Impedance Analysis Another method, **bioelectrical impedance analysis (BIA),** involves sending a small electrical current through the subject's body. The body's ability to conduct an electrical current reflects the total amount of water in the body. Generally, the more water, the more muscle and lean tissue. The amount of resistance to the current and the person's age, sex, and other physical characteristics are fed into a computer that calculates the total amount of lean and fat tissue. To obtain the most accurate readings, fasting for four hours prior to testing is recommended. BIA may not be as accurate for severely obese individuals.

Total Body Electrical Conductivity One of the newest (and most expensive) assessment techniques is **total body electrical conductivity (TOBEC),** which uses an electromagnetic force field to assess relative body fat. Although based on the same principle as impedance, this assessment requires much more elaborate, expensive equipment, and therefore is not practical for most people.

Although all of these methods can be useful, they also can be inaccurate and even harmful unless the testers are skillful and well trained. Before undergoing any procedure, make sure you understand the expense, potential for accuracy, risks, and training of the tester.

> **What do you think?**
>
> *Calculate your BMI using the formula provided. If possible, try to have your percentage of body fat tested with calipers or one of the other methods listed. Crosscheck your results by using the calculator found at the NHLBI website.* ✳ *Which value is most important to you? Why?* ✳ *How are they similar?*

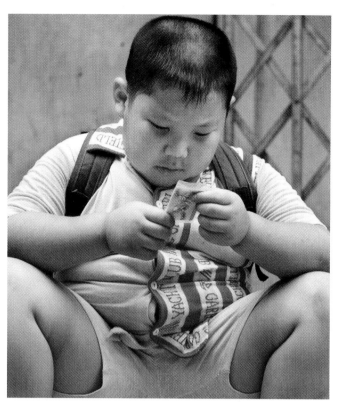

Obesity is increasing especially dramatically among children. Being overweight or obese from an early age can have devastating physical and emotional consequences.

Risk Factors for Obesity

In spite of massive efforts to keep Americans fit and in good health, obesity is the most common nutritional disorder in the United States, with rates that have increased dramatically among children and adults in recent decades.[18] The prevalence of obesity and overweight (defined as a BMI of 25 or higher) is generally higher among minorities, especially minority women. For example, 77.3 percent of African American females and 71.9 percent of Mexican American females

Girth and circumference measures A method of assessing body fat that employs a formula based on girth measurements of various body sites.

Soft-tissue roentgenogram A technique of body fat assessment in which radioactive substances are used to determine relative fat.

Bioelectrical impedance analysis (BIA) A technique of body fat assessment in which electrical currents are passed through fat and lean tissue.

Total body electrical conductivity (TOBEC) Technique using an electromagnetic force field to assess relative body fat.

Globesity: An Epidemic of Growing Proportions

It's not just Americans today who are bigger and less fit than at any time in history. A similar trend is emerging around the world in both developed and developing regions. In countries as diverse as the Czech Republic, Kuwait, and Jamaica, at least half of the population is overweight and 1 in 5 is obese. The highest obesity rate is in Samoa, where two-thirds of all women and half of all men are obese. Although rates in Canada and South America are slightly lower than in the United States, residents of the Americas as a whole are among the most overweight and obese in the world (see details by country in the figure).

While there is growing concern about the epidemic in adults, even more disturbing is the enormous jump in obesity rates among children. Rates of childhood obesity have increased 66% in the United States in the last decades. If that isn't bad enough, rates have increased a whopping 240% during the same period in Brazil.

Among the consequences is the parallel rise in type 2 diabetes in the global population; it is nearly 5 times more prevalent than it was 18 years ago. The dual impact of diabetes and obesity is sure to demand increasing attention to the global health consequences and disease burden.

Dietary excesses and sedentary lifestyles are key contributors to the increases in obesity. However, Donna Eberwine, editor of the Pan American Health Organization's *Perspectives in Health,* says "the growing body of public health literature on the 'globesity' epidemic places the bulk of the blame not on individuals but on globalization and development, with poverty as an exacerbating factor." As entire cultures move away from traditional diets, with raw fruits and vegetables and fewer fats, to diets heavy in highly processed, high-fat, and high-calorie fast food and packaged products, the same thing that happened to Americans during the move from the farms to cities is occurring. The world population is becoming supersized along with the products we consume.

Also contributing to the obesity epidemic is the increasingly sprawling environment in which people travel only by car, and walking or bicycling is difficult. Lack of health education about the risks of obesity also contributes to its increase.

The challenge is daunting. Nations must work together in the decades ahead to educate their populations, promote nutritious diets, and encourage physical activity.

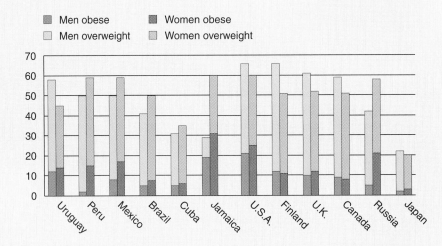

Percentage of Men and Women Who Are Overweight or Obese, by Country

Source: Figure reprinted with permission from *Perspectives in Health* 7, no. 3 © 2003, Pan American Health Organization.

---

are considered overweight or obese, while 57.3 percent of non-Hispanic white women fall into this category. Among men, 74.7 percent of Mexican American men and 60.7 percent of African American men are overweight or obese; 67.4 percent of white men are in this category.[19] These rates are especially noteworthy when compared to obesity trends in the rest of the world (see the Health in a Diverse World box).

The Surgeon General stated quite simply the cause of this epidemic of obesity: "Overweight and obesity result from an energy imbalance. This means eating too many calories and not getting enough exercise."[20] Clearly, environmental factors play a large role, especially factors that favor increased energy intake (consuming too much) and decreased energy expenditure (too little physical activity).

Key Environmental Factors

There is a long list of environmental factors that encourage us to increase our consumption, including the following.

- Bombardment with advertising designed to increase energy intake—ads for high-calorie foods at a low price, and promotion of larger portion sizes[21]
- Changes in the number of working women, which has led to greater use of restaurant meals, fast foods, and convenience foods[22]
- Bottle feeding of infants, which may increase energy intake relative to breast feeding[23]

Factors contributing to decreased energy expenditure include:

- The increasingly sedentary nature of many jobs.[24]
- Automated equipment and electronic communications, such as cell phones, remote controls, and other labor-saving devices[25]
- Spending more time in front of the computer and TV and playing video games[26]
- Fear of playing or being outside based on threat of violence
- Decline in physical education requirements in schools[27]
- Lack of community resources for exercise

What do you think?

In addition to those listed, can you think of other environmental factors that contribute to obesity?
✳ *What actions could you take to reduce your risk for each of these factors?*

Heredity

Are some people born to be fat? Several factors appear to influence why one person becomes obese and another remains thin; genes seem to interact with many of these factors.

Body Type and Genes In some animal species, the shape and size of the individual's body are largely determined by its parents' shape and size. Many scientists have explored the role of heredity in determining human body shape. You need only look at your parents and then glance in the mirror to see where you got your own body type. Children whose parents are obese also tend to be overweight. In fact, a family history of obesity increases one's chances of becoming obese by 25 to 30 percent.[28] Some researchers argue that obesity has a strong genetic determinant—it tends to run in families. They cite statistics that 80 percent of children who have two obese parents are also obese.[29] Genes play a significant role in how the body balances calories and energy. Also, by influencing the amount of body fat and fat distribution, genes can make a person more susceptible to gaining weight.

Twin Studies Studies of identical twins who were separated at birth and raised in different environments provide the strongest evidence yet that the genes a person inherits are a major factor in determining overweight, leanness, or average weight. Whether raised in family environments with fat or thin family members, twins with obese natural parents tend to be obese in later life.[30] According to another study, sets of identical twins who were separated and raised in different families and who ate widely different diets still grew up to weigh about the same.[31]

Although the exact mechanism remains unknown, it is believed that genes set metabolic rates, which influences how the body handles calories. Other experts believe that this genetic tendency may contribute as much as 25 to 40 percent of the reason for being overweight.[32]

Specific Obesity Genes? In the past decade, more and more research has pointed to the existence of a "fat gene." The most promising candidate is the *Ob* gene (for obesity), which is believed to disrupt the body's "I've had enough to eat" signaling system and may prompt individuals to keep eating past the point of being comfortably full. Research on Pima Indians, who have an estimated 75 percent obesity rate (nine out of ten are overweight), seems to point to an Ob gene that is a "thrifty gene." It is theorized that because their ancestors struggled through centuries of famine, their ancestors' basal metabolic rates slowed, which allowed them to store precious fat for survival. Survivors may have passed these genes on to their children, which would explain the lower metabolic rates found in Pimas today and their tendency toward obesity.[33] Scientists have found that they can manipulate mouse genes and construct an Ob gene that invariably leads to fatness in mice and the development of type 2 diabetes. Many suspect a human counterpart to this gene, but it has yet to be found. In addition, the (beta)-3 adrenergic-receptor gene has been identified in both human beings and mice. When mutated, it is thought to impede the body's ability to burn fat.[34]

Although the discovery of the Ob gene in mice has provided fertile ground for speculation, researchers have further refined their theories to focus on a protein that the Ob gene may produce, known as leptin, and a new leptin receptor in the brain. According to these studies, leptin is the chemical that signals the brain when you are full and need to stop eating.[35] Although obese people have adequate amounts of leptin and leptin receptors, they do not seem to work properly. However, it is not clear whether altering leptin levels would help in treating obesity.[36]

Other scientists have isolated a protein called *GLP-1*, which is known to slow down the passage of food through the intestines to allow the absorption of nutrients. When scientists injected GLP-1 into the brains of hungry rats, the rats stopped eating immediately.[37] It is speculated that leptin and GLP-1 might play complementary roles in weight control. Leptin and its receptors may regulate body weight over the long term and call on fast-acting appetite suppressants such as GLP-1 when necessary.

Hunger, Appetite, and Satiety

Theories abound concerning the mechanisms that regulate food intake. Some sources indicate that the hypothalamus (the part of the brain that regulates appetite) closely monitors levels of certain nutrients in the blood. When these levels fall, the brain signals us to eat. In the obese person, it is possible that the monitoring system does not work properly and the cues to eat are more frequent and intense than they are in people of normal weight.

(text continues on page 279)

Readiness for Weight Loss

To see how well your attitudes equip you for a weight-loss program, answer the questions that follow. For each question, circle the answer that best describes your attitude. As you complete each of the six sections, tally your score and analyze it according to the scoring guide.

I. GOALS, ATTITUDES, AND READINESS

1. Compared to previous attempts, how motivated are you to lose weight this time?

1	2	3	4	5
Not at all motivated	Slightly motivated	Somewhat motivated	Quite motivated	Extremely motivated

2. How certain are you that you will stay committed to a weight-loss program for the time it will take to reach your goal?

1	2	3	4	5
Not at all certain	Slightly certain	Somewhat certain	Quite certain	Extremely certain

3. Considering all outside factors at this time in your life—stress at work, family obligations, and so on—to what extent can you tolerate the effort required to stick to a diet?

1	2	3	4	5
Cannot tolerate	Can tolerate somewhat	Uncertain	Can tolerate well	Can tolerate easily

4. Think honestly about how much weight you hope to lose and how quickly you hope to lose it. Figuring a weight loss of one to two pounds per week, how realistic is your expectation?

1	2	3	4	5
Very unrealistic	Somewhat unrealistic	Moderately unrealistic	Somewhat realistic	Very realistic

5. While dieting, do you fantasize about eating a lot of your favorite foods?

1	2	3	4	5
Always	Frequently	Occasionally	Rarely	Never

6. While dieting, do you feel deprived, angry, and/or upset?

1	2	3	4	5
Always	Frequently	Occasionally	Rarely	Never

IF YOU SCORED

6 to 16: This may not be a good time for you to start a diet. Inadequate motivation and commitment and unrealistic goals could block your progress. Think about what contributes to your unreadiness, and consider changing these factors before undertaking a diet.

17 to 23: You may be close to being ready to begin a program but should think about ways to boost your readiness.

24 to 30: The path is clear: you can decide how to lose weight in a safe, effective way.

II. HUNGER AND EATING CUES

7. When food comes up in conversation or in something you read, do you want to eat, even if you are not hungry?

1	2	3	4	5
Never	Rarely	Occasionally	Frequently	Always

8. How often do you eat for a reason other than physical hunger?

1	2	3	4	5
Never	Rarely	Occasionally	Frequently	Always

9. Do you have trouble controlling your eating when your favorite foods are around the house?

1	2	3	4	5
Never	Rarely	Occasionally	Frequently	Always

IF YOU SCORED

3 to 6: You might occasionally eat more than you should, but it does not appear to be due to high responsiveness to environmental cues. Controlling the attitudes that make you eat may be especially helpful.

7 to 9: You may have a moderate tendency to eat just because food is available. Losing weight may be easier for you if you try to resist external cues and eat only when you are physically hungry.

10 to 15: Some or much of your eating may be in response to thinking about food or exposing yourself to temptations to eat. Think of ways to minimize your exposure to temptations so you eat only in response to physical hunger.

III. CONTROLLING OVEREATING

If the following situations occurred while you were on a diet, would you be likely to eat more or less immediately afterward and for the rest of the day?

10. Although you planned to skip lunch, a friend talks you into going out for a midday meal.

1	2	3	4	5
Would eat much less	Would eat somewhat less	Would make no difference	Would eat somewhat more	Would eat much more

11. You "break" your plan by eating a fattening, "forbidden" food.

1	2	3	4	5
Would eat much less	Would eat somewhat less	Would make no difference	Would eat somewhat more	Would eat much more

12. You have been following your diet faithfully and decide to test yourself by eating something you consider a treat.

1	2	3	4	5
Would eat much less	Would eat somewhat less	Would make no difference	Would eat somewhat more	Would eat much more

IF YOU SCORED

3 to 7: You recover rapidly from mistakes. However, if you frequently alternate between eating that is out of control and dieting very strictly, you may have a serious eating problem and should get professional help.

8 to 11: You do not seem to let unplanned eating disrupt your program. This is a flexible, balanced approach.

12 to 15: You may be prone to overeat after an event breaks your control or throws you off the track. Your reaction to these problem-causing events can be improved.

IV. BINGE EATING AND PURGING

13. Aside from holiday feasts, have you ever eaten a large amount of food rapidly and felt afterward that this eating incident was excessive and out of control?

2	0
Yes	No

14. If you answered yes to question 13, how often have you engaged in this behavior during the past year?

1	2	3	4	5	6
Less than once a month	About once a month	A few times a month	About once a week	About 3 times a week	Daily

(continued)

15. Have you purged (used laxatives or diuretics, or induced vomiting) to control your weight?

5	0
Yes	No

16. If you answered yes to question 15, how often have you engaged in this behavior during the past year?

1	2	3	4	5	6
Less than once a month	About once a month	A few times a month	About once a week	About 3 times a week	Daily

IF YOU SCORED

0: It appears that binge eating and purging are not problems for you.

2 to 11: Pay attention to these eating patterns. Should they arise more frequently, get professional help.

12 to 19: You show signs of having a potentially serious eating problem. See a counselor experienced in evaluating eating disorders right away.

V. EMOTIONAL EATING

17. Do you eat more than you would like to when you have negative feelings such as anxiety, depression, anger, or loneliness?

1	2	3	4	5
Never	Rarely	Occasionally	Frequently	Always

18. Do you have trouble controlling your eating when you have positive feelings—do you celebrate feeling good by eating?

1	2	3	4	5
Never	Rarely	Occasionally	Frequently	Always

19. When you have unpleasant interactions with others in your life, or after a difficult day at work, do you eat more than you'd like?

1	2	3	4	5
Never	Rarely	Occasionally	Frequently	Always

IF YOU SCORED

3 to 8: You do not appear to let your emotions affect your eating.

9 to 11: You sometimes eat in response to emotional highs and lows. Monitor this behavior to learn when and why it occurs, and be prepared to find alternate activities.

12 to 15: Emotional ups and downs can stimulate your eating. Try to deal with the feelings that trigger the eating and find other ways to express them.

VI. EXERCISE PATTERNS AND ATTITUDES

20. How often do you exercise?

1	2	3	4	5
Never	Rarely	Occasionally	Somewhat frequently	Frequently

21. How confident are you that you can exercise regularly?

1	2	3	4	5
Not at all confident	Slightly confident	Somewhat confident	Highly confident	Completely confident

22. When you think about exercise, do you develop a positive or negative picture in your mind?

1	2	3	4	5
Completely negative	Somewhat negative	Neutral	Somewhat positive	Completely positive

23. How certain are you that you can work regular exercise into your daily schedule?

1	2	3	4	5
Not at all certain	Slightly certain	Somewhat certain	Quite certain	Extremely certain

IF YOU SCORED

4 to 10: You're probably not exercising as regularly as you should. Determine whether attitude about exercise or your lifestyle is blocking your way, then change what you must and put on those walking shoes!

11 to 16: You need to feel more positive about exercise so you can do it more often. Think of ways to be more active that are fun and fit your lifestyle.

17 to 20: It looks as if the path is clear for you to be active. Now think of ways to get motivated.

After scoring yourself in each section of this questionnaire, you should be able to better judge your dieting strengths and weaknesses. Remember that the first step in changing eating behavior is to understand the conditions that influence your eating habits.

Source: Reprinted from "The Diet Readiness Test," in Kelly D. Brownell, "When and How to Diet," *Psychology Today,* June 1989, 41–46. Reprinted with permission from *Psychology Today* Magazine, copyright © 1989 (Sussex Publishers, Inc.).

Scientists distinguish between **hunger,** an inborn physiological response to nutritional needs, and **appetite,** a learned response to food that is tied to an emotional or psychological craving often unrelated to nutritional need. Obese people may be more likely than are thin people to satisfy their appetite and eat for reasons other than nutrition. However, the hypothesis that food tastes better to obese people, thus causing them to eat more, has largely been refuted.

In some instances, the problem with overconsumption may be more related to **satiety** than to appetite or hunger. People generally feel satiated, or full, when they have satisfied their nutritional needs and their stomach signals "no more." For undetermined reasons, obese people may not feel full until much later than thin people do. The leptin and GLP-1 studies seem to support this theory.

Setpoint Theory

Nutritional researchers William Bennett and Joel Gurin have developed the **setpoint theory,** which states that a person's body has a setpoint of weight at which it is programmed to be comfortable. If your setpoint is around 160 pounds, you will gain and lose weight fairly easily within a given range of that point. For example, if you gain 5 to 10 pounds on vacation, it will be fairly easy to lose that weight and remain around the 160-pound mark because the body actually tries to maintain this weight. Some people have equated this point with the **plateau** that dieters sometimes reach after losing a certain amount of weight. The setpoint theory proposes that after losing a predetermined amount of weight, the body will actually sabotage additional weight loss by slowing down metabolism. In extreme cases, the metabolic rate will decrease to a point at which the body will maintain its weight on as little as 1,000 calories per day.

Can a person change this predetermined setpoint? Proponents of this theory argue that it is possible to raise one's setpoint over time by continually gaining weight and failing to exercise. Conversely, reducing caloric intake and exercising regularly can gradually decrease one's setpoint. Exercise may be the most critical factor in readjusting setpoint, although diet may also be important.

The setpoint theory remains controversial. Perhaps its greatest impact was the sense of relief it provided for people who have lost weight, plateaued, and regained weight time and time again. It told them that their failure was not due to lack of willpower alone. The setpoint theory also prompted nutritional experts to look more carefully at popular methods of weight loss. If it is correct, an extremely low calorie diet isn't just dangerous; it may also cause the body to protect the dieter from starvation by slowing down metabolism, which makes weight loss even more difficult.

Hunger   An inborn physiological response to nutritional needs.

Appetite   A learned response that is tied to an emotional or psychological craving for food often unrelated to nutritional need.

Satiety   The feeling of fullness or satisfaction at the end of a meal.

Setpoint theory   A theory of obesity causation that suggests that fat storage is determined by a thermostatic mechanism in the body that acts to maintain a specific amount of body fat.

Plateau   That point in a weight loss program at which the dieter finds it difficult to lose more weight.

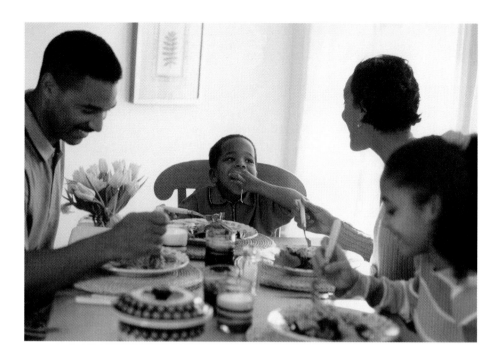

Many factors help determine body type, including heredity and genetic makeup, environmental factors, and learned eating patterns, many of which are connected to habits learned from family.

Endocrine Influence

Over the years, many people have attributed obesity to problems with their **thyroid gland.** They believed that an underactive thyroid impeded their ability to burn calories. However, most authorities agree that less than 2 percent of the obese population have a thyroid problem and can trace their weight problems to a metabolic or hormone imbalance.[38]

Psychosocial Factors

The relationship of weight problems to deeply rooted emotional insecurities, needs, and wants remains uncertain. Food often is used as a reward for good behavior in childhood. As adults face unemployment, broken relationships, financial uncertainty, fears about health and other problems, the bright spot in the day is often "what's on the table for dinner" or "we're going to that restaurant tonight." Again, the research underlying this theory is controversial. What is certain is that eating tends to be a focal point of people's lives, and the comfort foods of childhood may provide a salve for painful social pressures. Eating is essentially a social ritual associated with companionship, celebration, and enjoyment. For many people, the social emphasis on the eating experience is a

---

Thyroid gland   A two-lobed endocrine gland located in the throat region that produces a hormone that regulates metabolism.

Basal metabolic rate (BMR)   The energy expenditure of the body under resting conditions at normal room temperature.

---

major obstacle to successful weight control. Although some restaurants offer menu items designed to aid dieters, many people have difficulty choosing responsibly when confronted with an entire menu of delicious, fattening foods.

Metabolic Changes

Even when completely at rest, the body consumes a certain amount of energy. The amount of energy your body uses at complete rest is your **basal metabolic rate (BMR).** About 60 to 70 percent of all the calories you consume on a given day go to support your basal metabolism: heartbeat, breathing, maintaining body temperature, and so on. So if you consume 2,000 calories per day, 1,200 to 1,400 of those calories are burned without your doing any significant physical activity. But unless you exert yourself enough to burn the remaining 600 to 800 calories, you will gain weight.

Your BMR can fluctuate considerably, with several factors influencing whether it slows down or speeds up. In general, the younger you are, the higher your BMR, partly because in young people cells undergo rapid subdivision, which consumes a good deal of energy. BMR is highest during infancy, puberty, and pregnancy, when bodily changes are most rapid. BMR is also influenced by body composition. Muscle tissue is highly active—even at rest—compared to fat tissue. The more lean tissue you have, the greater your BMR; the more fat tissue you have, the lower your BMR. Men have a higher BMR than women do, at least partly because of their greater proportion of lean tissue.

Age is another factor. After age 30, BMR slows down by about 1 to 2 percent a year. Therefore, people over 30 commonly find that they must work harder to burn off an extra helping of ice cream than they did when in their teens. "Middle-aged spread," a reference to the tendency to put on weight later in life, is partly related to this change. A slower BMR, coupled with less activity and shifting priorities (family and career become more important than fitness), puts the weight of many middle-aged people in jeopardy.

In addition, the body has a number of self-protective mechanisms that signal BMR to speed up or slow down. For example, when you have a fever, the energy needs of your cells increase, which generates heat and speeds up your BMR. In starvation situations, the body protects itself by slowing down BMR to conserve precious energy. Thus, when people repeatedly resort to extreme diets, it is believed that their bodies reset their BMRs at lower rates. **Yo-yo diets,** in which people repeatedly gain weight and then starve themselves to lose it, are doomed to failure. When they resume eating after their weight loss, they have a BMR that is set lower, which makes it almost certain that they will regain the pounds they just lost. After repeated cycles of dieting and regaining weight, these people find it increasingly hard to lose weight and increasingly easy to regain it, so they become heavier and heavier.

According to a recent study by Kelly Brownell of Yale University, middle-aged men who maintained a steady weight (even if they were overweight) had a lower risk of heart attack than did men whose weight cycled up and down in a yo-yo pattern. Brownell found that smaller, well-maintained weight losses are more beneficial for reducing cardiovascular risk than are larger, poorly maintained weight losses.[39]

Lifestyle

Of all the factors affecting obesity, perhaps the most critical is the relationship between activity levels and calorie intake. Obesity rates are rising. But how can this be happening? Aren't more people exercising than ever before? Though the many advertisements for sports equipment and the popularity of athletes may give the impression that Americans love a good workout, the facts are not so positive. Data from a newly released National Health Interview Survey show that four in ten adults in the United States never engage in any exercise, sports, or physically active hobbies in their leisure time.[40] Women (43.2 percent) were somewhat more likely than men (36.5 percent) to be sedentary, a finding that was consistent across all age groups. Among both men and women, African American and Hispanic adults were more sedentary than were white adults.[41] Leisure-time physical activity also was strongly associated with level of education. About 72 percent of adults who never attended high school were sedentary; the statistics decline steadily to 45 percent among high school graduates and about 24 percent among adults with graduate-level college degrees.[42]

Do you know people who seemingly can eat whatever they want without gaining weight? With few exceptions, if you were to follow them around for a typical day, you would discover the reason. Even if their schedule does not include intense exercise, it probably includes a high level of activity.

Smoking Women who smoke tend to weigh 6 to 10 pounds less than nonsmokers do. After they quit, their weight generally increases to the level found among nonsmokers. Weight gain after smoking cessation may be partly due to nicotine's ability to raise metabolic rate. When smokers stop, they burn fewer calories. Another reason former smokers often gain weight is that they generally eat more to satisfy free-floating cravings.[43]

Gender and Obesity

Throughout a woman's life, issues of appearance and beauty are constantly in the foreground. Only recently have researchers begun to understand just how significant the quest for beauty and the perfect body really is.

Of increasing interest is an emerging problem seen in both young men and women, known as **social physique anxiety (SPA),** in which the desire to look good has a destructive and sometimes disabling effect on one's ability to function effectively in relationships and interactions with others. People suffering from SPA may spend a disproportionate amount of time fixating on their bodies, working out, and performing tasks that are ego centered and self-directed, rather than focusing on interpersonal relationships and general tasks.[44] Incessant worry about their bodies and their appearance permeates their lives. Overweight and obesity are clear risks for these people, and experts speculate that this anxiety may contribute to eating-disordered behaviors.

Researchers have determined that being severely overweight in adolescence may predetermine one's social and economic future—particularly for females. It was found that obese women complete about half a year less of schooling, are 20 percent less likely to get married, and earn $6,710 on average less per year than their slimmer counterparts. Obese women also have rates of household poverty 10 percent higher than those of women who are not overweight. In

Yo-yo diet Cycles in which people repeatedly gain weight, then starve themselves to lose weight. This lowers their BMR, which makes regaining weight even more likely.

Social physiqe anxiety (SPA) A desire to look good that has a destructive effect on a person's ability to function effectively socially.

contrast, the study found that overweight men are 11 percent less likely to be married than thinner men but suffer few adverse economic consequences.

It may be that women suffer such negative consequences because the social stigma of being overweight is more severe for women than for men. Women are also disadvantaged biologically when it comes to losing weight. Compared to men, they have a lower ratio of lean body mass to fatty mass, in part due to differences in bone size and mass, muscle size, and other variables. Muscle uses more energy than fat does. Because men have more muscle, they burn 10 to 20 percent more calories than women do during rest.[45] For all ages after sexual maturity, men have higher metabolic rates, which makes it easier for them to burn off excess calories. Women also face greater potential for weight fluctuation due to hormonal changes, pregnancy, and other conditions that increase the likelihood of weight gain. Also, as a group, men are more socialized into physical activity from birth. Strenuous activity in both work and play are encouraged for men, whereas women's roles have typically been more sedentary and required a lower level of caloric expenditure.

Not only are women more vulnerable to weight gain, but they also face pressures to maintain and/or lose weight that make them more likely to take dramatic measures. For example, eating disorders are more prevalent among women, and more women than men take diet pills.

However, men experience these pressures too. The male image is becoming more associated with the bodybuilder shape and size, and men are becoming more preoccupied with their own physical form. Thus eating disorders, exercise addictions, and other maladaptive responses are on the increase among men as well.

> ### What do you think?
> *Can you think of other reasons why men and women may differ in how much weight they gain and how easily they are able to lose it? ✳ What historical patterns may have contributed to this trend?*

Managing Your Weight

At some point in our lives, almost all of us will decide to go on a diet, and many will meet with mixed success. The problem is probably related to the fact that we think about losing weight in terms of dieting rather than in terms of adjusting lifestyle and eating behaviors. It is well documented that hypocaloric (low-calorie) diets produce only temporary losses and may actually lead to disordered binge eating or related problems.[46] While repeated bouts of restrictive dieting may be physiologically harmful, the sense of failure that we get

each time we try and fail can also exact far-reaching psychological costs.[47] Drugs and intensive counseling can contribute to positive weight loss, but even then, many people regain weight after treatment.

Keeping Weight Control in Perspective

Although experts say that losing weight simply requires burning more calories than are consumed, putting this principle into practice is far from simple. According to William W. Hardy, M.D., president of the Michigan-based Rochester Center for Obesity, to say weight control is simply a matter of pushing away from the table is ludicrous. Nature is a cheat. While it is true that "calories in minus calories out equals weight," people of the same age, sex, height, and weight can have differences of as much as 1,000 calories a day in resting metabolic rate (RMR). This may explain why one person's gluttony is another's starvation, even if it results in the same readout on the scale. And while people of normal weight average 25 billion to 35 billion fat cells, obese people can inherit a billowing 135 billion. A roll of the genetic dice adds more variety: at least 240 genes affect weight.[48] Also, factors such as depression, stress, culture, and available foods all affect obesity.

Weight loss is more difficult for some people and may require more supportive friends and relatives plus extraordinary efforts to prime the body for burning extra calories. Being overweight does not mean people are weak-willed or lazy. As scientists unlock the many secrets of genetic messengers that influence body weight and learn more about the role of certain foods in the weight loss equation, dieting may not be the same villain in the future that it is today.

Setting Realistic Goals

Rather than focusing on weight loss per se, health professionals emphasize the importance of psychological and physical health.[49] Modern weight-management programs incorporate the following goals.

- Establish tolerable, enjoyable, and stable eating and exercise patterns.
- Initially, focus on small gains and benefits to health and well-being. Later, focus on long-term functional improvements, improvements in energy, and reduced risk from disease.
- Establish maintainable goals.
- Make a lifetime commitment to a healthful lifestyle that includes exercise, prudent food choices, and stress management.
- Seek continued support from professionals and loved ones.
- Don't make food the central focus of your life. Learn to enjoy other activities that bring joy.
- Become a wise food consumer.

Understanding Calories

A *calorie* is a unit of measure that indicates the amount of energy we obtain from a particular food. One pound of body fat contains approximately 3,500 calories. So each time you consume 3,500 calories more than your body needs to maintain weight, you gain a pound. Conversely, each time your body expends an extra 3,500 calories, you lose a pound. So if you add a can of Coca-Cola or Pepsi (140 calories) to your daily diet and make no other changes in diet or activity, you would gain a pound in 25 days (3,500 calories ÷ 140 calories/day = 25 days). Conversely, if you walk for half an hour each day at a pace of 15 minutes per mile (172 calories burned), you would lose a pound in approximately 20 days (3,500 calories ÷ 172 calories/day = 20.3 days). The two ways to lose weight, then, are to lower calorie intake (through improved eating habits) and to increase exercise (thereby expending more calories).

Adding Exercise

Approximately 90 percent of the daily calorie expenditures of most people occurs as a result of the **resting metabolic rate (RMR).** Slightly higher than the BMR, the RMR includes the BMR plus any additional energy expended through daily sedentary activities such as food digestion, sitting, studying, or standing. Because lean muscle tissue appears to influence metabolic rates, increasing muscle mass may be a factor in burning calories throughout the day (see Chapter 11). The **exercise metabolic rate (EMR)** accounts for the remaining 10 percent of all daily calorie expenditures; it refers to the energy expenditure that occurs during physical exercise. For most of us, these calories come from light daily activities, such as walking, climbing stairs, and mowing the lawn. If we increase the level of physical activity to moderate or heavy, however, our EMR may be 10 to 20 times greater than typical RMRs and can contribute substantially to weight loss.

Increasing BMR, RMR, or EMR levels will help burn calories. An increase in the intensity, frequency, and duration of daily exercise levels can have significant impact on total calorie expenditure.

Physical activity makes a greater contribution to BMR when large muscle groups are used. The energy spent on physical activity is the energy used to move the body's muscles—the muscles of the arms, back, abdomen, legs, and so on—and the extra energy used to speed up heartbeat and respiration rate. The number of calories spent depends on three factors:

1. The amount of muscle mass moved
2. The amount of weight moved
3. The amount of time the activity takes

An activity involving both the arms and legs burns more calories than one involving only the legs. An activity performed by a heavy person burns more calories than one performed by a lighter person. And an activity performed for 40 minutes requires twice as much energy than one performed for only 20 minutes. Thus, obese people walking for 1 mile burn more calories than do slim people walking the same distance. It also may take overweight people longer to walk the mile, which means that they are burning energy for a longer time and therefore expending more overall calories than the thin walkers.

Changing Your Eating Habits

At any given time, many Americans are trying to lose weight. Given the hundreds of different diets and endless expert advice available, why do we find it so difficult?

Determining What Triggers an Eating Behavior Before you can change a behavior, you must first determine what causes it. Many people have found it helpful to keep a chart of their eating patterns: when they feel like eating, where they are when they decide to eat, the amount of time they spend eating, other activities they engage in during the meal (watching television or reading), whether they eat alone or with others, what and how much they consume, and how they felt before they took their first bite. If you keep a detailed daily log of eating triggers for at least a week, you will discover useful clues about what in your environment or your emotional makeup causes you to want food. Typically, these dietary triggers center on problems in everyday living rather than on real hunger pangs. Many people find that they eat compulsively when stressed. For other people, the same circumstances diminish their appetite, which causes them to lose weight.

Changing Your Triggers Once you recognize the factors that cause you to overeat, removing the triggers or substituting other activities for them will help you develop more sensible eating patterns. Here are some examples of substitute behaviors.

1. When eating dinner, turn off all distractions, including the television and radio.
2. Replace snack breaks or coffee breaks with exercise breaks.
3. Instead of gulping your food, chew each bite slowly and savor it.
4. Vary the time of day when you eat. Instead of eating by the clock, do not eat until you are truly hungry. Allow yourself only a designated amount of time for eating—but do not rush.

> **Resting metabolic rate (RMR)** The energy expenditure of the body under BMR conditions plus other daily sedentary activities.
>
> **Exercise metabolic rate (EMR)** The energy expenditure that occurs during exercise.

Tips for Sensible Weight Management

Rather than thinking about the best diet for you, the key to successful weight management is finding a sustainable way to control food that will work for you. Use the following strategies with a Behavior Change Contract to develop a weight management plan, and make changes in your diet and your activity level to create a plan that is right for you. Remember, you are making life-long changes that will result in weight loss. You are not going on a diet that you will quit someday.

MAKING A PLAN

- *Think of it as a way of life.* This is a way of improving your body and your health rather than a punishment or a diet. Remember that you are worth it.
- *Assess where you are.* Monitor your eating habits for 2 to 3 days; take careful note of the good things you are doing and the things that need improvement.

- *Set realistic goals.* No matter what you do, you may not have a perfect body. What do you realistically want to look like? How do you want to feel when you move? How do you want your clothes to feel on you? Set either a weight or a Body Mass Index (BMI) level that you want to achieve. Establish short-term goals on the way to the final goal.
- *Establish a plan.* What are three dietary changes you can make today? What exercise will you do tomorrow, the next day, and sustain for one week? Once you do one week, plot a course for two weeks. Jot down how you feel after each week's activity.
- *Be consistent.* Make a number of small changes in what you regularly eat and drink and in your daily activity levels. Make changes that you can stick with and that are comfortable for you (parking farther from a destination and walking, eating cereal and juice for breakfast, walking three days per week, and so on). Set a schedule and try to stick to it, with an alternative time each day in case your plans change. Always have a fallback option for your scheduled exercise.

- *Look for balance in what you do.* Remember that it's more about balance than about giving things up. If you must have that piece of pizza or chocolate cake, have it, but then do the extra exercise it takes to burn off the calories or limit caloric intake the next day. Remember that it's calories taken in and burned over time that makes the difference.
- *Stay positive.* A healthy lifestyle isn't about being bad or good; none of us is perfect. Focus on the positive steps you are taking and the healthy things you do each week rather than on the less healthy things.
- *Be patient and persistent.* You didn't develop a weight problem overnight. Don't expect instant results. Assess other gains that you make each week: gains in energy level, the fit of your clothes, and how you feel in your body.
- *Reward successes.* Set short-term goals, and reward yourself when you've reached them. If your first goal is to lose 10 pounds, reward yourself with something fun: new shoes, a new CD, whatever it takes to keep you motivated.

---

5. If you find that you generally eat all that you can cram on a plate, use smaller plates.
6. Stop buying high-calorie foods that tempt you to snack, or store them in an inconvenient place.

What do you think?

If you were going to try to lose weight, what strategies would you most likely choose? ❋ Which strategies offer the lowest health risk and the greatest chance for success? ❋ What factors might support or sabotage your weight-loss efforts?

Selecting a Nutritional Plan

Once you have discovered what factors tend to sabotage your weight-loss efforts, you will be well on your way to healthy weight control. To succeed, however, you must plan

for success. By setting goals that are unrealistic or too far in the future, you will doom yourself to failure. Do not try to lose 40 pounds in two months. Try, instead, to lose a healthy 1 to 2 pounds during the first week, and stay with this slow and easy regimen. Reward yourself when you lose pounds. If you binge and go off your nutrition plan, get right back on it the next day. Remember that you did not gain 40 pounds in eight weeks, so it is unrealistic to punish your body by trying to lose that amount of weight in such a short time.

Seek assistance from reputable sources in selecting a dietary plan that is nutritious and easy to follow. Registered dietitians, some physicians (not all doctors have a strong background in nutrition), health educators and exercise physiologists with nutritional training, and other health professionals can provide reliable information. Beware of people who call themselves nutritionists. There is no such official designation, which leaves the door open for just about anyone to call himself or herself a nutritional expert. Avoid weight-loss programs that promise quick miracle results.

CHANGING YOUR DIET

- *Be adventurous with your food choices.* Expand your usual meals and snacks to enjoy a wide variety of different options. Focus on the quality of the food rather than on the amount you get. Avoid buffets that allow you to replenish your plate several times.
- *Do not constantly deprive yourself of favorite foods or set unrealistic dietary rules or guidelines.* If you slip and eat something you shouldn't, be more careful in what you eat the next day. Balance over a week's time is important. Allow slips, and reward successes.
- *Be sensible with your knife and fork.* Enjoy all foods, just don't overdo. When you eat out, eat slowly, cut food into smaller pieces, and think about taking some home for tomorrow's lunch or dinner. Resist the urge to clean your plate. Share entrées with a friend, and order salads with dressings on the side.
- *Eat on a regular schedule.* Do not skip meals or let yourself get too hungry.
- *Eat breakfast.* This will prevent you from being too hungry and overeating at lunch.
- *Plan ahead, and be prepared for when you might get hungry.* Always have good food available when and where you get hungry.

CHANGING YOUR LEVEL OF ACTIVITY

- *Be active, and slowly increase activity.* If you stick to something, it will gradually take less and less effort to walk that mile, for example. Gradually increase your speed and/or the distance (see Chapter 11). Move more, sit less. If you find that you are always looking for a place to sit, consciously work toward standing or moving. Remember, every step counts. Purchasing an inexpensive pedometer and recording your daily steps are excellent ways to monitor and improve your level of activity.
- *Be creative with your physical activity.* Find activities that you really love, and stick to them. If you hate to walk in the rain but love to shop, walk in a covered mall and then shop! Try things you haven't tried before. Today, options such as yoga, pilates, dancing, swimming, skiing, and gardening are available.
- *Pick an activity that is inexpensive and does not require fancy equipment.* This means you will maintain your fitness program even when you are traveling away from home.
- *Find an exercise partner to help you get started and motivate you.* Don't pick your fittest friend. Find someone who is patient, understanding, and can take the time necessary to be a supporter. One of the worst mistakes you can make is to take your first bike ride with an avid bicyclist. You'll always feel like you can't keep up. Be patient with yourself. Choose other people who need help, and commit to helping them. It will also help you get through the difficult days until exercise is a part of your lifestyle.

Source: Adapted in part from Melinda Manore and Janice Thompson, "Table 15.3: Techniques to Help an Active Individual Identify and Maintain a Healthy Body Weight Throughout the Life Cycle," in *Sport Nutrition for Health and Performance* (Champaign, IL: Human Kinetics Publishing, 2000), 417.

For any weight-loss program, ask about the credentials of the adviser; assess the nutrient value of the prescribed diet; verify that dietary guidelines are consistent with reliable nutrition research; and analyze the suitability of the diet to your tastes, budget, and lifestyle. Any diet that requires radical behavior changes is doomed to failure. The most successful plans allow you to make food choices and do not ask you to sacrifice everything you enjoy. See the Consumer Health box on pages 286 and 287 and the New Horizons in Health box on page 288 for information on various popular diets and on low-carbohydrate diets in particular.

Considering Drastic Weight Loss Measures

When nothing seems to work, people often become willing to take significant risks in order to lose weight. Dramatic weight loss may be recommended in cases of extreme health risk. However, even in such situations, drastic dietary, pharmacological, or surgical measures should be considered carefully and discussed with several knowledgeable health professionals.

Drastic Diets Fasting, starvation diets, and other forms of **very low calorie diets (VLCDs)** have been shown to cause significant health risks. Typically, depriving the body of food for prolonged periods forces it to make adjustments to prevent the shutdown of organs. The body depletes its energy reserves to obtain necessary fuels. One of the first reserves the body turns to in order to maintain its supply of glucose is lean, protein tissue. As this occurs, weight is lost rapidly because protein contains only half as many calories per pound as fat. At the same time, significant water stores are lost. Over time, the body begins to run out of liver tissue, heart muscle, blood, and so on, since these readily available substances are burned to supply energy. Only after depleting the readily available proteins from these sources does the body

Very low calorie diets (VLCDs) Diets with caloric value of 400 to 700 calories per day.

Analyzing Popular Diets

In our ongoing quest to find an effective way to lose weight, Americans consider many seemingly reputable options. Are any of these diet plans really the miracles that they often claim to be? Don't count on it. Some are quite good, but others produce no long-term effects and may even be dangerous. Each year, "new and improved" versions of the same old dietary ploys surface in bookstores, where they sell millions of copies. Then there are reports of successes and dangers. And finally, professional groups jump into the fray to label

these diets as ineffective or dangerous. Just when we think we've seen the last of a fad, its authors re-invent themselves and capture our interest yet again. Dr. Kelly Brownell, noted obesity researcher at Yale University, describes this pattern: "When I get calls about the latest diet fad, I imagine a trick birthday cake candle that keeps lighting up and we have to keep blowing it out over and over again."

Virtually anyone can write a book making diet claims. Just because the authors have Ph.D.s or other credentials, they may not have expertise in the area that they write about. If they do have the expertise, they may base their arguments on un-

proven science or faulty scientific reasoning. Although health claims should only be published after solid research has proven the results repeatedly with different populations, this happens all too infrequently.

Below is a summary of some of the most popular diets and the consensus opinions of the U.S. Department of Agriculture, the American Heart Association, the Center for Science in the Public Interest, and several other professional groups and individuals regarding effectiveness and safety. For a detailed discussion of recent research into low-carbohydrate diets, see the New Horizons in Health box on page 288.

Book/Program and Author	Premise of the Diet	How It Claims to Work	Experts' Opinions	Comments
The Atkins Diet, Robert Atkins, M.D.	Says overweight people eat too many carbohydrates. High-protein diet allows you to eat all the protein you want (meat, eggs, cheese, and more) and restricts refined sugar, milk, white rice, and white flour.	Restrict carbohydrates and body goes into ketosis. In ketosis, body gets energy from ketones, little carbon fragments that are the fuel created by breakdown of fat stores. You feel less hungry.	Highly controversial. Low intake of fruits and vegetables a problem.	Possible side effects: nausea, fatigue, low blood pressure, elevated uric acid/kidney problems, bad breath, constipation, fetal harm if pregnant.
Dean Ornish Diet, Dean Ornish, M.D.	Diet and exercise are important. Watch *what* you eat; there are foods you should eat all of the time, some of the time, and none of the time. Less than 10% of your calories should come from fat. Eat lots of little meals.	Metabolism is a result of our ancestors. We need to change old metabolic patterns. Meditation is a part of this: when your soul is fed, you have less need to overeat.	Mostly positive for highly restrictive diet and healthy lifestyle regimen. Documented studies show heart blockage reversal. Drawbacks are that it is tough to stick to this diet, and new eating patterns must be learned. Only the most committed will stick to this rigid diet.	May be tough for all but strict vegans to adhere to this plan. Eating smaller, more frequent meals may be difficult. Otherwise a good model.
Eating Well for Optimum Health, Andrew Weil, M.D.	Eat less, exercise more. Take a more Eastern than Western approach. Avoid quick fixes, and set realistic goal of 1–2 pounds of weight loss per week. Balance the	Keeps it simple. Criticizes high-protein diets because of rise in cholesterol and calcium depletion. Moderation is a key.	A more holistic approach to dieting than most. Considers exercise and stress as factors.	May not be sustainable for those who are used to diets high in dairy or meat. Nutrition experts support this common-sense approach. The vegetarian emphasis is

begin to burn fat reserves. In this process, known as **ketosis,** the body adapts to prolonged fasting or carbohydrate depri-

> **Ketosis** A condition in which the body adapts to prolonged fasting or carbohydrate deprivation by converting body fat to ketones, which can be used as fuel for some brain activity.

vation by converting body fat to ketones, which can be used as fuel for some brain cells. Within about ten days after the typical adult begins a complete fast, the body will have used many of its energy stores and death may occur.

In very low-calorie diets, powdered formulas are usually given to patients under medical supervision. These formulas have daily values of 400 to 700 calories plus vitamin and mineral supplements. Although these diets may be beneficial for people who have failed at all conventional

Book/Program and Author	Premise of the Diet	How It Claims to Work	Experts' Opinions	Comments
Eating Well for Optimum Health, (continued)	amount and type of food. Describes meats as "flesh foods." Minimize dairy, and take a Mediterranean dietary approach.			substantiated as healthy by numerous studies.
The Pritikin Principle, Robert Pritikin	Concern not for calories, but for density of calories. Eat more foods that are not calorie dense, such as apples and oatmeal.	Fill up on foods that have fewer calories. Large volume of fiber and water will keep you full. Emphasis on vegetables, fruits, beans, unprocessed grains; exercise strongly recommended	Weight loss will occur but frequent feelings of hunger. Weight will usually creep back. Low in fat so healthy in general, except when taken to extreme or for certain groups of people.	Strict limitations of animal products a plus. Incorporates exercise and stress management. Not an easy plan to stick to.
The South Beach Diet, Arthur Agatston, M.D.	As with other low-carbohydrate diets, argues that carbohydrates are to blame for obesity.	Carbohydrates lead to overeating and cravings. Advocates combining small amounts of undesirable carbohydrates with vegetables and proteins.	As with other low-carbohydrate diets, research is still being conducted into effectiveness of this style of dieting.	Does not include recommendations to incorporate exercise into program, which is a key to any weight loss. Less restrictive on portion sizes than are other diets.
Sugar Busters, H. Leighton Steward, Morrison Bethea, M.D., Samuel Andrews MD, and Luis Balart, M.D.	Cut sugar to trim fat. Pay attention to portion size. Eliminate potatoes, corn, rice, bread, carrots, refined sugar, honey, soft drinks, and beer.	Glucose, insulin production theory: the more insulin produced, the more fat.	Most don't like this diet. When you gain weight, it doesn't matter where calories come from; it is total calorie intake that is most important.	You'll lose weight due to decreased calorie intake, but this is not a good long-term strategy.
Weight Watchers	Eat from food groups, tally points to monitor intake. Based on weight and dietary goals. Eat what you want, but use discretion in amount.	Based on calories in, calories out. Includes exercise and social support.	Life focus rather than diet focus. Has support of most national organizations. One of the most highly recommended diets.	Works well for many people, particularly those for whom social support is important.
The Zone, Barry Sears, Ph.D.	Offers a wellness philosophy to develop a metabolic state in which the body works efficiently. Recommends eating different calories than you do now and a small amount of protein. Identifies favorable versus unfavorable carbohydrates.	Claims that his percentages of fat, protein, and carbohydrates are the best ratios for health.	Superiority of given ratios is unsubstantiated by research. Mixed reviews from experts: easy to follow, but don't count on results. Some recommendations (eating high-fat ice cream) are questionable.	Not a lot of do's and don'ts. Dieters may find it easy to follow.

Source: United States Department of Agriculture, "The Great Nutrition Debate," 2000. www.usda.gov/cnpp/publications.html

weight-loss methods and who face severe health risks due to obesity, they never should be undertaken without strict medical supervision. Problems associated with fasting, VLCDs, and other forms of severe calorie deprivation include blood sugar imbalance, cold intolerance, constipation, decreased BMR, dehydration, diarrhea, emotional problems, fatigue, headaches, heart irregularity, ketosis, kidney infections and failure, loss of lean body tissue, weakness, and eventual weight gain due to the yo-yo effect and other variables.

Drug Treatment Experts reason that if obesity is a chronic disease, it should be treated as such and the treatment for most chronic diseases includes drugs.[50] The challenge is to develop an effective drug that can be used over time without adverse effects or abuse, and no such drug currently exists.

Getting the "Skinny" on Low-Carbohydrate Diets

In the past few years, low-carbohydrate diets have attracted millions of Americans with reports of massive, quick weight loss. Bookstores struggled to keep the latest edition of *The Atkins Diet, The South Beach Diet,* and other bestsellers on their shelves. The promise? Eliminate nearly all of the bread, pasta, sweets, and high-carbohydrate foods from your diet, eat red meat and other high-protein, high-fat foods until you are satisfied, and lose weight. Concerns were raised about the health effects of these diets. But when two major reports were published in *The New England Journal of Medicine* (NEJM) in May 2003 that seemed to support claims for safe, successful weight loss, sales of *Atkins* and other low-carbohydrate diet books and products sky-rocketed.

Many health professionals have spent the past 20 years describing low-carbohydrate diets as foolish, dangerous, ineffective, and unhealthy for many dieters. Should we suddenly believe that the scientific community has been wrong and start believing the hype? A careful reading of the relevant articles and their critiques reveals key points described here.

One NEJM study found that people on the high-protein, high-fat, low-carbohydrate Atkins diet lost twice as much as those on a standard low-fat diet recommended by most health organizations. Although the other study had similar initial weight-loss results, it found that Atkins dieters regained much of their weight by the end of the year. People just weren't able to maintain the weight loss.

In both studies, Atkins dieters had better levels of "good" cholesterol and triglycerides, or fats in the blood, than did non-dieters. There was no difference in "bad" cholesterol levels or blood pressure. About 40 percent of participants in each study dropped out early, which indicates that this diet isn't palatable for nearly half of all people.

A study released in April 2003 from the Stanford University Medical Center in conjunction with researchers at Yale University found that although these low-carbohydrate diets cause weight loss, the total calorie reduction and the duration of the reduction cause the loss, not the reduction in carbohydrate intake per se. The take-home message is that *any* low-calorie diet that a person can stay on long enough will have similar results.

These researchers summarized data from more than 107 diet studies. They concluded that we know little about the effect of these diets on people older than age 53 and that the long-term effectiveness of all of these diets remains in question. Interestingly, the Stanford researchers found no significant adverse effects from the low-carbohydrate diets on participants' glucose, insulin, cholesterol, or blood pressure levels, but noted that such effects might not have time to show up because the diets were so short in duration. Also, authors stressed that dieters who go overboard and eat high levels of animal fat and other fat-laden proteins could potentially increase levels of triglycerides and cholesterol in the body.

The health risks of being on these diets for prolonged periods of time remain in question. Known side effects of the diet include bad breath, fatigue, constipation, and nausea. Also possible are kidney damage in those who already have compromised kidneys and adverse effects on people with diabetes. In addition, eating a high-protein diet can increase your risk of osteoporosis because it causes calcium to be excreted from your bones. Metabolic imbalances, hypoglycemia and other imbalances are also hazards that may accompany these diets.

Sources: F. F. Samaha et al., "A Low-Carbohydrate as Compared with a Low-Fat Diet in Severe Obesity," *The New England Journal of Medicine* 348, no. 21 (2003): 2074–2081; G. D. Foster et al., "A Randomized Trial of Low-Carbohydrate Diet for Obesity," *The New England Journal of Medicine* 348, no. 21 (2003): 2082–2090; D. M. Bravata et al., "Efficacy and Safety of Low-Carbohydrate Diets," *The Journal of the American Medical Association* 289, no. 14 (2003): 1837–1850.

A classic example of a supposedly safe set of drugs that later were found to have dangerous side effects were Pondimen and Redux, known as *Fen Phen,* two of the most widely prescribed diet drugs in U.S. history.[51] When the drugs were found to damage heart valves and contribute to pulmonary hypertension, a massive recall and lawsuit occurred.

Here are other diet drugs that you should view with caution.

- Sibutramine. Suppresses appetite by inhibiting the uptake of serotonin. It works best with a reduced-calorie diet and exercise, but side effects are not to be taken lightly. They include dry mouth, headache, constipation, insomnia, and high blood pressure. Since many obese people have high blood pressure, this is an obvious concern.

- Orlistat (Xenical). Works by inhibiting the action of lipase, an enzyme that helps digest fats. About 30 percent of fats consumed pass through the system undigested, which leads to reduced overall caloric intake. Known side effects include oily spotting, gas with watery fecal discharge, fecal urgency, oily stools, frequent and often unexpected bowel movements, and possible deficiencies of fat soluble vitamins.[52]

- Over-the-Counter (OTC) Drugs. Only one OTC medication to help with weight loss has FDA approval. It contains *benzocaine* (in candy or gum form), which anesthetizes the tongue, thus reducing taste sensation. In 2000, the FDA recommended banning OTCs containing *phenylpropanolamine*, an appetite suppressant, due to problems with rapid pulse, insomnia, hypertension, irregular heartbeats, and kidney failure. The FDA is proceeding with steps to ban the ingredient completely.[53]

- Herbal Weight Loss Aids. St. John's Wort (SJW) and other substances that enhance serotonin and suppress appetite have been widely marketed for weight loss. Be aware that SJW is often combined with ephedrine, a stimulant found in certain cold and allergy pills and believed to cause heart attacks, seizures, and strokes.[54] Before you take any herbal medication, make sure you know its possible ingredients and their risks.

Surgery   When all else fails, a relatively permanent yet risky solution may lie in surgical stapling or tying off of the stomach. This procedure effectively reduces stomach size to hold only a few tablespoons of food. Patients can't eat enough calories, so they lose weight. Make no mistake about it, this procedure should be reserved only for the morbidly obese who face imminent health risks. Complications are many and include infections, nausea, vomiting, vitamin and mineral deficiencies, and dehydration. (Imagine really being thirsty and only being able to drink a few tablespoons of water at a time.) Lifelong medical and sometimes psychological monitoring is needed for those who have this procedure.

Liposuction is another surgical procedure for spot reducing. Although this technique has garnered much attention, it too is not without risk. Infections, severe scarring, and even death have resulted. Many people who have liposuction regain the fat or require multiple surgeries to repair lumpy, irregular surfaces from which the fat was removed.

Trying to Gain Weight

Although trying to lose weight poses a major challenge for many, a smaller group of Americans, for a variety of metabolic, hereditary, psychological, and other reasons, inexplicably start to lose weight or can't seem to gain weight no matter how hard they try. If you are one of these individuals, determining the reasons for your difficulty in gaining weight is a must. For example, among older adults, the senses of taste and smell may decline, which makes food taste differently and be less pleasurable. Visual problems and other disabilities may make meals more difficult to prepare, and dental problems may make it more difficult to eat. People who engage in extreme sports that require extreme nutritional supplementation may be at risk for nutritional deficiencies, which can lead to immune system problems and organ dysfunction, weakness that leads to falls and fractures, slower recovery from diseases, and a host of other problems.

Once you know what is causing a daily caloric deficit, there are steps you can take to gain extra weight.

- Eat at regularly scheduled times, whether you are hungry or not.
- Eat more. Obviously, you are not taking in enough calories to support whatever is happening in your body. Eat more frequently, spend more time eating, eat the high-calorie foods first if you fill up fast, and always start with the main course. Take time to shop, to cook, to eat slowly. Put extra spreads such as peanut butter, cream cheese, or cheese on your foods. Make your sandwiches with extra-thick slices of bread, and add more filling. Take second helpings whenever possible, and eat high-calorie snacks during the day.
- Supplement your diet. Add high-calorie drinks that have a healthy balance of nutrients.
- Try to eat with people you are comfortable with. Avoid people who you feel are analyzing what you eat or who make you feel like you should eat less.
- If you aren't exercising, exercise to increase your appetite. If you are exercising or exercising to extremes, moderate your activities until weight gain is evident.
- Avoid diuretics, laxatives, and other medications that cause you to lose body fluids and nutrients.
- Relax. Many people who are underweight operate at high gear most of the time. Slow down, get more rest, and control stress.

Body Image and Media Messages

Most of us think of the obsession with thinness as a recent phenomenon that began with supermodel Twiggy in the 1960s. Beyond a doubt, the thin look dominates fashion and the media. However, an obsession with being thin has been a part of our culture for decades. Anorexia nervosa, an eating disorder (see the next section), has been defined as a psychiatric illness since 1873. During the Victorian era, women wore corsets to achieve unrealistically tiny waists. By the 1920s, it was common knowledge that obesity was linked to poor health. The American Tobacco Company coined the phrase "reach for a Lucky instead of a sweet" to promote the idea that cigarettes dulled appetite.

Today more than ever before, underweight models and TV characters exemplify desirability and success, which delivers the subtle message that thin is in. In addition, public health warnings that being overweight increases risk for heart disease, certain cancers, and a number of other disorders can send a panic through people when their weight isn't what they think it should be. Being overweight has become socially unacceptable in many circles and something to be avoided at all costs, and Americans are looking for fast answers.

Some of these distorted views of self-image arise from misinterpreting height–weight charts, which makes some people strive for the lower readings stipulated for a light-boned person when determining their own normal weight. Sadly, increasing numbers of adolescents, teens, and adults

Are Super-Sized Meals Super-Sizing Americans?

Today, super-sized meals are the norm at many restaurants. Biscuits and gravy, huge steaks, and plate-filling meals are popular fare. Across the country, restaurants and food companies are piling it on as customers seek comfort food in large portions. Consider the 25-ounce prime rib for cowboys served at a local steak chain. At nearly 3,000 calories and 150 grams of fat for the meat alone, these dinners both slam shut arteries and add on pounds. Add a baked potato with sour cream and/or butter, a salad loaded with creamy salad dressing, and fresh bread with real butter, and the meal may surpass the 5,000-calorie mark and ring in at close to 300 grams of fat. This scale-tipping dinner exceeds what most adults should eat in two days!

And this is just the beginning. Soft drinks, once commonly served in 12-ounce sizes, now come in big gulps and 1-liter bottles. Cinnamon buns at local chains now come in giant, butter-laden,

700-calorie portions. What is the result? Super-sized portions consumed by super-sized Americans.

A quick glance at the fattening of Americans provides growing evidence of a significant health problem. According to Donna Skoda, a dietitian and chair of the Ohio State University Extension Service, "People are eating a ton of extra calories. For the first time in history, more people are overweight in America than are underweight. Ironically, although the U.S. fat intake has dropped in the past 20 years from an average of 40 to 33% of calories, the daily calorie intake has risen from 1,852 calories per day to over 2,000 per day. In theory, this translates into a weight gain of 15 pounds a year."

Skoda and others say that the main reason that Americans are gaining weight is that people no longer know what a normal serving size is. In a recent U.S. Department of Agriculture (USDA) survey, only 1% of the respondents could correctly identify the serving sizes recommended in the Food Guide Pyramid, the visual dietary aid developed by the USDA.

The National Heart, Lung, and Blood Institute, part of the National Institutes of

Health, has developed a "Portion Distortion" quiz that shows how today's portions compare to those of 20 years ago. You can test yourself online at http://hin.nhlbi.nih.gov/portion to see if you can recognize the differences between today's super-sized meals and those once considered normal. Just one example is the difference between an average cheeseburger 20 years ago (left photo) and the typical cheeseburger of today (right photo).

According to Carrie Wiatt, a Los Angeles dietitian and author of the recently released book *Portion Savvy,* a telling marker of the big-food trend is that restaurant plates have grown from an average of 9 to 13 inches in the past decade. Studies show that people eat 40–50% more than they normally would now that large portions are available.

These statistics alone are alarming. However, they are made worse by a growing trend toward sedentary lifestyles, increased use of technology and gadgetry, and computer-gazing among far too many Americans. The relationship between energy input and output is being knocked out of balance on both sides. Americans are taking in more calories and doing less

are so preoccupied with trying to look like size four models that they make themselves ill in their quest to be thin.

Eating Disorders

For an increasing number of people, particularly young women, an obsessive preoccupation with food develops into **anorexia nervosa,** a persistent, chronic eating disorder

characterized by deliberate food restriction and severe, life-threatening weight loss. **Bulimia nervosa,** or a variation known as **binge eating disorder (BED),** involves frequent bouts of binge eating followed by purging (self-induced vomiting), laxative abuse, or excessive exercise. In the United States more than 10 million people, 90 percent of whom are women, meet the established criteria for one of these disorders, and their numbers appear to be increasing.[55] Many more suffer from minor forms of these conditions—not enough for a true diagnosis, but dangerously close to the precipice that will ultimately lead to life-threatening results (Table 10.3 on page 292).

Anorexia Nervosa

Anorexia involves self-starvation motivated by an intense fear of gaining weight along with an extremely distorted body image. When anorexia occurs in childhood, failure to gain weight in a normal growth pattern may be the key indicator; later, this typically results in actual weight loss. Nearly 1 percent of girls in late adolescence meet the full criteria for anorexia; many others suffer from significant symptoms.

Anorexia nervosa   Eating disorder characterized by excessive preoccupation with food, self-starvation, and/or extreme exercising to achieve weight loss.

Bulimia nervosa   Eating disorder characterized by binge eating followed by inappropriate measures to prevent weight gain.

Binge eating disorder (BED)   Eating disorder characterized by recurrent binge eating, without excessive measures to prevent weight gain.

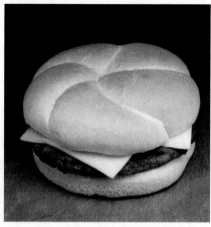

20 years ago

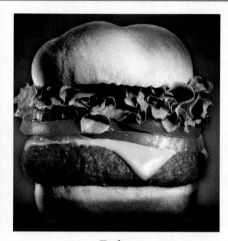

Today

to burn them off. Hence, an epidemic of obesity prevails and is getting worse. Younger and younger kids are eating more and more and picking up lifetime habits that will be hard to change. To reduce your own risk of super-sizing, follow these simple strategies.

- Avoid super-sizing anything. Order the smallest size available when dining out. Focus on taste, not quantity. Get used to eating less and to enjoying what you are eating.

- Chew your food, and avoid the urge to wash it down with high-calorie drinks. Take time, and let your fullness indicator have a chance to kick in while there is still time to quit.
- Serve food on a small or medium plate. Put those big platter-size dinner plates on the top shelf of your cupboard, and leave them there.
- Always order dressings, gravies, and sauces on the side. Sprinkle these added calories on carefully rather than

washing down your foods with them. Remember that a tablespoon of gravy could mean an hour on the treadmill to burn off its 200+ calories!

- If you order large muffins or bagels, share them with a friend, or bring only half with you and wrap up the rest. Carry a small zip-lock bag, and use it to take home part of those big portions for another day.
- Avoid appetizers in restaurants. Often they cost a lot, in terms of money, calories, and fat content.
- Share your dinner with a friend, and order a side salad for each of you. Alternatively, eat only half of your dinner, and save the rest for another day.
- Measure portions. Before ordering, ask for the size of servings, and always order a size smaller than you really want. When the server tells you it is a "rich dish" or "a lot of food," avoid it.
- Avoid buffets and all-you-can-eat establishments. Most of us can eat two to three times what we need—or more.

Source: Some statistics from J. Snow, "Are Super-Sized Meals Super-Sizing Americans?" *Corvallis Gazette Times,* May 24, 2000, Section C8.

Usually, people with anorexia lose weight through initial reduction in total food intake, particularly of high-calorie foods, but eventually they restrict their intake of almost all foods. What they do eat, they often purge through vomiting or using laxatives. Although they lose weight, people with anorexia never seem to feel thin enough and constantly identify body parts that they feel are too fat.

Bulimia Nervosa

People with bulimia often binge and then take inappropriate measures, such as secret vomiting, to lose the calories they have just acquired. Up to 3 percent of adolescents and young female adults are bulimic; males are one-tenth as likely as females to be bulimic. People with bulimia are also obsessed with their bodies, weight gain, and how they appear to others. Unlike those with anorexia, people with bulimia are often hidden from the public eye because their weight may vary only slightly or fall within a normal range. Also, treatment appears to be more effective for bulimia than for anorexia.

Binge Eating Disorder

Individuals with BED also binge like their bulimic counterparts, but they do not purge or take other excessive measures to lose the weight that they gain. Often they are clinically obese, and they tend to binge much more often than does the typical obese person who may consume too many calories but spaces his or her eating over a more normal daily eating pattern. To date, binge eating disorder is still under consideration as a psychiatric disorder.

Who's at Risk?

There's no simple explanation for why intelligent, often highly accomplished young people spiral downward into the destructive behaviors associated with eating disorders. Obsessive-compulsive disorder, depression, and anxiety all can play a role, as can a desperate need to win social approval or gain control of their lives through food.

Sufferers tend to be women from white middle-class or upper-class families in which there is undue emphasis

Table 10.3
DSM-IV Eating Disorder Criteria

Anorexia

According to the American Psychiatric Association's *Diagnostic and Statistical Manual of Mental Disorders,* 4th edition (*DSM-IV*), people who meet the criteria for anorexia nervosa experience all of the following symptoms:
- Refusal to maintain the minimum body weight for one's height and age
- Intense fear of gaining weight even though underweight
- Disturbed perception of one's body weight or size
- In post-pubescent women, the absence of at least three consecutive menstrual cycles. (In some women, the loss of periods precedes any significant weight loss.)

Bulimia

People with bulimia experience all of the following:
- Recurrent episodes of consuming a much larger amount of food than most people would during a similar time period (this is usually about two hours) and a sense of loss of control over eating during each episode
- Accompanying attempts to compensate for eating binges by vomiting, abusing laxatives or other drugs, or by fasting or excessive exercise
- Both the binge eating and purging occur at least twice a week for three months
- A negative perception of one's shape and weight

People with unhealthy or disordered eating patterns may show some or all of these signs:
- Excessive weight loss; preoccupation with food; intense fear of weight gain
- Obsession with clothing size, scales, and mirrors
- Refusal to eat with others; ritualistic eating
- Excessive exercise
- Moodiness; social withdrawal
- Frequent vomiting or use of laxatives
- Absent or irregular menstruation
- Excessive facial and body hair; hair loss
- Swollen salivary glands
- Broken blood vessels in the eyes

Sources: Reprinted with permission from the *Diagnostic and Statistical Manual of Mental Disorders,* 4th ed., Text Revision. Copyright 2000 American Psychiatric Association; E. Sohn, "The Roots of Anorexia," *U.S. News and World Report Guide to Family Health,* August 2003 © 2003 *U. S. News & World Report,* L. P. Reprinted with permission.

on achievement, body weight, and appearance. Contrary to popular thinking, however, eating disorders span social class, gender, race, and ethnic backgrounds and are present in countries throughout the world. In addition, increasing numbers of males suffer from various forms of eating disorders.

Some studies have shown possible associations between identical twins, and others have pointed to the large numbers of eating disordered persons who have a mother or sister with the disease. Many persons with disordered eating patterns also suffer from other problems: 50 percent are clinically depressed; 25 percent are alcoholics; and large numbers have other problems, such as compulsive stealing, gambling, or other addictions.

Treatment for Eating Disorders

Because eating disorders result from many factors, spanning many years of development, there are no quick or simple solutions. Treatment often focuses on reducing the threat to life; once the patient is stabilized, long-term therapy involves family, friends, and other significant people in the individ-

ual's life. Therapy focuses on the psychological, social, environmental, and physiological factors that have led to the problem. Finding a therapist who really understands the multidimensional aspects of the problem is a must. Therapy allows the patient to focus on building new eating behaviors, recognizing threats, building self-confidence, and finding other ways of dealing with life's problems. Support groups often help the family and the individual gain understanding and emotional support and learn self-development techniques designed to foster positive reactions and actions. Treatment of underlying depression also may be a focus.

> **What do you think?**
> *Which groups or individuals on your campus appear to be at greatest risk for eating disorders?* ✳ *What social factors might encourage this?* ✳ *Why do you think society tends to overlook eating disorders in males?* ✳ *What programs or services on your campus are available for someone with an eating disorder?*

Make It Happen!

Assessment: The Assess Yourself box on page 276 identifies six areas of importance in determining your readiness for weight loss. If you should lose weight to improve your health, understanding your attitudes about food and exercise will help you succeed in your plan.

Making a Change: In order to change your behavior, you need to develop a plan. Follow these steps.

1. Evaluate your behavior, and identify patterns and specific things you are doing. What can you change now? What can you change in the near future?
2. Select one pattern of behavior that you want to change.
3. Fill out a Behavior Change Contract. It should include your long-term goal for change, your short-term goals, the rewards you'll give yourself for reaching these goals, potential obstacles along the way, and strategies for overcoming these obstacles. For each goal, list the small steps and specific actions that you will take.
4. Chart your progress in a journal. At the end of a week, consider how successful you were in following

your plan. What helped you be successful? What made change more difficult? What will you do differently next week?

5. Revise your plan as needed. Are the short-term goals attainable? Are the rewards satisfying?

Example: Shannon had gained the "freshman 15" and wanted to put together a weight management plan. She assessed her readiness for weight loss and saw that her scores in certain areas highlighted areas that she needed to be aware of to succeed. She had never binged and purged (section IV), she had strong motivation (section I), and she already had an enjoyable, regular exercise program (section VI). However, Shannon also saw that she was not always aware of the eating cues and emotions that caused her to overeat (sections II, III, and V). Although she hadn't realized it, she tended to do most of her snacking while she was studying at night. No matter what else she had eaten during the day, she would end up eating candy and chips from the vending machines. Especially when she was anxious about an upcoming test or bored by her reading, she would eat even though she was already full.

Shannon made a plan for herself that would help her manage her snacking and be part of her weight loss program. She wanted to be conscious and aware of what she was eating and how it was contributing to her weight gain. Her first step was to buy some study snacks that were healthier choices than chips and candy, such as grapes and low-fat granola. Her next step was to make a commitment to think about how hungry she was before automatically starting to snack when she was studying. If she was snacking because she was bored or anxious, she would try to restrict her snack to a predetermined amount or to wait until she really was hungry. Shannon tried this plan for two weeks. At the end of two weeks she saw that she had lost 4 pounds. She decided she wanted to address another of her eating habits, which was ordering pizza with her roommates when they watched their favorite TV shows during the week. Even after she had eaten a full dinner, Shannon found herself eating two or three pieces of pizza in front of the TV. Shannon suggested to her roommates that, if they already had eaten dinner, they pop some popcorn to eat instead of the pizza. Not only was this healthier, but it cost less than having a pizza delivered.

Summary

* Overweight, obesity, and weight-related problems appear to be on the rise in the United States. Obesity is now defined in terms of fat content rather than in terms of weight alone.
* There are many different methods of assessing body fat. Body Mass Index (BMI) is one of the most commonly accepted measures of weight based on height. Body fat percentages more accurately indicate how fat or lean a person is.
* Many factors contribute to one's risk for obesity, including genetics, setpoint, endocrine influences, psychosocial factors, eating cues, lack of awareness, metabolic changes, lifestyle, and gender. Women often have considerably more difficulty losing weight.

* Exercise, dieting, diet pills, and other strategies are used to maintain or lose weight. However, sensible eating behavior and adequate exercise offer the best options.
* Eating disorders consist of severe disturbances in eating behaviors, unhealthy efforts to control body weight, and abnormal attitudes about body and shape. Anorexia nervosa, bulimia nervosa, and binge eating disorder are the three main eating disorders. Though prevalent among white women of upper- and middle-class families, eating disorders affect women of all backgrounds as well as a number of men.

Questions for Discussion and Reflection

1. Discuss the pressures, if any, you feel to improve your personal body image. Do these pressures come from media, family, friends, and other external sources, or from concern for your personal health?
2. What type of measurement would you choose in order to assess your fat levels? Why?
3. List the risk factors for obesity. Evaluate which seem to be most important in determining whether you will be obese in middle age.
4. Create a plan to help someone lose the "freshman 15" over the summer vacation. Assume that the person is male, 180 pounds, and has 15 weeks to lose the excess weight.
5. Differentiate among the three eating disorders. Then give reasons why females might be more prone to anorexia and bulimia than males are.

Accessing Your Health on the Internet

Visit the following Internet sites to explore further topics and issues related to personal health. To visit an organization's website, go to the Companion Website for *Health: The Basics, Sixth Edition* at www.aw-bc.com/donatelle, click on the book image, and select "Accessing Your Health on the Internet" from the navigation menu on the left.

1. ***American Dietetic Association.*** Includes recommended dietary guidelines and other current information about weight control.
2. ***Duke University Diet and Fitness Center.*** Includes information about one of the best programs in the country focused on helping people live healthier, fuller lives through weight control and lifestyle change.
3. ***Helping to End Eating Disorders (HEED).*** The website of an organization dedicated to fighting eating disorders and helping individuals through the ordeal. Includes a chatroom for people to exchange thoughts and share support.
4. ***Mayo Health O@sis.*** Summarizes many weight-control issues and concerns.
5. ***Shape Up America.*** Includes strategies and ideas for getting in shape and staying at your optimal weight.

Further Reading

Brownell, K., and K. Horgen. *Food Fight: The Inside Story of the Food Industry, America's Obesity Crisis, and What We Can Do about It.* New York: McGraw-Hill, 2003.

Director of the Yale Center for Eating and Weight Disorders, Brownell critiques the way that food is marketed and sold to children, and places much of the blame for childhood obesity on advertising and unhealthy foods being offered in schools.

Gaesser, G. *Big Fat Lies.* New York: Fawcett Columbine Press, 1997.

Excellent overview of leading theories on fat, obesity, and a host of related problems and issues. Also discusses potential weight-loss strategies that are "keepers" for life.

Piscatella, J. *The Fat-Gram Guide to Restaurant Food, 3rd ed.* New York: Workman Press, 2000.

Excellent guide to fast foods and restaurant fat content.

Price, D. *Healing the Hungry Self: The Diet-Free Solution to Lifelong Weight Management.* New York: Plume, 1998.

Interestingly written, realistic approach to weight control.

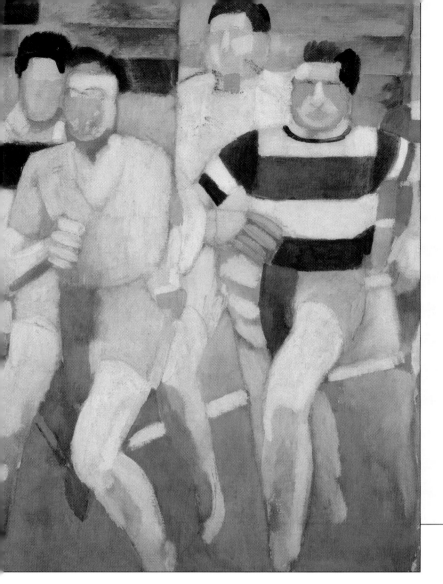

Personal Fitness

Improving Health through Exercise

11

Objectives

☀ Describe physical fitness and the benefits of regular physical activity, including improvements in cardiorespiratory fitness, muscular fitness, bone mass, weight control, stress management, mental health, and life span.

☀ Explain the components of an aerobic exercise program and how to determine the best frequency, intensity, and duration of exercise.

☀ Describe different stretching and strength exercises designed to improve flexibility.

☀ Compare the various types and benefits of resistance exercise programs.

☀ Summarize ways to prevent and treat common fitness injuries.

☀ Summarize the key components of a personal fitness program.

Now, the Fusionistas

By Mary Billard

In a spotless Manhattan exercise studio, 30 people are drenched in sweat, limbs shaking from a workout that mixes yoga, weight lifting, Pilates and a little ballet. Cut to a skier in the middle of a backcountry run, sailing off a cliff and then throwing his skis over his head in a 360 revolution, landing a trick usually confined to the terrain park. Or switch the channel to Fox Sports Net, where the latest Gen Y action show serves up a mix of sports, music from bands like Audioslave and travelogues on things like kiteboarding in Austria.

Bad news, sports fans. Just when extreme (or x-treme, for that matter) has gone mainstream, there's a new buzzword to learn: fusion. From Tahoe Longboards' Fusion 39, designed to combine the easy handling of a smaller skateboard with the turn-carving ability of a longer board, to Raw Distance Fusion golf balls (they promise a combination of distance and control) to the Cleveland Fusion, a women's football team, it's the hottest term for sporting-goods makers, athletes and gym owners looking for a little edge.

"We've gone past aerobics, past the boot camp classes," said Annbeth Eschbach, the chief executive and president of the Exhale spa, where the 30 sweating students were taking the hottest new class, a genre-busting mix of disciplines called Core Fusion by its creators.

Read the complete article online in the eThemes section of this book's website: www.aw-bc.com/donatelle.

Original article published November 21, 2003. Copyright © 2003 The New York Times. Reprinted with permission.

A century ago in the United States, simple survival meant performing physical labor on a daily basis. However, science and technology have transformed our lives. Today most adults in our country lead sedentary lifestyles and perform little physical labor or exercise.[1] The growing percentage of Americans who live sedentary lives has been linked to dramatic increases in the incidence of obesity, diabetes, and other chronic diseases.[2] More than 110 million Americans are overweight or obese, 50 million have high blood pressure, 17 million have diabetes (90 to 95 percent of whom are type 2 diabetics, which is associated with obesity and physical inactivity), approximately 16 million have "pre-diabetes,"[3] and 1.1 million suffer a heart attack in any given year.[4]

Regular physical activity improves more than 50 different physiological, metabolic, and psychological aspects of human life.[5] Now is an excellent time to develop exercise habits that will improve the quality and duration of your own life.

What Is Physical Fitness?

Physical fitness is the ability to perform moderate to vigorous physical activity on a regular basis without excessive fatigue. **Exercise training** is the systematic performance of exercise at a specified frequency, intensity, and duration to achieve a desired level of physical fitness.[6] Major health-related components of physical fitness include cardiorespiratory (aerobic) fitness, flexibility, muscular strength and endurance, and body composition. These components play a vital role in overall health (Table 11.1).

To be considered physically fit, you generally need to attain (and then maintain) certain minimum standards for each component that have been established by exercise physiologists and other fitness experts. Some people have physical limitations that make achieving one or more of these standards difficult. That doesn't mean they can't become physically fit. For example, a woman with limited flexibility due to arthritis in the knee and hip joints may be unable to jog without extreme pain. Yet, by exercising in a swimming pool, where the buoyancy of the water will relieve much of the stress on her joints, she can improve her range of motion. She can also develop muscular strength and cardiovascular fitness by "jogging" at the deep end of a swimming pool while wearing a flotation device. Similarly, a man who needs to use a wheelchair may be unable to run or walk a mile, as is required in some fitness tests, but can stay physically fit by playing wheelchair basketball.

Athletic skill is not a requirement for physical fitness— you do not have to possess the talents of an Olympic athlete to achieve health benefits from regular physical activity and exercise. Many healthy activities, such as walking, running, swimming, and cycling, require no special skill in order to be performed and enjoyed. Our definition of physical fitness should be adapted to address individual differences in capabilities. There are several different types of physical fitness.

Physical fitness The ability to perform regular moderate to vigorous physical activity without great fatigue.

Exercise training The systematic performance of exercise at a specified frequency, intensity, and duration to achieve a desired level of physical fitness.

Table 11.1
Major Components of Physical Fitness

Cardiorespiratory fitness	Ability to sustain moderate-intensity whole-body activity for extended time periods
Flexibility	Range of motion at a joint or series of joints
Muscular strength and endurance	Maximum force applied with single muscle contraction; ability to perform repeated high-intensity muscle contractions
Body composition	A composite of total body mass, fat mass, fat-free mass, and fat distribution

Source: From the American College of Sports Medicine, "ACSM Position Stand on the Recommended Quantity and Quality of Exercise for Developing and Maintaining Cardiorespiratory and Muscular Fitness and Flexibility in Adults," *Medicine and Science in Sports and Exercise* 30 (1998): 975–991.

What do you think?

Which of the key aspects of physical fitness do you currently possess? ✳ Which ones would you like to improve or develop? ✳ What types of activities could you do to improve your fitness level?

Benefits of Regular Physical Activity

Physical activity is any force exerted by skeletal muscles that results in energy usage above the level used when the body's systems are at rest.[7] Higher levels of physical activity reduce your risk of dying prematurely; developing diabetes, high blood pressure, and colon cancer; and experiencing depression and anxiety. Regular physical activity also:

- Helps control weight
- Builds and maintains healthy bones, muscles and joints
- Helps older adults become stronger and better able to move about without falling
- Promotes psychological well-being
- Reduces surgical risks
- Reduces complications from bone and joint disorders, respiratory disorders, etc.
- Helps immune functioning

A recent study shows that regular physical exercise (four hours a week or more) beginning in adolescence and continuing into adulthood can significantly reduce the risk of breast cancer in women age 40 and younger.[8] The recent Surgeon General's report on physical activity and health[9] indicates that physical activity need not be strenuous in order to achieve health benefits and that women and men of all ages benefit from a moderate amount of *daily* activity.

Fitness also benefits the nation. Researchers at the Centers for Disease Control and Prevention (CDC) have documented that physically active individuals have lower annual direct medical costs than inactive people do. The cost difference is $330 per person, and the potential savings if all inactive American adults become physically active could exceed $77 billion per year.[10] In spite of these benefits and the numerous health benefits from exercise, researchers estimate that "at best, no more than 20 percent and possibly less than 10 percent of adults in the United States, Australia, Canada, and England obtain sufficient regular physical activity at an intensity that imparts discernible health and fitness benefits."[11]

Improved Cardiorespiratory Fitness

Cardiorespiratory fitness refers to the ability of the circulatory and respiratory systems to supply oxygen to the body during sustained physical activity.[12] Regular exercise makes these systems more efficient by enlarging the heart muscle, enabling more blood to be pumped with each stroke, and increasing the number of *capillaries* (small arteries) in trained skeletal muscles, which supply more blood to working muscles. Exercise improves the respiratory system by increasing the amount of oxygen that is inhaled and distributed to body tissues.[13]

Reduced Risk of Heart Disease   Your heart is a muscle made up of highly specialized tissue. Because muscles become stronger and more efficient with use, regular exercise strengthens the heart, which enables it to pump more blood with each beat. This increased efficiency means that the heart requires fewer beats per minute to circulate blood throughout the body. A stronger, more efficient heart is better able to meet the ordinary demands of life.

Prevention of Hypertension   *Blood pressure* refers to the force exerted by blood against blood vessel walls that is generated by the pumping action of the heart. Hypertension, the medical term for abnormally high blood pressure, is a significant risk factor for cardiovascular disease and stroke. Regular physical activity can reduce blood pressure in people with normal blood pressure and in those with high blood pressure.[14] A recent study in Japan of sedentary volunteers with high blood pressure showed that adding 61 to 90 minutes of exercise per week to their lives significantly reduced their blood pressure, which shows that even small increases in activity can have benefits for hypertensives.[15]

Cardiorespiratory fitness   The ability of the heart, lungs, and blood vessels to supply oxygen to skeletal muscles during sustained physical activity.

Improved Blood Lipid and Lipoprotein Profile   Lipids are fats that circulate in the bloodstream and are stored in various places in the body. Regular exercise is known to reduce the levels of low-density lipoproteins (LDLs—"bad cholesterol") while increasing the number of high-density lipoproteins (HDLs—"good cholesterol") in the blood. Higher HDL levels are associated with lower risk for artery disease because they remove some of the bad cholesterol from artery walls and hence prevent clogging. The bottom line: Regular exercise lowers the risk of cardiovascular disease. (For more on cholesterol and blood pressure, see Chapter 12).

Improved Bone Mass

A common affliction among older adults is **osteoporosis,** a disease characterized by low bone mass and deterioration of bone tissue, which increase fracture risk. Osteoporosis is more common among women than among men for at least three reasons: Women live longer than men; they have lower peak bone mass than men; and they lose bone mass at rates nearly twice as great as men after age 35. These rates increase even more after menopause as women's estrogen levels decrease. The incidence of osteoporosis and fractures increases substantially with age in both women and men. In the United States alone, nearly 1.5 million osteoporosis-related fractures occur every year.[16]

Bone, like other human tissues, responds to the demands placed on it. Women (and men) have much to gain by remaining physically active as they age—bone mass levels are significantly higher among active than among sedentary women.[17] New research indicates that by "surprising" bone (by jumping and other sudden activities), young children may improve their bone density.[18] Regular weight-bearing exercise, when combined with a balanced diet containing adequate calcium, will help keep bones healthy.[19] See Chapter 15 for more information on risk factors for osteoporosis.

Improved Weight Control

Many people start exercising because they want to lose weight. Level of physical activity does have a direct effect on metabolic rate and even raises it for several hours following a vigorous workout. According to the American College of Sports Medicine (ACSM), if you want to lose weight through exercise alone without decreasing the amount of food you eat, you should exercise frequently (at least four days a week) for extended time periods (at least 50 minutes per workout).[20] An even more effective method for losing weight combines regular endurance-type exercises with a moderate decrease in food intake. Cutting daily caloric intake beyond

> **Osteoporosis**   A disease characterized by low bone mass and deterioration of bone tissue, which increase risk of fracture.

this range (severe dieting) actually decreases metabolic rate by up to 20 percent and makes weight loss more difficult.

A recent meta-analysis challenges the commonly held view that exercise alone is not a useful strategy for obesity reduction. Moderately obese white men who participated in daily exercise of moderate intensity (brisk walking) for 45 to 60 minutes per day, without decreasing their caloric intake, lost weight and made rapid improvements in cardiovascular fitness.[21] Regular exercise also reduced the incidence of heart disease and type 2 diabetes in these participants and reduced the overall death rate.[22]

Improved Health and Life Span

Prevention of Diabetes   Non–insulin-dependent diabetes (type 2 diabetes) is a complex disorder that affects millions of Americans, many of whom have no idea that they have the disease. (See Chapter 14.) Risk factors for diabetes include obesity, high blood pressure, and high cholesterol, as well as a family history of the disease.[23] Physicians suggest exercise combined with weight loss and healthy diet to manage diabetes. A recent large study found that for every 2,000 calories of energy expended during leisure-time activities, the incidence of diabetes was reduced by 24 percent. Perhaps the most encouraging finding was that the protective effect of exercise was greatest among those individuals who were at the highest risk.[24]

Longer Life Span   A landmark study conducted at the Institute for Aerobics Research in Texas found that exercise does increase longevity. More than 13,000 white men and women, ages 20 to 80, were followed for eight years. Participants were assigned fitness levels based on their age, sex, and results of exercise tests. The death rate in the least physically fit group was more than three times higher than that of the most fit group. How much physical activity was required to produce a difference? Sedentary participants who started taking a brisk 30- to 60-minute walk each day experienced significant increases in life expectancy.[25]

Improved Immunity to Disease   Recent research suggests that regular moderate exercise makes people less susceptible to disease, although this benefit may depend on whether they perceive exercise as pleasurable or stressful.[26] However, extreme exercise may actually be detrimental. For example, athletes engaging in marathon-type events or very intense physical training have an increased risk of colds and flu.[27] In a recent study of 2,300 marathon runners, those who ran more than 60 miles per week suffered twice as many upper respiratory tract infections as those who ran fewer than 20 miles per week.[28]

Just how exercise alters immunity is not well understood. We do know that brisk exercise temporarily increases the number of white blood cells (WBCs), the blood cells responsible for fighting infection. Generally speaking, the less

The Female Athlete Triad: When Exercise Becomes Obsession

In a quest to be thin and achieve the ideal body, many women, particularly those who are physically active, are at risk for a group of symptoms called the Female Athlete Triad. This often unrecognized disorder is a combination of three conditions: disordered eating, amenorrhea (lack of menstrual periods), and osteoporosis.

Disordered eating behaviors (anorexia, bulimia, or other forms of binging, purging, or restricted eating) combined with excessive exercise can lead to changes in normal body functions. If the disordered eating is prolonged or without effective intervention, serious calcium depletion, changes in body hormones, and other negative effects may cause weakening of bone and other problems. Severe cases can lead to disability or even death.

Although men can suffer from many of these symptoms, the problem tends to be much more common in females, particularly those in highly competitive sports that value self-discipline and perfection. Gymnasts, ice skaters, cross-country runners, swimmers, and ballet dancers are at the highest risk for the Female Athlete Triad.

Physical Warning Signs

Fatigue

Anemia

Tendency toward stress fractures and injury

Cold intolerance

Sore throat

Erosion of dental enamel from frequent vomiting

Abdominal pain and bloating

Constipation

Dry skin

Lightheadedness/fainting

Chest pain

Irregular or absent menstrual periods

Lanugo (fine, downy hair covering the body)

Changes in endurance, strength, or speed

Behavioral Warning Signs

Use of weight-loss products and/or laxatives

Depression

Decreased ability to concentrate

Excessive and compulsive exercise

Preoccupation with food and weight

Trips to bathroom during or after eating

Increasing self-criticism and hostility to self

The American College of Sports Medicine (ACSM) and other groups are noticing a growing incidence of the Female Athlete Triad in physically active girls and women who don't compete athletically but want to look and feel their best. A key is to pay attention and notice what is happening. If you wonder whether a friend or family member may be experiencing the symptoms of the Female Athlete Triad, ask her about her behavior. If symptoms are present, a multidisciplinary approach involving parents, coaches, friends, physicians, dietitians, and mental health professionals is warranted.

Sources: Brown University Health Services, "Nutrition: Eating Concerns: The Female Athlete Triad," 2002. www.brown.edu/Student_Services/Health_Services; Nebraska Cooperative Extension, "NEB Facts: The Female Athlete Triad," 1998. www.ianr.unl.edu/pubs/foods/nf361.htm

---

fit the person and the more intense the exercise, the greater the increase in WBCs.[29] After brief periods of exercise (without injury), the number of WBCs typically returns to normal levels within one to two hours. After exercise bouts lasting longer than 30 minutes, WBCs may be elevated for 24 hours or more before returning to normal levels.[30] An increased number of WBCs suggests greater immunity to disease and infection.

Improved Mental Health and Stress Management

People who engage in regular physical activity also notice psychological benefits. Regular vigorous exercise has been shown to burn off the chemical by-products released by the nervous system during normal response to stress. This reduces stress levels by accelerating the body's return to a balanced state. Regular exercise improves a person's physical appearance by toning and developing muscles and reducing body fat. Feeling good about personal appearance boosts self-esteem. At the same time, as people come to appreciate the improved strength, conditioning, and flexibility that accompany fitness, they often become less obsessed with physical appearance.[31] They learn new skills and develop increased abilities in favorite recreational activities, which also help improve self-esteem.

What do you think?

Among the many benefits to be derived from physical activity, which two are most important to you? Why? ✱ *After exercising regularly for several days, what benefits do you notice?*

Improving Cardiorespiratory Fitness

The number of walkers, joggers, bicyclists, step aerobics classes, and swimmers is tangible evidence of Americans' increased interest in cardiorespiratory fitness. The primary category of physical activity known to improve cardiorespiratory endurance is **aerobic exercise.** The term *aerobic* means "with oxygen" and describes any type of exercise, typically performed at moderate levels of intensity for extended periods of time, that increases your heart rate. A person said to be in good shape has an above-average **aerobic capacity**—a term used to describe the functional status of the cardiorespiratory system (i.e., heart, lungs, blood vessels). Aerobic capacity (commonly written as $VO_{2\ max}$) is defined as the maximum volume of oxygen consumed by the muscles during exercise.

To measure your maximal aerobic capacity, an exercise physiologist or physician typically will have you exercise on a treadmill. He or she will initially ask you to walk at an easy pace, and then, at set time intervals during this **graded exercise test,** will gradually increase the workload (i.e., a combination of running speed and the angle of incline of the treadmill). Generally, the higher your cardiorespiratory endurance level, the more oxygen you can transport to exercising muscles and the longer you can exercise without becoming exhausted. In other words, the higher the $VO_{2\ max}$ value, the higher your level of aerobic fitness.

You can test your own aerobic capacity by using either the 1.5-mile run or the 12-minute run endurance test described in the Assess Yourself box on page 303. However, do not take these tests if you are just starting to exercise.[32] Progress slowly through a walking/jogging program at low intensities before measuring your aerobic capacity with one of these tests. If you have any medical conditions, such as asthma, diabetes, heart disease, or obesity, consult your physician before beginning any exercise program.

Aerobic Fitness Programs

The most beneficial aerobic exercises are total body activities involving all the large muscle groups of your body, for exam-

- Exercise 3 to 5 days each week

- Warm up for 5 to 10 minutes before aerobic activity

- Maintain your exercise intensity for 30 to 45 minutes

- Gradually decrease the intensity of your workout, then stretch to cool down during the last 5 to 10 minutes

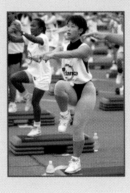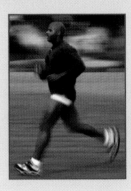

Figure 11.1
ACSM Guidelines for Aerobic Activity
Source: Reprinted with permission of the American College of Sports Medicine. © American College of Sports Medicine 2003.

ple, swimming, cross-country skiing, and rowing. If you have been sedentary for quite a while, simply initiating a physical activity program may be the hardest task you'll face. Don't be put off by the next-day soreness you are likely to feel. The key is to begin at a very low intensity, progress slowly. . . and stay with it! For example, if you want to start jogging, you'll need several weeks of workouts combining walking and jogging before you will reach a fitness level that enables you to jog continuously for 15 to 20 minutes. Adjust the frequency, intensity, and duration of your aerobic activity program to accommodate your cardiorespiratory fitness.

Determining Exercise Frequency If you are a newcomer to regular physical activity, try to exercise at least three times per week. If you exercise less frequently, you will achieve fewer health benefits. The Surgeon General recommends moderate amounts of *daily* physical activity.[33] As your fitness level improves, your goal should be to exercise 20 to 30 minutes per day, five days a week. Professionals now believe that any exercise contributes to cardiovascular and other health benefits. In fact, the health benefits derived from three 10-minute exercise bouts a day almost equal the effects of one 30-minute session.[34] Figure 11.1 provides the ACSM guidelines for healthy aerobic activity.

Determining Exercise Intensity Your aerobic exercise program should employ activities of moderate intensity that use

---

Aerobic exercise Any type of exercise, typically performed at moderate levels of intensity for extended periods of time (typically 20 to 30 minutes or longer), that increases heart rate.

Aerobic capacity The current functional status of a person's cardiovascular system; measured as $VO_{2\ max}$.

Graded exercise test A test of aerobic capacity administered by a physician, exercise physiologist, or other trained person; two common forms are the treadmill running test and the stationary bike test.

---

large muscle groups and can be maintained for prolonged periods of time. The measure of such a workout is your **target heart rate,** which is a percentage of your maximum heart rate (HR_{max}). To calculate target heart rate, subtract your age from 220. The result is your maximum heart rate. You determine your target heart rate by calculating a desired percentage of maximum heart rate, often 60 percent. Thus, if you are a 20-year-old female, your 60 percent target heart rate would be (220 − 20) × 0.60, or 120 beats per minute.

Heart rate reserve is another way to determine your target heart rate. First, subtract your resting heart rate (beats per minute after 10 minutes of complete rest) from your maximum heart rate. This is your heart rate reserve. Then take a percentage of this figure (often 60 percent) and add it to your resting heart rate. The result is your target heart rate.

People should exercise at an intensity of 40–50 to 85 percent of $VO_{2\ max}$ or 55–65 to 90 percent of HR_{max} for at least 20 to 60 minutes on at least three days per week. (The lower number in the range is for unfit or previously sedentary people. They should begin at this range with no more than 10 minutes of daily exercise two days a week.) From a health perspective, even activities such as gardening or housecleaning, done regularly for more than 60 minutes a day, can improve health.[35]

Once you know your target heart rate, you can take your pulse to determine how close you are to this value during your workout. As you exercise, lightly place your index and middle fingers (don't use your thumb) on your radial artery (inside your wrist, on the thumb side). Using a watch or clock, take your pulse for six seconds and multiply this number by 10 (just add a zero to your count) to get the number of beats per minute (bpm). Your pulse should be within a range of 5 bpm above or below your target heart rate. If necessary, adjust the pace or intensity of your workout to achieve your target heart rate.

A target heart rate of 70 percent of maximum is sometimes called the "conversational level of exercise" because you are able to talk with a partner while exercising.[36] If you are breathing so hard that talking is difficult, you are exercising too intensely. If you can sustain a conversational level of aerobic exercise for 20 to 30 minutes, you will improve your cardiorespiratory fitness.

Determining Exercise Duration   Duration refers to the number of minutes of activity performed during any one session. The ACSM and the CDC suggest that every adult engage in 30 minutes of continuous or intermittent (if intermittent, bouts of at least 10 minutes' duration) moderate-intensity physical activity most days of the week.[37] Activities that can contribute to this total include dancing; walking up stairs (instead of taking the elevator); gardening; raking leaves; as well as planned physical activities such as jogging, swimming, and cycling. One way to meet the CDC/ACSM recommendation is to walk 2 miles briskly.

The lower the intensity of your activity, the longer the duration you'll need to get the same caloric expenditure. For example, a 120-pound woman will burn 180 calories walking for one hour at 2.0 miles per hour, but will burn 330 calories if she walks for an hour at a pace of 4.5 miles per hour. A 180-pound man will expend 288 calories per hour of playing golf if he carries his clubs, but 805 calories per hour if he is cross-country skiing.[38] Aim to expend 300 to 500 calories per exercise session, with an eventual weekly goal of 1,500 to 2,000 calories. As you progress, add to your exercise load by increasing duration or intensity, but not both at the same time. From week to week, don't increase duration or intensity by more than 10 percent.

A program of repeated sessions of exercise over several months or years—exercise training—changes the way your cardiovascular system meets your body's oxygen requirements at rest and during exercise. Because many of the health benefits associated with cardiorespiratory fitness activities take about one year of regular exercise to achieve, don't expect improvements overnight.[39] However, any physical activity of low to moderate intensity will benefit your overall health almost from the start.

What do you think?

Calculate your maximum heart rate. Pick an intensity of exercise that suits your fitness level, for example, 60, 70, or 80 percent of your maximum heart rate. Using a familiar physical activity and monitoring your pulse, experiment by exercising at three different intensities. ✳ *Do you notice any difference in the way you feel while exercising?* ✳ *Afterward?*

Why Are Flexibility and Stretching Important?

Stretching and Well-Being

Who would guess that improved flexibility can give you a sense of well-being, help you deal with stress better, and stop your joints from hurting as much as they used to? But that's just what people who have improved their flexibility are saying. Stretching exercises have become the main route to improved flexibility. Today, they are extremely popular, both

---

Target heart rate   Calculated as a percentage of maximum heart rate (220 minus age); heart rate (pulse) is taken during aerobic exercise to check if exercise intensity is at the desired level (e.g., 60 percent of maximum heart rate).

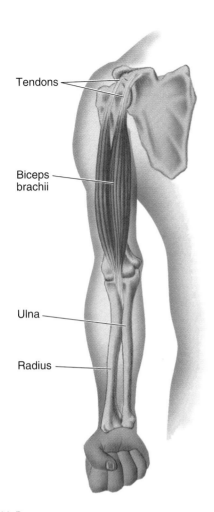

Figure 11.2
Muscles, Bones, and Tendons
Source: From S. A. Plowman and D. L. Smith, *Exercise Physiology for Health, Fitness, and Performance,* 2nd ed. (San Francisco: Benjamin Cummings, 2003).

because they work and because people can begin them at virtually any age and enjoy them for a lifetime. We'll look at three especially popular forms of exercise that focus on stretching and developing core muscle strength: yoga, tai chi, and Pilates.

Flexibility   The measure of the range of motion, or the amount of movement possible, at a particular joint.

Static stretching   Techniques that gradually lengthen a muscle to an elongated position (to the point of discomfort) and hold that position for 10 to 30 seconds.

Proprioceptive neuromuscular facilitation (PNF)
Techniques that involve the skillful use of alternating muscle contractions and static stretching in the same muscle.

A major objective of stretching exercises is to improve **flexibility,** a measure of the range of motion, or the amount of movement possible, at a particular joint. Improving range of motion through stretching exercises enhances efficiency, extent of movement, and posture. In addition, flexibility exercises have been shown to be effective in reducing the incidence and severity of lower back problems and muscle or tendon injuries that can occur during sports or everyday physical activities.[40] Improved flexibility can also mean less tension and pressure on joints, which results in less joint pain and joint deterioration.

Flexibility is enhanced by the controlled stretching of muscles and muscle attachments that act on a particular joint. Each muscle involved in a stretching exercise is attached to our skeleton by tendons. Figure 11.2 illustrates an example of the connection between muscle, bone, and tendons. The goal of stretching is to decrease the resistance of a muscle and its tendons to tension, that is, to reduce resistance to being stretched. Stretching exercises gradually result in greater flexibility. In stretching exercises a muscle or group of muscles is stretched to a point of slight discomfort, and that position is held for 10 to 30 seconds or more. For many people a regular stretching program enhances psychological as well as physical well-being.

Types of Stretching Exercises

In the language of exercise science, all of the commonly practiced stretching exercises fall into two major categories: static and proprioceptive neuromuscular facilitation (PNF).[41] **Static stretching** techniques involve the slow, gradual stretching of muscles and their tendons, then holding them at a point. During this holding period—the stretch—participants may feel a mild discomfort and a warm sensation in the muscles that are being stretched. Static stretching exercises involve specialized tension receptors in our muscles. When done properly, static stretching slightly lessens the sensitivity of tension receptors, which allows the muscle to relax and be stretched to greater length.[42] The stretch is followed by a slow return to the starting position. As discussed in the next section, the physical aspect of yoga and tai chi is largely composed of static techniques as are some of the exercises in Pilates programs.

The second major type of stretching exercise, **proprioceptive neuromuscular facilitation (PNF),** is relatively new. While PNF techniques have been shown to be superior to other stretching techniques for improving flexibility, they are, unfortunately, quite complex in their original form. A certified athletic trainer or physical therapist may be required to help in performing PNF exercises correctly; however, several have been simplified to the point that they can be performed with an exercise partner or even alone. PNF techniques involve contraction of a muscle followed by a stretch.

Self-Assessment of Cardiorespiratory Endurance

After you have exercised regularly for several months, you might want to assess your cardiorespiratory endurance level. Find a local track, typically one-quarter mile per lap, to perform your test. You may either run or walk for 1.5 miles and measure how long it takes to reach that distance, or run or walk for 12 minutes and determine the distance you covered in that time. Use the chart below to estimate your cardiorespiratory fitness level based upon your age and sex. Note that women have lower standards for each fitness category because they have higher levels of essential fat than men do.

Age*	1.5-Mile Run (min:sec)		12-Minute Run (miles)	
	Women (min:sec)	Men (min:sec)	Women (miles)	Men (miles)
Good				
15–30	<12:00	<10:00	>1.5	>1.7
35–50	<13:30	<11:30	>1.4	>1.5
55–70	<16:00	<14:00	>1.2	>1.3
Adequate for most activities				
15–30	<13:30	<11:50	>1.4	>1.5
35–50	<15:00	<13:00	>1.3	>1.4
55–70	<17:30	<15:30	>1.1	>1.3
Borderline				
15–30	<15:00	<13:00	>1.3	>1.4
35–50	<16:30	<14:30	>1.2	>1.3
55–70	<19:00	<17:00	>1.0	>1.2
Need extra work on cardiovascular fitness				
15–30	>17:00	>15:00	<1.2	<1.3
35–50	>18:30	>16:30	<1.1	<1.2
55–70	>21:00	>19:00	<0.9	<1.0

*Cardiorespiratory fitness declines with age.

If you are now at the Good level, congratulations! Your emphasis should be on maintaining this level for the rest of your life. If you are now at lower levels, set realistic goals for improvement.

Source: Reprinted by permission from Edward T. Howley and B. Don Franks, *Health Fitness Instructor's Handbook, 3rd ed.* (Champaign, IL: Human Kinetics Publishers, 1992), 85.

Yoga, Tai Chi, and Pilates

Three major styles of exercise that include stretching have become practiced widely in the United States and other Western countries. **Yoga** originated in India about 5,000 years ago. **Tai chi** is an ancient Chinese form of exercise that, like yoga, combines stretching, balance, coordination, and meditation. Yoga and tai chi are excellent for improving flexibility and muscular coordination. **Pilates** combines stretching with movement against resistance, which is aided by devices such as tension springs or heavy rubber bands. All three of these popular exercise programs include a joining of mind and body as a result of intense concentration on breathing and body position.

Yoga A variety of Indian traditions geared toward self-discipline and the realization of unity; includes forms of exercise widely practiced in the West today that promote balance, coordination, flexibility, and meditation.

Tai chi An ancient Chinese form of exercise widely practiced in the West today that promotes balance, coordination, stretching, and meditation.

Pilates Exercise programs that combine stretching with movement against resistance, aided by devices such as tension springs and heavy bands.

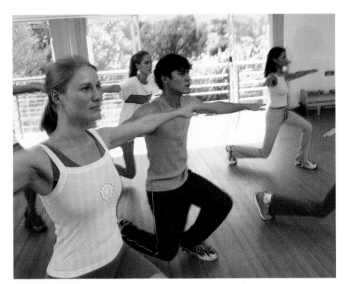

Yoga and other styles of exercise that strengthen core body muscles also enhance flexibility and lower stress levels.

Yoga has become one of the most popular fitness and static stretching activities. It blends the mental and physical aspects of exercise, a union of mind and body that participants find rewarding and satisfying. Done regularly, its combination of mental focus and physical effort improves vitality, posture, agility, and coordination.

The practice of yoga focuses attention on controlled breathing as well as purely physical exercise. In addition to its mental dimensions, yoga incorporates a complex array of static stretching exercises expressed as postures (asanas). More than 200 postures exist, but only about 50 are commonly practiced. During a session participants move to different asanas and hold them for 30 seconds or more. Yoga not only enhances flexibility, but it also has the great advantage of being flexible itself. Asanas and combinations of asanas can be changed and adjusted for young and old and to accommodate people with physical limitations or disabilities. Asanas can also be combined to provide even conditioned athletes with challenging sessions.

A typical yoga session will move the spine and joints through their full range of motion. Yoga postures lengthen, strengthen, and balance musculature, which leads to increased flexibility, stamina, and strength. Many people report an increased sense of general well-being too.

There are many styles of yoga. Three of the most popular are:

- *Iyengar yoga* focuses on precision and alignment in the poses. Standing poses are basic to this style, and poses often are held longer than in other styles of yoga.
- *Ashtanga yoga* in its pure form is based on a specific flow of poses that creates internal heat. The copious sweating that results is said to have a cleansing effect. Power yoga, a style growing in popularity, is a derivative of Ashtanga yoga.

- *Bikram's yoga* is similar to power yoga but does not incorporate a specific flow of poses. Literally the hottest yoga going, it is performed in temperatures of 100°F, or even a bit higher.

Tai chi is an exercise regimen that is designed to increase range of motion and flexibility while reducing muscular tension. Based on Chi Kung, a Taoist philosophy dedicated to spiritual growth and good health, tai chi was developed about 1000 A.D. by monks to defend themselves against bandits and warlords. It involves a series of positions called *forms* that are performed continuously.

Compared to yoga and tai chi, Pilates is the new kid on the exercise block. It was developed by Joseph Pilates who came from Germany to New York in 1926. Shortly after his arrival, he introduced his exercise methodology, which emphasizes flexibility, coordination, strength, and tone. Pilates differs in part from yoga and tai chi in that it includes a component designed to increase strength. The method consists of a sequence of carefully performed movements. Some are carried out on specially designed equipment, while others are performed on mats. Each exercise stretches and strengthens the muscles involved and has a specific breathing pattern associated with it. A Pilates class will focus on strengthening specific muscle groups and use equipment that provides resistance.

What do you think?

Why is it so important to have good flexibility throughout life? ✻ *Describe some situations in which improved flexibility would help you perform daily activities with less effort.* ✻ *What actions can you take to become more flexible?*

Designing Your Own Stretching Exercise Program: General Guidelines

If participation in formal exercise classes isn't for you, you can easily design your own stretching exercise program. Figure 11.3 shows a selection of exercises that will stretch the major muscle groups of your body and can be used as a warm-up for other physical activities and exercise programs such as jogging and tennis.

A program of regular stretching exercise doesn't need to take a great deal of time and doesn't require expensive equipment. You can reap the benefits of stretching with just two or three 10-minute sessions per week. Start off slowly with a five-minute session for the first week, then add a 5-minute session each week, until you reach a schedule and comfort level that suit you. A hefty program would consist of five 30-minute sessions each week. Sessions get longer as you slowly increase the time you hold a particular stretch and how many times you repeat each type of stretch.

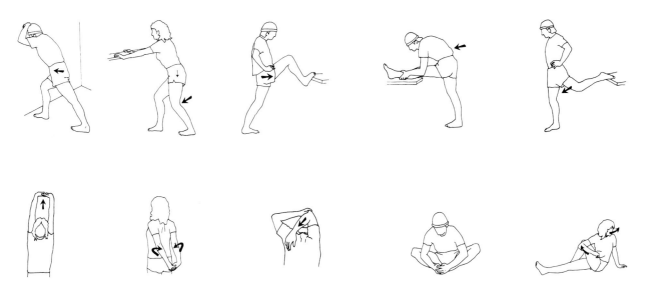

Figure 11.3

Stretching Exercises to Improve Flexibility

Use these stretches as part of your warm-up and cool-down. Hold each stretch for 10 to 30 seconds and repeat four times for each limb. After only a few weeks of regular stretching, you'll begin to see more flexibility.

Source: Drawings from B. Anderson, *Stretching, 20th Anniversary Revised Edition.* © 2000 Shelter Publications, Box 279, Bolinas, CA 94924.

Improving Muscular Strength and Endurance

To get a sense of what resistance training is about, do a resistance exercise. Start by holding your right arm straight down by your side, then turn your hand palm up and bring it up toward your shoulder. That's a resistance exercise: using a muscle, your biceps, to move a resistance, which in this case, is just the weight of your hand—not very much resistance. (See Figure 11.2.) Resistance training usually involves more weight or tension than this, but unlike flexibility training, resistance training is usually equipment intense. You don't get to look like Arnold Schwarzenegger doing these exercises empty handed. Free weights such as dumbbells and barbells and all sorts of tension-producing machines are usually part of resistance training. It's not just bodybuilding that uses this type of exercise either. Fitness programs and many sports employ resistance training to improve strength and endurance; many rehabilitation programs for recovery from injuries to muscles and joints are designed around resistance exercises.

Strength and Endurance

In the field of resistance training, **muscular strength** refers to the amount of force a muscle or group of muscles is capable of exerting. The most common way to assess strength in a resistance exercise program is to measure the **one repetition maximum (1-RM),** which is the maximum amount of weight a person can move one time in a particular exercise. For example, 1-RM for the simple exercise done at the begin-

ning of this section is the maximum weight you lift to your shoulder one time. **Muscular endurance** is the ability of muscle to exert force repeatedly without fatiguing. If you can perform the exercise described earlier holding a 5-pound weight in your hand and lifting ten times, you will have greater endurance than someone who attempts that same exercise but is only able to lift the weight seven times.

Some resistance programs are designed primarily for increasing strength; others are aimed more at increasing endurance. Winning an Olympic weight-lifting event depends on the amount of weight that is lifted in just a few seconds. Endurance doesn't play a large role. Conversely, a soccer event lasts much longer and requires enormous endurance but less strength than does weight lifting. In football, strength and endurance are both important. Training for endurance uses smaller weights but repeats an exercise more times than does training for strength. If you were endurance training for performing the hand-to-shoulder exercise used as an example (called a curl in weight-training circles), you might hold a 5-pound weight in each hand and curl 15 times per exercise segment. In training for strength, 40-pound weights might be used for a five-time curl.

Muscular strength The amount of force that a muscle is capable of exerting.

One repetition maximum (1-RM) The amount of weight/resistance that can be lifted or moved once, but not twice; a common measure of strength.

Muscular endurance A muscle's ability to exert force repeatedly without fatiguing.

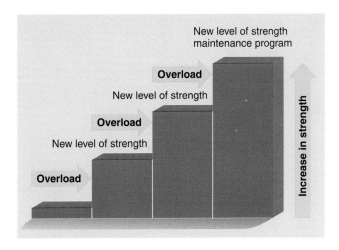

Figure 11.4

The Overload Principle

The overload principle contributes to an increase in strength. Notice that once the muscle has adapted to the original overload, a new overload must be placed on the muscle for subsequent strength gains to result.

Source: P. A. Sienna, *One Rep Max: A Guide to Beginning Weight Training,* Fig. 2.1, 8. © 1989 Wm. C. Brown Communications, Inc., Dubuque, IA. Reprinted by permission of Times Mirror Higher Education Group, Inc., Dubuque, IA. All rights reserved.

Principles of Strength Development

An effective **resistance exercise program** involves three key principles: tension, overload, and specificity of training.[43]

The Tension Principle   The key to developing strength is to create tension within a muscle or group of muscles. Tension is created by resistance provided by weights such as barbells or dumbbells, specially designed machines, or the weight of the body.

The Overload Principle   The overload principle is the most important of our three key principles. Overload doesn't mean forcing a muscle or group of muscles to do too much, which could result in injuries. Rather, overload in resistance training requires muscles to do more than they are used to doing. Everyone begins a resistance training program with

---

Resistance exercise program   A regular program of exercises designed to improve muscular strength and endurance in the major muscle groups.

Hypertrophy   Increased size (girth) of a muscle.

Isometric muscle action   Force produced without any resulting joint movement.

Concentric muscle action   Force produced while the muscle is shortening.

---

an initial level of strength. To become stronger, you must regularly create a degree of tension in your muscles that is greater than you are accustomed to. This overload will cause your muscles to adapt to a new level. As your muscles respond to a regular program of overloading by getting larger, they become stronger. Figure 11.4 illustrates how a continual process of overload and adaptation to the overload improves strength.

Remember that resistance training exercises cause microscopic damage (tears) to muscle fibers, and the rebuilding process that increases the size and capacity of the muscle takes 24 to 48 hours. Thus, resistance training exercise programs should include at least one day of rest and recovery between workouts before overloading the same muscles again.

The Specificity of Training Principle   According to the specificity principle, the effects of resistance exercise training are specific to the muscles being exercised. Only the muscle or muscle group that you exercise responds to the demands placed upon it. For example, if you regularly do curls, the muscles involved—your biceps—will become larger and stronger, but the other muscles in your body won't change.

Gender Differences in Weight Training

The results of resistance training in men and women are quite different. Women normally don't develop the muscles to the same extent that men do. The main reason for this difference is that men and women have different levels of the hormone testosterone in their blood. Before puberty, testosterone levels are similar for both boys and girls. During adolescence, testosterone levels in boys increase dramatically, about ten-fold, while testosterone levels in girls remain unchanged. Muscles will become larger **(hypertrophy)** as a result of resistance training exercise; typically this change is not as dramatic in women as it is in men. To enhance muscle bulk, some bodybuilders (both men and women) take synthetic hormones (anabolic steroids) that mimic the effects of testosterone. However, using anabolic steroids is a dangerous and illegal practice. (See Chapter 7.)

Types of Muscle Activity

Your skeletal muscles act in three different ways: isometric, concentric, and eccentric.[44] (See Figure 11.5.) In **isometric muscle action,** force is produced through tension and muscle contraction, not movement. Figure 11.5(a) shows an isometric contraction. A **concentric muscle action,** shown in Figure 11.5(b), causes joint movement and a production of force while the muscle shortens. The empty-hand curl we did at the beginning of this section is a concentric exercise, with joint movement occurring at the elbow. In general, concentric muscle actions produce movement in a direction opposite to the downward pull of gravity.

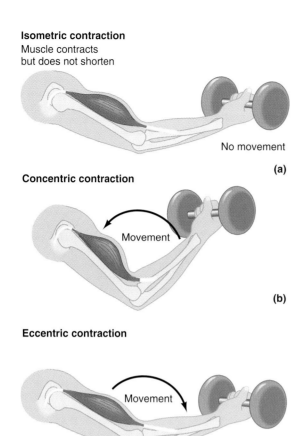

Isometric contraction
Muscle contracts
but does not shorten

No movement

(a)

Concentric contraction

Movement

(b)

Eccentric contraction

Movement

(c)

Figure 11.5
Isometric, Concentric, and Eccentric Muscle Actions
Source: S. Powers and E. Howley, *Exercise Physiology: Theory and Application to Fitness and Performance* (Madison, WI: Brown and Benchmark, 1997).

Eccentric muscle action describes the ability of a muscle to produce force while lengthening. Typically, eccentric muscle actions occur when movement is in the same direction as the pull of gravity. Once you've brought a weight up during a curl, an eccentric muscle action would be to lower your hand and the weight back to their original position. Figure 11.5(c) demonstrates an eccentric muscle action.

Methods of Providing Resistance

There are four commonly used resistance exercise methods: body weight, fixed, variable, and accommodating resistance devices.

Body Weight Resistance (Calisthenics)
Strength and endurance training doesn't always have to rely on equipment. You can use your own body weight to develop skeletal muscle fitness. Calisthenics use part or all of your body weight to offer resistance during exercise. While less effective than other resistance methods in developing large muscle mass and strength, calisthenics are quite adequate for improving general muscular fitness and generally sufficient to improve muscle tone and maintain a level of muscular strength.

Fixed Resistance
Fixed resistance exercises provide a constant amount of resistance throughout the full range of movement. Barbells, dumbbells, and some types of machines provide fixed resistance because their weight, or the amount of resistance, does not change during an exercise. Fixed resistance equipment has the potential to strengthen all the major muscle groups in the body.

One advantage of dumbbells and barbells is that they are relatively inexpensive. Fixed resistance exercise machines are commonly available at college recreation/fitness facilities, health clubs, and many resorts and hotels.

Variable Resistance
Variable resistance equipment alters the resistance encountered by a muscle during a movement, so that the effort by the muscle is more consistent throughout the full range of motion. Variable resistance machines, such as Nautilus and Bowflex, are typically single-station devices; a person stays on the same machine throughout the whole series of exercises. Other types of machines, such as Soloflex, have multiple stations; the person using them moves from one machine to another. While some of these machines are expensive and too big to move easily, others are affordable and more portable. Many forms of variable resistance devices are sold for home use.

Accommodating Resistance Devices
These devices adjust the resistance according to the amount of force generated by the person using the equipment. The exerciser performs at maximal level of effort, while the exercise machine controls the speed of the exercise. The machine is set to a particular speed, and muscles being exercised must move at a rate faster than or equal to that speed in order to encounter resistance.[45]

The Benefits of Strength Training

You may wonder about the benefits associated with strength training beyond that of simply getting stronger. It turns out that regular strength training has many other benefits as well. It can reduce the occurrence of lower back pain and joint and muscle injuries. It can also postpone loss of muscle tissue due to aging and a sedentary lifestyle, and help prevent osteoporosis.

Strength training enhances muscle definition and tone and improves personal appearance. This, in turn, enhances self-esteem. Strength training even has a hidden benefit: Muscle tissue burns calories faster than most other tissues do, even when it is resting. So, increasing your muscle mass can help you lose pounds and maintain a healthy weight.

> **Eccentric muscle action**   Force produced while the muscle is lengthening.

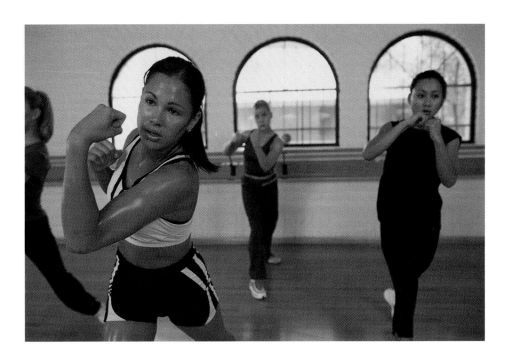

Cardio kickboxing is just one of many activities that can improve fitness and provide health benefits.

Getting Started

When beginning a resistance exercise program, always consider your age, fitness level, and personal goals. Strength training exercises are done in a *set,* or a single series of multiple repetitions using the same resistance. For both men and women under the age of 50, the ACSM recommends working major muscle groups with one set of eight to ten different exercises two to three days per week.[46] Weight loads should be at a level to allow up to 8 to 12 repetitions. Very unfit people should decrease weight loads and complete 10 to 15 repetitions. Remember, experts suggest allowing at least one day of rest and recovery between workouts.

> **What do you think?**
> *What types of resistance equipment are currently available to you?* ✻ *Based on what you've read, what actions can you take to increase your muscular strength?* ✻ *Muscular endurance?* ✻ *How would you measure your improvement?*

Body Composition

Body composition is the fourth and final component of a comprehensive fitness program. Body composition parameters that can be influenced by regular physical activity include total body mass, fat mass, fat-free mass, and regional fat distribution.[47] Body composition differs significantly for women and men, since women have a higher percentage of body fat and a significantly lower percentage of fat-free mass (such as muscle and bone) and bone mineral density.[48]

The most successful weight-loss programs combine diet and exercise effectively. When participating in endurance training programs for the purpose of losing weight, total body mass and fat mass generally decrease, while fat-free mass remains constant. If your main reason for exercising is to lose weight, combine healthy eating habits with at least three workouts per week that expend 250 to 300 kilocalories per session (at least 30 to 45 minutes of continuous low-to-moderate intensity activity, depending on your body weight) in order to see significant reductions in your total body mass and fat mass.[49]

Fitness Injuries

Overtraining is the most frequent cause of injuries associated with fitness activities and affects up to 20 percent of all athletes. Enthusiastic but out-of-shape beginners often injure themselves by doing too much too soon. Experienced athletes develop *overtraining syndrome* by engaging in systematic and progressive increases in training without getting enough rest and recovery time. Eventually, performance begins to decline, and training sessions become increasingly difficult. Adequate rest, good nutrition (including replenishing carbohydrates), and rehydration are important to sustain or improve fitness levels. Pay attention to your body's warning signs. To avoid injuring a particular muscle group or body part, vary your fitness activities throughout the week to give muscles and joints a rest. Set appropriate short-term and long-term training goals. Establishing realistic but challenging fitness goals can help you stay motivated without overdoing it. Overtraining injuries occur most often in repetitive activities like skiing, running, bicycling, and step aerobics. However, use common sense, and you're likely to remain injury-free.

Causes of Fitness-Related Injuries

There are two basic types of injuries stemming from fitness-related activities: overuse and traumatic. **Overuse injuries** occur because of cumulative, day-after-day stresses placed on tendons, bones, and ligaments during exercise. The forces that occur normally during physical activity are not enough to cause a ligament sprain or muscle strain. But when these forces are applied on a daily basis for weeks or months, they can result in an injury. Common sites of overuse injuries are the leg, knee, shoulder, and elbow joints.

Traumatic injuries occur suddenly and violently, typically by accident. Examples include broken bones, torn ligaments and muscles, contusions, and lacerations. Some traumatic injuries occur quickly and are difficult to avoid—for example, spraining your ankle by landing on another person's foot after jumping up for a rebound in basketball. If your traumatic injury causes a noticeable loss of function and immediate pain or pain that does not go away after 30 minutes, you should have a physician examine it.

Prevention

Your exercise clothing is more than a fashion statement—smart choices can help you prevent injuries. For some types of physical activity, you need clothing that allows body heat to dissipate—for example, light-colored nylon shorts and mesh tank top while running in hot weather. For other types, you need clothing that retains body heat without getting you sweat-soaked—for example, layers of polypropylene and/or wool clothing while cross-country skiing.

Appropriate Footwear   When you purchase running shoes, look for several key components. Biomechanics research has revealed that running is a collision sport—that is, with each stride, the runner's foot collides with the ground with a force three to five times the runner's body weight.[50] The 150-pound runner who takes 1,000 strides per mile applies a cumulative force to his or her body of 450,000 pounds per mile. The force not absorbed by the running shoe is transmitted upward into the foot, leg, thigh, and back. Our bodies are able to absorb forces such as these but may be injured by the cumulative effects of repetitive impacts (e.g., running 40 miles per week). Therefore, the ability of running shoes to absorb shock is critical.

The midsole of a running shoe must absorb impact forces but must also be flexible. To evaluate the flexibility of the midsole, hold the shoe between the index fingers of your right and left hand. When you push on both ends of the shoe with your fingers, the shoe should bend easily at the midsole. If the force exerted by your index fingers cannot bend the shoe, its midsole is probably too rigid and may irritate your Achilles tendon, among other problems.[51] Other basic characteristics of running shoes include a rigid plastic insert within the heel of the shoe (known as a heel counter) to control the movement of your heel; a cushioned foam pad surrounding the heel of the shoe to prevent Achilles tendon irritation; and a removable thermoplastic innersole that customizes the fit of the shoe by using your body heat to mold it to the shape of your foot. Shoes are the runner's most essential piece of equipment, so carefully select appropriate footwear before you start a running program.

Shoe companies also sell cross-training shoes to help combat the high cost of having to buy separate pairs of running shoes, tennis shoes, weight-training shoes, and so on. Although the cross-training shoe can be used for several different fitness activities by the novice or recreational athlete, a distance runner who runs 25 or more miles per week needs a pair of specialty running shoes to prevent injury.

Appropriate Exercise Equipment   Some activities require special protective equipment to reduce chances of injury. Eye injuries can occur in virtually all fitness-related activities, although some activities are more risky than others. As many as 90 percent of the eye injuries resulting from racquetball and squash could be prevented by wearing appropriate eye protection—for example, goggles with polycarbonate lenses.[52] Nearly 100 million people in the United States ride bikes for pleasure, fitness, or competition. Head injuries used to account for 85 percent of all deaths from bicycle accidents; however, bike helmets have significantly reduced the number of skull fractures and facial injuries.[53] Look for helmets that meet the standards established by the American National Standards Institute and the Snell Memorial Foundation.

> **What do you think?**
> *Given your activity level, what injury risks are you exposed to on a regular basis?* ✳ *What changes can you make in your equipment and clothing to reduce your risk?*

Common Overuse Injuries

Body movements in physical activities such as running and bicycling are highly repetitive, so participants are susceptible to overuse injuries. In fitness activities, the joints of the lower extremities (foot, ankle, knee, and hip) tend to be injured more frequently than the upper-extremity joints (shoulder, elbow, wrist, and hand). Three of the most common overuse injuries are plantar fasciitis, shin splints, and runner's knee.

> **Overuse injuries**   Injuries that result from the cumulative effects of day-after-day stresses placed on tendons, muscles, and joints.
>
> **Traumatic injuries**   Injuries that are accidental in nature and occur suddenly and violently (e.g., fractured bones, ruptured tendons, and sprained ligaments).

Plantar Fasciitis   Plantar fasciitis is an inflammation of the plantar fascia, a broad band of dense, inelastic tissue (fascia) that runs from the heel to the toe on the bottom of the foot. The main function of the plantar fascia is to protect the nerves, blood vessels, and muscles of the foot from injury. Repetitive weight-bearing movements such as walking and running can inflame the plantar fascia. Common symptoms are pain and tenderness under the ball of the foot, at the heel, or at both locations.[54] The pain of plantar fasciitis is particularly noticeable during the first steps out of bed in the morning. If not treated properly, this injury may progress to the point that weight-bearing exercise is too painful to endure. Uphill running is not advised, because each uphill stride severely stretches (and thus irritates) the already inflamed plantar fascia. This injury can often be prevented by regularly stretching the plantar fascia prior to exercise and by wearing athletic shoes with good arch support and shock absorbency. Stretch the plantar fascia by slowly pulling all five toes upward toward your head, holding for 10 to 15 seconds, and repeating this three to five times on each foot prior to exercise.

Shin Splints   A general term for any pain that occurs below the knee and above the ankle is *shin splints*. This broad description includes more than 20 different medical conditions. Problems range from stress fractures of the tibia (shin bone) to severe inflammation in the muscles of the lower leg, which can interrupt the flow of blood and nerve supply to the foot. The most common type of shin splints occurs along the inner side of the tibia and is usually a combination of muscle irritation and irritation of the tissues that attach the muscles to the bone in this region. Typically, there is pain and swelling along the middle third of the posteromedial tibia in the soft tissues, not the bone.

Sedentary people who start a new weight-bearing exercise program are at the greatest risk for shin splints, though well-conditioned aerobic exercisers who rapidly increase their distance or pace may also develop them.[55] Running is the most frequent cause of shin splints, but people who do a great deal of walking (e.g., mail carriers, servers in restaurants) may also develop this injury.

To help prevent shin splints, wear athletic shoes with good arch support and shock absorbency. If the pain continues, see your physician. You may be advised to substitute a non–weight-bearing activity, such as swimming, during your recovery period.

Runner's Knee   *Runner's knee* describes a series of problems involving the muscles, tendons, and ligaments about the knee. The most common problem identified as runner's knee is abnormal movement of the kneecap, which irritates the cartilage on the back side of the kneecap as well as nearby tendons and ligaments.[56] Women experience this more often than men.

The main symptom of this kind of runner's knee is the pain experienced when downward pressure is applied to the kneecap after the knee is straightened fully. Additional symptoms may include swelling, redness, tenderness around the kneecap, and a dull, aching pain in the center of the knee.[57] If you have these symptoms, your physician will probably recommend that you stop running for a few weeks and reduce daily activities that compress the kneecap (e.g., exercise on a stair-climbing machine or doing squats with heavy resistance) until you no longer feel any pain.

Treatment

First-aid treatment for virtually all personal fitness injuries involves **RICE: r**est, **i**ce, **c**ompression, and **e**levation. *Rest,* the first component of this treatment, is required to avoid further irritation of the injured body part. *Ice* is applied to relieve pain and constrict the blood vessels to stop any internal or external bleeding. Never apply ice cubes, reusable gel ice packs, chemical cold packs, or other forms of cold directly to your skin. Instead, place a layer of wet toweling or elastic bandage between the ice and your skin. Ice should be applied to a new injury for approximately 20 minutes every hour for the first 24 to 72 hours. *Compression* of the injured body part can be accomplished with a 4- or 6-inch-wide elastic bandage; this applies indirect pressure to damaged blood vessels to help stop bleeding. Be careful, though, that the compression wrap does not interfere with normal blood flow. A throbbing, painful hand or foot indicates that the compression wrap should be loosened. *Elevation* of the injured extremity above the level of your heart also helps to control internal or external bleeding by making the blood flow upward to reach the injured area.

Exercising in the Heat or Cold

Heat stress, which includes several potentially fatal illnesses resulting from excessive core body temperatures, should be a concern whenever you exercise in warm, humid weather. In these conditions, your body's rate of heat production can exceed its ability to cool itself.

You can help prevent heat stress by following certain precautions. First, proper acclimatization to hot and/or humid climates is essential. The process of heat acclimatization, which increases your body's cooling efficiency, requires about 10 to 14 days of gradually increased activity in the hot environment. Second, avoid dehydration by replacing the fluids you lose during and after exercise. Third, wear clothing appropriate for your activity and the environment. And finally, use common sense—for example, on an 85-degree,

---

RICE   Acronym for the standard first-aid treatment for virtually all traumatic and overuse injuries: **r**est, **i**ce, **c**ompression, and **e**levation.

---

80 percent humidity day, postpone your usual lunchtime run until the cool of evening.

The three different heat stress illnesses are progressive in severity: heat cramps, heat exhaustion, and heat stroke. **Heat cramps** (heat-related muscle cramps), the least serious problem, can usually be prevented by warm-ups, adequate fluid replacement, and a diet that includes the electrolytes lost during sweating (sodium and potassium). (For general information on cramps, see the next section.) **Heat exhaustion** is caused by excessive water loss resulting from prolonged exercise or work. Symptoms of heat exhaustion include nausea, headache, fatigue, dizziness and faintness and, paradoxically, goosebumps and chills. If you are suffering from heat exhaustion, your skin will be cool and moist. Heat exhaustion is actually a mild form of shock in which the blood pools in the arms and legs away from the brain and major organs of the body, which causes nausea and fainting. **Heat stroke,** often called sunstroke, is a life-threatening emergency with a 20 to 70 percent death rate.[58] Heat stroke occurs during vigorous exercise when the body's heat production significantly exceeds its cooling capacities. Body core temperature can rise from normal (98.6°F) to 105°F to 110°F within minutes after the body's cooling mechanism shuts down. With no cooling taking place, rapidly increasing core temperatures can cause brain damage, permanent disability, and death. Common signs of heat stroke are dry, hot, and usually red skin; very high body temperature; and a very rapid heart rate.

If you experience any of the symptoms mentioned here, stop exercising immediately, move to the shade or a cool spot to rest, and drink large amounts of cool fluids. Be aware that heat stress can strike in situations in which the danger is not obvious. Serious or fatal heat strokes may result from prolonged sauna or steam baths, prolonged immersion in a hot tub or spa, or by exercising in a plastic or rubber head-to-toe "sauna suit."[59]

What are the best fluids to drink? In comparing participants' performance during exercise sessions lasting less than one hour, the ACSM found little difference between plain water versus sports drinks (drinks containing carbohydrates and electrolytes).[60] However, a recent study suggests otherwise. In a laboratory study requiring intense stationary bicycling (50 minutes of high-level activity followed by a 9- to 12-minute "sprint to the finish"), subjects' cycling performance improved by 6 percent when they drank enough water to replace 80 percent of the fluid they lost as sweat—but by 12 percent when they consumed a similar amount of a sports drink.[61]

Remember that dehydration of only 1 to 2 percent of body weight quickly affects physiological function and performance. Dehydration of greater than 3 percent of body weight increases the risk of heat cramps, heat exhaustion, and heat stroke.[62] During intense exercise lasting longer than one hour, the ACSM recommends drinking fluids that contain 4 percent to 8 percent carbohydrates (to delay muscular fatigue) and a small amount of sodium (to improve taste and promote fluid retention). Fluid intake *following* physical

activity is also important to prevent dehydration—be sure to drink at least a pint of fluid for every pound of body weight lost during your exercise session.

When you exercise in cool weather, **hypothermia**—a potentially fatal condition resulting from abnormally low body core temperature, which occurs when body heat is lost faster than it is produced—may result. Temperatures need not be frigid for hypothermia to occur; it can also result from prolonged, vigorous exercise in 40°F to 50°F temperatures, particularly if there is rain, snow, or a strong wind.

In mild cases of hypothermia, as body core temperature drops from the normal 98.6°F to about 93.2°F, you will begin to shiver. Shivering increases body temperature by using the heat given off by muscle activity. During this first stage of hypothermia, you may also experience cold hands and feet, poor judgment, apathy, and amnesia.[63] Shivering ceases as body core temperatures drop to between 87°F and 90°F, a sign that the body has lost its ability to generate heat. Death usually occurs at body core temperatures between 75°F and 80°F.

To prevent hypothermia, pay attention to weather conditions, don't exercise alone, dress in layers, and avoid dehydration.[64]

Preventing Cramps

Although most of us have experienced the quick, intense pain of muscle cramps, they are poorly understood. According to the overexertion theory of muscle cramps, when a muscle gets tired, the numerous muscle fibers that compose the muscle fail to contract in a synchronized rhythm, probably due to overstimulation from the nerves that trigger the muscles to contract.[65]

Cramps are a problem for those who exercise and perspire heavily. Drinking enough fluids before, during, and after such activity is important. On a daily basis, drink enough fluids so you have to urinate every two to four hours. Your urine should be pale, and there should be lots of it. During extended exercise, it is recommended that you drink as

---

Heat cramps   Muscle cramps that occur during or following exercise in warm or hot weather.

Heat exhaustion   A heat stress illness caused by significant dehydration resulting from exercise in warm or hot conditions; frequent precursor to heat stroke.

Heat stroke   A deadly heat stress illness resulting from dehydration and overexertion in warm or hot conditions; can cause body core temperature to rise from normal to 105°F to 110°F in just a few minutes.

Hypothermia   Potentially fatal condition caused by abnormally low body core temperature.

Table 11.2
Picking Your Workout Machine

Machine	Workout	For the Best Workout
Exercise Rider	Upper body: Fair Lower body: Fair Learning curve: Easy	Experiment with seat heights until you find one that's comfortable. Make sure your legs don't bend more than 90 degrees at the bottom phase of the motion, which can be hard on the knees. Then, as you straighten, don't arch your spine backward; that stresses your lower back.
Rowing	Upper body: Excellent Lower body: Excellent Learning curve: Hard	Don't hyperextend your back as you finish your stroke. Keep your elbows tight to your body to best strengthen your arms.
Ski	Upper body: Excellent Lower body: Excellent Learning curve: Hard	Perfect arm movements first, then the leg actions, then put it all together; it usually takes a few sessions. One habit to avoid: constantly leaning against the hop pad to hold yourself upright.
Stair-Climber	Upper body: Poor Lower body: Excellent Learning curve: Hard	Keep your posture upright, your steps shallow (no deeper than 6 inches), and your weight off your arms.
Treadmill	Upper body: Poor Lower body: Excellent Learning curve: Easy	Start on the flat as a warm-up, gradually increase speed and incline (to 10 percent), then wind down to a slow, flat walk.
Stationary Bike	Upper body: Poor Lower body: Excellent Learning curve: Easy	Adjust the seat so your leg is almost fully extended when the pedal is at its lowest. Then just start pumping.

Source: Adapted by permission of Time Inc. Health from Karmen Butterer, "Picking Your Dream Machine," *Health* (September 1995): 48. © 1995.

much as you can tolerate, ideally 8 ounces every 15 to 20 minutes.[66]

Although calcium plays a role in muscle contraction and people with a tendency to have cramps are often calcium deficient, exercise physiologists question the validity of the low calcium theory. However, because calcium has many health benefits, experts continue to recommend it for anyone who has a tendency toward cramping.

Lack of sodium is another possible factor. If you exercise a lot and sweat a lot, you will lose sodium through sweat, may develop a sodium imbalance, and experience cramps. This is mostly likely to occur in extreme sports such as Ironman triathlons or 100-mile trail runs, particularly in athletes who have consumed only plain water (not sodium-containing food or beverages) during the event.[67] Many health-conscious athletes restrict their salt intake on a regular basis in an attempt to keep blood pressure under control, but clearly there is a risk in doing so.

Although paying attention to the above nutrients is important to avoid cramping, it is probably more important to make sure that muscles are warmed up, and that muscles are not strained beyond their limit.

If you get cramps, what should you do? Generally massage, stretching, putting pressure on the muscle that is cramping, and deep breathing are useful remedies.

Planning a Fitness Program

Identify Your Fitness Goals

Before you start a fitness program, analyze your personal needs, limitations, physical activity likes and dislikes, and daily schedule. Your specific goal may be to achieve (or maintain) healthy levels of body fat, cardiovascular fitness, muscular strength and endurance, or flexibility and mobility.

Once you become committed to regular physical activity and exercise, you will observe gradual improvements in your functional abilities and note progress toward your goals. Perhaps your most vital goal will be to become committed to fitness for the long haul—to establish a realistic schedule of diverse exercise activities that you can maintain and enjoy throughout your life.

Design Your Program

What type of fitness program is best suited to your needs? The amount and type of exercise required to yield beneficial results vary with the age and physical condition of the exerciser. Men over age 40 and women over age 50 should consult their physicians before beginning any fitness program.

Good fitness programs are designed to improve or maintain cardiorespiratory fitness, flexibility, muscular strength and endurance, and body composition. A comprehensive program might include a warm-up period of easy walking followed by stretching activities to improve flexibility, selected strength development exercises, an aerobic activity for 20 minutes or more, and a cool-down period of gentle flexibility exercises.

Choose an aerobic activity you think you will like. Many people find cross training—alternate-day participation in two or more aerobic activities (i.e., jogging and swimming)—less monotonous than long-term participation in only one activity. Cross training also strengthens a variety of muscles and thus helps you avoid overuse injuries.

Jogging, walking, cycling, rowing, step aerobics, and cross-country skiing are all excellent activities for developing cardiovascular fitness. Most universities have recreation centers where students can use stair-climbing machines, stationary bicycles, treadmills, rowing machines, and ski-simulators. Table 11.2 describes various workout machines and provides tips for their use.

Taking Charge

Make It Happen!

Assessment: Complete the Assess Yourself box on page 303 to determine your current cardiorespiratory endurance level. Your results may indicate that you should start taking steps to improving this component of your physical fitness.

Making a Change: In order to change your behavior, you need to develop a plan. Follow these steps.

1. Evaluate your behavior, and identify patterns and specific things you are doing. What can you change now? What can you change in the near future?
2. Select one pattern of behavior that you want to change.
3. Fill out a Behavior Change Contract. It should include your long-term goal for change, your short-term goals, the rewards you'll give yourself for reaching these goals, potential obstacles along the way, and strategies for overcoming these obstacles. For each goal, list the small steps and specific actions that you will take.

4. Chart your progress in a journal. At the end of a week, consider how successful you were in following your plan. What helped you be successful? What made change more difficult? What will you do differently next week?
5. Revise your plan as needed. Are the short-term goals attainable? Are the rewards satisfying?

Example: Chris decided to measure how long it took him to run 1.5 miles around the school track to determine his level of cardiorespiratory endurance. It took him 14.5 minutes, which, as a 20 year old, put him into the borderline category. Chris had played sports in high school and considered himself in good physical shape. However, he realized he had stopped exercising regularly in his freshman year when he didn't make the baseball team.

Chris decided to start by incorporating more activity into his daily routine. He tended to drive even to places that he could walk or bicycle to as easily. His friends had invited him to join in the pick-up basketball games they played on Saturday afternoons, but he had turned them down in order to play Playstation with his roommate. Chris filled out a Behavior Change Contract with a goal of riding his bicycle the three miles each way to campus three times a week and to play basketball every Saturday. If he did this consistently every week, he would reward himself with a new CD. After a month of this increased activity, Chris already was feeling more fit and was ready to add another aerobic activity. With winter weather coming, he thought he should add an indoor activity. He started swimming laps at the school pool. He realized he was making excuses not to go, though, because he found swimming boring. Chris switched to using a stair-climber machine, which he could do while reading *Sports Illustrated* or watching ESPN. He was able to stick to doing this three times a week and made a commitment to go a fourth time whenever he missed his Saturday basketball game.

Summary

✳ The physiological benefits of regular physical activity include reduced risk of heart attack, hypertension, and diabetes; and improved blood lipid profile, skeletal mass, weight control, immunity to disease, mental health and stress management, and physical fitness. Regular activity can also increase life span.

✳ An aerobic exercise program improves cardiorespiratory fitness. Exercise frequency begins with three days per week and eventually moves up to five. Exercise intensity involves working out at target heart rate. Exercise duration should increase to 30 to 45 minutes; the longer the exercise period, the more calories burned, and the greater the improvement in cardiovascular fitness.

✳ Flexibility exercises should involve static stretching exercises performed in sets of four or more repetitions held for 10 to 30 seconds on at least two to three days a week.

✳ The key principles for developing muscular strength and endurance are the tension principle, the overload principle, and the specificity of training principle. The different types of muscle actions include isometric, concentric, and eccentric. Resistance training programs include body weight resistance (calisthenics), fixed resistance, variable resistance, and accommodating resistance devices.

✳ Fitness injuries generally are caused by overuse or trauma; the most common ones are plantar fasciitis, shin splints, and runner's knee. Proper footwear and equipment can help prevent injuries. Exercise in the heat or cold requires special precautions.

✳ Planning a fitness program involves setting goals and designing a program to achieve these goals.

Questions for Discussion and Reflection

1. How do you define physical fitness? What are the key components of a physical fitness program? What might you need to consider when beginning a fitness program?
2. How would you determine the proper intensity and duration of an exercise program? How often should exercise sessions be scheduled?
3. Why is stretching vital to improving physical flexibility?
4. Identify at least four physiological and psychological benefits of physical fitness. What is the significance of the latest fitness report from the Surgeon General's Office? How might it help more people realize the benefits of physical fitness?
5. Describe the different types of resistance employed in an exercise program. What are the benefits of each type of resistance?
6. Your roommate has decided to start running first thing in the morning in an effort to lose weight, tone muscles, and improve cardiorespiratory fitness. What advice would you give to make sure your roommate begins properly and doesn't get injured?
7. What key components would you include in a fitness program for yourself?

Accessing Your Health on the Internet

Visit the following Internet sites to explore further topics and issues related to personal health. To visit an organization's website, go to the Companion Website for *Health: The Basics, Sixth Edition* at www.aw-bc.com/donatelle, click on the book image, and select "Accessing Your Health on the Internet" from the navigation menu on the left.

1. *ACSM Online.* A link with the American College of Sports Medicine and all their resources.
2. *American Council on Exercise.* Information on exercise and disease prevention.
3. *The American Medical Association's Health Insight.* Provides a fitness assessment and guidelines to help you develop your own fitness program.
4. *Just Move.* The American Heart Association's fitness website has the latest information on heart disease and exercise, plus a guide to local, regional, and national fitness events.
5. *National Strength and Conditioning Association.* A resource for personal trainers and others interested in conditioning and fitness.

Further Reading

Fahey, T. D. *Super Fitness for Sports, Conditioning, and Health.* Boston: Allyn & Bacon, 2000.

A brief guide to developing fitness that emphasizes training techniques for improving sports performance.

Powers, S. K., and S. L. Dodd. *Total Fitness and Wellness, 3rd ed.* San Francisco: Benjamin Cummings, 2003.

A complete guide to improving all areas of fitness, including being a smart health consumer, interviews with fitness specialists, and the links between nutrition and fitness.

Schlosberg, S. *The Ultimate Workout Log: An Exercise Diary and Fitness Guide.* Boston: Houghton Mifflin, 1999.

A six-month log that also provides fitness definitions, training tips, and motivational quotes.

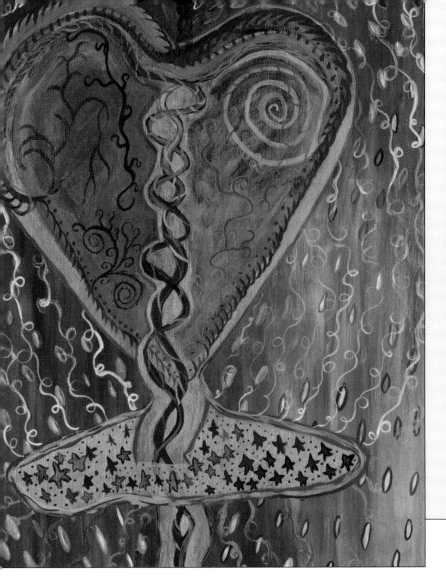

12

Cardiovascular Disease

Reducing Your Risk

Objectives

* Discuss the incidence, prevalence, and outcomes of cardiovascular disease in the United States, including its impact on society.

* Describe the anatomy and physiology of the heart and circulatory system and the importance of healthy heart function.

* Review major types of heart disease, factors that contribute to

their development, diagnostic and treatment options, and the importance of fundamental lifestyle modifications aimed at prevention.

* Discuss controllable risk factors for cardiovascular disease, including smoking, cholesterol and triglycerides, certain infectious organisms, diet and obesity, exercise, hypertension, diabetes mellitus, and stress. Examine your own risk

profile and determine which risk factors you can and cannot control.

* Discuss the issues surrounding cardiovascular disease risk and disease burden in women.

* Discuss methods of diagnosing and treating cardiovascular disease, and evaluate the importance of being a wise health care consumer.

The New York Times
In the News

Blow a Gasket, for Your Heart

By Eric Nagourney

Studies have suggested that people who have a lot of anger may be at higher risk for cardiovascular disease, but a new report finds that the relationship may not be so clear.

For men who express some of that anger, the researchers say, the risks may be lower.

Writing in the current issue of *Psychosomatic Medicine,* the researchers report that among the men studied (more than 23,000 over two years) those with moderate expressions of anger had about half the risk of nonfatal heart attacks as those with low expression of anger. The rate of strokes was also lower.

"It is a more complex picture than has been perhaps previously posed," said the lead author of the study, Dr. Patricia Mona Eng, who conducted the study as a researcher at the Harvard School of Public Health.

The study was based on information generated by the Health Professionals Follow-Up Study, a continuing look at the health of more than 50,000 men, including dentists, veterinarians and pharmacists.

The men who participated in the anger study were asked in a survey to describe how they handled anger.

Read the complete article online in the eThemes section of this book's website: www.aw-bc.com/donatelle.

Despite the many medical advances we enjoy, diseases of the heart and cardiovascular system continue to be a significant health threat in the United States (Figure 12.1). In fact, **cardiovascular disease (CVD)** remains the leading single cause of death around the world.

An Epidemiological Overview

In 2000, CVD accounted for almost 40 percent of all deaths in the United States, nearly 1 out of every 2.5. This is nearly three times the rate of the second leading killer, cancer, and more than the number of deaths caused by all other diseases combined. Of the more than 2.4 million deaths from all causes every year in the United States, CVD is listed as a primary or contributing cause of death on more than 1.4 million death certificates.[1] To realize just how serious CVD is, consider the following points.[2]

- More than 2,600 Americans die of CVD each day, an average of one death every 33 seconds. That's more than 945,000 deaths per year.
- Many of these fatalities are **sudden cardiac deaths,** which means that these Americans die from sudden, abrupt

---

Cardiovascular disease (CVD) Term encompassing a variety of diseases of the heart and blood vessels.

Sudden cardiac death Death that occurs as a result of sudden, abrupt loss of heart function.

---

loss of heart function (cardiac arrest), either instantly or shortly after symptoms occur. Most of these deaths result from coronary heart disease (CHD). In fact, between 400,000 and 460,000 people—nearly half of all victims of heart attack—die from CHD in an emergency room or before they get to a hospital. People who attempt to perform cardiac resuscitation are sometimes riddled with guilt when they fail to save a life. However, many such deaths are due to sudden heart stoppage or slowing that even the most heroic efforts could not prevent.

- CVD claims nearly 11,000 more lives each year than the next five leading causes of death combined.
- Almost 150,000 Americans killed by CVD are under age 65.
- The year 2000 death rates from CVD were 397.6 for white males, 509.6 for African American males, 285.8 for white females, and 397.1 for African American females. (The rate is per 100,000 of population.)
- From 1990 to 2000, death rates from CVD declined by 17 percent. However, because of increases in the total population, the number of actual CVD deaths increased 2.5 percent.
- If all forms of major CVD were eliminated, life expectancy would rise by almost seven years.
- The probability at birth of eventually dying of CVD is 47 percent; from cancer, 22 percent; from accidents, 3 percent; from diabetes, 2 percent; and from HIV, 0.7 percent.

Note that these statistics do not include the effects of CVD experienced by people who must live with the disease.

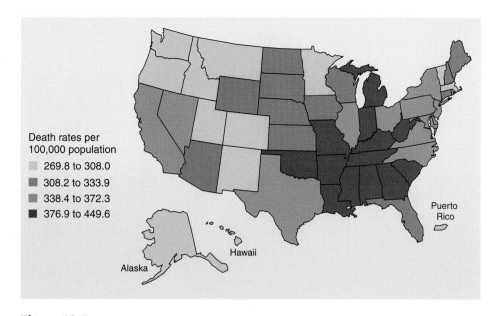

Figure 12.1

1999 Total Cardiovascular Disease Age-Adjusted Death Rates by State

Source: American Heart Association, *Heart Disease and Stroke Statistics—2003 Update* (Dallas, TX: American Heart Association, 2003). © 2003 American Heart Association. Reproduced by permission.

Today, nearly 61 million Americans live with one of the major categories of CVD. Many do not know they have a serious problem.[3] Nearly 13 million of them have a history of heart attack, angina pectoris (chest pain), or both.[4] In spite of major improvements in medication, surgery, and other health care procedures, the prognosis for many of these individuals is not good.[5]

- Twenty-five percent of women and 38 percent of men will die within one year after an initial heart attack.
- People who survive the acute stages of a heart attack have a chance of illness and death that is 1.5 to 15 times higher than that of the general population, depending on their sex and clinical outcomes. The risk of another heart attack, sudden death, angina pectoris, heart failure, or stroke is substantial.
- Within six years after a recognized heart attack, 18 percent of men and 35 percent of women will have another heart attack, 7 percent of men and 6 percent of women will experience sudden death, and about 22 percent of men and 46 percent of women will be disabled with heart failure. About two-thirds of heart attack patients won't make a complete recovery, but 88 percent of those under age 65 will be able to return to their usual work.
- CHD will permanently disable 19 percent of the U.S. labor force.

Although it is impossible to place a monetary value on human life, the economic burden of cardiovascular disease on our society is staggering— more than $351.8 billion estimated in 2003.[6] This figure includes the cost of physician and nursing services, hospital and nursing home services, medications, and lost productivity resulting from disability. By comparison, in 2002 the estimated cost of all cancers and their treatment was $202 billion. As Americans live longer, these numbers will continue to increase, which will result in a tremendous burden on the health care system. Some Americans think CVD can be cured with a bypass or other surgical procedure, after which life simply returns to normal. However, the effects of CVD can be far reaching and take a toll on quality of life.

The best line of defense against CVD is to prevent it from developing in the first place. How can you reduce your risk? Take steps now to change certain behaviors. For example, controlling high blood pressure and reducing intake of saturated fats and cholesterol are two things you can do to lower your chances of heart attack. You can lower your blood pressure by maintaining your weight, decreasing your intake of sodium, exercising, not smoking, and changing your lifestyle to reduce stress. You can also monitor the levels of fat and cholesterol in your blood and adjust your diet to prevent arteries from becoming clogged (see the Assess Yourself box on page 320).

Having combinations of risk factors seems to increase overall risk by a factor greater than those of the combined risks. Happily, the converse is also true: reducing several risk factors can have a dramatic effect. Understanding how your cardiovascular system works will help you understand your risks and how to reduce them.

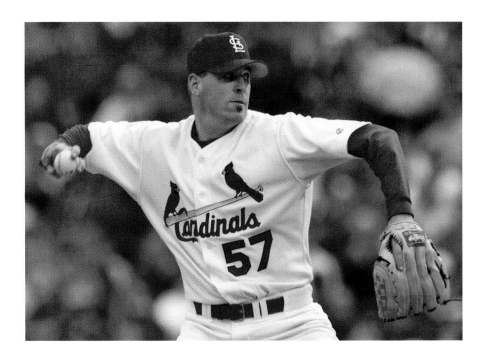

Cardiovascular disease can affect even the youngest and most fit people. Daryl Kile, a 33-year-old professional baseball player, died suddenly from atherosclerosis. It was discovered after his death that two of the main arteries in his heart were 80 to 90 percent blocked. His heart was also enlarged, weighing 20 percent more than normal.

What do you think?

Consider what happens when people who suffer a heart attack survive. ✳ *What unique challenges do they face?* ✳ *What difficulties might they encounter at home, at work, and in leisure time?* ✳ *What might it be like to live in fear that your heart might give out or a problem could crop up at any time?* ✳ *What support services are available for coping with the unique anxieties faced by CVD survivors and their families?*

Understanding the Cardiovascular System

The **cardiovascular system** is the network of elastic tubes through which blood flows as it carries oxygen and nutrients to all parts of the body. It includes the *heart, arteries, arterioles*

Cardiovascular system   A complex system consisting of the heart and blood vessels. It transports nutrients, oxygen, hormones, and enzymes throughout the body and regulates temperature, the water levels of cells, and the acidity levels of body components.

Atria   The two upper chambers of the heart that receive blood.

Ventricles   The two lower chambers of the heart that pump blood through the blood vessels.

(small arteries), and *capillaries* (minute blood vessels). It also includes *venules* (small veins) and *veins,* the blood vessels though which blood flows as it returns to the heart and lungs.

The Heart: A Mighty Machine

The heart is a muscular, four-chambered pump, roughly the size of your fist. It is a highly efficient, extremely flexible organ that manages to contract 100,000 times each day and pumps the equivalent of 2,000 gallons of blood to all areas of the body. In a 70-year lifetime, an average human heart beats 2.5 billion times. This number is significantly higher for hearts that must work to keep people moving who are out of shape and overweight.

Under normal circumstances, the human body contains approximately 6 quarts of blood. This blood transports nutrients, oxygen, waste products, hormones, and enzymes throughout the body. Blood also regulates body temperature, cellular water levels, and acidity levels of body components, and aids in bodily defense against toxins and harmful microorganisms. An adequate blood supply is essential to health and well-being.

The heart has four chambers that work together to recirculate blood constantly throughout the body (Figure 12.2). The two upper chambers of the heart, called **atria,** or *auricles,* are large collecting chambers that receive blood from the rest of the body. The two lower chambers, known as **ventricles,** pump the blood out again. Small valves regulate the steady, rhythmic flow of blood between chambers and prevent inappropriate backwash. The *tricuspid valve* (located between the right atrium and the right ventricle), the *pulmonary (pulmonic) valve* (between the right ventricle and the pulmonary artery), the *mitral valve* (between the left atrium and left ventricle),

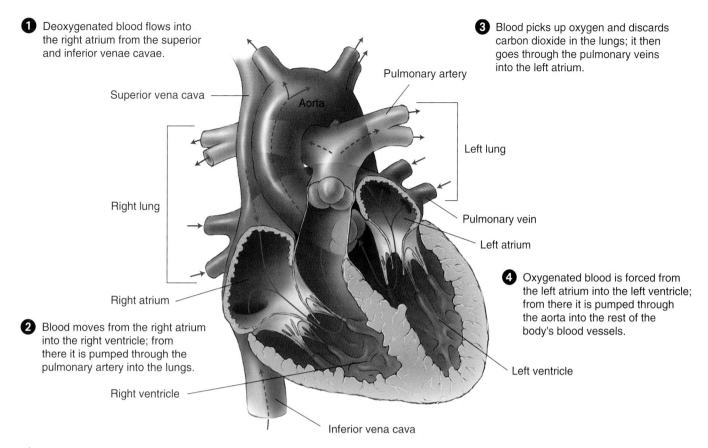

① Deoxygenated blood flows into the right atrium from the superior and inferior venae cavae.

③ Blood picks up oxygen and discards carbon dioxide in the lungs; it then goes through the pulmonary veins into the left atrium.

Pulmonary artery

Superior vena cava

Aorta

Left lung

Right lung

Pulmonary vein

Left atrium

Right atrium

④ Oxygenated blood is forced from the left atrium into the left ventricle; from there it is pumped through the aorta into the rest of the body's blood vessels.

② Blood moves from the right atrium into the right ventricle; from there it is pumped through the pulmonary artery into the lungs.

Right ventricle

Left ventricle

Inferior vena cava

Figure 12.2
Anatomy of the Heart

and the *aortic valve* (between the left ventricle and the aorta) permit blood to flow in only one direction.

Heart Function   Heart activity depends on a complex interaction of biochemical, physical, and neurological signals. Here are the basic steps involved in heart function.

1. Deoxygenated blood enters the right atrium after having been circulated through the body.
2. From the right atrium, blood moves to the right ventricle and is pumped through the pulmonary artery to the lungs, where it receives oxygen.
3. Oxygenated blood from the lungs then returns to the left atrium of the heart.
4. Blood from the left atrium is forced into the left ventricle.
5. The left ventricle pumps blood through the aorta to all body parts.

Different types of blood vessels are required for different parts of this process. **Arteries** carry blood away from the heart—except for pulmonary arteries, which carry deoxygenated blood to the lungs, where the blood picks up oxygen and gives off carbon dioxide. As they branch off from the heart, the arteries divide into smaller blood vessels called **arterioles,** and then into even smaller blood vessels called **capillaries.** Capillaries have thin walls that permit the exchange of oxygen, carbon dioxide, nutrients, and waste

products with body cells. The carbon dioxide and waste products are transported to the lungs and kidneys through **veins** and venules (small veins).

For the heart to function properly, the four chambers must beat in an organized manner. Your heartbeat is governed by an electrical impulse that directs the heart muscle to move when the impulse moves across it, which results in a sequential contraction of the four chambers. This signal starts in a small bundle of highly specialized cells, the **sinoatrial node (SA node),** located in the right atrium. The SA

(text continues on page 322)

Arteries   Vessels that carry blood away from the heart to other regions of the body.

Arterioles   Branches of the arteries.

Capillaries   Minute blood vessels that branch out from the arterioles; their thin walls allow for the exchange of oxygen, carbon dioxide, nutrients, and waste products among body cells.

Veins   Vessels that carry blood back to the heart from other regions of the body.

Sinoatrial node (SA node)   Node serving as a form of natural pacemaker for the heart.

Find Your Cholesterol Plan

The following two-step program will guide you through the National Cholesterol Education Program's new treatment guidelines. The first step helps you establish your overall coronary risk; the second uses that information to determine your low-density lipoprotein (LDL) treatment goals and how to reach them.

You'll need to know your blood pressure, your total LDL and high-density lipoprotein (HDL) cholesterol levels, and your triglyceride and fasting glucose levels. If you're not sure of those numbers, ask your doctor and, if necessary, schedule an exam to get them. (Everyone should have a complete lipid profile every 5 years, starting at age 20.)

STEP 1: TAKE THE HEART-ATTACK RISK TEST

This test will identify your chance of having a heart attack or dying of coronary disease in the next 10 years. (People with previously diagnosed coronary disease, diabetes, aortic aneurysm, or symptomatic carotid- or peripheral-artery disease already face more than a 20% risk; they can skip the test and go straight to Step 2.) The test uses data from the Framingham Heart Study, the world's longest-running study of cardiovascular risk factors. The test is limited to established, major factors that are measured easily.

Circle the point value for each of the risk factors shown at right and below.

AGE

Years	Women	Men
20–34	−7	−9
35–39	−3	−4
40–44	0	0
45–49	3	3
50–54	6	6
55–59	8	8
60–64	10	10
65–69	12	11
70–74	14	12
75–79	16	13

TOTAL CHOLESTEROL

Mg/dL	Age 20–39 Women	Age 20–39 Men	Age 40–49 Women	Age 40–49 Men	Age 50–59 Women	Age 50–59 Men	Age 60–69 Women	Age 60–69 Men	Age 70–79 Women	Age 70–79 Men
<160	0	0	0	0	0	0	0	0	0	0
160–199	4	4	3	3	2	2	1	1	1	0
200–239	8	7	6	5	4	3	2	1	1	0
240–279	11	9	8	6	5	4	3	2	2	1
280+	13	11	10	8	7	5	4	3	2	1

HIGH-DENSITY LIPOPROTEIN (HDL) CHOLESTEROL

Mg/dL	Women and Men
60+	−1
50–59	0
40–49	1
<40	2

SYSTOLIC BLOOD PRESSURE (THE HIGHER NUMBER)

Mm/Hg	Untreated Women	Untreated Men	Treated Women	Treated Men
<120	0	0	0	0
120–129	1	0	3	1
130–139	2	1	4	2
140–159	3	1	5	2
>159	4	2	6	3

SMOKING

Age 20–39 Women	Age 20–39 Men	Age 40–49 Women	Age 40–49 Men	Age 50–59 Women	Age 50–59 Men	Age 60–69 Women	Age 60–69 Men	Age 70–79 Women	Age 70–79 Men
9	8	7	5	4	3	2	1	1	1

TOTAL YOUR POINTS

Now find your total point score in the men's or women's column at right, then locate your 10-year risk in the far-right column.

Women's Score	Men's Score	Your 10-Year Risk
< 20	< 12	< 10%
20–22	12–15	10%–20%
> 22	> 15	> 20%

STEP 2: FIND YOUR LOW-DENSITY LIPOPROTEIN (LDL) TREATMENT PLAN

Consult the table below to learn how your overall coronary risk affects whether you need to lower your LDL cholesterol level and, if you do, by how much. First, locate your coronary risk in the left-hand column. (That's based on the 10-year heart-attack risk that you just calculated as well as your coronary risk factors and any heart-threatening diseases you may have.) Then look across that row to see whether you should make lifestyle changes and take cholesterol-lowering medication, based on your current LDL level.

Coronary-Risk Group	Start lifestyle changes if your LDL level is . . .[1]	Add drugs if your LDL level is . . .
Very High 1. Ten-year heart-attack or risk of 20% or more or 2. history of coronary heart disease, diabetes, peripheral-artery disease, carotid-artery disease, or aortic aneurysm.	100 mg/dL or higher. (Aim for an LDL under 100.) Get retested after three months.	130 or higher. (Drugs are optional if your LDL is between 100 and 130.)
High 1. Ten-year heart-attack risk of 10% to 20% and 2. two or more major coronary risk factors.[2]	130 or higher. (Aim for an LDL under 130.) Get retested after three months.	130 or higher, and lifestyle changes don't achieve your LDL goal in three months.
Moderately High 1. Ten-year heart-attack risk under 10% and 2. two or more major coronary risk factors.[2]	Same as above.	160 or higher, and lifestyle changes don't achieve your LDL goal in three months.[3]
Low to Moderate 1. One or no major coronary risk factors.[2, 4]	160 or higher. (Aim for an LDL under 160.) Get retested after three months.	190 or higher, and lifestyle changes don't achieve your LDL goal in three months. (Drugs are optional if your LDL is between 160 and 189.)

1. People who have the metabolic syndrome should make lifestyle changes, even if their LDL level alone doesn't warrant it. You have the metabolic syndrome if you have three or more of these risk factors: HDL under 40 in men, 50 in women; systolic blood pressure of 130 or more or diastolic pressure of 85 or more; fasting glucose level of 110–125; triglyceride level of 150 or more; and waist circumference over 40 inches in men, 35 inches in women. People with the syndrome should limit their carbohydrate intake, get up to 30–35% of their calories from total fat (more than usually recommended), and make the other lifestyle changes, including restriction of saturated fat.

2. The major coronary risk factors are cigarette smoking; coronary disease in a father or brother before age 55 or a mother or sister before age 65; systolic blood pressure of 140 or more, a diastolic pressure of 90 or more, or being on drugs for hypertension; and an HDL level under 40. If your HDL is 60 or more, subtract one risk factor. (High LDL is a major factor, of course, but it's already figured into the table.)
3. While the goal is to get LDL under 130, the use of drugs in these people usually isn't worthwhile, even if lifestyle steps fail to achieve that goal.
4. People in this group usually have less than 10% 10-year risk. Those who have higher risk should ask their doctor whether they need more aggressive treatment than shown here.

node serves as a natural pacemaker for the heart.[7] People with a damaged SA node must often have a mechanical pacemaker implanted to ensure the smooth passage of blood through the sequential phases of the heartbeat.

The average adult heart at rest beats 70 to 80 times per minute, although a well-conditioned heart may beat only 50 to 60 times per minute to achieve the same results. When overly stressed, a heart may beat more than 200 times per minute, particularly in an individual who is overweight or out of shape. A healthy heart functions more efficiently and is less likely to suffer damage from overwork.

Types of Cardiovascular Disease

There are several different types of cardiovascular disease:

* Atherosclerosis (fatty plaque buildup in the arteries)
* Coronary heart disease (CHD)
* Chest pain (angina pectoris)
* Irregular heartbeat (arrhythmia)
* Congestive heart failure (CHF)
* Congenital and rheumatic heart disease
* Stroke (cerebrovascular accident)

Prevention and treatment of these diseases range from changes in diet and lifestyle to medications and surgery.

Atherosclerosis

Arteriosclerosis is a general term for thickening and hardening of the arteries, a condition that underlies many cardiovascular health problems. **Atherosclerosis** is actually a type of arteriosclerosis and is characterized by deposits of fatty substances, cholesterol, cellular waste products, calcium, and *fibrin* (a clotting material in the blood) in the inner lining of the artery. The resulting buildup is referred to as **plaque.**[8] Often, atherosclerosis is called *coronary artery disease* because of the resultant damage to coronary arteries.

Atherosclerotic plaque appears primarily in large and medium-sized arteries and can block blood flow to the heart, brain, or extremities. Plaque may be present throughout a person's lifetime; the earliest formation, known as a fatty streak, is fairly common in infants and young children.[9]

Arteriosclerosis A general term for thickening and hardening of the arteries.

Atherosclerosis Condition characterized by deposits of fatty substances, cholesterol, cellular waste products, calcium, and fibrin in the inner lining of an artery.

Plaque Buildup of deposits in the arteries.

Early Theories Initially, it was thought that plaque developed in response to injury and tended to collect at sites of injury. Many scientists believed that the process of plaque buildup begins when the protective inner lining of the artery *(endothelium)* becomes damaged, and fats, cholesterol, and other substances in the blood aggregate in these damaged areas. High blood pressure surges, elevated cholesterol and triglyceride levels in the blood, and cigarette smoking were the main suspects in causing this injury to artery walls. As a result of national campaigns aimed at reducing dietary fats, millions of people cut down on animal fat and dairy products. However, despite massive lifestyle changes and the use of cholesterol-lowering drugs, CVDs continue to be the leading cause of death in the United States, Europe, and most of Asia.[10]

Inflammatory Risks Today, scientists are beginning to view the formation of atherosclerotic lesions in a new way, with a vastly expanded list of possible causes. Many experts believe that atherosclerosis is an *inflammatory* disease, with numerous factors contributing to plaque formation.[11] Among these culprits are elevated and modified levels of low-density lipoprotein (LDL), free radicals caused by cigarette smoking, high blood pressure, diabetes mellitus, certain infectious microorganisms, and a combination of these and other factors.[12] The bottom line is that although elevated cholesterol levels continue to be significant in approximately 50 percent of patients with CVD,[13] other factors also need to be considered, particularly those that inflame and injure the interior of artery walls.[14] See the New Horizons in Health box for more on recent research into the role of inflammation in CVD.

Syndrome X, or Metabolic Syndrome According to Gerald Reaven, an endocrinologist at Stanford University, and other researchers, when people consume too many calories, particularly carbohydrates, their bodies eventually become insulin resistant. This means that their cells resist (or don't work properly in) handling blood glucose levels. Consequently, insulin and blood sugar levels remain high over time. Reaven describes how these dynamics can cause a cluster of metabolic problems that raise the risk of heart disease.[15]

Further research into metabolic syndrome has led to the conclusion that risk factors for the syndrome are, in addition to glucose intolerance, obesity with excess fat centered in the abdomen, high blood pressure, high levels of triglycerides, and low levels of high-density lipoprotein (HDL, the "good" cholesterol). Those people who have metabolic syndrome are at increased risk of CVD, and their condition should be monitored closely by their health care provider. It is particularly important for them to lose excess weight and manage their glucose levels.[16]

Coronary Heart Disease

Of all the major cardiovascular diseases, CHD is the greatest killer. In fact, this year well more than 1.1 million people

New Factors in CVD Risk: C-Reactive Proteins and Homocysteine

Is it time to forget the cholesterol and fat in your diet altogether and focus on other risks? Probably not. However, researchers are investigating new factors that may contribute to CVD risk as much as that juicy steak or high-fat ice cream.

A growing number of studies have examined inflammation in the walls of your blood vessels as a possible contributor to heart attacks and strokes. (This inflammation is implicated in atherosclerosis, the process in which fatty deposits build up in the lining of the arteries.) Pathogens such as the herpes simplex virus and the *Helicobacter pylori* and Chlamydia bacteria are among the agents that may cause such an inflammatory reaction. *C-Reactive Protein (CRP)* is a protein that increases when the body is subjected to inflammation from some form of attack. We may be able to predict who might be at risk for CVD based on tests that measure the presence of CRP when it appears in connection with this inflammatory response.

A high sensitivity assay for CRP (hs-CRP test) is already widely available. According to a joint statement by the Centers for Disease Control and Prevention and the American Heart Association, there appears to be solid evidence that the higher your hs-CRP levels, the higher your risk of having a heart attack and the lower your survival rate after a heart attack. Further research indicates that if you have high levels of hs-CRP *and* elevated LDL cholesterol levels, your risk may be increased. In fact, some studies indicate that CRP may be a greater risk than elevated LDL cholesterol. However, these studies do not have adequate controls and are not population-based, so results must be considered inconclusive and the true association between hs-CRP and new cardiovascular events not yet firmly established. Generally, these professional organizations advise that the test is probably not necessary if your other risk factors for CVD are small, but that it might be a good idea if you have several risk factors. Although not yet firmly established, the consensus is that an hs-CRP level lower than 1.0 mg/L is a low risk, an hs-CRP level of 1–3.0 mg/L is an average risk, and if your hs-CRP level is 3.0 mg/L or higher, you may have a high risk.

Another substance that has been implicated in increased risk for CVD is *homocysteine*, an amino acid normally present in the blood. Some studies have indicated that high levels of homocysteine may be related to higher risk of coronary heart disease, stroke, and peripheral vascular disease. In fact, it is theorized that homocysteine may work in much the same way as CRP by inflaming the inner lining of arteries and promoting fat deposits on the damaged walls and development of blood clots. However, a causal link has not been established between homocysteine and CVD.

Folic acid and other B vitamins such as B_6 and B_{12} help break down homocysteine in the body, so many have jumped on the folic acid bandwagon as a preemptive action against CVD risk. Because conclusive evidence of risk reduction from folic acid is not available, authorities such as the American Heart Association do not recommend taking folic acid supplements. A healthy, balanced diet that includes at least 5 servings of fruits and vegetables a day is the best preventive action for now. Citrus fruits, tomatoes, vegetables, and grain products that are fortified with folic acid are good sources of the recommended 400 micrograms.

Sources: American Heart Association, "Inflammation, Heart, Disease, and Stroke: The Role of C-Reactive Protein" and "Homocysteine, Folic Acid, and Cardiovascular Disease," 2003. www.americanheart.org; P. Ridker et al., "Comparison of C-Reactive Protein and Low-Density Lipoprotein Cholesterol Levels in Prediction of First Cardiovascular Events," *The New England Journal of Medicine* 347, no. 20 (2002): 1557–1565; D. M. Lloyd-Jones et al., "C-Reactive Protein in the Prediction of Cardiovascular Events," *The New England Journal of Medicine* 348, no. 11 (2003): 1059–1061.

will suffer from a heart attack, and more than 40 percent of them will die.[17] Those of you raised on a weekly dose of TV doctor programs will recognize *Code Blue* as the term for a **myocardial infarction (MI),** or **heart attack.** A heart attack involves an area of the heart that suffers permanent damage because its normal blood supply has been interrupted. This condition is often brought on by a **coronary thrombosis,** or blood clot in a coronary artery, or through an atherosclerotic narrowing that blocks an artery. When blood does not flow readily, there is a corresponding decrease in oxygen flow. If the heart blockage is extremely minor, an otherwise healthy heart will adapt over time by utilizing small blood vessels to reroute blood through other areas. This

Myocardial infarction (MI) Heart attack.

Heart attack A blockage of normal blood supply to an area in the heart.

Coronary thrombosis A blood clot occurring in a coronary artery.

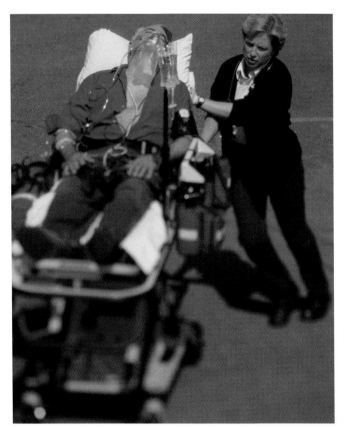

Forty percent of heart attack victims die within the first hour, so immediate treatment is vital to the patient's survival.

What do you think?

What risk factors might typical college-age students have for plaque formation? ✳ What information should new CVD prevention guidelines include if the new theories discussed in this section prove true?

Angina Pectoris

Atherosclerosis and other circulatory impairments often reduce the heart's oxygen supply, a condition known as **ischemia.** People with ischemia often suffer from varying degrees of **angina pectoris,** or chest pain. In fact, an estimated 2.5 million men and 4.1 million women suffer mild to crushing forms of chest pain each day.[18] Many people experience short episodes of angina whenever they exert themselves physically. Symptoms range from a slight feeling of indigestion to a feeling that the heart is being crushed. Generally, the more serious the oxygen deprivation, the more severe the pain. Although angina pectoris is not a heart attack, it does indicate underlying heart disease.

Currently, there are several methods of treating angina. In mild cases, rest is critical. The most common treatments for more severe cases are drugs that affect (1) the supply of blood to the heart muscle or (2) the heart's demand for oxygen. Pain and discomfort are often relieved with *nitroglycerin,* a drug used to relax (dilate) veins, which thereby reduces the amount of blood returning to the heart and lessens its workload. Patients whose angina is caused by spasms of the coronary arteries often take *calcium channel blockers,* drugs that prevent calcium atoms from passing through coronary arteries and causing heart contractions. They also appear to reduce blood pressure and slow heart rates. *Beta blockers,* the other major type of drugs used to treat angina, control potential overactivity of the heart muscle.

Arrhythmias

Over 4 million Americans experience some type of **arrhythmia,** an irregularity in heart rhythm.[19] A person who complains of a racing heart in the absence of exercise or anxiety may be experiencing *tachycardia,* the medical term for abnormally fast heartbeat. On the other end of the continuum is *bradycardia,* or abnormally slow heartbeat. When a heart goes into **fibrillation,** it beats in a sporadic, quivering pattern that results in extreme inefficiency in moving blood through the cardiovascular system. If untreated, fibrillation may be fatal.

Not all arrhythmias are life threatening. In many instances, excessive caffeine or nicotine consumption can trigger an arrhythmia episode. However, severe cases may require drug therapy or external electrical stimulus to prevent serious complications.

system, known as **collateral circulation,** is a form of self-preservation that allows an affected heart muscle to cope with the damage.

When heart blockage is more severe, however, the body is unable to adapt on its own, and outside lifesaving support is critical. The hour following a heart attack is the most crucial period—more than 40 percent of heart attack victims die within this time. These sudden deaths are caused by cardiac arrest that usually results from *ventricular fibrillation,* or irregular, inefficient heartbeats.

Collateral circulation Adaptation of the heart to partial damage accomplished by rerouting needed blood through unused or underused blood vessels while the damaged heart muscle heals.

Ischemia Reduced oxygen supply to the heart.

Angina pectoris Chest pain occurring as a result of reduced oxygen flow to the heart.

Arrhythmia An irregularity in heartbeat.

Fibrillation A sporadic, quivering pattern of heartbeat that results in extreme inefficiency in moving blood through the cardiovascular system.

Congestive Heart Failure

When the heart muscle is damaged or overworked and lacks the strength to keep blood circulating normally through the body, its chambers are often taxed to the limit. **Congestive heart failure (CHF)** affects more than 5 million Americans and dramatically increases risk of premature death.[20] The heart muscle may be injured by a number of health conditions, including rheumatic fever, pneumonia, heart attack, or other cardiovascular problems. In some cases, the damage is due to radiation or chemotherapy treatments for cancer. These weakened muscles respond poorly, which impairs blood flow out of the heart through the arteries. The return flow of blood through the veins begins to back up, which causes congestion in body tissues. This pooling of blood enlarges the heart and decreases the amount of blood that can be circulated. Fluid begins to accumulate in other body areas, such as the vessels in the legs and ankles or the lungs, which causes swelling or difficulty in breathing. Today, CHF is the single most frequent cause of hospitalization in the United States.[21] If untreated, congestive heart failure can be fatal. However, most cases respond well to treatment that includes *diuretics* (water pills) to relieve fluid accumulation; drugs, such as *digitalis,* that increase the pumping action of the heart; and drugs called *vasodilators* that expand blood vessels and decrease resistance, which allows blood to flow more easily and makes the heart's work easier.

Congenital and Rheumatic Heart Disease

Approximately 1 out of every 125 children is born with some form of **congenital heart disease** (disease present at birth). These forms may be relatively minor, such as slight *murmurs* (low-pitched sounds caused by turbulent blood flow through the heart) that result from valve irregularities, which some children outgrow. Other congenital problems involve serious complications in heart function that can be corrected only with surgery. Their underlying causes are unknown but may be related to hereditary factors; maternal diseases, such as rubella, that occur during fetal development; or chemical intake (particularly alcohol) by the mother during pregnancy. Because of advances in pediatric cardiology, the prognosis for children with congenital heart defects is better than ever.

Rheumatic heart disease can cause similar heart problems in children. It is attributed to rheumatic fever, an inflammatory disease that may affect many connective tissues of the body, especially those of the heart, joints, brain, or skin, and is caused by an unresolved *streptococcal infection* of the throat (strep throat). In a small number of cases, this infection can lead to an immune response in which antibodies attack the heart as well as the bacteria. Many of the 96,000 annual operations on heart valves in the United States are related to rheumatic heart disease.[22]

Stroke

Like heart muscle, brain cells must have a continuous adequate supply of oxygen in order to survive. A **stroke** (also called a *cerebrovascular accident*) occurs when the blood supply to the brain is interrupted. Strokes may be caused by a **thrombus** (a clot in a blood vessel), an **embolus** (a clot that is floating in the bloodstream), or an **aneurysm** (a weakening in a blood vessel that causes it to bulge and, in severe cases, burst). Figure 12.3 illustrates these blood vessel disorders. When any of these events occur, oxygen deprivation kills brain cells, which do not have the capacity to heal or regenerate. Some strokes are mild and cause only temporary dizziness or slight weakness or numbness. More serious interruptions in blood flow may cause speech impairments, memory problems, and loss of motor control.

Other strokes affect parts of the brain that regulate heart and lung function and kill within minutes. Stroke killed 167,661 Americans in 2003 and accounted for 1 in 14.5 of our total deaths, surpassed only by CHD and cancer.[23] Each year, about 700,000 people experience new or recurrent stroke, which averages out to one person suffering a stroke every 45 seconds, and one person dying as a result of a stroke every 3.3 minutes.[24] Each year, about 40,000 more women than men have a stroke, largely because women's average life expectancy is greater than men's.

About one in ten major strokes is preceded (days, weeks, or months before) by **transient ischemic attacks (TIAs),** brief interruptions of the blood supply to the brain that cause only

---

Congestive heart failure (CHF)   An abnormal cardiovascular condition that reflects impaired cardiac pumping and blood flow; pooling blood leads to congestion in body tissues.

Congenital heart disease   Heart disease that is present at birth.

Rheumatic heart disease   A heart disease caused by untreated streptococcal infection of the throat.

Stroke   A condition occurring when the brain is damaged by disrupted blood supply.

Thrombus   Clot in a blood vessel.

Embolus   Clot that is forced through the circulatory system.

Aneurysm   A weakened blood vessel that may bulge under pressure and, in severe cases, burst.

Transient ischemic attack (TIA)   Brief interruption of the blood supply to the brain that causes only temporary impairment; often an indicator of impending major stroke.

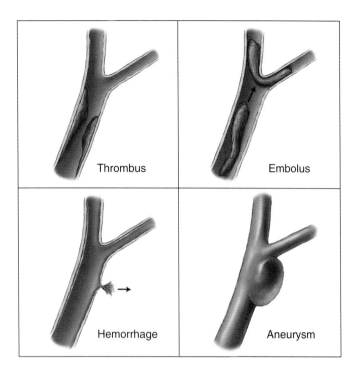

Figure 12.3
Common Blood Vessel Disorders

temporary impairment. TIAs are often indications of an impending stroke. Warning signs of stroke include:

- Sudden weakness or numbness of the face, arm, or leg on one side of the body
- Sudden dimness or loss of vision, particularly in only one eye
- Loss of speech, or trouble talking or understanding speech
- Sudden, severe headaches with no known cause
- Unexplained dizziness, unsteadiness, or sudden falls, especially with any of the previously listed symptoms

If you experience any of these symptoms, or if you are with someone who does, seek medical help immediately. The earlier treatment starts, the more effective it will be.

One of the greatest medical successes in recent years has been the decline in fatality rates from strokes, a rate that has dropped by one-third in the United States since the 1980s and continues to fall. Improved diagnostic procedures, better surgical options, clot-busting drugs injected soon after a stroke has occurred, and acute care centers specializing in stroke treatment and rehabilitation have all been factors. Increased awareness of risk factors for stroke, especially high blood pressure, and an emphasis on prevention have also helped. It is estimated that more than half of all remaining strokes could be avoided if more people followed the recommended preventive standards.

Reducing Your Risk for Cardiovascular Diseases

Factors that increase the risk for cardiovascular problems fall into two categories: those we can control and those we cannot. Fortunately, we can take steps to minimize many risk factors.

Risks You Can Control

Avoid Tobacco   As early as 1984, the Surgeon General of the United States asserted that smoking was the greatest risk factor for heart disease. Today, one in five deaths from CVD is directly related to smoking.[25] Generally, the more a person smokes, the greater the risk for heart attack or stroke. The risk for CVD is 70 percent greater for smokers than for nonsmokers. Smokers who have a heart attack are more likely to die suddenly (within one hour) than are nonsmokers. Evidence also indicates that chronic exposure to environmental tobacco smoke (passive smoking) increases the risk of heart disease by as much as 30 percent. About 35,000 nonsmokers die each year from heart disease that resulted from exposure to environmental smoke.[26]

How does smoking damage the heart? There are two plausible explanations. One theory states that nicotine increases heart rate, heart output, blood pressure, and oxygen use by heart muscles. Because the carbon monoxide in cigarette smoke displaces oxygen in heart tissue, the heart is forced to work harder to obtain sufficient oxygen. The other theory states that chemicals in smoke damage the lining of the coronary arteries, which allows cholesterol and plaque to accumulate more easily. This additional buildup constricts the vessels, which increases blood pressure and causes the heart to work harder.

When people stop smoking, regardless of how long or how much they've smoked, their risk of heart disease declines rapidly.[27] Three years after quitting, the risk of death from heart disease and stroke for people who smoked a pack a day or less is almost the same as for people who never smoked. Quitting today will also raise your HDL levels, which reduces your risks even further (see the next section).[28]

Cut Back on Saturated Fats and Cholesterol   How concerned should you be about the amount of fat and cholesterol in your diet? Very concerned. In fact, according to recent evidence, cholesterol risks may be greater than ever for Americans. When dietary experts from the National Heart, Lung and Blood Institute (NHLBI) met recently to prepare their *Third Report on Detection, Evaluation, and Treatment of Cholesterol National Guidelines,* they gave Americans a wake-up call by drastically reducing the levels of cholesterol that are considered acceptable. These guidelines not only show that cholesterol levels are out of control in the United States, but also indicate that the numbers of people needing cholesterol-cutting drugs may be three times what we originally thought. In fact, nearly 36 million people in the United States—one-fifth of all adults—may require medications to avoid cardiovascular problems.[29]

Why all of the fuss about fats and cholesterol? Diets high in saturated fats are known to raise cholesterol levels, send the body's blood-clotting system into high gear, and make the blood more viscous in just a few hours, which increases the risk of heart attacks or stroke. Studies indicate that fatty foods apparently trigger production of *factor VII*, a blood-clotting substance. Switching to a low-fat diet greatly reduces the risk of clotting.

A fatty diet also increases the amount of cholesterol in the blood, which contributes to atherosclerosis. In past years, cholesterol levels between 200 to 240 milligrams per 100 milliliters of blood (mg/dL) were considered normal. Recent research indicates that levels between 180 and 200 mg/dL are more desirable and that 150 mg/dL levels would be even better to reduce CVD risks.[30] See Table 12.1.

However, it isn't just the total cholesterol level that you should be concerned about. Cholesterol comes in two main varieties: **low-density lipoprotein (LDL)** and **high-density lipoprotein (HDL).** LDL, often referred to as "bad" cholesterol, is believed to build up on artery walls. In contrast, HDL, or "good" cholesterol, appears to remove cholesterol from artery walls and thus serves as a protector. In theory, if LDL levels get too high or HDL levels too low, largely because of too much saturated fat in the diet, a lack of physical exercise, high stress levels, or genetic predisposition, cholesterol will accumulate inside arteries and lead to cardiovascular problems. Scientists now believe that other factors also may increase CVD risk. A component of HDL known as apo A-II may be the most important element of the HDL makeup. The more a person has of this protective protein, the lower the risk for CVD seems to be.[31]

The goal is to control the ratio of HDL to total cholesterol by lowering LDL levels, raising HDL, or both. Regular exercise and a healthy diet low in saturated fat continue to be the best methods for maintaining healthy ratios. However, if dietary efforts and exercise do not reduce total cholesterol or LDL, several medications are available that may help.

Triglycerides, another type of fat in the blood, also appears to promote clogged arteries. As people get older, heavier, or both, their triglyceride and cholesterol levels tend to rise. Although some CVD patients have elevated triglyceride levels, a causal link between high triglyceride levels and CVD has yet to be established. It may be that high triglyceride levels do not directly cause atherosclerosis but, rather, are among the abnormalities that speed its development.

Current guidelines suggest that you should reduce intake of saturated fat (obtained mostly from animal products) to *less than 7 percent of your total daily caloric expenditures* and minimize your consumption of *trans*-fat (see Chapter 9) found in partially hydrogenated products such as margarine, many fast foods, and many packaged foods. By cutting your intake of saturated fats and *trans*-fats, experts from the NHLBI believe that you can reduce your LDL levels by as

much as 10 percent.[32] In addition, NHLBI experts indicate that you should consume fewer than 200 mg per day of cholesterol, which is found mainly in eggs and meat. Doing so may result in reductions in LDL by as much as 5 percent.[33]

While it is wise to cut back on saturated fat, be aware that some fat is necessary to overall health. Ironically, the consumption of too many low-fat or fat-free foods, such as salad dressings and other products, may actually contribute to the escalating problem of obesity in America. According to top researchers, it is better to eat foods with olive oil, canola oil, and other monounsaturated fats than to consume

---

Table 12.1
Classification of LDL, Total, and HDL Cholesterol (mg/dL) and Recommended Levels for Adults

LDL Cholesterol

<100	Optimal
100–129	Near optimal/above optimal
130–159	Borderline high
160–189	High
≥190	Very high

Total Cholesterol

<200	Desirable
200–239	Borderline high
≥240	High

HDL Cholesterol

<40	Low
≥60	High

Triglycerides

<150	Normal
150–199	Borderline high
200–499	High
≥500	Very high

Source: National Heart, Lung, and Blood Institute, *Detection, Evaluation, and Treatment of High Blood Cholesterol in Adults* (NIH Publication No. 02-5215), 2002. www.nhlbi.nih.gov/guidelines/cholesterol/atp3_rpt.htm

---

Low-density lipoproteins (LDLs) Compounds that facilitate the transport of cholesterol in the blood to the body's cells.

High-density lipoproteins (HDLs) Compounds that facilitate the transport of cholesterol in the blood to the liver for metabolism and elimination from the body.

Triglycerides The most common form of fat in the body; excess calories are converted into fat and stored as body fat.

low-fat or no-fat products. (For a complete discussion of this topic, see Chapter 9.) Of course, all fat intake should be in moderation.

Monitor Your Cholesterol Levels   In order to get an accurate assessment of your total cholesterol and LDL and HDL levels, you should have a *lipoprotein analysis*. This analysis requires that you not eat or drink anything for 12 hours prior to the test and that a reputable health care provider do the analysis. The LDL level is derived using a standard formula:

$$LDL = total\ cholesterol - HDL - (triglycerides \div 5)$$

For example, if the level of total cholesterol is 200, the level of HDL 45, and the level of triglycerides 150, the LDL level would be 125 ($200 - 45 - 30$).

In general, LDL is more closely associated with cardiovascular risks than is total cholesterol. However, most authorities agree that looking only at LDLs ignores the positive effects of HDL. Perhaps the best method of evaluating risk is to examine the *ratio* of HDL to total cholesterol or the percentage of HDL in total cholesterol. If the percentage of HDL is less than 35, the risk increases dramatically.

Change Lifestyle to Reduce Your Risk   Of the more than 100 million Americans who need to worry about their cholesterol levels, almost half, particularly those at the low to moderate risk levels, should be able to reach their LDL and HDL goals though lifestyle changes alone. People who are at higher risk or those for whom lifestyle modifications make no difference may need to take cholesterol-lowering drugs while they continue modifying their lifestyle.

Maintain a Healthy Weight   No question about it—body weight plays a role in CVD. Researchers are not certain whether high-fat, high-sugar, high-calorie diets are a direct risk for CVD or whether they invite risk by causing obesity, which strains the heart and forces it to push blood through the many miles of capillaries that supply each pound of fat. A heart that has to continuously move blood through an overabundance of vessels may become damaged. People who are overweight are more likely to develop heart disease and stroke even if they have no other risk factors. If you're overweight, losing even 5 to 10 pounds can make a significant difference of as much as 5 percent LDL reduction,[34] especially if you're an "apple" (thicker around your upper body and waist) rather than a "pear" (thicker around your hips and thighs). Your waist measurement divided by your hip measurement should be less than 0.9 (for men) and less than 0.8 (for women). (See Chapter 10 on weight control).[35]

Modify Other Dietary Habits   The NHLBI guidelines recommend the following dietary modifications to reduce CVD risk.

- Consume 5 to 10 mg per day of *soluble fiber* from sources such as fruits, vegetables, oat bran, and legumes. (See Chapter 9.) Even this small dietary modification may result in another 5 percent drop in LDL levels.
- Consume about 2 grams per day of *plant sterols* or sterol derivatives from substances such as Benecol or Take Control margarine. These are the first widely available sources of sterols, but more will be on the market soon. This has the potential to reduce LDL by another 5 percent.
- Although less widely supported by rigorous research findings, many experts believe that consuming at least 25 grams of soy protein from various soy foods, instead of dairy sources, could reduce LDL by 5 percent.

Exercise Regularly   According to all available evidence, inactivity is a definite risk factor for CVD.[36] The good news is that you do not have to be an exercise fanatic to reduce your risk. Even modest levels of low-intensity physical activity—walking, gardening, housework, dancing—are beneficial if done regularly and over the long term. Exercise can increase HDL, lower triglycerides, and reduce coronary risk in several ways. For more information, see Chapter 11.

Making the above modifications could reduce LDL levels by as much as 35 percent. This reduction is similar to the reduction one could expect to achieve by taking any of the statin drugs typically prescribed.

Control Diabetes   The NHLBI guidelines underscore the unique difficulties and risks of CVD for people with diabetes. Diabetics who have taken insulin for a number of years have a greater chance of developing CVD. In fact, CVD is the leading cause of death among diabetic patients. Because overweight people have a higher risk for diabetes, distinguishing between the effects of the two conditions is difficult. Diabetics also tend to have elevated blood fat levels, increased atherosclerosis, and a tendency toward deterioration of small blood vessels, particularly in the eyes and extremities. However, through a prescribed regimen of diet, exercise, and medication, diabetics can control much of their increased risk for CVD (see Chapter 14).

Control Your Blood Pressure   **Hypertension** refers to sustained high blood pressure. If it cannot be attributed to any specific cause, it is known as **essential hypertension.** Approximately 90 percent of all cases of hypertension fit this category. **Secondary hypertension** refers to hypertension caused by specific factors, such as kidney disease, obesity, or tumors of the adrenal glands. In general, the higher your blood pressure, the greater your risk for CVD.

Hypertension   Sustained elevated blood pressure.

Essential hypertension   Hypertension that cannot be attributed to any cause.

Secondary hypertension   Hypertension caused by specific factors, such as kidney disease, obesity, or tumors of the adrenal glands.

Hypertension is known as the "silent killer" because it usually has no symptoms. Although it affects one in four adult Americans, 31.6 percent of them don't know they have the condition, and only one-third of those who are aware of it have it under control.[37] Common forms of treatment are dietary changes (reducing salt and calorie intake), weight loss (when appropriate), diuretics and other medications (only when prescribed by a physician), regular exercise, and the practice of relaxation techniques and effective coping and communication skills.

Blood pressure is measured in two parts and is expressed as a fraction—for example, 110/80, or 110 over 80. Both values are measured in *millimeters of mercury* (mm Hg). The first number refers to **systolic pressure,** the pressure being applied to the walls of the arteries when the heart contracts and pumps blood to the rest of the body. The second value is **diastolic pressure,** the pressure applied to the walls of the arteries during the heart's relaxation phase. During this phase, blood is reentering the chambers of the heart, which is preparing for the next heartbeat.

Normal blood pressure varies depending on weight, age, and physical condition. It also varies for different groups of people, such as women and minorities. As a rule, men have a greater risk for high blood pressure than women have until age 55, when their risks become about equal. At age 75 and over, women are more likely to have high blood pressure than are men.[38] If your blood pressure exceeds 140 over 90, you need to take steps to lower it. See Table 12.2 for a summary of blood pressure classifications.

Manage Stress   Some scientists have noted a relationship between CVD risk and a person's stress level, behavior habits, and socioeconomic status. These factors may affect established risk factors. For example, people under stress may start smoking or smoke more than they otherwise would.[39] Other studies have challenged the apparent link between emotional stress and heart disease. Although it was once widely assumed that the Type A personality, who suffers from high stress levels, was a time bomb ticking toward a heart attack, this theory has not been proven clinically.

Researcher–physician Robert S. Eliot demonstrated that approximately one of five people has an extreme cardiovascular reaction to stressful stimulation. These people experience alarm and resistance so strongly that when they are under stress, their bodies produce large amounts of stress chemicals. The chemicals, in turn, cause tremendous changes in the cardiovascular system, including remarkable increases in blood pressure. These people are called *hot reactors.* Although their blood pressure may be normal when they are not under stress, it increases dramatically in response to even small amounts of everyday stress.

Cold reactors are those who are able to experience stress (even to live as Type A personalities) without showing harmful cardiovascular responses. Cold reactors may internalize stress, but their self-talk and perceptions about the

Table 12.2
Blood Pressure Classifications

Classification	Systolic Reading (mm Hg)		Diastolic Reading (mm Hg)
Normal	<120	and	<80
Prehypertension	120–139	or	80–89
Stage 1 Hypertension	140–159	or	90–99
Stage 2 Hypertension	≥160	or	or≥100

Note: If systolic and diastolic readings fall into different categories, treatment is determined by the highest category. Readings are based on the average of 2 or more properly measured, seated readings on each of 2 or more health care provider visits.
Source: National Heart, Blood, and Lung Institute, *The Seventh Report of the Joint National Committee on Prevention, Detection, Evaluation, and Treatment of High Blood Pressure* (NIH Publication No. 03-5233) (Bethesda, MD: National Institutes of Health, May 2003).

stressful events lead them to a nonresponse state in which their cardiovascular system remains virtually unaffected.[40] Some research indicates that people who have an underlying predisposition toward a toxic core personality (in other words, who are chronically hostile and hateful) may be at greatest risk for a CVD event. A recent study funded by the NHLBI found that impatience and hostility, two key components of the Type A behavior pattern, increase young adults' risk of developing high blood pressure. Other related factors, such as competitiveness, depression, and anxiety, did not appear to increase risk. The research was the first to study these factors as a group, rather than individually and has clear implications for prevention.[41]

What do you think?
What is your resting heart rate? You can find out by taking your pulse. Gently press the pads of your first two fingers against the inside of your wrist, just below the base of your thumb. Sit quietly, and count the number of beats that occur during a 10-second period. Multiply the number of beats by 6. Repeat the process. ✱ *How does your heart rate compare to that of your friends?*

Systolic pressure   The upper number in the fraction that measures blood pressure; it indicates pressure on the walls of the arteries when the heart contracts.

Diastolic pressure   The lower number in the fraction that measures blood pressure; it indicates pressure on the walls of the arteries during the relaxation phase of heart activity.

Disparity in CVD Risk

Cardiovascular disease is not an equal opportunity disease. In fact, when it comes to risk of attack and eventual mortality, there are huge disparities based on gender, race, and age. Consider the following.

- African American and Mexican American women have a higher risk of CVD than do white women of comparable socioeconomic status (SES). The striking differences by both ethnicity and SES underscore the critical need to improve screening, early detection, and treatment of CVD-related conditions for African American and Mexican American women, as well as for women of lower SES in all ethnic groups.
- Among American Indians/Alaskan Natives age 18 and older, 63.7% of men and 61.4% of women have one or more CVD risk factors (hypertension, current cigarette smoking, high blood cholesterol, obesity, or diabetes). If data on physical activity had been included in this analysis, the prevalence of risk factors would have been much higher.
- In 2002, the prevalence of CVD was 30% for white males and 40.5% for African American males (more than 10% higher) at all ages and stages of

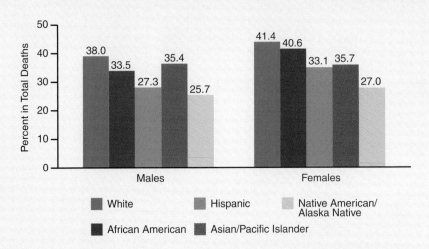

Deaths from Cardiovascular Disease in the United States: 2000 Final Data
Source: American Heart Association, *Heart Disease and Stroke Statistics—2003 Update.* (Dallas, TX: American Heart Association, 2003). © American Heart Association.

life. The rate for Mexican Americans was 28.8%.
- In 2002, the prevalence of CVD was 23.8% for white females, 39.6% for African American females, and 26.6% for Mexican American females.
- African Americans are 60% more likely to suffer a stroke than are whites, and two and one half times more likely to die from a stroke.
- A family history of diabetes, gout, high blood pressure, or high cholesterol increases one's risk of heart disease. African Americans are more likely to

have these familial risk factors, which increases their overall chances for CVD.
- Cholesterol levels higher than 200 milligrams per milliliter (mg/dL) in those age 20 and over are found in:
  - 53% of non-Hispanic white females
  - 47% of non-Hispanic African American females
  - 43% of Mexican Americans
  - 28% of Indian/Alaskan Natives
  - 27% of Asian/Pacific Islanders

Source: American Heart Association, *Heart Disease and Stroke Statistics—2003 Update* (Dallas, TX: American Heart Association, 2003).

Risks You Cannot Control

There are, unfortunately, some risk factors for CVD that we cannot prevent or control. The most important are the following:

- *Heredity.* A family history of heart disease appears to increase the risk significantly. Whether the increase is due to genetics or environment is unresolved.
- *Age.* Seventy-five percent of all heart attacks occur in people over age 65. The risk for CVD increases with age for both sexes.
- *Gender.* Men are at greater risk for CVD until about age 60. Women under 35 have a fairly low risk unless they have

high blood pressure, kidney problems, or diabetes. Using oral contraceptives and smoking also increase the risk. Hormonal factors appear to reduce risk for women, although after menopause or after estrogen levels are otherwise reduced (e.g., because of hysterectomy), women's LDL levels tend to go up, which increases their chances for CVD. (For more on the gender factor, see the next section.)
- *Race.* African Americans have a 45 percent greater risk for hypertension and thus a greater risk for CVD than whites. In addition, African Americans are less likely to survive a heart attack.

The Health in a Diverse World box describes the impact of race, gender, and age on CVD risk.

Women and Cardiovascular Disease

Although men tend to have more heart attacks and to suffer them earlier in life than do women, some interesting trends in survivability have emerged. In 1999, CVD claimed the lives of 445,692 men and a surprising 503,927 women. Why do more men have heart attacks but more women die of them? Why do some studies say that women have about the same mortality rate after MI and others indicate there are vast differences, supported by actual numbers?[42] Although we understand the mechanisms that cause heart disease in men and women (or at least we think we do!), their experiences in the health care system, their reactions to life-threatening diseases, and a host of other technological and environmental factors may play a role in these statistics.

Risk Factors for Heart Disease in Women

Premenopausal women are unlikely candidates for heart attacks, except for those who suffer from diabetes, high blood pressure, kidney disease, or a genetic predisposition to high cholesterol levels. Family history and smoking can also increase the risk.

The Role of Estrogen   Once her estrogen production drops with menopause, a woman's chance of developing CVD rises rapidly. A 60-year-old woman has the same heart attack risk as a 50-year-old man. By her late 70s, a woman has the same heart attack risk as a man her age. To date, much of this changing risk has been attributed to the aging process, but the role of estrogen remains unclear. Early studies of various **hormone replacement therapies (HRTs)** indicated that HRT might reduce the risk of CVD by as much as 12 to 25 percent. However, newer findings throw a huge wrench in what was previously believed to be the CVD-risk-reducing powers of HRT. Even when their total blood cholesterol levels are higher than men's, however, women may be at less risk because they typically have a higher percentage of HDL.[43] (See the Women's Health/Men's Health box on page 332.)

But that's only part of the story. It's true that women age 25 and over tend to have lower cholesterol levels than men of the same age. But when they reach 45, things change. Most men's cholesterol levels become more stable,

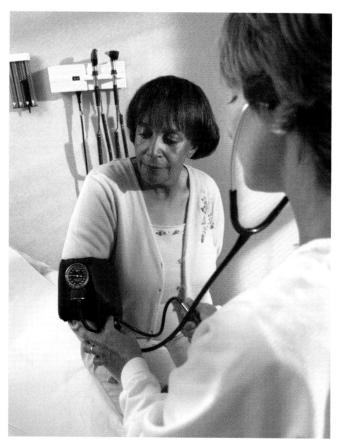

Women at risk for heart disease need to have their blood pressure and other CVD risk factors carefully monitored.

while both LDL and total cholesterol levels in women start to rise. And the gap widens further beyond age 55.[44]

Before age 45, women's total blood cholesterol levels average below 220 mg/dL. By the time she is 45 to 55, the average woman's blood cholesterol rises to between 223 and 246 mg/dL. Studies of men have shown that for every 1 percent drop in cholesterol, there is a 2 percent decrease in CVD risk.[45] If this holds true for women, prevention efforts focusing on dietary interventions and exercise may significantly help postmenopausal women.

Disparities in Treatment and Research in Women

During the past decade, research has suggested three main reasons for the widespread neglect of the signs of heart disease in women:

1. Physicians may be gender-biased in their delivery of health care and tend to concentrate on women's reproductive organs rather than on the whole woman.

Hormone replacement therapies (HRTs)   Therapies that replace estrogen in postmenopausal women.

CVD Protection or Increased Risk? The Hormone Controversy

For decades, the prevailing wisdom was that taking hormones during and after menopause would not only reduce hot flashes, but also provide protection against CVD in women. The rate of CVD only increases in women after menopause. This leads experts to believe that by keeping hormone levels high after menopause, CVD risk would be controlled. Although scientists didn't really know why this apparent relationship existed, they began to prescribe hormones to millions of women. The results of a major study in the mid-1990s, the Post-menopausal Estrogen/Progestin Intervention (PEPI) Trial, seemed to give doctors the proof they needed that hormone replacement therapy (HRT) lowered CVD risk by raising levels of HDL and decreasing LDL. This led to widespread promotion of HRT as a panacea for CVD risk by professional organizations, doctors, educators, and the community at large. Other studies seemed to confirm these facts, and women moved to take HRT in unprecedented numbers, some 38% of all postmenopausal women in the most recent data.

Women choose to take HRT for various reasons. Although reduction of CVD risk has been one of the factors, most women take HRT because it is the most effective treatment for menopausal symptoms such as hot flashes, night sweats, sexual dysfunction and vaginal dryness, insomnia, and hair loss. For women experiencing these problems, short-term use of HRT to get them through the years when the symptoms are most disruptive may seem worth any small risk. Other women took HRT because it has been shown to reduce the risk of bone fractures and osteoporosis, another major threat to older women's health.

NEW FINDINGS RAISE QUESTIONS

Today, results from several new studies provide growing evidence that the advice to take HRT to prevent CVD was not only inaccurate, but also may have been deadly for some of those who followed it. Consider the following.

- The 1998 Heart and Estrogen/ Progestin Replacement Study (HERS), a large-scale randomized, controlled clinical trial, showed that after four years on HRT, there was no difference in heart attack rates and higher rates of coronary death for those on HRT compared to those taking a placebo. Perhaps the most alarming results of HERS indicated a 52% increase in cardiovascular events in the first year for those taking HRT.

- The 2000 Estrogen Replacement and Atherosclerosis Trial, the first study to use angiographic images to assess the effects of HRT and Estrogen Replacement Therapy (ERT) on women with pre-existing coronary disease, showed no effect on disease progression with hormone replacement.

- In the spring of 2000, investigators conducting the huge Women's Health Initiative (WHI) study stirred even more controversy. Researchers announced that they had noted an alarming trend in their data that suggested that women on HRT in the study were experiencing a small but unacceptable increase in heart attacks, blood clots in the lungs (pulmonary embolism) and legs (deep vein thrombosis), and stroke. Although the study was scheduled to continue until 2005, these results caused the researchers to stop this portion of the study and send warning letters to women in the trial

2. Physicians tend to view male heart disease as a more severe problem because medical training has traditionally focused on it as a "male" problem.
3. Women decline major procedures more often than men do.

Other explanations for diagnostic and therapeutic difficulties encountered by women with heart disease include the following:[46]

- Delay in diagnosing a possible heart attack
- The complexity involved in interpreting chest pain in women
- Typically less aggressive treatment of women who are heart attack victims
- Their older age, on average, and greater frequency of other health problems

- The fact that women's coronary arteries are often smaller than men's, which makes surgical or diagnostic procedures more difficult technically
- Their increased incidence of postinfarction angina and heart failure

In addition, symptoms of heart attack often differ for women and men, which makes it more difficult for a woman to determine whether to go to the doctor. Instead of the classic symptom of chest-crushing pain, women often experience shortness of breath, fatigue, and jaw pain, stretched out over hours rather than minutes. While there is considerable debate over whether inequities exist in treatment of CVD in men compared to women, at least one study suggests that any disparities may reflect overtreatment of men rather than undertreatment of women.[47]

informing them of the possible risk. One version of HRT, known as Prempro, appeared to pose a greater risk than others.

WHAT ARE THE IMPLICATIONS FOR CONSUMERS?

Should a woman toss out her hormones based on the WHI results? Generally, experts recommend that if you are over-weight, have high cholesterol, or have a family history of heart disease, you may already be at increased risk for CVD, and it may be prudent to look for alternatives.

It should be noted that these increased risks apply to women on HRT, not on es-trogen alone. They also do not apply to women who had hysterectomies and were on HRT. The decision to use ERT or HRT is complex and should be made in consultation with knowledgeable health care providers and after reviewing the latest information from reputable sources. The most important thing to take away from the WHI findings is that HRT does not seem to prevent or improve cardio-vascular risks, so no woman should take it to protect against heart attacks or stroke.

New information about the effects of estrogen alone, or various levels of

How great is the risk? Scientists indicate that if 10,000 women took HRT for one year:

The number of women with. . . .	Would increase by	Would decrease by
Breast cancer	8[1]	
Heart attack	7	
Stroke	8	
Pulmonary embolism	8[2]	
Venous thrombosis	10[2]	
Colorectal cancer		6[3]
Hip fracture		5

1. Risk appears after 4 years of use.
2. Risk is greatest in first 2 years of use.
3. Benefit appears after 3 years of use.

HRT, may become available soon. If you have questions about these studies or want additional information, the references below are valuable sources of information.

Sources: The Postmenopausal Estrogen/Progestin Intervention (PEPI) Trial: The Writing Group for the PEPI Trial, "Effects of Estrogen or Estrogen/Progestin Regimens on Heart Disease Risk Factors in Menopausal Women," *The Journal of the American Medical Association* 273 (1995): 199–208; L. Mosca, et al., "Hormone Replacement Therapy and Cardiovascular Disease," *Circulation* 104 (2001): 499; S. Hulley et al., "Randomized Trial of Estrogen Plus Progestin for Secondary Prevention of Coronary Heart Disease in Postmenopausal Women" (Heart and Estrogen/Progestin Replacement Study [HERS] Research Group), *The Journal of the American Medical Association* 280 (1998): 605–613; Writing Group for the Women's Health Initiative Investigators, "Risks and Benefits of Estrogen Plus Progestin in Healthy Postmenopausal Women," *The Journal of the American Medical Association* 288, no. 3 (2002); U.S. Preventive Services Task Force, Agency for Healthcare Research and Quality, "Recommendation and Rationale, Hormone Replacement Therapy for Primary Prevention of Chronic Conditions," October 2002. www.ahrq .gov/clinic/3rduspstf/hrt/hrtrr.htm; C. Runowics, "A Clearer Picture of HRT," *Health News* 8, no. 9 (September 2002): 1–4.

Another important difference in the treatment of CVD is the effectiveness of drugs. Medications used to break up clots and stabilize erratic heartbeats are less effective in women than in men. Beta-blockers, used to reduce blood pressure, take longer to metabolize in women, affecting dose regulation.

The traditional view that heart disease is primarily a male problem has carried over into research as well. A well-publicized example was a study suggesting that aspirin could help prevent heart attacks—based entirely on its effects in 22,000 male doctors. To address such concerns, the National Institutes of Health has launched a 15-year, $625 million study of 140,000 postmenopausal women known as the Women's Health Initiative (WHI), which focuses on the leading causes of death and disease. Researchers hope to determine how a healthy lifestyle and increased medical attention can help prevent women's heart disease, as well as cancer and osteoporosis.

What do you think?

How do men and women differ in their experiences related to CVD? ✱ Why do you think women's risks largely were ignored until fairly recently? ✱ What actions do you think individuals can take to help improve the situation for both men and women? ✱ What actions can communities and medical practitioners take?

New Weapons Against Heart Disease

The victim of a heart attack today has many options that were not available a generation ago. Medications can strengthen heartbeat, control arrhythmias, remove fluids in case of congestive heart failure, and relieve pain. New surgical procedures are saving many lives.

Techniques of Diagnosing Heart Disease

Several techniques are used to diagnose heart disease, including electrocardiogram, angiography, and positron emission tomography scans. An **electrocardiogram (ECG)** is a record of the electrical activity of the heart. In an ECG, patients may undergo a stress test, such as walking or running on a treadmill while their hearts are monitored. A more accurate method of testing for heart disease is **angiography** (often referred to as *cardiac catheterization*), in which a needle-thin tube called a *catheter* is threaded through heart arteries, a dye is injected, and an X ray is taken to discover which areas are blocked. A more recent and even more effective method of measuring heart activity is **positron emission tomography scan (PET scan),** which produces three-dimensional images of the heart as blood flows through it. During a PET scan, a patient receives an intravenous injection of a radioactive tracer. As the tracer decays, it emits positrons that are picked up by the scanner and transformed by a computer into color images of the heart. Other tests include the following.

- *Radionuclide imaging* (includes tests such as the thallium test, MUGA scan, and acute infarct scintigraphy). These procedures involve injecting substances called radionuclides into the bloodstream. Computer-generated pictures can then show them in the heart. These tests can reveal how well the heart muscle is supplied with blood, how well the heart's chambers are functioning, and which part of the heart has been damaged by a heart attack.
- *Magnetic resonance imaging* (MRI or NMR). The MRI test uses powerful magnets to look inside the body. Computer-generated pictures can show the heart muscle and help physicians identify damage from a heart attack, diagnose congenital heart defects, and evaluate disease of larger blood vessels such as the aorta.
- *Digital cardiac angiography* (DCA or DSA). DCA is a modified form of computer-aided imaging that records pictures of the heart and its blood vessels.

Angioplasty versus Bypass Surgery

Coronary bypass surgery has helped many patients who have suffered coronary blockages or heart attacks. In coronary bypass surgery, a blood vessel is taken from another site in the patient's body (usually the *saphenous vein* in the leg or the *internal mammary artery*) and implanted to bypass blocked arteries and transport blood. Bypass patients typically spend four to seven days in the hospital to recuperate. The average cost of the procedure itself is well more than $50,000, and the additional intensive care treatments and follow-ups often result in total medical bills of $125,000. Death rates are generally much lower at medical centers where surgical teams and intensive care teams see large numbers of patients.[48]

Another procedure called **angioplasty** (sometimes called *balloon angioplasty*) carries fewer risks and may be more effective than bypass surgery in selected cases. As in angiography, a thin catheter is threaded through blocked heart arteries. The catheter has a balloon at the tip, which is inflated to flatten fatty deposits against the artery walls; this allows blood to flow more freely. Angioplasty patients are generally awake but sedated during the procedure and spend only one or two days in the hospital after treatment. Most people can return to work within five days. In about 30 percent of patients, the treated arteries become clogged again within six months. Some patients may undergo the procedure as many as three times within a five-year period. Some surgeons argue that given angioplasty's high rate of recurrence, bypass may be a more effective treatment.

Research suggests that in many instances, drug treatments may be just as effective as invasive surgical techniques in prolonging life. But it is critical that doctors follow an aggressive drug treatment program and that patients comply with it.

Aspirin for Heart Disease: Can It Help?

Research indicates that low doses of aspirin (80 mg daily or every other day) are beneficial to heart patients because of its blood-thinning properties. Aspirin has even been advised

---

Electrocardiogram (ECG)   A record of the electrical activity of the heart.

Angiography   A technique for examining blockages in heart arteries.

Positron emission tomography scan (PET scan)   Method for measuring heart activity by injecting a patient with a radioactive tracer that is scanned electronically to produce a three-dimensional image of the heart and arteries.

Coronary bypass surgery   A surgical technique whereby a blood vessel is implanted to bypass a clogged coronary artery.

Angioplasty   A technique in which a catheter with a balloon at the tip is inserted into a clogged artery; the balloon is inflated to flatten fatty deposits against artery walls, which allows blood to flow more freely.

---

as a preventive strategy for people with no current heart disease symptoms. However, major problems associated with aspirin use are gastrointestinal intolerance and a tendency for some people to have difficulty with blood clotting; these factors may outweigh aspirin's benefits in some cases. People taking aspirin face additional risks from emergency surgery or if accidental bleeding occurs. Although the findings concerning aspirin and heart disease are still inconclusive, the research seems promising.[49]

Thrombolysis

Whenever a heart attack occurs, prompt action is vital. When a coronary artery gets blocked, the heart muscle doesn't die immediately, but time determines how much damage occurs. If the victim reaches an emergency room and is diagnosed fast enough, a form of reperfusion therapy called **thrombolysis** can be performed. Thrombolysis involves injecting an agent such as tissue plasminogen activator to dissolve the clot and restore some blood flow, which thereby reduces the amount of tissue that dies from ischemia. These drugs must be administered within one to three hours after a heart attack for best results.

> **What do you think?**
>
> *With all the new diagnostic procedures, treatments, and differing philosophies about prevention and intervention techniques, how can health consumers ensure that they will get the best treatment?* ✳ *Where can they go for information?* ✳ *Why might patients need a "health advocate" who can help them get through the system?*

Cardiac Rehabilitation

Every year, nearly 1 million people survive heart attacks. More than 7 million more have unstable angina, and about 650,000 undergo bypass surgery or angioplasty. Heart failure is the most common discharge diagnosis for hospitalized Medicare patients and the fourth most common diagnosis among all patients hospitalized in the United States. Most of these patients are eligible for cardiac rehabilitation (including exercise training and health education classes on good nutrition and CVD risk management) and need only a doctor's prescription for these services. However, many Americans do not have access to these programs. Even larger numbers are finding it difficult to afford such programs in light of skyrocketing costs for prescription drugs. While some patients must choose between home health care and cardiac rehabilitation, others stay away from such programs because of cost, transportation, or other factors. Perhaps the biggest deterrent is fear of having another attack due to exercise. However, the benefits of cardiac rehabilitation (including increased stamina

and strength and faster recovery) far outweigh the risks when these programs are run by certified health professionals.[50]

Personal Advocacy and Heart-Smart Behaviors

People who suspect they have CVD are often overwhelmed and frightened. Where should they go for diagnosis? What are the best treatments? Answering these questions becomes even more difficult if they are upset, scared, or tend to listen unquestioningly to doctors' orders. If you or a loved one must face a CVD crisis, it is important to act with knowledge, strength, and assertiveness. These suggestions will help.

1. *Know your rights as a patient.* Ask about the risks and costs of various diagnostic tests. Some procedures, particularly angiography, may pose significant risks for people who are elderly, who have a history of minor strokes, or have had chemotherapy or other treatments that could have damaged their blood vessels. Ask for test results and an explanation of any abnormalities.
2. *Find out about informed consent procedures, living wills, durable power of attorney, organ donation, and other legal issues before you become sick.* Having someone shove a clipboard in your face and ask you whether life support can be terminated in case of a problem is one of the great horrors of many people's hospital experiences. Be prepared.
3. *Ask about alternative procedures.* If possible, seek a second opinion at a different health care facility (in other words, get at least two opinions from doctors who are not in the same group and who cannot read each other's diagnoses). New research indicates that doctors may not use drug treatments as aggressively as they could and that medications may be as effective as major bypass or open heart surgeries. Ask, ask, and ask again. Remember, it is your life, and there is always the possibility that another treatment will be better for you.
4. *Remain with your loved one as his or her personal advocate.* If your loved one is weak and unable to ask questions, ask the questions yourself. Inquire about new medications, tests, and potentially risky procedures that may be undertaken during the course of treatment or recovery. If you feel your loved one is being removed from intensive care or other closely monitored areas prematurely, ask whether the hospital is taking this action to comply with DRGs (diagnosis-related groups, or established limits of treatment for certain conditions) and whether this action is warranted. Most hospitals have waiting areas or special rooms so family members can stay close to a patient. Exercise your right to this option.

> **Thrombolysis** Injection of an agent to dissolve clots and restore some blood flow, thereby reducing the amount of tissue that dies from ischemia.

What to Do in the Event of a Heart Attack

Because heart attacks are so frightening, we would prefer not to think about them. However, knowing how to act in an emergency could save your life or that of somebody else.

KNOW THE WARNING SIGNS OF A HEART ATTACK

- Uncomfortable pressure, fullness, squeezing, or pain in the center of the chest that lasts two minutes or longer
- Jaw pain and/or shortness of breath
- Pain spreading to the shoulders, neck, or arms
- Dizziness, fatigue, fainting, sweating, and/or nausea

Not all these warning signs occur in every heart attack. For instance, women's heart attacks tend to show up as shortness of breath, fatigue, and jaw pain, stretched out over hours rather than minutes. If some of these symptoms do appear, however, don't wait. Get help immediately!

KNOW WHAT TO DO IN AN EMERGENCY

- Find out which hospitals in your area have 24-hour emergency cardiac care.
- Determine (in advance) the hospital or medical facility that's nearest your home and office, and tell your family and friends to call this facility in an emergency.
- Keep a list of emergency rescue service numbers next to your telephone and in your pocket, wallet, or purse.
- If you have chest or jaw discomfort that lasts more than two minutes, call the emergency rescue service. Do not drive yourself to the hospital.

BE A HEART SAVER

- If you're with someone who is showing signs of a heart attack and the warning signs last for two minutes or longer, act immediately.
- Expect a denial. It's normal for a person with chest discomfort to deny the possibility of anything as serious as a heart attack. Don't take no for an answer, however. Insist on taking prompt action.
- Call the emergency rescue service or get to the nearest hospital emergency room that offers 24-hour emergency cardiac care.
- Give CPR (mouth-to-mouth breathing and chest compression) if it's necessary and if you're properly trained to do it.

Source: American Heart Association, *Heart and Stroke Facts* (Dallas, TX: American Heart Association, 2002).

5. *Monitor the actions of health care providers.* To control costs, some hospitals are hiring nursing aides and other personnel who may lack the training that registered nurses have in handling patients with CVD. Ask about the patient-to-nurse ratio, and make sure that people monitoring you or your loved ones have appropriate credentials.

6. *Be considerate of your care provider.* One of the most stressful jobs any person can be entrusted with is care of a critically ill person. Although questions are appropriate and your emotions are running high, be as tactful and considerate as possible. Nurses often carry a disproportionate responsibility for the care of patients during critical times. They are often forced to carry a higher than necessary patient load. Try to remain out of their way, ask questions as necessary, and report any irregularities in care to the supervisor.

7. *Be patient with the patient.* The pain, suffering, and fears associated with a cardiac event often cause otherwise nice people to act in not-so-nice ways. Be patient and helpful, and allow time for the person to rest. Talk with the patient about his or her feelings, concerns, and fears. Do not ignore these concerns in order to ease your own anxieties.

Taking Charge

Make It Happen!

Assessment: The Assess Yourself box on page 320 evaluates your risk of heart disease and the status of your LDL cholesterol. Based on your results and the advice of your physician, you may need to take steps to reduce your cholesterol level and risk of CVD.

Making a Change: In order to change your behavior, you need to develop a plan. Follow these steps.

1. Evaluate your behavior, and identify patterns and specific things you are doing. What can you change now? What can you change in the near future?

2. Select one pattern of behavior that you want to change.

3. Fill out a Behavior Change Contract. It should include your long-term goal for change, your short-term

goals, the rewards you'll give yourself for reaching these goals, potential obstacles along the way, and strategies for overcoming these obstacles. For each goal, list the small steps and specific actions that you will take.

4. Chart your progress in a journal. At the end of a week, consider how successful you were in following your plan. What helped you be successful? What made change more difficult? What will you do differently next week?

5. Revise your plan as needed. Are the short-term goals attainable? Are the rewards satisfying?

Example: Nathan knew that his father had a history of heart disease, so he knew it was important to monitor his own risk. Using the results from his most recent checkup, he completed the self-assessment. Although his initial score for ten-year risk of heart attack (in step one of the assessment) was less than 10 percent, the combination of two major coronary risk factors (high systolic blood pressure and family history of CVD) with an LDL level of 140 showed in step 2 of the assessment that he needed to start making some lifestyle changes. At 6 feet in height, he weighed 220 pounds, which he discovered is close to obese according to the Body Mass Index calculations. He decided to manage his weight through exercise and improved eating habits. He also expected a modified diet would help lower his cholesterol levels.

Nathan's first step was to keep track of everything he normally ate for a week. When he analyzed his food journal, he saw that he rarely ate breakfast, which made him more likely to grab a doughnut later in the morning and a big lunch. He bought some whole wheat, high-fiber cereal and skim milk and started getting up 15 minutes earlier so he had time to eat his healthy breakfast. For the days when he didn't feel like eating cold cereal, he bought some five-minute oatmeal that also had healthy fiber and nutrients. Nathan found that he was not as tempted by the doughnuts and other unhealthy snacks during the day, and that he didn't overeat as much at lunch. He even had more energy during the day. As he started to lose weight, he felt more able to begin a moderate exercise program. All of these changes—losing weight, eating more fiber and less fat, and adding some exercise to his life—made Nathan confident that his next checkup with his doctor would show a lower LDL level and, perhaps, lower blood pressure. When Nathan is in a healthier range on these measures, he plans to buy himself a new DVD player.

Summary

※ Cardiovascular disease (CVD) incidence and prevalence rates have changed considerably in the past 50 years. Certain segments of the population have disproportionate levels of risk.

※ The cardiovascular system consists of the heart and circulatory system and is a carefully regulated, integrated network of vessels that supply the body with the nutrients and oxygen necessary to perform daily functions.

※ CVDs include atherosclerosis, heart attack, angina pectoris, arrhythmias, congestive heart failure, congenital and rheumatic heart disease, and stroke. These combine to be the leading cause of death in the United States today.

※ Many risk factors for CVD can be controlled, such as cigarette smoking, high blood fat and cholesterol levels, hypertension, lack of exercise, high-fat diet, obesity, diabetes, and emotional stress. Some risk factors, such as age, gender, and heredity, cannot be controlled. Many of these factors have a compounded effect when combined. Dietary changes, exercise, weight reduction, and attention to lifestyle risks can greatly reduce susceptibility to CVD.

※ Women face a unique challenge in controlling their risk for CVD, particularly after menopause, when estrogen levels are no longer sufficient to be protective.

※ New methods developed for treating heart blockages include coronary bypass surgery and angioplasty. Also, drugs such as beta blockers and calcium channel blockers can reduce high blood pressure and treat other symptoms. Research has provided important clues on how to best prevent or reduce risk of CVD today. Recognizing your own risks and acting now to reduce risk are important elements of lifelong cardiovascular health.

Questions for Discussion and Reflection

1. Trace the path of a drop of blood from the time it enters the heart until it reaches the extremities.

2. List the different types of CVD. Compare and contrast their symptoms, risk factors, prevention, and treatment.

3. What are the major indicators that CVD poses a particularly significant risk to people of your age? To the elderly? To people from selected minority groups?

4. Discuss the role that exercise, stress management, dietary changes, medical checkups, sodium reduction, and other factors can play in reducing risk for CVD. What role may chronic infections play in CVD risk?

5. Discuss why age is such an important factor in women's risk for CVD. What can be done to decrease women's risk in later life?

6. Describe some of the diagnostic and treatment alternatives for CVD. If you had a heart attack today, which treatment would you prefer? Explain why.

Accessing Your Health on the Internet

Visit the following Internet sites to explore further topics and issues related to personal health. To visit an organization's website, go to the Companion Website for *Health: The Basics, Sixth Edition* at www.aw-bc.com/donatelle, click on the book image, and select "Accessing Your Health on the Internet" from the navigation menu on the left.

1. *American Heart Association.* Home page for the leading private organization dedicated to heart health. This site provides information, statistics, and resources regarding cardiovascular care, including an opportunity to test your own risk for CVD.

2. *Johns Hopkins Cardiac Rehabilitation Homepage.* Information about prevention of heart disease and rehabilitation from CVD from one of the best cardiac care centers in the United States. Includes information about programs to help individuals stop smoking, lose weight, lower blood pressure and blood cholesterol, and reduce emotional stress.

3. *National Heart, Lung and Blood Institute.* A valuable resource for information on all aspects of cardiovascular health and wellness.

4. *U.S. National Library of Medicine: Health Services/ Technology Assessment Text.* Provides access to numerous databases of health care documents outlining procedures for clinicians and patients. Choose the database for the Agency for Health Care Policy and Research (AHCPR) to review various guidelines regarding all forms of cardiac care.

Further Reading

American Heart Association. *Heart and Stroke Facts.* Dallas, TX: American Heart Association.

An annual overview providing facts and figures concerning CVD in the United States. Supplement provides key statistics about current trends and future directions in treatment and prevention.

Gersh, Bernard, and Michael Wood, eds. *The Mayo Clinic Heart Book.* New York: William Morrow, 2000.

Pashkow, Frederic, and Charlotte Libov. *The Women's Heart Book.* New York: Hyperion, 2001.

Gersh and Pashkow provide overviews of heart disease in America, including risk factors, trends, and options for patients.

McCrum, Robert. *My Year Off: Recovering after a Stroke.* New York: Broadway Books, 1999.

The chronicle of a young man's recovery from a severe stroke.

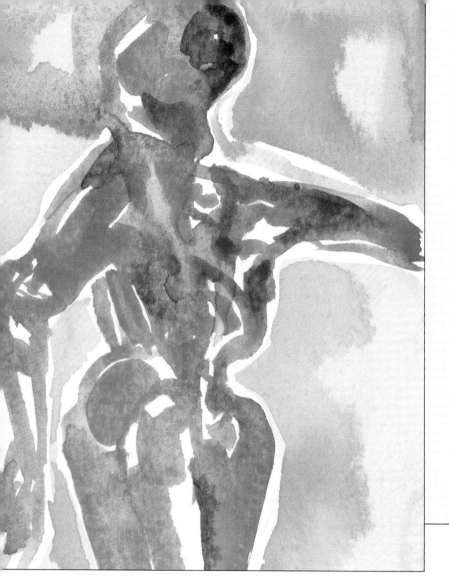

Cancer

Reducing Your Risk

Objectives

✳ Define cancer and discuss how it develops.

✳ Discuss the causes of cancer, including biological causes, occupational and environmental hazards, lifestyle, psychological factors, chemicals in foods, viruses, and medical factors.

✳ Describe the different types of cancer and the risks they pose to people at different ages and stages of life.

✳ Explain the importance of understanding and responding appropriately to self-exams, medical exams, and symptoms related to different types of cancer. Explain the importance of early detection.

✳ Discuss cancer detection and treatment, including radiation therapy, chemotherapy, immunotherapy, and other common methods of detection and treatment.

339

Hair Styling, Plus Cancer Education

By Richard Perez-Pena

The daily banter at Michou Hair Care goes far beyond hair. It encompasses a new job, an unfaithful boyfriend, a pair of sexy but painful shoes, a coveted day care slot.

Yet even by this anything-goes standard, the direction Micheline Edouard takes the conversation, between clipping and relaxing her clients' curls, is unorthodox. "You use the flat of your fingers, dear, not your fingertips, and you go in circles," she explained to a customer, demonstrating on a model of a breast. "And you need to get regular mammograms."

At about 25 salons in Brooklyn with mostly black clienteles, stylists like Ms. Edouard have added breast cancer education to their regular fare, with training from the Arthur Ashe Institute for Urban Health.

The Ashe Institute hopes to tap into the secret identity of a neighborhood salon, part social club, part counseling center, part bulletin board, a place where women can air their concerns away from men.

Ruth C. Browne, executive director of the Ashe Institute, said the experiment was conceived in response to the fact that black people remain significantly less likely than whites to get preventive care like cancer screenings.

Read the complete article online in the eThemes section of this book's website: www.aw-bc.com/donatelle.

As few as 50 years ago, a diagnosis of cancer was usually a death sentence. Health professionals could only guess at the cause, and treatments were often as deadly as the disease itself. Because we had no idea how a person "got" cancer, fears about possible infection led to ostracism and bigotry aimed at people who desperately needed support.

Today we know that there are multiple causes of cancer, and very few are linked to any type of infectious agent. Early detection and vast improvements in technology have dramatically improved the prognosis for most cancer patients. We also know that there are many actions we can take individually and as a society to prevent cancer. Knowing the facts about cancer, recognizing your risk, and taking action to reduce your risk are important steps in the battle.

An Overview of Cancer

During 2003, approximately 556,500 Americans died of cancer and more than 1.3 million new cases were diagnosed. Cancer is the second leading cause of death, exceeded only by heart disease, in the United States.[1] Put into perspective, this means that each day of the year more than 1,500 people die of some form of cancer. One of four deaths in the United States is from cancer; of these, one-third of the cancers were related to poor nutrition, physical inactivity, obesity, and other lifestyle factors, which means they could have been preventable.[2] However, it is important to note that although more than 1.3 million people will be diagnosed with cancer

in a year, nearly 6 in 10 will be alive five years after diagnosis. Many will be considered "cured," meaning that they have no subsequent cancer in their bodies five years after diagnosis and can expect to live a long and productive life.[3]

When adjusted for normal life expectancy (factors such as dying of heart disease, accidents, etc.), a relative five-year survival of 62 percent is seen for all cancers. Although survival rates are useful in monitoring progress in early detection and treatment, they do not represent those cured permanently, since cancers can recur after five years. Some cancers that only a few decades ago presented a very poor outlook are often cured today: acute lymphocytic leukemia in children, Hodgkin's disease, Burkitt's lymphoma, Ewing's sarcoma (a form of bone cancer), Wilms' tumor (a kidney cancer in children), testicular cancer, and osteogenic (bone) sarcoma are among the most remarkable indicators of progress.

Variations in Rates

While cancer strikes people of all ages, races, cultures, and socioeconomic levels, some Americans are at greater risk. Overall, African Americans are more likely to develop cancer than persons of any other racial and ethnic group. The most current data indicates that in 2003, incidence rates were 703.6 per 100,000 African Americans and 568.2 per 100,000 whites; 393.1 per 100,000 Hispanics; 408.9 per 100,000 Asian/Pacific Islanders; and 277.1 per 100,000 Alaska Natives and American Indians.[4] Cancer sites for which African Americans have significantly higher incidence and mortality rates include the esophagus, uterus, cervix, stomach, liver, prostate, and larynx. African Americans are 33 percent more likely to die of cancer than whites and more than twice as likely to die of cancer than are Hispanics, Asian/Pacific Islanders, and American Indians. Researchers at the National Cancer Institute believe that these differences are due more to African Americans' lower average socioeconomic status and generally more limited access to health care than to any inherent physical characteristics.[5] Some findings indicate that certain cancers are simply more common in different races.

Cancer incidence and mortality rates within other minority groups, such as Hispanics, are often lower (sometimes by as much as 25 percent or more) than those of white or African Americans. Due to Hispanics' low average socioeconomic status, we might expect that they would have cancer rates similar to those of African Americans. But Hispanics seem to be "protected" from high rates. Why? No one knows for sure, but the answer may lie in differences in diet, exercise patterns, or other culturally influenced behaviors. Because cancer risk is strongly associated with lifestyle and behavior, differences in ethnic and cultural groups can provide clues to factors involved in its development. Culturally influenced values and belief systems can also affect whether a person seeks care, participates in screenings, or follows recommended treatments. Socioeconomic factors such as lack of health insurance or lack of transportation to treatment centers can lead to late diagnosis and poor survival.

What Is Cancer?

Cancer is the name given to a large group of diseases characterized by the uncontrolled growth and spread of abnormal cells.[6] Think of a healthy cell as a small computer programmed to operate in a particular fashion. Under normal conditions, healthy cells are protected by a powerful overseer, the immune system, as they perform their daily functions of growing, replicating, and repairing body organs. When something interrupts normal cell programming, however, uncontrolled growth and abnormal cellular development result in a new growth of tissue serving no physiological function, which is called a **neoplasm.** This neoplasmic mass often forms a clumping of cells known as a **tumor.**

Not all tumors are **malignant** (cancerous); in fact, most are **benign** (noncancerous). Benign tumors are generally harmless unless they grow in such a fashion that they obstruct or crowd out normal tissues. A benign tumor of the brain, for instance, is life threatening if it grows enough to restrict blood flow and cause a stroke. The only way to determine whether a given tumor or mass is malignant is through **biopsy,** or microscopic examination of cell development.

Benign and malignant tumors differ in several key ways. Benign tumors generally consist of ordinary-looking cells enclosed in a fibrous shell or capsule that prevents their spreading to other body areas. Malignant tumors are usually not enclosed in a protective capsule and can therefore spread to other organs. This process, known as **metastasis,** makes some forms of cancer particularly aggressive in their ability to overcome the body's defenses. By the time they are diagnosed, malignant tumors have frequently metastasized throughout the body, which makes treatment extremely difficult. Unlike benign tumors, which merely expand to take over a given space, malignant cells invade surrounding tissue and emit clawlike protrusions that disturb the RNA and DNA within normal cells. Disrupting these substances, which control cellular metabolism and reproduction, produces **mutant cells** that differ in form, quality, and function from normal cells. Assess your own cancer risk by completing the Assess Yourself box on page 344.

What Causes Cancer?

After decades of research, most cancer epidemiologists believe that cancers are, at least in theory, preventable and that many could be avoided by suitable choices in lifestyle and environment.[7] Many specific causes of cancer are believed to be known, the most important of which are smoking, obesity, and a few organic viruses (Figure 13.1 on page 342). However, a large proportion of global variation in common cancers, such as cancer of the breast, prostate, colon, and rectum, remain unexplained.[8] Most research supports the idea that cancer is caused by both *external* factors (chemicals, radiation, viruses, and lifestyle) and *internal* factors (hormones, immune conditions, and inherited mutations). Causal factors may act together or in sequence to promote cancer development.[9] We do not know why some people have malignant cells in their body and never develop cancer, while others may take ten years or more to develop the disease.

Cancer   A large group of diseases characterized by the uncontrolled growth and spread of abnormal cells.

Neoplasm   A new growth of tissue that serves no physiological function and results from uncontrolled, abnormal cellular development.

Tumor   A neoplasmic mass that grows more rapidly than surrounding tissue.

Malignant   Very dangerous or harmful; refers to a cancerous tumor.

Benign   Harmless; refers to a noncancerous tumor.

Biopsy   Microscopic examination of tissue to determine if a cancer is present.

Metastasis   Process by which cancer spreads from one area to different areas of the body.

Mutant cells   Cells that differ in form, quality, or function from normal cells.

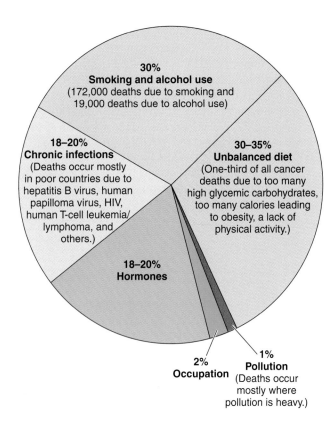

Figure 13.1

Factors Believed to Contribute to Global Causes of Cancer

Sources: S. Heacht et al., *Public Session/Panel Discussion* (Portland, OR: Linus Pauling Institute International Conference on Diet and Optimum Health, May 2001); American Cancer Society, *Cancer Facts and Figures 2003* (Atlanta: American Cancer Society, 2003).

Anyone can develop cancer; however, most cases affect adults beginning in middle age. In fact, nearly 80 percent of cancers are diagnosed at age 55 and over. Cancer researchers refer to one's *cancer risk* when they assess risk factors. *Lifetime risk* refers to the probability that an individual, over the course of a lifetime, will develop cancer or die from it. In the United States, men have a lifetime risk of about one in two; women have a lower risk of one in three.[10] *Relative risk* is a measure of the strength of the relationship between risk factors and a particular cancer. Basically, relative risk compares your risk if you engage in certain known risk behaviors with that of someone who does not engage in such behaviors. For example, if you are a male and you smoke, you may have a

---

Carcinogens   Cancer-causing agents.

Oncogenes   Suspected cancer-causing genes present on chromosomes.

Protooncogenes   Genes that can become oncogenes under certain conditions.

Oncologists   Physicians who specialize in the treatment of malignancies.

20-fold relative risk over a nonsmoker of developing lung cancer; this mean that your chances of getting lung cancer are about 20 times greater than the chances of a nonsmoker.[11]

Cellular Change/Mutation Theories

One theory of cancer development proposes that cancer results from spontaneous error that occurs during cell reproduction. Perhaps cells that are overworked or aged are more likely to break down, which causes genetic errors that result in mutant cells.

Another theory suggests that cancer is caused by some external agent or agents that enter a normal cell and initiate the cancerous process. Numerous environmental factors, such as radiation, chemicals, hormonal drugs, immunosuppressant drugs (drugs that suppress the normal activity of the immune system), and other toxins, are considered possible **carcinogens** (cancer-causing agents); perhaps the most common carcinogen is the tar in cigarettes. The greater the dose or exposure to environmental hazards, the greater the risk of disease. People who are forced to work, live, and pass through areas that have high levels of environmental toxins may be at greater risk for several types of cancers.[12]

A third theory came out of research on certain viruses that are believed to cause tumors in animals. This research led to the discovery of **oncogenes,** suspected cancer-causing genes that are present on chromosomes. Although oncogenes are typically dormant, scientists theorize that certain conditions, such as age, stress, and exposure to carcinogens, viruses, and radiation, may activate them. Once activated, they grow and reproduce in an out-of-control manner.

Scientists are uncertain whether only people who develop cancer have oncogenes or whether we all have **protooncogenes,** genes that can become oncogenes under certain conditions. Many **oncologists** (physicians who specialize in the treatment of malignancies) believe that the oncogene theory may lead to a greater understanding of how individual cells function and bring us closer to developing effective treatments.

Many factors are believed to contribute to cancer development. Combining risk factors can dramatically increase a person's risk for cancer.

Risks for Cancer—Lifestyle

Over the years, researchers have found that people who engage in certain behaviors show a higher incidence of cancer. In particular, diet, sedentary lifestyle (and resultant obesity), consumption of alcohol and cigarettes, stress, and other lifestyle factors seem to play a role. Likewise, colon and rectal cancer occur more frequently among persons with a high-fat, low-fiber diet; in those who don't eat enough fruits and vegetables; and in those who are inactive. See Chapter 9 for information about certain dietary risks related to cancer and the role of supplements in preventing cancer. More research is needed to pinpoint the mechanisms that act in the body to increase the odds of cancer. For now, there is compelling evidence that certain actions are clearly associated with a greater-than-average risk of developing diseases.

Smoking and Cancer Risk   Of all of the risk factors for cancer, smoking is among the greatest. In the United States, tobacco is responsible for nearly one in five deaths annually. Tobacco use accounts for at least 30 percent of all cancer deaths and 87 percent of all lung cancer deaths.[13] Over the five decades since British and American epidemiologists have singled out tobacco as a culprit in lung cancer and other diseases, tar levels in British cigarettes have declined dramatically, as has the prevalence of smoking in general. As a result, the lung cancer rate for British men under age 55 has fallen by two-thirds since 1955, which places it among the lowest in the developed world.[14] In the last 20 years, America's rates have shown a similar decline. Lung cancer rates among men are still increasing in most developing countries and in Eastern Europe, however, where consumption of cigarettes remains high and is still increasing in some areas.[15]

Most authorities have believed that cigarettes cause only cancers of the lung, pancreas, bladder and kidney, and (synergistically with alcohol) of the larynx, mouth, pharynx, and esophagus. However, more recent evidence indicates that several other types of cancer are related to tobacco. Most notably, cancer of the stomach, liver, and cervix seem to be directly related to long-term smoking.[16]

Obesity and Cancer Risk   It is difficult to sort through the accumulated evidence about the role of nutrients, obesity, sedentary lifestyle, and related variables. Nevertheless, a body of research has emerged that seems to point (albeit not with absolute certainty) to a link between cancer and obesity. What is clear: Cancer is more common among people who are overweight, and risk increases as obesity increases. This evidence for a link is strongest for postmenopausal breast cancer and cancers of the endometrium, gallbladder, and kidney, but obesity is also implicated in other cancers. For women, cancers of the cervix and ovaries are added to this list; for men, cancers of the colon and prostate seem to be related to obesity and/or diet. The following facts provide evidence for this obesity/cancer link:[17]

- The relative risk of breast cancer in postmenopausal women is 50 percent higher for obese women.
- The relative risk of colon cancer in men is 40 percent higher for obese men.
- The relative risks of gallbladder and endometrial cancer are five times higher in obese individuals compared to individuals with healthy weight.
- Some studies have shown a positive association between obesity and cancers of the kidney, pancreas, rectum, esophagus, and liver.
- Obesity is believed to alter complex interactions among diet, metabolism, physical activity, hormones, and growth factors.

Biological Factors

Early theorists believed that we inherit a genetic predisposition toward certain forms of cancer.[18] Cancers of the breast, stomach, colon, prostate, uterus, ovaries, and lungs appear to run in families. For example, a woman runs a much higher risk of breast cancer if her mother or sisters (primary relatives) have had the disease, particularly if they had it at a young age. Hodgkin's disease and certain leukemias show similar familial patterns. Can we attribute these patterns to genetic susceptibility or to the fact that people in the same families experience similar environmental risks? To date, the research in this area is inconclusive. Recent research conducted by the University of Utah indicates that a gene for breast cancer exists. A rare form of eye cancer does appear to be passed genetically from mother to child. It is possible that we can inherit a tendency toward a cancer-prone, weak immune system or, conversely, that we can inherit a cancer-fighting potential. But the complex interaction of hereditary predisposition, lifestyle, and environment on the development of cancer makes it a challenge to determine a single cause.

Gender also affects the likelihood of developing certain forms of cancer. For example, breast cancer occurs primarily among females, although men do occasionally get breast cancer. Obviously, factors other than heredity and familial relationships affect which sex develops a particular cancer. In the 1950s, for example, women rarely contracted lung cancer. But with increases in the number of women who smoke and the length of time they have smoked, lung cancer rates have soared to become the leading cause of cancer death in women. However, while gender plays a role in certain cases of cancer, other variables such as lifestyle are probably more significant.

Reproductive and Hormonal Risks for Cancer   The effects of reproductive factors on breast and cervical cancer have been well documented. Pregnancy and estrogen supplementation in the form of oral contraceptives or hormone replacement therapy (HRT) increase a woman's risk of breast cancer. Late menarche, early menopause, early first childbirth, and high parity (having many children) have been shown to reduce a woman's risk of breast cancer. A higher risk of endometrial cancer is also associated with HRT.[19]

Breast cancer incidence is much higher in most Western countries than in developing countries. This is partly—and perhaps largely—accounted for by dietary effects (consuming a diet high in calories and fat), combined with later first childbirth, lower parity (having fewer children), shorter breastfeeding, and higher obesity rates.[20]

Occupational and Environmental Factors

Overall, workplace hazards account for only a small percentage of all cancers. However, various substances are known to cause cancer when exposure levels are high or prolonged.

(text continues on page 346)

Cancer: Assessing Your Personal Risk

Although the evidence is pretty clear that there are some types of cancer that you may be predisposed to due to genetic, biological, and/or environmental causes, there are many more that may be, at least in part, prevented through lifestyle behavior changes and risk reduction strategies. If you carefully assess your individual risk, you can then make behavior changes that will make you less susceptible to the various cancers. By answering each of the following questions, you will have an indicator of your susceptibility. Of course, no single instrument can serve as a complete risk

assessment or diagnostic guide. These questions merely serve as the basis for personal introspection and thoughtful planning about ways to reduce your risk.

Read each question and circle the number to indicate your response. Be honest and accurate in order to get the most complete understanding of your cancer risk. Individual scores for specific questions should not be interpreted as a precise measure of relative risk, but the totals in each section give a general indication of your risk.

SECTION 1: BREAST CANCER

	Yes	No
1. Do you check your breasts at least monthly using breast self-examination (BSE) procedures?	1	2
2. Do you look at your breasts in the mirror regularly and check for any irregular indentations/lumps, discharge from the nipples, or other noticeable changes?	1	2
3. Has your mother, sister, or daughter been diagnosed with breast cancer?	2	1
4. Have you ever been pregnant?	1	2
5. Have you had a history of lumps or cysts in your breasts or underarms?	2	1

Total Points _____

SECTION 2: SKIN CANCER

	Yes	No
1. Do you spend a lot of time in the sun, either at work or at play?	2	1
2. Do you use sunscreens with an SPF rating of 15 or more when you are in the sun?	1	2
3. Do you use tanning beds or sun booths regularly to maintain a tan?	2	1
4. Do you examine your skin once a month and check any moles or other irregularities, particularly in hard-to-see areas such as your back, genitals, neck, and under your hair?	1	2
5. Do you purchase and wear sunglasses that adequately filter out harmful sun rays?	1	2

Total Points _____

SECTION 3: CANCERS OF THE REPRODUCTIVE SYSTEM

MEN	Yes	No
1. Do you examine your penis regularly for unusual bumps or growths?	1	2
2. Do you perform regular testicular self-examination?	1	2
3. Do you have a family history of prostate or testicular cancer?	2	1
4. Do you practice safer sex and wear condoms with every sexual encounter?	1	2
5. Do you avoid exposure to harmful environmental hazards such as mercury, coal tars, benzene, chromate, and vinyl chloride?	1	2

Total Points _____

WOMEN	Yes	No
1. Do you have a regularly scheduled Pap test?	1	2
2. Have you been infected with the human papillomaviruses, Epstein-Barr virus, or other viruses believed to increase cancer risk?	2	1
3. Has your mother, sister, or daughter been diagnosed with breast, cervical, uterine, or ovarian cancer (particularly at a young age)?	2	1
4. Do you practice safer sex and use condoms with every sexual encounter?	1	2
5. Are you obese, taking estrogen, and/or consuming a diet that is very high in saturated fats?	2	1

Total Points _____

SECTION 4: CANCERS IN GENERAL

	Yes	No
1. Do you smoke cigarettes on most days of the week?	2	1
2. Do you consume a diet that is rich in fruits and vegetables?	1	2
3. Are you obese and/or do you lead a primarily sedentary lifestyle?	2	1
4. Do you live in an area with high air pollution levels and/or work in a job where you are exposed to several chemicals on a regular basis?	2	1
5. Are you careful about the amount of animal fat in your diet and substitute olive oil or canola oil for animal fat whenever possible?	1	2
6. Do you limit your overall consumption of alcohol?	1	2
7. Do you eat foods rich in lycopene (such as tomatoes) and antioxidants?	1	2
8. Are you "body aware" and alert for changes in your body?	1	2
9. Do you have a family history of ulcers or of colorectal cancer, stomach cancer, or other digestive system cancers?	2	1
10. Do you try to avoid unnecessary exposure to radiation, cell phone emissions, and microwave emissions?	1	2

Total Points _____

ANALYZING YOUR SCORES

Take a careful look at each question for which you received a 2 score. Are there any areas in which you received mostly 2s? Did you receive total points of 6 or higher in Sections 1–3? Did you receive total points of 11 or higher in Section 4? If so, you have at least one identifiable risk. The higher the score, the more risks you may have. However, rather than focusing just on your score, focus on which items you might change. Review the suggestions throughout this chapter, and list actions that you could take right now that might help you reduce your risk for these cancers. Plan a course of action that you can continue in the months ahead, and use the Behavior Change Contract to put these plans into action.

One of the most common occupational carcinogens is asbestos, a fibrous material once widely used in the construction, insulation, and automobile industries. Nickel, chromate, and chemicals such as benzene, arsenic, and vinyl chloride have definitively been shown to be carcinogens for humans. Also, people who routinely work with certain dyes and radioactive substances may have increased risks for cancer. Working with coal tars, as in the mining profession, or working near inhalants, as in the auto painting business, is hazardous. So is working with herbicides and pesticides, although the evidence is inconclusive for low-dose exposures. Several federal and state agencies are responsible for monitoring such exposures and ensuring that businesses comply with standards designed to protect workers.

Radiation: Ionizing and Non-Ionizing   Ionizing radiation (IR)—radiation from X rays, radon, cosmic rays, and ultraviolet (UV) radiation (primarily ultraviolet B, or UVB, radiation)—is the only form of radiation proven to cause human cancer. (See the section on skin cancer.) Incidents such as the Chernobyl accident in the 1980s focused attention on the potential risks of ionizing radiation. Evidence that high-dose IR causes cancer comes from studies of atomic bomb survivors, patients receiving radiotherapy, and certain occupational groups (for example, uranium miners). Virtually any part of the body can be affected by IR, but bone marrow and the thyroid are particularly susceptible. Radon exposures in homes can increase lung cancer risk, especially in cigarette smokers. To reduce the risk of harmful effects, diagnostic medical and dental X rays are set at the lowest dose levels possible.[21] Although non-ionizing radiation produced by radio waves, cell phones, microwaves, computer screens, televisions, electric blankets, and other products has been a topic of great concern in recent years, research has not proven excess risk to date.

Social and Psychological Factors

Many researchers claim that social and psychological factors play a major role in determining whether a person gets cancer. Stress has been implicated in increased susceptibility to several types of cancers. By reducing stress levels in your daily life, you may, in fact, lower your risk for cancer. A number of therapists have even established preventive treatment centers where the primary focus is on being happy and thinking positive thoughts. However, to date, no controlled studies have proven that laughter or positive thoughts can reduce cancer risks.

Although medical personnel are skeptical of overly simplistic solutions, we cannot rule out the possibility that negative emotional states contribute to disease. People who are under chronic, severe stress or who suffer from depression or other persistent emotional problems show higher rates of cancer than do their healthy counterparts. Sleep disturbances, diet, or a combination of factors may weaken the body's immune system and increase the susceptibility to cancer.

Although psychological factors may play a part in cancer development, exposure to substances such as tobacco and alcohol are far more important. The American Cancer Society states that cigarette smoking is responsible for 30 percent of all cancer deaths—and 87 percent of all lung cancer deaths. Heavy consumption of alcohol has been related to cancers of the mouth, larynx, throat, esophagus, and liver. These cancers show up even more frequently in people whose heavy drinking is accompanied by smoking. The negative effects of smoking are not just concerns for the active smoker. Every year, environmental (passive) tobacco smoke (ETS) causes an estimated 3,000 deaths from lung cancer, 40,000 deaths from heart disease, up to 300,000 respiratory problems, and countless deaths among nonsmokers. Cancers of the mouth and throat pose significant risks for smokers.[22]

Chemicals in Foods

Among the food additives suspected of causing cancer is *sodium nitrate,* a chemical used to preserve and give color to red meat. Research indicates that the actual carcinogen is not sodium nitrate but *nitrosamines,* substances formed when the body digests the chemical. Sodium nitrate has not been banned, primarily because it kills the bacterium *Clostridium botulinum,* which causes the highly virulent food-borne disease botulism. It should also be noted that the bacteria found in the human intestinal tract may contain more nitrates than a person could ever take in from eating cured meats or other nitrate-containing food products. Nonetheless, concern about the carcinogenic properties of nitrates has led to the introduction of meats that are nitrate-free or contain reduced levels of the substance.

Much of the concern about chemicals in foods centers on the possible harm caused by pesticide and herbicide residues. Although some of these chemicals cause cancer at high doses in experimental animals, the very low concentrations found in some foods are well within established government safety levels. Continued research regarding pesticide and herbicide use is essential, and the continuous monitoring of agricultural practices is necessary to ensure a safe food supply. Scientists and consumer groups stress the importance of a balance between chemical use and the production of quality food products. Prevention efforts should focus on policies to protect consumers, develop low-chemical pesticides and herbicides, and reduce environmental pollution. See Table 13.1 for more information on preventing cancer through diet and lifestyle.

Viral Factors

The chances of becoming infected with a "cancer virus" are very remote. However, several forms of virus-induced cancers have been observed in laboratory animals, and there is some indication that human beings display a similar tendency toward virally transmitted cancers. For example, the *herpes-related*

Table 13.1

Preventing Cancer through Diet and Lifestyle

Type	Decreases Risk	Increases Risk	Preventable by Diet
Lung	Vegetables, fruits	Smoking; some occupations	33–50%
Stomach	Vegetables, fruits; food refrigeration	Salt; salted foods	66–75%
Breast	Vegetables, fruits	Obesity; alcohol	33–50%
Colon/rectum	Vegetables; physical activity	Meat; alcohol; smoking	66–75%
Mouth/throat	Vegetables, fruits; physical activity	Salted fish; alcohol; smoking	33–50%
Liver	Vegetables	Alcohol; contaminated food	33–66%
Cervix	Vegetables, fruits	Smoking	10–20%
Esophagus	Vegetables, fruits	Deficient diet; smoking; alcohol	50–75%
Prostate	Vegetables	Meat or meat fat; dairy fat	10–20%
Bladder	Vegetables, fruits	Smoking; coffee	10–20%

Here are some tips issued by a panel of cancer researchers:

- Avoid being underweight or overweight, and limit weight gain during adulthood to less than 11 pounds.
- If you don't get much exercise at work, take a 1-hour brisk walk or similar exercise daily, and exercise vigorously for at least 1 hour a week.
- Eat 8 or more servings a day of cereals and grains (such as rice, corn, breads, and pasta), legumes (such as peas), roots (such as beets, radishes, and carrots), tubers (such as potatoes), and plantains (including bananas).
- Eat 5 or more servings a day of a variety of other vegetables and fruits.
- Limit consumption of refined sugar.
- Limit alcoholic drinks to less than 2 a day for men and 1 for women.
- Limit intake of red meat to less than 3 ounces a day, if eaten at all.
- Limit consumption of salted foods and use of cooking and table salt. Use herbs and spices to season foods.

Sources: World Cancer Research Fund, American Institute for Cancer Research.

viruses may be involved in the development of some forms of leukemia, Hodgkin's disease, cervical cancer, and Burkitt's lymphoma. The *Epstein-Barr virus,* associated with mononucleosis, may also contribute to cancer; cervical cancer has been linked to *human papillomavirus,* the virus that causes genital warts.[23] *Helicobacter pylori,* a chronic gastric bacterium that causes ulcers, is a major factor in the development of stomach cancer.[24]

Many scientists believe that selected viruses help to provide an *opportunistic* environment for subsequent cancer development. It is likely that a combination of immunological bombardment by viral or chemical invaders and other risk factors substantially increases the risk of cancer.

Medical Factors

Some medical treatments increase the risk of cancer. One famous example is the prescription drug *diethylstilbestrol (DES),* widely used from 1940 to 1960 to control problems with bleeding during pregnancy and reduce the risk of miscarriage. Not until the 1970s did the dangers of this drug became apparent. Although DES caused few side effects in the

millions of women who took it, their daughters were found to have an increased risk for cancer of the reproductive organs. Some scientists claim that estrogen replacement therapy (ERT) in postmenopausal women is dangerous because it increases the risk for uterine cancer. Others believe that the benefits of estrogen outweigh its risks. Chemotherapy to treat one cancer may increase the risks of the patient's developing other forms of cancer.

What do you think?

How do we determine whether a given factor is a risk factor for a disease? ✳ *Although a direct causal relationship between lung cancer and smoking has not been proved, the evidence supporting such a relationship is strong. Must a clearly established causal link exist before consumers are warned about risk?* ✳ *Can you think of apparent dietary risks for cancer that seemed conclusive but have since been refuted?* ✳ *How does the consumer know what to believe?*

What's New in Cancer Research, Prevention, and Treatment?

THE LATEST ON FIBER

Although fiber has been downplayed recently as a protective agent against colon and other forms of cancer, don't throw out that bran muffin just yet. A study of more than 68,000 women found that dietary fiber—particularly from breakfast cereals—can significantly decrease the risk of heart attacks by improving cholesterol levels, lowering blood sugar, boosting sensitivity to insulin, and lowering the risk of blood clotting. A previous study of men showed similar results. Also, while some recent studies questioned fiber's benefits for cancer prevention, many experts doubt that these findings should outweigh all the previous studies that indicate it does indeed reduce risk. In short, the scientific community is unsure of the fiber–cancer link but quite sure that the benefits in other areas more than justify a healthy high-fiber, low-fat diet.

ALCOHOL AND CANCER

Heavy drinking is associated with an increased risk for several cancers—notably, cancer of the mouth, esophagus, pharynx, larynx, liver, and pancreas. An analysis of multiple studies found that having two alcoholic drinks per day (any type of alcohol) increased a woman's chances of developing breast cancer by nearly 25 percent. The reasons for this are unclear, but researchers speculate that alcohol influences the metabolism of estrogen and that prolonged exposure to high levels of estrogen increases breast cancer risk, particularly for women on hormone replacement therapy (HRT). The effect of one drink per day is controversial, although most experts feel that one daily drink does not increase risk. But, before you toss out all of your alcohol, you should know that there is increasing evidence that a glass of red wine, with its antioxidant potential and HDL-boosting potential, seems to protect against heart disease.

NEW METHODS OF DETECTION

Several new methods of breast cancer detection are on the horizon.

- Blood tests. Researchers from the John Wayne Cancer Center in Santa Monica are developing biological markers that would identify microscopic tumors as they travel through the blood, before they are large enough to be picked up on conventional tests.
- "Pap test for the breast." Similar to the Pap test, which checks fluids from the cervix for abnormal cells, this newer test analyzes fluids from the breasts' milk ducts (where most tumors originate). It may be widely available soon. This test would pick up cancerous cells in their earliest, most treatable stages.
- Better breast scans. Researchers at the University of Chicago and elsewhere are developing better computer programs to point out questionable spots on mammograms and better, more reliable machines such as MRI machines.

Sources: American Dietetic Association, "Position Paper: Health Implications of Dietary Fiber," *Journal of the American Dietetic Association* (July 2002); "Fiber and Colon Cancer. . . . Again," *Nutrition Action Healthletter* (July–August 2003); H. Peters et al., "Dietary Fibre and Colorectal Adema in a Colorectal Cancer Early Detection Program," *The Lancet* 361, no. 9368 (2003): 1391. "The Facts about Drinking and Your Health," *Johns Hopkins Medical Health Letter—Health after 50* 12, no. 5 (2000): 4–6.

Types of Cancers

As mentioned earlier, the term *cancer* refers not to a single disease but to hundreds of different diseases. They are grouped into four broad categories based on the type of tissue from which the cancer arises.

Classifications of Cancer

- *Carcinomas.* Epithelial tissues (tissues covering body surfaces and lining most body cavities) are the most common sites for cancers. Carcinomas of the breast, lung, intestines, skin, and mouth are examples. These cancers affect the outer layer of the skin and mouth as well as the mucous membranes. They metastasize through the circulatory or lymphatic system initially and form solid tumors.
- *Sarcomas.* Sarcomas occur in the mesodermal, or middle, layers of tissue—for example, in bones, muscles, and general connective tissue. They metastasize primarily via the blood in the early stages of disease. These cancers are less common but generally more virulent than carcinomas. They also form solid tumors.
- *Lymphomas.* Lymphomas develop in the lymphatic system—the infection-fighting regions of the body—and metastasize through the lymphatic system. Hodgkin's disease is an example. Lymphomas also form solid tumors.
- *Leukemias.* Cancer of the blood-forming parts of the body, particularly the bone marrow and spleen, is called leukemia. A nonsolid tumor, leukemia is characterized by an abnormal increase in the number of white blood cells.

Trained oncologists determine the seriousness and general prognosis of a particular cancer. Once laboratory results and clinical observations have been made, cancers are rated by level and stage of development. Those diagnosed as "carcinoma in situ" are localized and often curable. Cancers with higher level or stage ratings have spread farther and are less likely to be cured. Figure 13.2 shows the most common cancer sites and the number of annual deaths from each type.

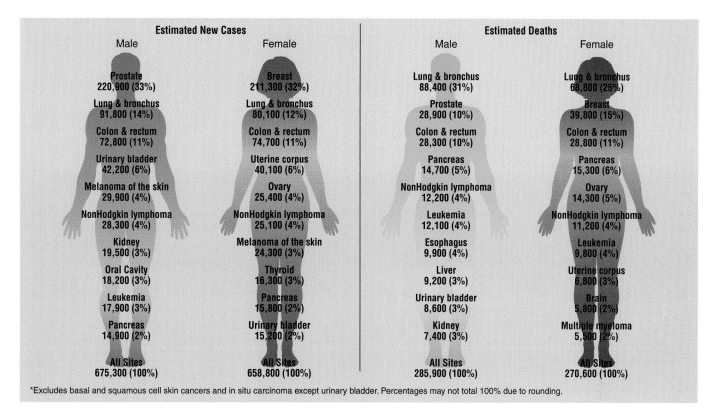

Figure 13.2

Leading Sites of New Cancer Cases and Deaths—2003 Estimates

Source: Reprinted by permission of the American Cancer Society, *Cancer Facts and Figures 2003*
(Atlanta: American Cancer Society, 2003).

Lung Cancer

Although lung cancer rates have dropped among white males during the past decade, the rate among white females and African American males and females continues to be a pervasive threat. Lung cancer killed an estimated 157,200 people in 2003. Since 1987, more women have died each year from lung cancer than from breast cancer, which for more than 40 years had been the major cause of cancer deaths in women. Today, lung cancer continues to be the leading cancer killer for both men and women.[25] As smoking rates have declined over the past 30 years, however, we have seen significant declines in male lung cancer. But these rates are not dropping as quickly among women. Another cause for concern is that although fewer adults are smoking, tobacco use among youth is again on the rise.

Symptoms of lung cancer include a persistent cough, blood-streaked sputum, chest pain, and recurrent attacks of pneumonia or bronchitis. Treatment depends on the type and stage of the cancer. Surgery, radiation therapy, and chemotherapy are all options. If the cancer is localized, surgery is usually the treatment of choice. If it has spread, surgery is combined with radiation and chemotherapy. Unfortunately, despite advances in medical technology, survival rates for lung cancer have improved only slightly over the past decade. Just 15 percent of lung cancer patients live five or more years after diagnosis. These rates improve to 49 percent with early detection, but only 15 percent of lung cancers are discovered in their early stages.[26]

Prevention Smokers, especially those who have smoked for more than 20 years, and people who have been exposed to industrial substances such as arsenic and asbestos or to radiation from occupational, medical, or environmental sources are at the highest risk for lung cancer. The American Cancer Society estimated that in 2003, more than 440,000 cancer deaths were caused by tobacco use and an additional 20,000 cancer deaths were related to alcohol use, frequently in combination with tobacco use.[27] Exposure to sidestream cigarette smoke, known as *environmental tobacco smoke* or *ETS,* increases the risk for nonsmokers. Researchers theorize that 90 percent of all lung cancers could be avoided if people did not smoke. Substantial improvements in overall prognosis have been noted in smokers who quit at the first signs of precancerous cellular changes and allow their bronchial linings to return to normal.

Breast Cancer

About one out of eight women will develop breast cancer at some time in her life. Although this oft-repeated ratio has frightened many women, it represents lifetime risk. Thus, not until the age of 80 does a woman's risk of breast cancer rise to one in eight.[28] Here is the risk at earlier ages:

- Birth to age 39: 1 in 227
- Ages 40 to 59: 1 in 25
- Ages 60 to 79: 1 in 15
- Birth to death: 1 in 8

In 2003, approximately 211,300 women in the United States were diagnosed with invasive breast cancer for the first time. In addition, 55,700 new cases of *in situ* breast cancer, typically Ductal Carcinoma In Situ (DCIS), a more localized cancer, were diagnosed. The increase in detection of DCIS is a direct result of earlier detection through mammographies.[29] In the same year, about 1,500 new cases of breast cancer were diagnosed in men. About 39,800 women (and 400 men) died, which makes breast cancer the second leading cause of cancer death for women.[30] According to the most recent data, mortality rates went down dramatically from 1990 to 1998, with the largest decrease in younger women, both white and African Americans.[31] The decline in rates may be due to earlier diagnosis and improved treatment.

Numerous studies have shown that early detection saves lives and increases treatment options. The earliest signs of breast cancer are usually observable on mammograms, often before lumps can be felt. However, mammograms are not foolproof. Hence, regular breast self-examination and careful attention to subtle body changes are important. If a mammogram detects a suspicious mass, a biopsy is performed to provide a more definitive assessment.

Once breast cancer has grown to where it can be palpated, symptoms may include persistent breast changes, such as a lump in the breast or surrounding lymph nodes, thickening, dimpling, skin irritation, distortion, retraction or scaliness of the nipple, nipple discharge, or tenderness. Breast pain is commonly due to noncancerous conditions, such as fibrocystic breasts, and is not usually a first symptom. However, any time pain or tenderness persists in the breast or underarm area, it is a good idea to seek medical attention.

Risk Factors   The incidence of breast cancer increases with age. Although there are many possible risk factors, those that are supported by research include:[32]

- Personal or family history of breast cancer (primary relatives, such as mother, daughter, sister)
- Biopsy-confirmed atypical hyperplasia (excessive increase in the number of cells)
- Long menstrual history (menstrual periods that started early and ended late in life)
- Obesity after menopause
- Recent use of oral contraceptives or postmenopausal estrogens
- Never having children, or having a first child after age 30
- Consuming two or more drinks of alcohol per day
- Higher education and socioeconomic status

Factors that need more rigorous research before being firmly established as risks include:

- Consuming a diet high in saturated fats
- Exposure to pesticides and other chemicals
- Weight gain, especially after menopause
- Physical inactivity
- Genetic predisposition through BRCA1 and BRCA2 genes. (Genes appear to account for approximately 5 percent of all cases of breast cancer. Screening for these genes is recommended for women with a family history of breast cancer, when counseling is available.)

Although risk factors are useful indicators, they do not always predict individual susceptibility. However, because of increased awareness, better diagnostic techniques, and improved treatments, breast cancer patients have a better chance of surviving today. The five-year survival rate for people with localized breast cancer (which includes all women living five years after diagnosis, whether the patient is in remission, disease-free, or under treatment) has risen from 72 percent in the 1940s to 97 percent today. These statistics vary dramatically, however, based on when the cancer is first detected. If the cancer has spread to surrounding tissue, the five-year survival rate is 78 percent. If it has spread to distant parts of the body, these rates fall to 23 percent. If the breast cancer has not spread at all, the survival rate approaches 100 percent. Survival after a diagnosis of breast cancer continues to decline beyond five years. Seventy-three percent of women diagnosed with breast cancer survive 10 years, and 59 percent survive 15 years.[33]

Prevention   A study of the role of exercise in reducing the risk for breast cancer generated much excitement in the scientific community. The study, which involved 1,090 women who were 40 or younger (545 with breast cancer and 545 without), analyzed subjects' exercise patterns since they began menstruating. The risk of those who averaged four hours of exercise a week since menstruation was 58 percent lower than that of women who did no exercise at all. More good news: subjects did not have to be avid joggers to have reduced risk. Their exercise included team sports, individual sports, dance, exercise classes, swimming, walking, and a variety of other activities. Researchers speculate that exercise may protect women by altering the production of the ovarian hormones estrogen and progesterone during menstrual cycles.

Other research has shown that vigorous athletics can delay the onset of menstruation and halt ovulation in some women. A woman's cumulative exposure to the sex hormones is associated with breast cancer risk.[34] Exercise can increase muscle mass and decrease body fat, which also lowers risk.[35]

Regular self-examination (Figure 13.3) and mammography are the best ways to detect breast cancer early. The American Cancer Society offers guidelines for how often women should get mammograms and other cancer checkups

How to Examine Your Breasts

Do you know that 95% of breast cancers are discovered first by women themselves? And that the earlier the breast cancer is detected, the better the chance for a complete cure? Of course, most lumps or changes are not cancer. But you can safeguard your health by making a habit of examining your breasts once a month—a day or two after your period, or, if you're no longer menstruating, on any given day. And, if you notice anything changed or unusual—a lump, thickening, or discharge—contact your doctor right away.

How to Look for Changes

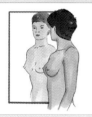

Step 1
Sit or stand in front of a mirror with your arms at your side. Turning slowly from side to side, check your breasts for
- changes in size or shape
- puckering or dimpling of the skin
- changes in size or position of one nipple compared to the other

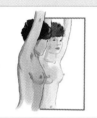

Step 2
Raise your arms above your head and repeat the examination in Step 1.

Step 3
Gently press each nipple with your fingertips to see if there is any discharge.

How to Feel for Changes

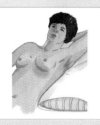

Step 1
Lie down and put a pillow or folded bath towel under your left shoulder. Then place your left hand under your head. (From now on you will be feeling for a lump or thickening in your breasts.)

Step 2
Imagine that your breast is divided into quarters.

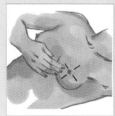

Step 3
With the fingers of your right hand held together, press firmly but gently, using small circular motions to feel the inner, upper quarter of your left breast. Start at your breastbone and work toward the nipple. Also examine the area around the nipple. Now do the same for the lower, inner portion of your breast.

Step 4
Next, bring your arm to your side and feel under your left armpit for swelling.

Step 5
With your arm still down, feel the upper, outer part of your breast, starting with your nipple and working outward. Examine the lower, outer quarter in the same way.

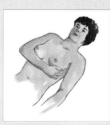

Step 6
Now place the pillow under your right shoulder and repeat all the steps, using your left hand to examine your right breast.

Figure 13.3
Breast Self-Examination
Follow these instructions for breast self-examination (BSE), the ten-minute habit that could save your life.

(Table 13.2 on page 352). All women, no matter their age, should be in the habit of breast self-examination every month. International differences in breast cancer incidence correlate with variations in diet, especially fat intake, although a causal role for dietary factors has not been firmly established. Sudden weight gain has also been implicated.

Treatment Today, people with breast cancer (like those with nearly any type of cancer) have many treatment options to choose from. It is important to thoroughly check out a physician's track record and his or her philosophy on the best treatment. Is the physician's recommendation consistent with that of major cancer centers in the country? Check out the doctor's credentials and the experiences of patients who have seen this doctor, as well as the surgeon who will perform your biopsy and other surgical techniques. If possible, seek a facility that has a significant number of breast cancer patients, does many surgeries, is regarded as a teaching facility for new oncologists, has the latest and greatest in terms of technology, and is highly regarded by past patients. Cancer support groups can provide invaluable information and advice. Treatments range from a lumpectomy to radical mastectomy to various combinations of radiation or chemotherapy. Seek more than one opinion before making a decision.

Colon and Rectum Cancers

Colorectal cancers (cancers of the colon and rectum) continue to be the third most common cancer in both men and women, with more than 147,500 cases diagnosed in 2003.[36] Although colon cancer is the third most common cancer in men and women, many people are unaware of their risk. In its early stages, colorectal cancer has no symptoms. Bleeding from the rectum, blood in the stool, and changes in bowel habits are the major warning signals. People who are over age 40, who are obese, who have a family history of colon and rectum cancer, a personal or family history of polyps (benign growths) in the colon or rectum, or inflammatory bowel problems, such as colitis, run an increased risk. Other possible risk factors include a diet high in fat or low in fiber, smoking, physical inactivity, high alcohol consumption, and low intake of fruit and vegetables. Studies have suggested that ERT and aspirin may reduce colorectal risk.[37]

Because colorectal cancer tends to spread slowly, the prognosis is quite good if it is caught in the early stages. Early screening can detect and remove precancerous polyps and diagnose disease at early, more treatable stages. Beginning at age 50, people at average risk should have a fecal occult blood test annually, flexible sigmoidoscopy every five years, or, preferably, both. Treatment often consists of radiation or surgery. Chemotherapy, although not used extensively in the past, is today a possibility. A permanent *colostomy,* the creation of an abdominal opening to eliminate body wastes, is seldom required.

Table 13.2
Recommendations for the Early Detection of Cancer in Asymptomatic People

Site	Recommendation
Cancer-Related Checkup	For individuals undergoing periodic health examinations, a cancer-related checkup should include health counseling and, depending on a person's age, might include examination for cancers of the thyroid, oral cavity, skin, lymph nodes, testes, and ovaries, as well as for some nonmalignant diseases.
Breast	Women 40 and older should have an annual mammogram and an annual clinical breast exam (CBE) performed by a health care professional, and should perform monthly breast self-examination (BSE). Ideally, the CBE should occur before the scheduled mammogram.
	Women ages 20–39 should have a clinical breast exam performed by a health care professional every 3 years and should perform monthly breast self-examination.
Colon and Rectum	Beginning at age 50, men and women should follow one of the examination schedules below: <ul><li>A fecal occult blood (FOBT) test every year, or</li><li>A flexible sigmoidoscopy (FSIG) every five years, or</li><li>Annual fecal occult blood test and flexible sigmoidoscopy every five years.*</li><li>A double-contrast barium enema every 5 to 10 years.</li><li>A colonoscopy every 10 years.</li></ul>
Prostate	The American Cancer Society recommends that both the prostate-specific antigen (PSA) blood test and the digital rectal examination be offered annually, beginning at age 50, to men who have a life expectancy of at least 10 more years.
	Men at high risk (African-American men and men with a strong family history of one or more first-degree relatives diagnosed with prostate cancer at an early age) should begin testing at age 45.
	Information should be provided to patients about what is known and what is uncertain about the benefits and limitations of early detection and treatment of prostate cancer, so that they can make an informed decision.
Uterus	**Cervix:** Screening should begin approximately 3 years after a woman begins having vaginal intercourse, but no later than 21 years of age. Screening should be done every year with Pap tests or every 2 years using liquid-based tests. At or after age 30, women who have had 3 normal tests in a row may get screened every 2–3 years, unless they have certain risk factors, such as HIV infection or a weak immune system.
	Endometrium: The American Cancer Society recommends that all women should be informed about the risks and symptoms of endometrial cancer, and strongly encouraged to report any unexpected bleeding or spotting to their physicians. Annual screening for endometrial cancer with endometrial biopsy beginning at age 35 should be offered to women with or at risk for hereditary nonpolyposis colon cancer (HNPCC).

*Combined testing is preferred over either annual FOBT or FSIG every 5 years alone. People who are at moderate or high risk for colorectal cancer should talk with a doctor about a different testing schedule.

Source: American Cancer Society, *Cancer Facts and Figures 2003* (Atlanta: American Cancer Society, 2003). Reprinted with permission.

Prostate Cancer

Cancer of the prostate gland is the most common type of cancer in males today, after skin cancer. In 2003, 220,000 new cases of prostate cancer were diagnosed, and from these, about 28,900 men would die.[38]

From 1980 to 1990, prostate cancer incidence rates increased by 65 percent, largely because of earlier diagnosis in men without symptoms. This was accomplished by increased use of **prostate-specific antigen (PSA)** blood test screenings and increased public awareness.[39] Today, prostate cancer rates are declining due to improved diagnosis and treatment, although rates remain more than twice as high among African American men than white men.

Most signs of prostate cancer are nonspecific—that is, they mimic the signs of infection or enlarged prostate. Symptoms include weak or interrupted urine flow; difficulty starting or stopping the urine flow; the need to urinate frequently; pain or difficulty in urinating; blood in the urine; and pain in the lower back, pelvis, or upper thighs. Many men mistake these symptoms for infections or normal aging, and delay seeking treatment.

Incidence of prostate cancer increases with age; more than 75 percent of all cases are diagnosed in men over age 65, although increasing numbers of young men seem to be

> **Prostate-specific antigen (PSA)** An antigen found in prostate cancer patients.

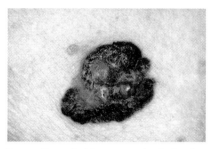 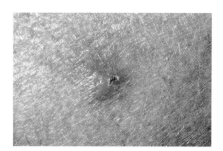 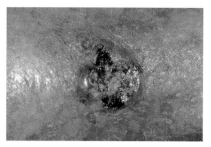

Prevention of skin cancer includes keeping a careful watch for any new pigmented growths and for changes to any moles. Melanoma symptoms, as shown in the left photo, include scalloped edges, asymmetrical shapes, discoloration, and an increase in size. Basal cell carcinoma and squamous cell carcinoma (middle and right photos) should be brought to your physician's attention but are not as deadly as melanoma.

affected. African Americans have the highest prostate cancer rates in the world. The disease is most common in north-western Europe and North America, but rare in the Near East, Africa, Central America, and South America. There seems to be a slightly increased risk if a family member has the disease, but it is unclear whether this is due to genetic or environmental factors. Recent genetic studies suggest that strong familial predisposition may be responsible for 5 to 10 percent of prostate cancers.[40] International studies suggest that dietary fat may also be a factor.

Fortunately, 83 percent of all prostate cancers are detected while they are still in the local or regional stages and tend to progress slowly. Five-year survival rates in these early stages is 100 percent. Because most men develop the disease in their late 60s and early 70s, it is likely that they will die of other causes first. For this reason, some health care groups question the cost effectiveness and necessity of prostate surgeries and other costly procedures that may have little real effect on life expectancy. Over the past 20 years, the survival rate for all stages combined has increased from 67 percent to 96 percent, largely due to earlier diagnosis and improved treatment.

Every man over age 40 should have an annual digital rectal prostate examination. In addition, the American Cancer Society recommends that men aged 50 and older have an annual PSA test. If either result is suspicious, further evaluation in the form of transrectal ultrasound is recommended.[41]

Skin Cancer: Sun Worshipers Beware

If you are one of the millions of people who try to get a "healthy tan" each year, think again. As the primary cause of more than 1.3 million cases of skin cancer in the United States this year, many of which will disfigure or permanently change the person's appearance, the sun may just be the skin's public enemy number one. Skin cancer is the most common cancer in the United States today and accounts for nearly 2 percent of all cancer deaths.[42]

Although most people don't die from the highly treatable *basal* or *squamous cell* skin cancers, the highly virulent **malignant melanoma** has become the most frequent cancer in women ages 25 to 29 and runs second only to breast cancer in women ages 30 to 34. Rates of melanoma are ten times higher among whites than African Americans. In 2003, 9,800 people died of skin cancer. Of those, 7,600 died of melanoma and 2,200 died of other forms of skin cancer.[43]

In spite of these grisly statistics, more than 60 percent of all Americans 25 years and under report that they are "working on a tan" at some point during the year. Fewer than one in three sunbathers bothers to wear UVB-thwarting sunscreen lotions. Are tanning booths safer than natural sunlight? No. Tanning lamps emit large amounts of UV radiation that are at least two to three times more powerful than the ultraviolet A (UVA) rays that occur naturally from the sun. In fact, according to experts at the American Academy of Dermatology, a single 15 to 30 minute salon session exposes the body to the same amount of harmful UV light as an entire day at the beach.[44] See the Skills for Behavior Change box on the next page for strategies to stay safe in the sun.

Many people do not know what to look for when examining themselves for skin cancer. Basal and squamous cell carcinomas can be a recurrent annoyance, showing up most commonly on the face, ears, neck, arms, hands, and legs as warty bumps, colored spots, or scaly patches. Bleeding, itchiness, pain, or oozing are other symptoms that warrant attention. Surgery may be necessary to remove them, but they are seldom life-threatening. In striking contrast is the insidious melanoma, an invasive killer that quickly spreads to regional organs and throughout the body and accounts for more than 75 percent of all skin cancer deaths. Risks increase dramatically among whites after age 20.[45] Often, melanoma starts as a normal-looking mole but quickly develops abnormal characteristics. A simple *ABCD* rule outlines the warning signs of melanoma:

- *Asymmetry*—One half of the mole does not match the other half.
- *Border irregularity*—The edges are uneven, notched, or scalloped.

Malignant melanoma   A virulent cancer of the melanin (pigment-producing portion) of the skin.

Tips for Sun Worshipers

Planning on working on your suntan? Before heading out, consider these facts.

TANNING AND THE ANATOMY OF A BURN

Ultraviolet A (UVA) and B (UVB) rays tan, burn, and age the skin. Tanning is how the skin protects itself from damage. UVA rays darken melanin grains in the epidermis, the skin's top layer. After a few days, newly pigmented skin cells, stimulated by both UVA and UVB rays, migrate to the surface. UVA rays are weaker than UVB rays, but more of them penetrate the dermis, or deepest layer of skin. Over time, exposure can break down collagen and lead to wrinkles and other signs of aging. UVB radiation is the main cause of burns and skin cancer. These shorter-wavelength rays have more energy than UVA rays and damage cells in the epidermis.

TIME OF DAY

How long you're in the sun matters, but so does time of day. Burning is more likely between 10:00 A.M. and 3:00 P.M., when the atmosphere filters out less ultraviolet (UV) energy.

CLOUD COVER

Clouds let 80% of UV rays through and increase exposure by scattering the rays. It's important to protect your skin even on cloudy days.

PEAK PROTECTION

At high altitudes more UV rays get through, and snow reflects 80% of sunlight. Wear protective clothing and a high-SPF (sun protection factor) sunscreen.

IN THE WATER

UV rays can burn parts of your body that are under water, so use waterproof sunscreen. Wearing a shirt while swimming and wading is advisable, because UV rays reflected off water and sand intensify exposure.

SUNGLASSES

Shades not only cut glare, but also reduce the risk of UV-caused cataracts.

WHAT TO WEAR

An ordinary t-shirt has an effective SPF of only 6 to 8, which drops to 4 or 5 when wet. The more opaque the material, the fewer UV rays get through. Color, however, doesn't affect the number of UV rays that penetrate the fabric. Special sun-blocking clothing has an SPF of 30 or more.

SUNSCREEN TIPS

Apply an SPF 15 or higher sunscreen to the entire body 30 minutes before going out. Use at least a full ounce. Reapply even "waterproof" sunscreen if you're in the water longer than 80 minutes, towel off, or perspire heavily. Recent reports have highlighted the potential harmful effects of one active ingredient in some sunscreens, oxybenzone, particularly after repeated applications. The concern is based on the fact that this chemical is absorbed in the body and may have long-term negative effects.

STAY ALERT

Avoid alcohol use on hot, sunny days. It can make you so sleepy that you doze off in the sun, or it can numb the first warning signs of sunburn.

Sources: Adapted by permission from "A Sun Worshiper's Guide," *U.S. News & World Report,* June 24, 1996. Basic data from the American Academy of Dermatology, American Optometric Association, Sun Precautions, Inc.; "The Active Ingredients in Sunscreen: Is It Safe?" *Health-facts* 23 (1998): 5.

- *Color*—Pigmentation is not uniform. Melanoma may vary in color from tan to deeper brown, reddish black, black, or deep bluish black.
- *Diameter*—The diameter is greater than 6 millimeters (about the size of a pea).

If you notice any of these symptoms, consult a physician promptly.

Skin cancer is one of the most preventable forms of cancer. Key strategies to reduce risk include limiting exposure to the sun, particularly at midday; wearing hats, protective clothing, and sunglasses; and using sunscreen with an adequate sun protection factor (SPF).

Treatment of skin cancer depends on its seriousness. Surgery is performed in 90 percent of all cases. Radiation therapy, *electrodesiccation* (tissue destruction by heat), and *cryosurgery* (tissue destruction by freezing) are also common forms of treatment. For melanoma, treatment may involve surgical removal of the regional lymph nodes, radiation, or chemotherapy.

Testicular Cancer

Testicular cancer is one of the most common types of solid tumors found in young adult males. Those between the ages of 17 and 34 are at greatest risk. There has been a steady increase in tumor frequency over the past several years in this age group.[46] Although the cause of testicular cancer is unknown, several risk factors have been identified. Males with undescended testicles appear to be at greatest risk, and some studies indicate a genetic influence.

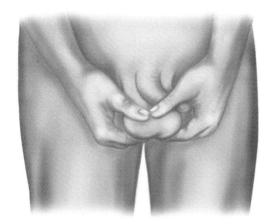

Figure 13.4

Testicular Self-Examination

Examine each testicle by placing the index and middle fingers of each hand on the underside of the testicle and the thumbs on top. Gently roll the testicle between your thumbs and fingers. If a suspicious lump or thickening is found, consult a doctor immediately. Perform the exam after a bath or shower, when the heat causes the testicles to descend and the scrotal skin to relax.

In general, testicular tumors first appear as a painless enlargement of the testis or thickening in testicular tissue. Because this enlargement is often painless, it is extremely important that all young men practice regular testicular self-examination (Figure 13.4).

Ovarian Cancer

Ovarian cancer is the fourth leading cause of cancer death for women; it killed 14,300 in 2003.[47] Because its symptoms are often nonspecific, ovarian cancer frequently goes undiagnosed in its early stages. The most common sign is enlargement of the abdomen (or a feeling of bloating) in women over age 40. Other symptoms include vague digestive disturbances, such as persistent gas and stomachache, fatigue, pain during intercourse, unexplained weight loss, unexplained changes in bowel or bladder habits, urinary frequency, and incontinence. (Abnormal vaginal bleeding is rarely a symptom.)

The risk for ovarian cancer increases with age and peaks in women's late 70s. Women who have never had children are twice as likely to develop ovarian cancer as are those who have. This is because the main risk factor appears to be exposure to the reproductive hormone estrogen. Women who have multiple pregnancies or use oral contraceptives, both of which inhibit estrogen, are at lower risk. In addition, having one or more primary relatives (mother, sisters, grandmothers) who have had the disease appears to increase risk. With the exception of Japan, the highest incidence rates are reported in the industrialized countries of the world. Research

indicates that mutations in the BRCA1 and BRCA2 genes may increase risk.[48] Another genetic syndrome, hereditary non-polyposis colon cancer (HNPCC) has also been linked to increased risk.

Prevention An early Yale University study indicated that diet may play a role in ovarian cancer.[49] When comparing 450 Canadian women who had newly diagnosed ovarian cancer with 564 demographically similar, healthy women, researchers found that the women without ovarian cancer had a diet lower in saturated fat. For every 10 grams of saturated fat a woman ate per day, her risk of ovarian cancer rose 20 percent. Conversely, women who lowered their saturated fat consumption by 10 grams a day experienced a 20 percent drop in risk. Every 10 grams of vegetable fiber (but not fruit or cereal fiber) added to a woman's daily menu lowered her risk by 37 percent. The study also found that each full-term pregnancy lowered risk by about 20 percent, and each year of oral contraceptive use lowered it by 5 to 10 percent. So, should you get pregnant or start taking birth control pills to reduce risk? No. However, these results, particularly when combined with cardiovascular studies and other health information, provide yet another reason to eat plenty of vegetables and cut down on your fat intake.

To protect yourself, annual thorough pelvic examinations are important. Pap tests, although useful in detecting cervical cancer, do not reveal ovarian cancer. Women over age 40 should have a cancer-related checkup every year. Transvaginal ultrasound and a tumor marker, CA125, may assist in diagnosis but are not recommended for routine screening.[50] If you have any symptoms of ovarian cancer and they persist, see your doctor promptly.

Uterine Cervical and Uterine Corpus (Endometrium) Cancer

In 2003, an estimated 12,200 new cases of uterine cervix and 40,100 cases of uterine corpus (endometrium) cancer were diagnosed in the United States. Most uterine cancers develop in the body of the uterus, usually in the endometrium (lining). The rest develop in the cervix, located at the base of the uterus. The overall incidence of early-stage uterine cancer—that is, cervical cancer—has increased slightly in recent years in women under age 50.[51] In contrast, invasive, later-stage forms of the disease appear to be decreasing. This may be due to more regular screenings of younger women using the **Pap test,** a procedure in which cells taken from the cervical region are examined for abnormal cellular activity. Although the Pap test is very effective for detecting early-stage cervical cancer, it is less effective for detecting cancers

Pap test A procedure in which cells taken from the cervical region are examined for abnormal cellular activity.

of the uterine lining and not effective at all for detecting cancers of the fallopian tubes or ovaries.[52]

Risk factors for cervical cancer include early age of first intercourse, multiple sex partners, cigarette smoking, and certain sexually transmitted diseases, such as the herpesvirus and the human papillomavirus. For endometrial cancer, a history of infertility, failure to ovulate, obesity, and treatment with tamoxifen or unopposed estrogen therapy appear to be major risk factors.[53]

Early warning signs of uterine cancer include bleeding outside the normal menstrual period or after menopause, or persistent unusual vaginal discharge. These symptoms should be checked by a physician immediately.[54]

Cancer of the Pancreas

The incidence of cancer of the pancreas, known as a "silent" disease, has increased substantially during the last 25 years to 30,700 cases in 2003.[55] Chronic inflammation of the pancreas, diabetes, cirrhosis, and a high-fat diet may contribute to its development. Smokers have double the risk of nonsmokers.[56] Unfortunately, pancreatic cancer is one of the worst cancers to get. Only 4 percent of patients live more than five years after diagnosis, usually because the disease is well advanced by the time there are any symptoms.

Leukemia

Leukemia is a cancer of the blood-forming tissues that leads to proliferation of millions of immature white blood cells. These abnormal cells crowd out normal white blood cells (which fight infection), platelets (which control hemorrhaging), and red blood cells (which carry oxygen to the cells). As a result, symptoms such as fatigue, paleness, weight loss, easy bruising, repeated infections, nosebleeds, and other forms of hemorrhaging occur. In children, these symptoms can appear suddenly.[57]

Leukemia can be acute or chronic and can strike both sexes and all age groups. Although many people think of it as a childhood disease, leukemia struck many more adults (30,600) than children (2,000) in 2003.[58] Chronic leukemia can develop over several months and have few symptoms. The five-year survival rate for patients with chronic lymphocytic leukemia, one of the most common types, had increased to 73.1 percent by 2003.

Magnetic resonance imaging (MRI) A device that uses magnetic fields, radio waves, and computers to generate an image of internal tissues of the body for diagnostic purposes without the use of radiation.

Computerized axial tomography (CAT scan) A machine that uses radiation to view internal organs not normally visible on X rays.

Facing Cancer

While heart disease mortality rates have declined steadily over the past 50 years, cancer mortality has increased consistently in the same period. Based on current rates, about 83 million Americans—or one in three of us now living—will eventually develop cancer. Many factors have contributed to the rise in cancer mortality, but the increased incidence of lung cancer—a largely preventable disease—is probably the most important. Despite these gloomy predictions, recent advancements in diagnosis and treatment have reduced much of the fear and mystery that once surrounded cancer.

Detecting Cancer

The earlier cancer is diagnosed, the better the prospect for survival. Several high-tech tools have been developed to detect cancer. They include the following.

- New high-technology diagnostic imaging techniques have replaced exploratory surgery for some cancer patients. In **magnetic resonance imaging (MRI),** a huge electromagnet detects hidden tumors by mapping the vibrations of the various atoms in the body on a computer screen.
- **Computerized axial tomography scanning (CAT scan)** uses X rays to examine parts of the body. In both of these painless, noninvasive procedures, cross-section pictures can reveal a tumor's shape and location more accurately than conventional x-ray films.
- *Prostatic ultrasound* (a rectal probe using ultrasonic waves to produce an image of the prostate) is being investigated as a means to increase the early detection of prostate cancer. Prostatic ultrasound has been combined with a blood test for PSA, an antigen found in prostate cancer patients.

Such medical techniques, along with regular self-examinations and checkups, play an important role in the early detection and secondary prevention of cancer. Table 13.3 shows the seven warning signals of cancer. Make sure you know which symptoms to watch for, and follow the recommendations for self-exams and medical checkups in Table 13.2.

New Hope in Cancer Treatments

Although cancer treatments have changed dramatically over the past 20 years, surgery, in which the tumor and surrounding tissue are removed, is still common. Today's surgeons tend to remove less surrounding tissue than previously and to combine surgery with either **radiotherapy** (the use of radiation) or **chemotherapy** (the use of drugs) to kill cancerous cells.

Radiation works by destroying malignant cells or stopping cell growth. It is most effective in treating localized cancer masses. Unfortunately, in the process of destroying malignant cells, radiotherapy also destroys some healthy cells. It may also increase the risk for other types of cancers. Despite these qualifications, radiation continues to be one of the most common and effective forms of treatment.

When cancer has spread throughout the body, it is necessary to use some form of chemotherapy. Currently, more than 50 different anticancer drugs are in use, some of which have excellent records of success. A chemotherapeutic regimen of four anticancer drugs combined with radiotherapy has resulted in remarkable survival rates for some cancers, including Hodgkin's disease. Ongoing research will result in new drugs that are less toxic to normal cells and more potent against tumor cells. Current research indicates that some tumors may actually be resistant to certain forms of chemotherapy and that the treatment drugs do not reach the core of the tumor. Scientists are working to circumvent resistance and make tumor cells more vulnerable.

Whether used alone or in combination, radiotherapy and chemotherapy have side effects, including extreme nausea, nutritional deficiencies, hair loss, and general fatigue. Long-term damage to the cardiovascular system and other body systems can be significant. It is important to discuss these matters fully with doctors when making treatment plans.

Substances found in nature, such as taxol (originally found in Pacific Yew trees), are being synthesized in laboratories and tested on a variety of cancers. Other compounds, including those derived from sea urchins, are rich in resources for anticancer drugs.

Today, researchers are targeting cancer as a genetic disease that is brought on by some form of mutation, either inherited or acquired. Promising treatments focus on stopping the cycle of these mutant cells, targeting toxins through monoclonal antibodies, and rousing the immune system to be more effective. Other treatments are being pursued on many fronts, including *tamoxifen* as an alternative to chemotherapy for breast cancer; *cancer-fighting vaccines* that alert the body's immune defenses to healthy cells that have turned cancerous; *gene therapy;* compounds that inhibit angiogenesis, the process by which tumors form new blood vessels; and *neoadjuvant chemotherapy* (giving chemotherapy to shrink the cancer and then removing it surgically).

Talking with Your Doctor about Cancer

Anytime cancer is suspected, people react with anxiety, fear, and anger. Emotional distress is sometimes so intense that they are unable to make critical health care decisions. If you find it difficult to talk to your doctor on a routine exam, imagine how hard it would be to discuss life-or-death options. Before you arrive at the doctor's office, prepare a list of questions. Remember, your health care provider should be your partner and help you make the best decisions for yourself.

If the diagnosis is cancer, here are some suggestions for questions to ask:

- What kind of cancer do I have? What stage is it in? Based on my age and stage, what prognosis do I have?
- What are my treatment choices? Which do you recommend? Why?
- What are the benefits of each kind of treatment?
- What are the long- and short-term risks and possible side effects?
- Would a clinical trial be appropriate for me? (Clinical trials are research studies designed to answer specific questions and to find better ways to prevent or treat cancer. Often new cancer-fighting treatments are used.)

If surgery is recommended, you may want to ask:

- What kind of operation will it be, and how long will it take? What form of anesthesia will be used? How many similar procedures has this surgeon done in the past month? What is his or her success rate?
- How will I feel after surgery? If I have pain, how will you help me?
- Where will the scars be? What will they look like? Will they cause disability?

Radiotherapy   The use of radiation to kill cancerous cells.

Chemotherapy   The use of drugs to kill cancerous cells.

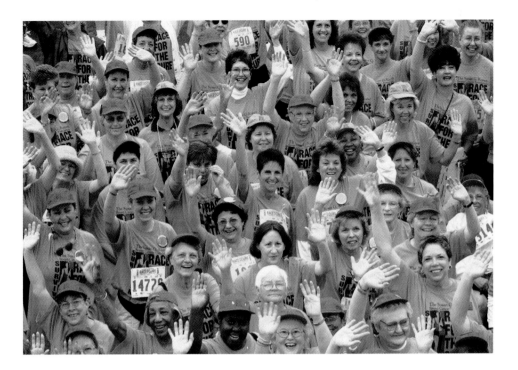

Cancer survivors can live long and healthy lives. Some, such as these breast cancer survivors and their supporters, take place in walkathons, races, and other activities to raise money for cancer research and treatment and to raise public awareness about prevention.

- Will I have any activity limitations after surgery? What kind of physical therapy, if any, will I have? When will I get back to normal activities?

If radiation is recommended, you may want to know:

- Why do you think this treatment is better than my other options?
- How long will I need to have treatments, and what will the side effects be in the short and long term? What body organs or systems may be damaged?
- What can I do to take care of myself during therapy? Are there services available to help me?
- What is the long-term prognosis for people my age with my type of cancer who are using this treatment?

Questions to ask about chemotherapy include:

- Why do you think this treatment is better than my other options?
- Which drug combinations pose the fewest risks and most benefits?
- What are the short- and long-term side effects on my body?
- What are my options?

Before you begin any form of cancer therapy, it is imperative to be a vigilant and vocal consumer. Read and seek information from cancer support groups. Check the skills of your surgeon, your radiation therapist, and your doctor in terms of clinical experience and interpersonal interactions.

Life After Cancer

Heightened public awareness and an improved prognosis have made the cancer experience less threatening and isolating than it once was. While you may hear stories of recovering cancer patients experiencing job discrimination and being unable to obtain health or life insurance, these cases are decreasing. Several states have even enacted legislation to prevent insurance companies from canceling policies or instituting other forms of discrimination. Health insurance can be obtained through large employers. Because large companies spread the insurance risk among many employees, insurance companies accept new employees without underwriting.

In fact, assistance for the cancer patient is more readily available than ever. Cancer support groups, cancer information workshops, and low-cost medical consultation are just a few of the forms of assistance now offered in many communities. The national breast cancer coalition and other groups have successfully lobbied Congress to increase cancer research dollars. As a result, government funding has increased substantially over the past decade. The battle for funds continues. Increasing efforts in cancer research, improvements in diagnostic equipment, and advances in treatment provide hope for the future.

Make It Happen!

Assessment: The Assess Yourself box on page 344 identifies certain behaviors that can contribute to increased cancer risks. If you have identified particular behaviors that may be putting you at risk, consider steps you can take to change these behaviors and improve your future health.

Making a Change: In order to change your behavior, you need to develop a plan. Follow these steps.

1. Evaluate your behavior, and identify patterns and specific things you are doing. What can you change now? What can you change in the near future?
2. Select one pattern of behavior that you want to change.
3. Fill out a Behavior Change Contract. It should include your long-term goal for change, your short-term goals, the rewards you'll give your- self for reaching these goals, potential obstacles along the way, and strategies for overcoming these ob- stacles. For each goal, list the small steps and specific actions that you will take.
4. Chart your progress in a journal. At the end of a week, consider how successful you were in following your plan. What helped you be suc- cessful? What made change more difficult? What will you do differ- ently next week?
5. Revise your plan as needed. Are the short-term goals attainable? Are the rewards satisfying?

Example: Keisha's assessment showed that, while she was taking pre- cautions to reduce her cancer risk in most areas, she was not doing what she should about her breast cancer risk. Her score in this area was 8, be- cause she did not regularly examine her breasts, her mother had been diag- nosed with breast cancer two years ago, and she had never been pregnant. Keisha decided she needed to learn how to examine her breasts and to make a plan to ensure she did it every month. After studying this textbook's illustrations, she made an appointment with her gynecologist. While she was there, she asked the doctor to confirm that she was doing the examination correctly.

Next, Keisha decided that she would spend the first ten minutes of her morning once a month to do the exam and that she would give herself a re- ward for each month that she exam- ined herself on schedule. On her way to campus after doing the exam, she would treat herself to a latte and a scone. After she stuck with her sched- ule for six months in a row, she would buy herself a new outfit. She also re- solved to talk to her younger sister, who was also at risk, about the impor- tance of the exam.

Summary

* Cancer is a group of diseases characterized by uncon- trolled growth and spread of abnormal cells. These cells may create tumors. Benign (noncancerous) tumors grow in size but do not spread; malignant (cancerous) tumors spread to other parts of the body.
* Several causes of cancer have been identified. Lifestyle factors include smoking and obesity. Biological factors in- clude inherited genes and gender. Occupational and envi- ronmental hazards are carcinogens present in people's home or work environments. Chemicals in foods that may act as carcinogens include preservatives and pesti- cides. Viral diseases that may lead to cancer include her- pes, mononucleosis, and human papillomavirus (which causes genital warts). Medical factors include certain drug therapies given for other conditions that may elevate the chance of cancer. Combined risk refers to a combination of the above factors, which tends to compound the risk for cancer.
* There are many different types of cancer, each of which poses different risks, depending on a number of factors. Common cancers include lung, breast, colon and rectum, prostate, skin, testicular, ovarian, uterine, and pancreatic cancers, as well as leukemia.
* Early diagnosis improves survival rate. Self-exams for breast, testicular, and skin cancer and knowledge of the seven warning signals of cancer aid early diagnosis.
* New types of cancer treatments include various combina- tions of radiotherapy, chemotherapy, and immunotherapy.

Questions for Discussion and Reflection

1. What is cancer? How does it spread? What is the difference between a benign and a malignant tumor?
2. List the likely causes of cancer. Do any of them put you at greater risk? What can you do to reduce your risk? What risk factors do you share with family members? With friends?
3. What are the symptoms of lung, breast, prostate, and testicular cancer? What can you do to reduce your risk of developing these cancers or increase your chances of surviving them?
4. What are the differences between carcinomas, sarcomas, lymphomas, and leukemia? Which is the most common? Least common?
5. Why are breast and testicular self-exams important for women and men? What could be the consequences of not doing these exams regularly?
6. Discuss the seven warning signals of cancer. What could signal that you have cancer instead of a minor illness? How soon should you seek treatment for any of the warning signs?

Accessing Your Health on the Internet

Visit the following Internet sites to explore further topics and issues related to personal health. To visit an organization's website, go to the Companion Website for *Health: The Basics, Sixth Edition* at www.aw-bc.com/donatelle, click on the book image, and select "Accessing Your Health on the Internet" from the navigation menu on the left.

1. *American Cancer Society.* Home page for the leading private organization dedicated to cancer prevention. This site provides information, statistics, and resources regarding cancer.
2. *International Cancer Information Center.* Sponsored by the National Cancer Institute, this site is designed to be a comprehensive information resource on cancer for patients and health professionals.
3. *National Cancer Institute.* Check here for information on clinical trials and the Physician Data Query (PDQ), a comprehensive database of cancer treatment information.
4. *National Women's Health Information Center (NWHIC).* Provides a wealth of information about cancer in women. Cosponsored by the National Cancer Institute.
5. *Oncolink.* Sponsored by the University of Pennsylvania Cancer Center, this site seeks to educate cancer patients and their families by offering information on support services, cancer causes, screening, prevention, and common questions.

Further Reading

American Cancer Institute Journal, published monthly.

> *Focuses on current risk factors, prevention, and treatment research in the area of cancer.*

American Cancer Society. *Cancer Facts and Figures.* Atlanta, GA: published annually.

> *A summary of major facts relating to cancer. Provides information on incidence, prevalence, symptomology, prevention, and treatment. Available through local divisions of the American Cancer Society.*

American Cancer Society. *A Breast Cancer Journey: Your Personal Guidebook, 2nd ed.* Atlanta: American Cancer Society, 2004.

> *Contains up-to-date information on treatments, medicines, reconstructive surgery, and complementary and alternative options. Also includes information for caregivers, family, and friends.*

Nutrition and Cancer Journal, published monthly.

> *Focuses on etiological aspects of various dietary factors and research on risks for cancer development. Also includes current research on dietary factors and prevention.*

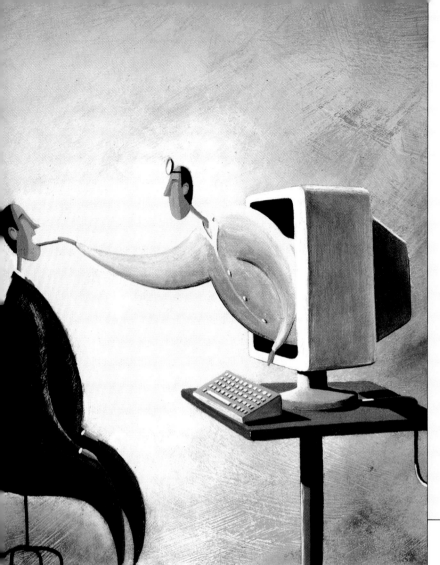

Infectious and Noninfectious Conditions

Risks and Responsibilities

Objectives

* Discuss the risk factors for infectious diseases.

* Describe the most common pathogens infecting humans today.

* Explain how your immune system works to protect you and what factors may make it less effective.

* Explain the major emerging and resurgent diseases affecting humans; discuss why they are increasing in incidence and what actions are being taken to reduce risks.

* Discuss the various sexually transmitted infections, their means of transmission, and actions that can be taken to prevent their spread.

* Discuss human immunodeficiency virus and acquired immune deficiency syndrome, trends in infection and treatment, and the impact on special populations, such as women and members of the international community.

* Discuss the chronic lung diseases, common neurological disorders, diabetes and other digestion-related disorders, and the varied musculoskeletal diseases.

The New York Times

In the News

H.I.V. Secrecy Is Proving Deadly

By Howard Markel

With the progress in the medical treatment for HIV over the past decade, unsafe sexual practices have risen and prevention efforts stalled.

And when it comes to being infected with HIV, the truth still remains shrouded in secrecy.

Today, many public health experts say that failure to disclose HIV infection to partners, whether unintentionally or intentionally, is a significant but underreported factor in the continued spread of the virus in the United States.

The Centers for Disease Control and Prevention estimates that as many as 33 percent of the 900,000 Americans infected with the virus may not know it.

Dr. Robert Klitzman, a psychiatrist, and Dr. Ronald Bayer, an ethicist, both professors at Columbia, have explored the prevailing range of views and practices concerning HIV disclosure in a newly published book, *Mortal Secrets: Truth and Lies in the Age of AIDS.*

Using oral history interviews, the book explores the sexual practices of 49 men and 28 women in New York City.

Read the complete article online in the eThemes section of this book's website: www.aw-bc.com/donatelle.

Original article published November 25, 2003. Copyright © 2003 The New York Times. Reprinted with permission.

Every moment of every day, you are in contact with microscopic organisms that have the ability to cause illness or even death. These disease-causing agents, known as **pathogens,** are found in air and food and on nearly every object or person with whom you come in contact. Although new varieties of pathogens arise all the time, scientific evidence indicates that many have existed for as long as there has been life on the planet. Fossil evidence shows that infections, cancer, heart disease, and a host of other ailments afflicted the earliest human beings. At times, infectious diseases wiped out whole groups of people through epidemics such as the Black Death, or bubonic plague, which killed half the population of Europe in the 1300s. A pandemic, or global epidemic, of influenza killed more than 20 million people in 1918, while strains of tuberculosis and cholera continue to cause premature death throughout the world.

In spite of our best efforts to eradicate them, these diseases are a continuing menace to all of us. The news isn't all bad, however. Even though we are bombarded by potential pathogenic threats, our immune systems are remarkably adept at protecting us. *Endogenous microorganisms* are those that live in peaceful coexistence with their human host most of the time. For people in good health and whose immune systems are functioning properly, endogenous organisms are usually harmless. But in sick people or those with weakened immune systems, these normally harmless pathogenic organisms can cause serious health problems.

Exogenous microorganisms are organisms that do not normally inhabit the body. When they do, however, they are apt to produce an infection and/or illness. The more easily these pathogens can gain a foothold in the body and sustain themselves, the more **virulent,** or aggressive, they may be in causing disease. However, if your immune system is strong, you will often be able to fight off even the most virulent attacker. Several factors influence your susceptibility to disease.

Assessing Your Disease Risks

Most diseases are **multifactorial diseases**—that is, they are caused by the interaction of several factors from inside and outside the person. For a disease to occur, the *host* must be *susceptible,* which means that the immune system must be in a weakened condition; an *agent* capable of transmitting a disease must be present; and the *environment* must be hospitable to the pathogen in terms of temperature, light, moisture, and other requirements. Other risk factors also apparently increase or decrease susceptibility. Figure 14.1 summarizes the body's defenses against invasion.

Pathogen   A disease-causing agent.

Virulent   Strong enough to overcome host resistance and cause disease.

Multifactorial disease   Disease caused by interactions of several factors.

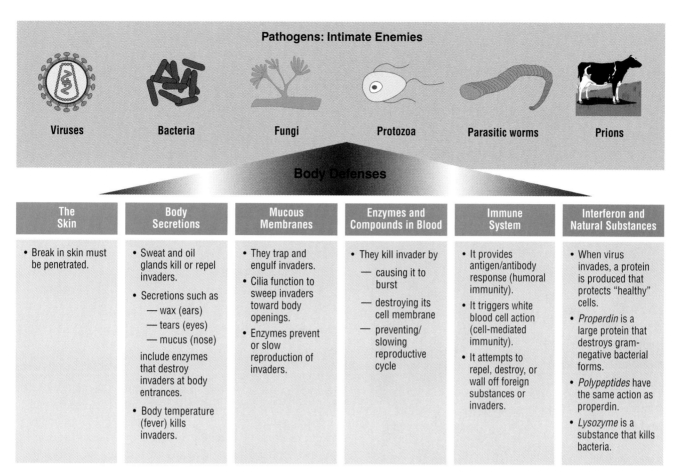

Figure 14.1
The Body's Defenses Against Disease-Causing Pathogens

Risk Factors You Can't Control

Unfortunately, some risk factors are beyond our control. Here are some of the most common.

Heredity   Perhaps the single greatest factor influencing longevity is the longevity of a person's parents. Being born into a family in which heart disease, cancer, or other illnesses are prevalent seems to increase risk. Still other diseases are caused by direct chromosomal inheritance. For example, **sickle-cell anemia,** an inherited blood disease that primarily affects African Americans, is often transmitted to the fetus if both parents carry the sickle-cell trait. It is often unclear whether hereditary diseases occur as a result of inherited chromosomal traits or inherited insufficiencies in the immune system.

Aging   After age 40 we become more vulnerable to most of the chronic diseases. Moreover, as we age, our immune systems respond less efficiently to invading organisms, thus increasing risk for infection and illness. The same flu that produces an afternoon of nausea and diarrhea in a younger person may cause days of illness or even death in an older

person. The very young are also at risk for many diseases, particularly if they are not vaccinated against them.

Environmental Conditions   Unsanitary conditions and the presence of drugs, chemicals, and hazardous pollutants and wastes in food and water probably have a great effect on our immune systems. It is well documented that poor environmental conditions can weaken **immunological competence**—the body's ability to defend itself against pathogens.

Organism Resistance   Some organisms, such as the food-borne organism **botulism,** are particularly virulent, and even tiny amounts may make the most hardy of us ill. Other

> **Sickle-cell anemia**   Genetic disease commonly found among African Americans; results in organ damage and premature death.
>
> **Immunological competence**   Ability of the immune system to defend the body from pathogens.
>
> **Botulism**   A resistant food-borne organism that is extremely virulent.

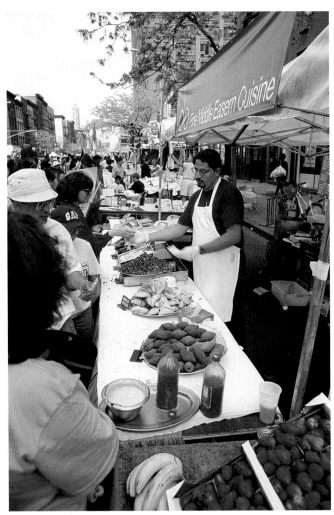

Airborne pathogens can be transmitted easily and unknowingly, so special precautions must be taken to ensure the health and safety of patrons of food markets and other public places.

organisms have mutated and are resistant to the body's defenses as well as to other conventional treatments designed to protect against them. Still other, newer pathogens pose unique challenges for our immune systems—ones that our bodily defenses are ill adapted to fight.

Risk Factors You Can Control

The good news is that we all have some degree of personal control over many risk factors for disease. Too much stress, inadequate nutrition, a low physical fitness level, lack of sleep, misuse or abuse of legal and illegal substances, poor personal

---

Autoinoculation Transmission of a pathogen from one part of the body to another.

Interspecies transmission Transmission of disease from humans to animals or from animals to humans.

---

hygiene, high-risk behaviors, and other variables significantly increase the risk for a number of diseases. Various chapters of this text discuss these variables. Several factors influence our individual susceptibility to various diseases. Those we have the most control over, via lifestyle decisions and behaviors, are noted on the following list with an asterisk (*)[1]:

- Dosage, virulence, and portal of entry of agent
- Age at time of infection
- Preexisting level of immunity*
- Nature and vigor of immune response*
- Genetic factors controlling immune response
- Nutritional status*
- Preexisting diseases*
- Personal habits: smoking, alcohol, exercise, drugs*
- Dual infection or superinfection with other agents
- Psychological factors (e.g., motivation, emotional status, and so on)*

Types of Pathogens and Routes of Transmission

Pathogens enter the body in several ways. They may be transmitted by *direct contact* between infected persons, such as during sexual relations, kissing, or touching, or by *indirect contact,* such as by touching an object the infected person has had contact with. The hands are probably the greatest source of infectious disease transmission. You may also **autoinoculate** yourself, or transmit a pathogen from one part of your body to another. For example, you may touch a sore on your lip that is teeming with viral herpes, then transmit the virus to your eye when you scratch your itchy eyelid.

Pathogens are also transmitted by *airborne contact*—you can breathe in air that carries a particular pathogen—or by *food-borne infection* if you eat something contaminated by microorganisms. Recent episodes of food poisoning from *Salmonella* bacteria found in certain foods and *E. coli* bacteria found in undercooked beef have raised concerns about the safety of the U.S. food supply. As a direct result of these concerns, food labels now caution consumers to cook meats thoroughly, wash utensils, and take other food-handling precautions.

Your best friend may be the source of *animal-borne pathogens.* Dogs, cats, livestock, and wild animals can spread numerous diseases through their bites or feces or by carrying infected insects into living areas and transmitting diseases either directly or indirectly. Although **interspecies transmission** of diseases (diseases passed from humans to animals and vice versa) is rare, it does occur. *Waterborne diseases* are transmitted directly from drinking water and indirectly from foods washed or sprayed with contaminated water. These pathogens can also invade your body if you wade or swim in contaminated streams, lakes, or reservoirs. Pathogens may also transmit *insect-borne diseases* via mosquitoes, ticks, and other hosts that spread disease through sucking or biting.

Mothers may transmit diseases *perinatally* to an infant in the womb or as the baby passes through the vagina during birth.

We can categorize pathogens into six major types: bacteria, viruses, fungi, protozoa, parasitic worms, and prions.

Bacteria

Bacteria are single-celled organisms that are plantlike in nature but lack chlorophyll (the pigment that gives plants their green coloring). There are three major types of bacteria: cocci, bacilli, and spirilla. Bacteria can be viewed under a standard light microscope.

Although there are several thousand species of bacteria, only approximately 100 cause diseases in humans. In many cases, it is not the bacteria themselves that cause disease but rather the poisonous substances, called **toxins,** that they produce. The following are the most common bacterial infections.

Staphylococcal Infections   **Staphylococci** are normally present on our skin at all times and usually cause few problems. But when there is a cut or break in the **epidermis,** or outer layer of the skin, staphylococci may enter and cause a localized infection. If you have ever suffered from acne, boils, styes (infections of the eyelids), or infected wounds, you have probably had a staph infection. Although most such infections are readily defeated by your immune system, resistant forms of staph bacteria are on the rise. These bacteria must be treated with heavy doses of antibiotics and pose serious risks to those infected.

At least one staph-caused disorder, **toxic shock syndrome,** is potentially fatal. Although most cases of toxic shock syndrome have occurred in menstruating women, the disease was first reported in 1978 in children and continues to be reported in people recovering from wounds, surgery, or other injury. To reduce the likelihood of toxic shock syndrome, take the following precautions: (1) avoid superabsorbent tampons except during the heaviest menstrual flow; (2) change tampons at least every four hours; and (3) use napkins at night instead of tampons.

Streptococcal Infections   At least five types of the **streptococcus** microorganism are known to cause bacterial infections. Group A streptococcus causes the most common diseases, such as streptococcal pharyngitis (strep throat) and scarlet fever.[2] Group B streptococcus can cause illness in newborn babies, pregnant women, the elderly, and adults with other illnesses such as diabetes or liver disease.[3]

Pneumonia   In the early twentieth century, **pneumonia** was one of the leading causes of death in the United States. This lung disease is characterized by chronic cough, chest pain, chills, high fever, fluid accumulation, and eventual respiratory failure. One of the most common forms of pneumonia is caused by bacterial infection and responds readily to antibiotic treatment in the early stages. Other forms are caused by viruses, chemicals, or other substances in the lungs and are

more difficult to treat. Although medical advances have reduced the overall incidence of pneumonia, it continues to be a major threat in the United States and throughout the world. Vulnerable populations include the poor, the elderly, and those already suffering from other illnesses.[4]

Legionnaires' Disease   This bacterial disorder gained widespread publicity in 1976, when several Legionnaires at the American Legion convention in Philadelphia contracted the disease and died before the invading organism was isolated and effective treatment devised. Although it is not well known, the water-borne nature of Legionnaires' Disease has led to several recent outbreaks in the United States.[5] The symptoms are similar to those of pneumonia, which sometimes makes identification difficult. In people whose resistance is lowered, particularly the elderly, delayed identification can have serious consequences.

Tuberculosis   A major killer in the United States during the early twentieth century, **tuberculosis (TB)** was largely controlled in America by 1950 due to improved sanitation, isolation of infected persons, and treatment with drugs such as *rifampin* or *isoniazid*. But though many health professionals assumed that TB had been conquered, that appears not to be the case. During the past 20 years, several factors have led to an epidemic rise in the disease: deteriorating social conditions, including overcrowding and poor sanitation; failure to isolate active cases of TB; a weakening of public health infrastructure, which has led to less funding for screening; and migration of TB to the United States through international travel. In 2002, there were more than 15,075 active cases of TB in the United States.[6] More than one-half of all TB cases in the U.S. in 2002 occurred in foreign-born individuals.[7] Newer

---

Bacteria   Single-celled organisms that may cause disease.

Toxins   Poisonous substances produced by certain microorganisms that cause various diseases.

Staphylococci   Round, gram-positive bacteria, usually found in clusters.

Epidermis   The outermost layer of the skin.

Toxic shock syndrome   A potentially life-threatening bacterial infection that is most common in menstruating women who use tampons.

Streptococci   Round bacteria, usually found in chain formation.

Pneumonia   Disease of the lungs characterized by chronic cough, chest pain, chills, high fever, and fluid accumulation; may be caused by bacteria, viruses, chemicals, or other substances.

Tuberculosis (TB)   A disease caused by bacterial infiltration of the respiratory system.

strains of multiple drug-resistant TB make this epidemic potentially more devastating than previous outbreaks.

Although increases in the incidence of TB in the United States are troubling, U.S. statistics pale by comparison to the staggering TB burden in the global population. Assuming no significant improvements in prevention and control between now and 2020, the World Health Organization (WHO) estimates that 1 billion people will acquire new TB infection, 200 million will develop active disease, and 70 million will die.[8]

TB is caused by bacterial infiltration of the respiratory system that results in a chronic inflammatory reaction in the lungs. Airborne transmission via the respiratory tract is the primary and most efficient mode of transmitting TB. People with active cases can transmit the disease while talking, coughing, sneezing, or singing. Fortunately, TB is fairly difficult to catch, and prolonged exposure, rather than single exposure, is the typical mode of infection. Only about 20 to 30 percent of people exposed to an active case will become infected.[9] Symptoms include persistent coughing, weight loss, fever, and spitting up blood. A simple skin test will indicate infection, and treatments are effective for most nonresistant cases. Many people have a form of latent TB in which the bacteria are present in the body but the person is symptom-free and not infectious. Most of these people never develop active TB, unless their immune system becomes compromised.

Periodontal Diseases Diseases of the tissue around the teeth, called **periodontal diseases,** affect three out of four adults over age 35. Improper tooth care, including lack of flossing and poor brushing habits, and the failure to obtain professional dental care lead to increased bacterial growth, caries (tooth decay), and gum infections. If left untreated, permanent tooth loss may result.

What do you think?

Why do you think we are experiencing global increases in diseases such as TB? ✳ *Should we be concerned about diseases in other countries?* ✳ *Do we have an obligation to help the world's population in their struggle against these diseases?* ✳ *What policies, programs, and services might help?*

Periodontal diseases   Diseases of the tissue around the teeth.

Viruses   Minute parasitic microbes that live inside another cell.

Interferon   A protein substance produced by the body that aids the immune system by protecting healthy cells.

Endemic   Describing a disease that is always present to some degree.

Viruses

Viruses are the smallest pathogens, approximately 1/500th the size of bacteria. Because of their tiny size, they are visible only under an electron microscope and were not identified until the twentieth century.[10] More than 150 viruses are known to cause diseases in humans, although their role in various cancers and chronic diseases is still unclear.

Essentially, a virus consists of a protein structure that contains either *ribonucleic acid (RNA)* or *deoxyribonucleic acid (DNA)*. Incapable of carrying out the normal cell functions of respiration and metabolism, a virus cannot reproduce on its own and can exist only in a parasitic relationship with the cell it invades.

Viral diseases can be difficult to treat because many viruses can withstand heat, formaldehyde, and large doses of radiation with little effect on their structure. Drug treatment for viral infections is also limited. Drugs powerful enough to kill viruses generally kill the host cells too, although some medications block stages in viral reproduction without damaging host cells.

When exposed to certain viruses, the body produces a protein substance known as **interferon.** Interferon does not destroy the invading microorganisms but sets up a protective mechanism to aid healthy cells in their struggle against the invaders. Although interferon research is promising, it should be noted that not all viruses stimulate interferon production.

The Common Cold Colds are responsible for more days lost from work and more uncomfortable days spent at work than any other ailment.[11] Caused by any number of viruses (some experts claim there may be more than 200 different viruses responsible for the common cold), colds are **endemic** (always present to some degree) among people throughout the world. In the course of a year, Americans suffer more than 1 billion colds. Otherwise healthy people carry cold viruses in their noses and throats most of the time. These viruses are held in check until the host's resistance is lowered. It is possible to "catch" a cold—from the airborne droplets of another person's sneeze or from skin-to-skin or mucous membrane contact—though recent studies indicate that the hands are the greatest avenue for transmitting colds and other viruses.[12] Although many people believe that a cold results from exposure to cold weather or from getting chilled or overheated, experts believe that such things have little or no effect on cold development. Stress, allergy disorders that affect the nasal passages, and menstrual cycles do, however, appear to increase susceptibility.[13]

The best rule of thumb is to keep your resistance level high. Sound nutrition, adequate rest, stress reduction, and regular exercise appear to be the best bets in helping fight off infection. Avoid people with newly developed colds (colds appear to be most contagious during the first 24 hours of onset). If you contract a cold, bed rest, plenty of fluids, and aspirin to relieve pain and discomfort are the tried-and-true remedies for adults. Children should not take aspirin for

Body Piercing and Tattooing: Risks to Health

A look around almost any college campus reveals many examples of the widespread trend of body piercing and tattooing, also referred to as "body art." People are getting their ears and bodies pierced in record numbers, in such places as the eyebrows, tongues, lips, noses, navels, nipples, genitals, and just about any place possible. Many view the trend as a fulfillment of a desire for self-expression, as this University of Wisconsin–Madison student points out: "The nipple [ring] was one of those things that I did as a kind of empowerment, claiming my body as my own and refuting the stereotypes that people have about me. . . . The tattoo was kind of a lark and came along the same lines and I like it too. . . . [T]hey both give me a secret smile." Whatever the reason, tattoo artists are doing a booming business in both tattooing and the "art" of body piercing.

However, health professionals cite several concerns over health risks. The most common health-related problems associated with tattoos and body piercing include skin reactions, infections, and scarring. The average healing times for piercings depend on the size of the insert, location, and the person's overall health. Facial and tongue piercings tend to heal more quickly than areas not commonly exposed to open air or light and which are often teeming with bacteria, such as the genitals. Because the hands are great germ transmitters, "fingering" pierced areas poses a significant risk for infection.

Of even greater concern is the potential transmission of dangerous pathogens that any puncture of the human body exacerbates. The use of unsterile needles—which can cause serious infections and can transmit HIV, hepatitis B (HBV) and hepatitis C (HCV), tetanus, and a host of other diseases—poses a very real risk. (Actress Pamela Anderson claims to have contracted HCV from sharing a tattoo needle with her ex-husband Tommy Lee.) Body piercing and tattooing are performed by unlicensed "professionals" who generally have learned their trade from other body artists. Laws and policies regulating body piercing and tattooing vary greatly by state. While some states don't allow tattoo and body-piercing parlors, others may regulate them carefully, and still others provide few regulations and standards by which parlors have to abide. Standards for safety usually include minimum age of use, standards of sanitation, use of aseptic techniques, sterilization of equipment, informed risks, instructions for skin care, record keeping, and recommendations for dealing with adverse reactions. Because of the lack of standards regulating this business and the potential for transmission of dangerous pathogens, anyone who receives a tattoo, body piercing, or permanent makeup tattoo cannot donate blood for one year.

If you opt for tattooing or body piercing, remember the following points:

✔ Look for clean, well-lit work areas, and ask about sterilization procedures.

✔ Before having the work done, watch the artist at work. Tattoo removal is expensive and often impossible. Make sure the tattoo is one you can live with for years.

✔ Immediately before piercing or tattooing, the body area should be carefully sterilized. The artist should put on new latex gloves and touch nothing else while working.

✔ Packaged, sterilized needles should be used only once and then discarded. A piercing gun should not be used because it cannot be sterilized properly.

✔ Only jewelry made of noncorrosive metal, such as surgical stainless steel, niobium, or solid 14-karat gold, is safe for new piercing.

✔ Leftover tattoo ink should be discarded after each procedure. Do not allow the artist to reuse ink that has been used for other customers.

✔ If any signs of pus, swelling, redness, or discoloration persist, remove the piercing object and contact a physician.

Sources: U.S. Food and Drug Administration, Center for Food Safety and Applied Nutrition, "Tattoos and Permanent Makeup," Office of Cosmetics and Colors Fact Sheet, 2000, www.cfsan.fda.gov/~dms/cos-204.html; M. L. Armstrong and K. P. Murphy, "Adolescent Tattooing and Body Piercing," *The Prevention Researcher* (Integrated Research Services, Eugene, Oregon) 5, no. 3 (1998): 5.

---

colds or the flu because this could lead to *Reye's syndrome,* a potentially fatal disease.

Influenza   In otherwise healthy people, **influenza,** or flu, is usually not serious. Symptoms, including headaches, fatigue, aches and pains, fever, and coldlike ailments, generally pass quickly. However, in combination with other disorders or among the elderly, those with respiratory or heart disease, or children under age five, the flu can be very serious. Contrary to common belief, the flu is primarily a respiratory disease. You cannot have a "stomach flu." Nausea, vomiting, and diarrhea are extremely rare with the flu, except in small children. The period of November through March is the typical flu season.[14]

To date, three major varieties of flu virus have been discovered, with many different strains existing within each variety. The "A" form of the virus is generally the most virulent, followed by the "B" and "C" varieties. If you contract one form of flu you may develop immunity to it, but you will not necessarily be immune to other forms of the disease. Little can be done to treat flu patients once the infection has become established. Some vaccines have proved effective

---

Influenza   A common viral disease of the respiratory tract.

against certain strains of flu virus, but they are totally ineffective against others. In spite of minor risks, it is recommended that people over age 65, pregnant women, people with heart or lung disease, and those with certain other illnesses be vaccinated. In fall of 2003, an inhaled vaccine called FluMist was released for use with healthy, nonpregnant adults up to age 49. Because the vaccine contains a weakened version of the live virus, people who receive the vaccine may pose a risk to anyone with a weakened immune system who is around them. More investigation into the risks are needed.

Infectious Mononucleosis   Initial symptoms of mononucleosis, or mono, include sore throat, fever, headache, nausea, chills, and pervasive weakness/fatigue. As the disease progresses, lymph nodes may enlarge, and jaundice, spleen enlargement, aching joints, and body rashes may occur.

Caused by the *Epstein-Barr virus,* mono is readily detected through a *monospot test,* a blood test that measures the percentage of specific forms of white blood cells. Because many viruses are caused by transmission of body fluids, many people once believed that young people contracted mono through kissing (hence its nickname, "the kissing disease"). Although this is still considered a possible cause, mono is not believed to be highly contagious. It does not appear to be easily spread through normal, everyday personal contact.

Treatment of mono is often a lengthy process that involves bed rest, balanced nutrition, and medications. Gradually, the body develops immunity to the disease, and the person returns to normal activity.

Hepatitis   One of the most highly publicized viral diseases is **hepatitis,** a virally caused inflammation of the liver. Hepatitis symptoms include fever, headache, nausea, loss of appetite, skin rashes, pain in the upper right abdomen, dark yellow (with brownish tinge) urine, and jaundice (yellowing of the whites of the eyes and the skin). In some regions of the United States and among certain segments of the population, hepatitis has reached epidemic proportions. Internationally, viral hepatitis is a major contributor to acute and chronic liver disease and accounts for high morbidity and mortality. Currently, there are seven known forms, with the following three indicating the highest rate of incidence (see the Centers for

Disease Control and Prevention [CDC] website for further information on the types not discussed here).

- *Hepatitis A (HAV).* HAV is contracted from eating food or drinking water contaminated with human excrement. Each year, more than 150,000 people in the United States are infected, typically through something in the household, sexual contact, day care attendance, or international travel. Fortunately, people with HAV do not become chronic carriers.[15]
- *Hepatitis B (HBV).* This disease, spread primarily through body fluids, particularly during unprotected sex, can lead to chronic liver disease or liver cancer. However, it can also be contracted via sharing needles when injecting drugs, or passed by an infected mother to her baby during birth. One of the fastest growing sexually transmitted infections (STIs) in the United States, with more than 300,000 new cases per year, HBV infection is more prevalent than human immunodeficiency virus (HIV). More than 1.2 million people are chronic carriers.[16] Most people recover within six months, although some become chronic carriers.
- *Hepatitis C (HCV).* HCV infections are on an epidemic rise in many regions of the world, as resistant forms are emerging. Currently, it is estimated that there are 150,000 new cases of HCV in the United States each year, with more than 4 million people infected.[17] More than 85 percent of those infected develop chronic infections; if the infection is left untreated, the person may develop cirrhosis of the liver, liver cancer, or liver failure. Liver failure due to chronic HCV is the leading cause of liver transplants in the United States.[18] Some cases can be traced to blood transfusions or organ transplants.

In the United States, hepatitis continues to be a major threat in spite of a safe blood supply and massive efforts at education about hand washing (HAV) and safer sex (primarily HBV). Treatment of all forms of viral hepatitis is somewhat limited.

Measles   Measles is a viral disorder that often affects young children. Symptoms, appearing about ten days after exposure, include an itchy rash and a high fever. **German measles (rubella)** is a milder viral infection that is believed to be transmitted by inhalation, after which it multiplies in the upper respiratory tract and passes into the bloodstream. It causes a rash, especially on the upper extremities. It is not generally a serious health threat and usually runs its course in three to four days. The major exceptions to this rule are newborns and pregnant women. Rubella can damage a fetus, particularly during the first trimester, by creating a condition known as congenital rubella in which the infant may be born blind, deaf, cognitively impaired, or with heart defects. Immunization has reduced the incidence of both measles and German measles. Infections in children not immunized against measles can lead to fever-induced problems such as rheumatic heart disease, kidney damage, and neurological disorders.

Hepatitis   A virally caused disease in which the liver becomes inflamed, which produces symptoms such as fever, headache, and jaundice.

Measles   A viral disease that produces symptoms including an itchy rash and a high fever.

German measles (rubella)   A milder form of measles that causes a rash and mild fever in children and may cause damage to a fetus or a newborn baby.

Other Pathogens

Fungi   Hundreds of species of **fungi,** multicellular or unicellular primitive plants, inhabit our environment. Many fungi are useful, providing such foodstuffs as edible mushrooms and some cheeses. But some species of fungi can produce infections. *Candidiasis* (a vaginal yeast infection), athlete's foot, ringworm, and jock itch are examples of fungal diseases. Keeping the affected area clean and dry plus treatment with appropriate medications will generally bring prompt relief.

Protozoa   Protozoa are microscopic, single-celled organisms that are generally associated with tropical diseases such as African sleeping sickness and malaria. Although these pathogens are prevalent in nonindustrialized countries, they are largely controlled in the United States. The most common protozoal disease in the United States is *trichomoniasis,* which we will discuss later in this chapter's section on STIs. A common water-borne protozoan disease in many regions of the country is *giardiasis.* People who drink or are exposed to the *Giardia* pathogen may suffer intestinal pain and discomfort weeks after infection. Protection of water supplies is the key to prevention.

Parasitic Worms   Parasitic worms are the largest of the pathogens. Ranging in size from the small pinworms typically found in children to the relatively large tapeworms found in all warm-blooded animals, most parasitic worms are more a nuisance than a threat. Of special note today are the worm infestations associated with eating raw fish in Japanese sushi restaurants. Cooking fish and other foods to temperatures sufficient to kill the worms and their eggs can prevent this.

Prions   A **prion,** or unconventional virus, is a self-replicating, protein-based *agent* that can infect humans and other animals. Believed to be the underlying cause of spongiform diseases such as "mad cow disease," this agent systematically destroys brain cells. We will say more about prion-based diseases later in this chapter.

Your Body's Defenses: Keeping You Well

Although all the pathogens just described pose a threat if they take hold in your body, the chances that they will do so are actually quite small. First, they must overcome a number of effective barriers, many of which were established in your body before you were born.

Physical and Chemical Defenses

Perhaps our most critical early defense system is the skin. Layered to provide an intricate web of barriers, the skin allows few pathogens to enter. **Enzymes,** complex proteins manufactured by the body that appear in body secretions such as sweat, provide additional protection; they destroy microorganisms on skin surfaces by producing inhospitable pH levels. Microorganisms that flourish at a selected pH will be weakened or destroyed as these changes occur. A third protection is our frequent slight elevations in body temperature, which create an inhospitable environment for many pathogens. Only when cracks or breaks occur in the skin can pathogens gain easy access to the body.

The linings of the body provide yet another protection. Mucous membranes in the respiratory tract and other linings of the body trap and engulf invading organisms. *Cilia,* hairlike projections in the lungs and respiratory tract, sweep invaders toward body openings, where they are expelled. Tears, nasal secretions, earwax, and other secretions found at body entrances contain enzymes designed to destroy or neutralize pathogens. Finally, any organism that manages to breach such initial lines of defense faces a formidable specialized network of defenses thrown up by the immune system.

The Immune System: Your Body Fights Back

Immunity is a condition of being able to resist a particular disease by counteracting the substance that produces the disease. Any substance capable of triggering an immune response is called an **antigen.** An antigen can be a virus, a bacterium, a fungus, a parasite, or a tissue or cell from another individual. When invaded by an antigen, the body responds by forming substances called **antibodies** that are matched to the specific antigen much as a key is matched to a lock. Antibodies belong to a mass of large molecules known as *immunoglobulins,* a group of nine chemically distinct protein substances, each of which plays a role in

---

Fungi   A group of plants that lack chlorophyll and do not produce flowers or seeds; several microscopic varieties are pathogenic.

Protozoa   Microscopic, single-celled organisms.

Parasitic worms   The largest of the pathogens, most of which are more a nuisance than a threat.

Prions   A self-replicating protein-based agent that systematically destroys brain cells.

Enzymes   Organic substances that cause bodily changes and destruction of microorganisms.

Antigen   Substance capable of triggering an immune response.

Antibodies   Substances produced by the body that are individually matched to specific antigens.

---

neutralizing, setting up for destruction, or actually destroying antigens.

Once an antigen breaches the body's initial defenses, the body begins a process of antigen analysis. It considers the size and shape of the invader, verifies that the antigen is not part of the body itself, and then produces a specific antibody to destroy or weaken the antigen. This process, which is much more complex than described here, is part of a system called *humoral immune responses*. Humoral immunity is the body's major defense against many bacteria and bacterial toxins.

Cell-mediated immunity is characterized by the formation of a population of lymphocytes that can attack and destroy the foreign invader. These lymphocytes constitute the body's main defense against viruses, fungi, parasites, and some bacteria. Key players in this immune response are specialized groups of white blood cells known as *macrophages* (a type of phagocytic, or cell-eating, cell) and *lymphocytes,* other white blood cells in the blood, lymph nodes, bone marrow, and certain glands.

Two forms of lymphocytes in particular, the *B-lymphocytes* (B-cells) and *T-lymphocytes* (T-cells), are involved in the immune response. There are different types of B-cells, named according to the area of the body in which they develop. Most are manufactured in the soft tissue of the hollow shafts of the long bones. T-cells, in contrast, develop and multiply in the thymus, a multilobed organ that lies behind the breastbone. T-cells assist the immune system in several ways. *Regulatory T-cells* help direct the activities of the immune system and assist other cells, particularly B-cells, to produce antibodies. Dubbed "helper T's," these cells are essential for activating B-cells, other T-cells, and macrophages. Another form of T-cell, known as the "killer T" or "cytotoxic T," directly attacks infected or malignant cells. Killer T-cells enable the body to rid itself of cells that have been infected by viruses or transformed by cancer; they are also responsible for the rejection of tissue and organ grafts. The third type of T-cell, "suppressor T," turns off or suppresses the activity of B-cells, killer T-cells, and macrophages. Suppressor T-cells circulate in the bloodstream and lymphatic system where they neutralize or destroy antigens, thus enhancing the effects of the immune response and helping to return the activated immune system to normal levels. After a successful attack on a pathogen, some of the attacker T- and B-cells are preserved as *memory T-* and *B-cells* that enable the body to quickly recognize and respond to subsequent attacks by the same kind of organism at a later time. Thus, macrophages, T- and B-cells, and antibodies are the key factors in mounting an immune response.

Referred pain Pain that is present at one point, but whose source is elsewhere.

Once people have survived infectious diseases, they become immune to those diseases, which means that in all probability they will not develop them again. Upon subsequent attack by the disease-causing microorganism, their memory T- and B-cells are quickly activated to come to their defense.

Autoimmune Diseases Although white blood cells and the antigen–antibody response generally work in our favor by neutralizing or destroying harmful antigens, the body sometimes makes a mistake and targets its own tissue as the enemy, builds up antibodies against that tissue, and attempts to destroy it. This is known as *autoimmune disease* (*auto* means "self"). Common autoimmune disorders are rheumatoid arthritis, systemic lupus erythematosus (SLE), and myasthenia gravis.

In some cases, the antigen–antibody response completely fails to function. The result is a form of *immune deficiency syndrome*. Perhaps the most dramatic case of this syndrome was the "bubble boy," a youngster who died in 1984 after living his short life inside a sealed-off environment designed to protect him from all antigens. A much more common immune system disorder is *acquired immune deficiency syndrome (AIDS),* which we will discuss later in this chapter.

Fever

If an infection is localized, pus formation, redness, swelling, and irritation often occur. These symptoms indicate that the invading organisms are being fought systematically. Another indication is the development of a fever, or a rise in body temperature above the norm of 98.6°F. Fever is frequently caused by toxins secreted by pathogens that interfere with the control of body temperature. Although this elevated temperature is often harmful to the body, it is also believed to act as a form of protection. Raising body temperature by even one or two degrees provides an environment that destroys some disease-causing organisms. A fever also stimulates the body to produce more white blood cells, which destroy more invaders.

Pain

Although we do not usually think of pain as a defense mechanism, it is a response to injury, and it plays a valuable role in the body's response to invasion. Pain may be either *direct pain,* caused by the stimulation of nerve endings in an affected area, or **referred pain,** meaning that it is present in one place although the source is elsewhere. Most pain responses are accompanied by inflammation. Pain tends to be the earliest sign that an injury has occurred and often causes the person to slow down or stop the activity that was aggravating the injury, thereby protecting against further damage. Because it is often one of the first warnings of disease, persistent pain should not be overlooked or masked with short-term pain relievers.

Vaccines: Bolstering Your Immunity

Recall that once people have been exposed to a specific pathogen, subsequent attacks will activate their memory T- and B-cells, thus giving them immunity. This is the principle on which **vaccination** is based.

A vaccine consists of killed or attenuated (weakened) versions of a disease-causing microorganism, or an antigen that is similar to but less dangerous than the disease antigen. It is administered to stimulate the person's immune system to produce antibodies against future attacks—without actually causing the disease. Vaccines are given orally or by injection, and this form of artificial immunity is termed **acquired immunity,** in contrast to **natural immunity,** which a mother passes to her fetus via their shared blood supply.

Depending on the virulence of the organism, vaccines containing live, attenuated, or dead organisms are given for a variety of diseases. In some instances, if a person is already weakened by other health problems, vaccination may provoke an actual mild case of the disease. Figure 14.2 on page 372 shows the recommended schedule for childhood vaccinations.

Emerging and Resurgent Diseases

Although our immune systems are remarkably adept at responding to many challenges, they are threatened by an army of microbes that is so diverse, virulent, and insidious that the invaders appear to be gaining ground. According to the WHO's *World Health Report* issued in 2002, trends such as the aging of the population (the young and old are particularly vulnerable), the urbanization of developing countries, poverty, environmental pollution, globalization of the food supply, and crumbling health care systems bode very badly for the future.[19] As international travel increases (more than 1 million people per day cross international boundaries), with germs transported from remote regions of developing countries to huge urban centers within a matter of hours, the likelihood of infection by microbes previously unknown on U.S. soil increases. Table 14.1 identifies major contributors to the emergence and resurgence of infectious diseases.

Tiny Microbes: Lethal Threats

Today's arsenal of antibiotics appears to be increasingly ineffective. Penicillin-resistant strains of diseases are on the rise as microbes become able to outlast and outsmart even the best of our antibiotic weapons.[20] Old scourges are back, and new ones are emerging.

"Mad Cow Disease"   The American beef industry has been the subject of a great amount of media attention, with the first confirmed case of *bovine spongiform encephalitis* (BSE, or "mad cow disease") being detected in December 2003. BSE may be linked to a disease in humans known as *new variant Creutzfeldt-Jakob disease* (NvCJD).[21] Both disorders are invariably fatal brain diseases with unusually long incubation periods measured in years, and both are caused by unconventional transmittable agents known as *prions*.

BSE is thought to have been transmitted when cows were fed a protein-based substance (slaughterhouse leftovers from sheep and other cows) to help them put on weight and grow faster. Failure to treat this protein by-product sufficiently to kill the BSE organism allowed it to infect the cows. The disease is believed to be transmitted to humans through the meat of these slaughtered cows. The resultant variant of BSE in humans, known as NvCJD disease and characterized by progressively worsening neurological damage and possible death, was noted in ten people in England and linked by some studies to the BSE-diseased cows. It should be noted that this link has not yet been scientifically verified.[22]

A related prion-caused disease, *chronic wasting disease,* has been found in deer and is similar to BSE. Studies are underway investigating the implications of this disease for human health.

Dengue and Dengue Hemorrhagic Fever   Transmitted by mosquitoes, **dengue** viruses are the most widespread insect-borne viruses in the world. Today, dengue is found on most continents, and more than one half of all United Nations member states are threatened.[23] Dengue symptoms include flulike nausea, aches, and chronic fatigue and weakness. As urban areas become increasingly infected with mosquitoes, nearly 1.5 billion people, including about 600 million children, are at risk. Each year, it is estimated that more than 100 million people are infected, and more than 8,000 die.[24] A more serious form of the disease, **dengue hemorrhagic fever,** can kill children in 6 to 12 hours, as the virus causes capillaries to leak and spill fluid and blood into surrounding tissue. Dengue is on the rise in the United States, largely because of increased international travel.

Vaccination   Inoculation with killed or weakened pathogens or similar, less dangerous antigens in order to prevent or lessen the effects of some disease.

Acquired immunity   Immunity developed during life in response to disease, vaccination, or exposure.

Natural immunity   Immunity passed to a fetus by its mother.

Dengue   A disease transmitted by mosquitoes, which causes flulike symptoms.

Dengue hemorrhagic fever   A more serious form of dengue.

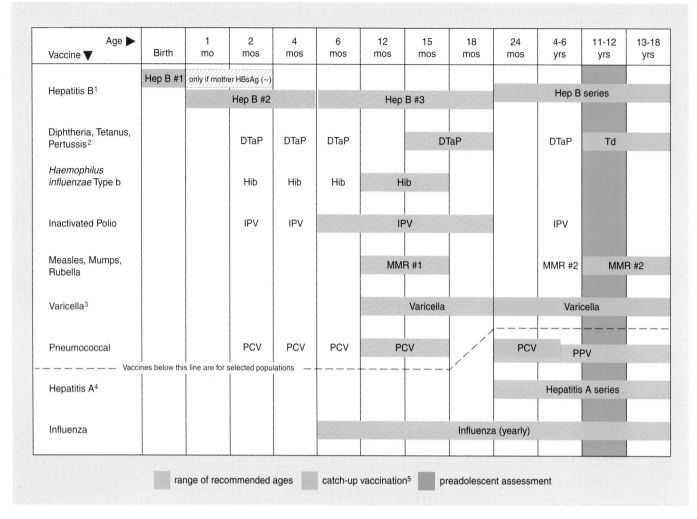

Figure 14.2

Recommended Childhood and Adolescent Immunization Schedule, 2003

1. Mothers who have tested positive for hepatitis B (HBV) should consult their doctors about their infant's vaccinations.

2. Tetanus and diphtheria toxoids (Td) are recommended at age 11–12 years if at least 5 years have elapsed since the last dose of tetanus and diphtheria vaccines. Subsequent routine Td boosters are recommended every 10 years.

3. Varicella is recommended at any visit or after age 12 months for children who lack a reliable history of chicken pox. Susceptible persons over 13 years should receive 2 doses, given at least 4 weeks apart.

4. Hepatitis A (HAV) vaccine is recommended for use in selected states and regions and for certain high-risk groups; consult your physician.

5. "Catch-up vaccination" indicates age groups that warrant special effort to administer any missed vaccines.

Source: Centers for Disease Control and Prevention, "Recommended Childhood and Adolescent Immunization Schedule," *Morbidity and Mortality Report* 52, no. 4 (2003): Q1–Q4.

Ebola Hemorrhagic Fever (Ebola HF) Another emerging disease, Ebola HF is a severe, often fatal disease in humans and nonhuman primates (monkeys, gorillas, and chimpanzees). Although much about Ebola HF is unknown, researchers believe that the virus is animal-borne and normally occurs in animal hosts that are native to the African continent.[25] The virus is spread via direct contact with blood and/or secretions, and possibly through the air. With an incubation period of 2 to 21 days, the course of the disease is quick and characterized by fever, headache, joint and muscle aches, sore throat, and weakness, followed by diarrhea, vomiting, stomach pain, and internal and external bleeding.[26] Although there have been no known cases of human transmission in the United States, several outbreaks have occurred

Table 14.1
Factors Contributing to Emergent/Resurgent Disease Spread and Possible Solutions

Contributing Factors	Possible Solutions
Hardier bugs: tiny size, adaptability, resistant strains, misuse of antibiotics	Increased pharmaceutical efforts, new drug development, selective use of new drugs; improved vaccination rates; funding of new research
Failure to prioritize public health initiatives on national level	Increased government funding; improved efforts aimed at prevention and intervention (Less than 1 percent of the federal budget goes to prevention programs.)
Explosive population growth: resource degradation, overcrowding, land use atrocities, increased urbanization	Population control, wise use of natural resources, environmental controls, reduced deforestation, and increased pollution prevention efforts
International travel	Education or risk reduction; restrictions related to unvaccinated populations; improved air quality and venting on commercial airlines
Human behaviors, particularly intravenous (IV) drug use and risky sexual behavior	Education about risky behaviors; incentives for improved behaviors; increased personal motivation
Vector management failures: widespread overuse/misuse of pesticides and antimicrobial agents that hasten resistance	Management of pesticide use; focus on pollution prevention; regulation; enforcement of laws
Food and water contamination; globalization of food supply and centralized processing	Control of population growth; animal controls; food controls; improved environmental legislation; food safety; pollution prevention
Complacency and apathy	Education—develop "we" mentality rather than "me" mentality
Poverty	Government support; international aid for vaccination programs, early diagnosis, and treatment; care for disadvantaged
War and mass refugee migration, famine, disasters	Government intervention; international aid
Aging of population	Support for prevention/intervention against controllable age-related health problems
Irrigation, deforestation, and reforestation projects that alter habitats of disease-carrying insects and animals	Improved techniques for conservation; responsible use of resources; policies and programs that protect environment
Increased human contact with tropical rainforests and other wilderness habitats that are reservoirs for insects and animals that harbor unknown infectious agents	Increased regulation to reduce human impact; more research to improve interactions between humans and environment

Sources: Author, plus information from U.S. Department of Health and Human Services, Centers for Disease Control and Prevention, "Emerging Infectious Diseases: A Strategy for the 21st Century," 2001. www.cdc.gov/ncidod/emergplan

in various regions of Africa. In 1995, an Ebola HF outbreak in Zaire killed 245 of the 316 people infected, thus forcing strict government-enforced quarantine of the entire region. Subsequent infections in other regions of the world have caused increasing concern. Fortunately, Ebola HF is not as prevalent worldwide as dengue fever.

Cryptosporidium In 1993, the intestinal parasite *Cryptosporidium*, or crypto, infected the municipal water supply of Milwaukee, Wisconsin. The result was the largest waterborne protozoan disease outbreak ever recognized in this country; it caused many deaths and sickened hundreds of thousands of people with acute diarrhea. Exactly how the water supply became infected remains in question; however, the fact that humans, birds, and animals can carry the infective agent and be highly contagious suggests many possible routes. Today crypto is one of the most common waterborne diseases in the United States.

Escherichia coli O157:H7 *Escherichia coli O157:H7* is one of more than 170 types of *E. coli* bacteria that can infect humans. Commonly called *E. coli O157:H7,* it produces a lethal toxin and can cause severe illness or death. Eating ground beef that is rare or undercooked is a common way of becoming infected. Drinking unpasteurized milk or juices and drinking or swimming in sewage-contaminated water or public pools can also cause infection via ingestion of feces that contain *E. coli.* In 2003, several children were infected at a fair in Oregon when they petted infected farm animals and did not wash their hands. Recent findings indicate that simple changes in the way cattle are fed prior to slaughter may reduce the growth of *E. coli* in cattle stomachs.

Cholera Cholera, an infectious disease transmitted through fecal contamination of food or water supplies, has been rare in the United States since the early 1900s. Recent epidemic outbreaks in the Western Hemisphere (more than 900,000 cases), however, have started to affect the United States. Efforts to control cholera may be increasingly difficult as international travel and trade increase.

Hantavirus Transmitted via rodent feces, this virus was responsible for many deaths in the southwestern United States in 1994 before experts were able to identify the culprit. Victims were believed to have come into contact with this organism through breathing the virus-laden dust in rodent-infested homes. Within hours, victims showed serious symptoms as their lungs filled with fluid; they subsequently experienced respiratory collapse and died. Today, cases of hantavirus have been noted in more than 20 states, and vaccines are being developed to counteract it.

Bioterrorism: The New Global Threat The idea of using infectious microorganisms as weapons is not new. In fact, in the English wars with Native Americans, blankets impregnated with scabs from patients with smallpox were traded to Native Americans in hopes of causing disease.[27] The threat of deliberate spreading of deadly microorganisms is a topic of much discussion among today's world leaders, particularly after the instances of anthrax delivered via the mail following the September 11, 2001, terrorist attacks. For more on those biological threats considered to pose the greatest risk, see the Bioterrorism box on page 90 in Chapter 4.

Sexually Transmitted Infections

Sexually transmitted infections (STIs) have been with human beings since earliest recorded history. Today, there are more than 20 known types of STIs. Once referred to as venereal diseases and then as sexually transmitted diseases, the current terminology is more reflective of the number and types of these communicable diseases. More virulent strains and more antibiotic-resistant forms spell trouble for at-risk populations in the days ahead.

A report issued by the CDC in 2000 indicated that there were 16.2 million new occurrences of STIs in 1999, an increase of more than 3.5 million since 1988.[28] Although exact numbers are not available for each STI, the number of cases did increase for several in 2001 after years of decline. Syphilis was among those showing the greatest increase.[29] According to Felicia Stewart of the Kaiser Family Health Foundation, "[T]here is no indication that STIs are coming rapidly under control. . . . In fact, people vastly underestimate risks and fail to take precautions. A . . . Kaiser survey found that just 14% of men and 8% of women felt at risk for STIs, even though at least one third will get one."[30]

> **Sexually transmitted infections (STIs)** Infectious diseases transmitted via some form of intimate, usually sexual, contact.

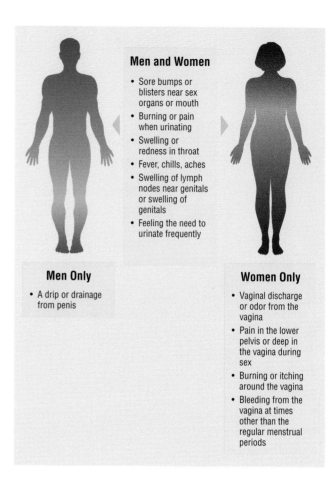

Men and Women
- Sore bumps or blisters near sex organs or mouth
- Burning or pain when urinating
- Swelling or redness in throat
- Fever, chills, aches
- Swelling of lymph nodes near genitals or swelling of genitals
- Feeling the need to urinate frequently

Men Only
- A drip or drainage from penis

Women Only
- Vaginal discharge or odor from the vagina
- Pain in the lower pelvis or deep in the vagina during sex
- Burning or itching around the vagina
- Bleeding from the vagina at times other than the regular menstrual periods

Figure 14.3
Signs or Symptoms of an STI

Early symptoms of an STI are often mild (Figure 14.3). Left untreated, some of these infections can have grave consequences, such as sterility, blindness, central nervous system destruction, disfigurement, and even death. Infants born to mothers carrying the organisms for these infections are at risk for a variety of health problems. As with many communicable diseases, much of the pain, suffering, and anguish associated with STIs can be eliminated through education, responsible action, simple preventive strategies, and prompt treatment.

Possible Causes: Why Me?

Several reasons have been proposed to explain the present high rates of STIs. The first relates to the moral and social stigma associated with these infections. Shame and embarrassment often keep infected people from seeking treatment. Unfortunately, they usually continue to be sexually active, thereby infecting unsuspecting partners. People who are uncomfortable discussing sexual issues may also be less likely to use and ask their partners to use condoms to protect against STIs and pregnancy.

Another reason proposed for the STI epidemic is our culture's casual attitude about sex. Bombarded by media hype that glamorizes easy sex, many people take sexual partners without considering the consequences. Others are pressured into sexual relationships they don't really want. Generally, the more sexual partners a person has, the greater the risk for contracting an STI. Evaluate your own attitude about STIs by completing the Assess Yourself box on page 376.

Ignorance—about the infections, their symptoms, and the fact that someone can be asymptomatic (symptom-free) but still infected—is also a factor. A person who is infected but asymptomatic can unknowingly spread an STI to an unsuspecting partner, who may, in turn, ignore or misinterpret any symptoms. By the time either partner seeks medical help, he or she may have infected several others.

Modes of Transmission

STIs are generally spread through some form of intimate sexual contact. Sexual intercourse, oral–genital contact, hand–genital contact, and anal intercourse are the most common modes of transmission. More rarely, pathogens for STIs are transmitted from mouth to mouth or through contact with fluids from body sores. Although each STI is a different infection caused by a different pathogen, all STI pathogens prefer dark, moist places, especially the mucous membranes lining the reproductive organs. Most of them are susceptible to light, excess heat, cold, and dryness, and many die quickly on exposure to air. (A toilet seat is not a likely breeding ground for most bacterial or viral STIs!) Although most STIs are passed on by sexual contact, other kinds of close contact, such as sleeping on sheets used by someone who has pubic lice, may also infect you. Like other communicable infections, STIs have both pathogen-specific incubation periods and periods of time during which transmission is most likely, called periods of communicability.

Chlamydia

Chlamydia, a disease that often presents no symptoms, tops the list of the most commonly reported infections in the United States. Chlamydia infects about 800,000 people annually in the United States, the majority of them women.[31] Public health officials believe that the actual number of cases is probably closer to 3 or 4 million because these figures represent only those cases reported. College students account for more than 10 percent of infections, and these numbers seem to be increasing yearly.

The name of the disease is derived from the Greek verb *chlamys,* meaning "to cloak," because, unlike most bacteria, *Chlamydia* bacteria can live and grow only inside other cells. Although many people classify chlamydia as either *nonspecific* or *nongonococcal urethritis (NGU),* a person may have NGU without having the organism for chlamydia.

In males, early symptoms may include painful and difficult urination, frequent urination, and a watery, puslike discharge from the penis. Symptoms in females may include a yellowish discharge, spotting between periods, and occasional spotting after intercourse. However, many chlamydia victims display no symptoms and therefore do not seek help until the disease has done secondary damage. Females are especially likely to be asymptomatic; more than 70 percent do not realize they have the disease until secondary damage occurs.

The secondary damage resulting from chlamydia is serious in both sexes. Men can suffer damage to the prostate gland, seminal vesicles, and bulbourethral glands as well as arthritislike symptoms and damage to the blood vessels and heart. In women, chlamydia-related infection can injure the cervix or fallopian tubes, which causes sterility, and can damage the inner pelvic structure, which leads to pelvic inflammatory disease (PID). If an infected woman becomes pregnant, she has a high risk for miscarriage and stillbirth. *Chlamydia* may also be responsible for one type of **conjunctivitis,** an eye infection that affects not only adults but also infants, who can contract the disease from an infected mother during delivery. Untreated conjunctivitis can cause blindness. If detected early, chlamydia is easily treatable with antibiotics.

What do you think?
Even though many college students have heard about the risks of STIs and AIDS, why do so many fail to use condoms and take other precautions?
* *What actions could be taken to make more of your friends heed the warnings about STIs?*

Pelvic Inflammatory Disease

Pelvic inflammatory disease (PID) is a term used to describe a number of infections of the uterus, fallopian tubes, and ovaries. Although PID often results from an untreated STI, especially chlamydia or gonorrhea, it is not actually an STI. Several nonsexual factors increase the risk of PID, particularly excessive vaginal douching, cigarette smoking, and substance abuse.

In the United States, PID affects 11 percent of women of reproductive age. Approximately 1 million women experience PID each year, and 20 percent require hospitalization for treatment.[32] Symptoms vary but generally include acute

(text continues on page 378)

Chlamydia   Bacterially caused STI of the urogenital tract.

Conjunctivitis   Serious inflammation of the eye caused by any number of pathogens or irritants; can be caused by STDs such as chlamydia.

Pelvic inflammatory disease (PID)   Term used to describe various infections of the female reproductive tract.

Sexually Transmitted Infections: Attitude and Belief Scale

The following quiz will help you evaluate whether your beliefs and attitudes about STIs lead you to take risks that increase your risk of infection.

DIRECTIONS

Indicate that you believe the following items are true or false by circling the T or the F. Then consult the answer key that follows.

1. You can usually tell whether someone is infected with an STI, especially HIV infection.   T   F

2. Chances are that if you haven't caught an STI by now, you probably have a natural immunity and won't get infected in the future.   T   F

3. A person who is successfully treated for an STI needn't worry about getting it again.   T   F

4. So long as you keep yourself fit and healthy, you needn't worry about STIs.   T   F

5. The best way for sexually active people to protect themselves from STIs is to practice safer sex.   T   F

6. The only way to catch an STI is to have sex with someone who has one.   T   F

7. Talking about STIs with a partner is so embarrassing that it's better not to raise the subject and instead hope the other person will.   T   F

8. STIs are mostly a problem for people who have numerous sex partners.   T   F

9. You don't need to worry about contracting an STI as long as you wash yourself thoroughly with soap and hot water immediately after sex.   T   F

10. You don't need to worry about contracting AIDS if no one you know has ever come down with it.   T   F

11. When it comes to STIs, it's all in the cards. Either you're lucky, or you're not.   T   F

12. The time to worry about STIs is when you come down with one.   T   F

13. As long as you avoid risky sexual practices, such as anal intercourse, you're pretty safe from STIs.   T   F

14. The time to talk about safer sex is before any sexual contact occurs.   T   F

15. A person needn't be concerned about an STI if the symptoms clear up on their own in a few weeks.   T   F

ANSWER KEY

1. False. While some STIs have telltale signs, such as the appearance of sores or blisters on the genitals or disagreeable genital odors, others do not. Several STIs, such as chlamydia, gonorrhea (especially in women), internal genital warts, and even HIV infection in its early stages cause few if any obvious signs or symptoms. You often cannot tell whether your partner is infected with an STI. Many of the nicest-looking and best-groomed people carry STIs, often unknowingly. The only way to know whether a person is infected with HIV is by means of an HIV-antibody test.

2. False. If you practice unprotected sex and have not contracted an STI to this point, count your blessings. The thing about good luck is that it eventually runs out.

3. False. Sorry. Successful treatment does not render immunity against reinfection. You still need to take precautions to avoid reinfection, even if you have had an STI in the past and were successfully treated. If you answered true to this item, you're not alone. About one in five college students polled in a recent survey of more than 5,500 college students across Canada believed that a person who gets an STI cannot get it again.

4. False. Even people in prime physical condition can be felled by the tiniest of microbes that cause STIs. Physical fitness is no protection against these microscopic invaders.

5. True. If you are sexually active, practicing safer sex is the best protection against contracting an STI.

6. False. STIs can also be transmitted through nonsexual means, such as by sharing contaminated needles or, in some cases, through contact with disease-causing organisms on towels and bed sheets or even toilet seats.

7. False. Because of the social stigma attached to STIs, it's understandable that you may feel embarrassed about raising the subject with your partner. But don't let embarrassment prevent you from taking steps to protect your own and your partner's welfare.

8. False. It stands to reason that people who are sexually active with numerous partners stand a greater chance that one of their sexual partners will carry an STI. Nevertheless, all it takes is one infected partner to pass along an STI to you, even if he or she is the only partner you've had, or even if the two of you had sex only once. STIs are a potential problem for anyone who is sexually active.

9. False. While washing your genitals immediately after sex may have some limited protective value, it is no substitute for practicing safer sex.

10. False. You can never know whether you may be the first among your friends and acquaintances to become infected. Moreover, symptoms of HIV infection may not appear for years after initial infection with the virus, so you may have sexual contacts with people who are infected but don't know it and who are capable of passing along the virus to you. You, in turn, may then pass it along to others, whether or not you are aware of any symptoms.

11. False. Nonsense. While luck may play a part in determining whether you have a sexual contact with an infected partner, you can significantly reduce your risk of contracting an STI.

12. False. The time to start thinking about STIs (thinking helps, but worrying only makes you more anxious than you need be) is now, not after you have contracted an infection. Some STIs, like herpes and AIDS, cannot be cured. The only real protection you have against them is prevention.

13. False. Any sexual contact between the genitals, or between the genitals and the anus, or between the mouth and genitals, is risky if one of the partners is infected with an STI.

14. True. Unfortunately, too many couples wait until they have commenced sexual relations to have "a talk." By then it may already be too late to prevent the transmission of an STI. The time to talk is before any intimate sexual contact occurs.

15. False. Several STIs, notably syphilis, HIV infection, and herpes, may produce initial symptoms that clear up in a few weeks. But while the early symptoms may subside, the infection is still at work within the body and requires medical attention. Also, as noted previously, the infected person is capable of passing along the infection to others, regardless of whether noticeable symptoms were ever present.

INTERPRETING YOUR SCORE

First, add up the number of items you got right. The higher your score, the lower your risk. The lower your score, the greater your risk. A score of 13 correct or better may indicate that your attitudes toward STIs would probably decrease your risk of contracting them. Yet, even one wrong response on this test may increase your risk of contracting an STI. You should also recognize that attitudes have little effect on behavior unless they are carried into action. Knowledge alone isn't sufficient to protect yourself from STIs. You need to ask yourself how you are going to put knowledge into action by changing your behavior to reduce your chances of contracting an STI.

Source: Jeffrey S. Nevid with Fern Gotfried, *Choices: Sex in the Age of STDs* (Boston: Allyn and Bacon, 1995), 10–13. © Copyright 1995 by Allyn and Bacon. Reprinted by permission.

inflammation of the pelvic cavity, severe pain in the lower abdomen, menstrual irregularities, fever, nausea, painful intercourse, tubal pregnancies, and severe depression.[33] Major consequences of untreated PID are infertility, ectopic pregnancy, chronic pelvic pain, and recurrent upper genital infections. Risk factors include young age at first sexual intercourse, multiple sex partners, high frequency of sexual intercourse, and change of sexual partners within the past 30 days. Regular gynecological examinations and early treatment for STI symptoms reduce risk.

Gonorrhea

One of the most common STIs in the United States, **gonorrhea** is surpassed only by chlamydia in number of cases. The Institute of Medicine estimates that there are more than 800,000 cases per year and that large numbers go unreported.[34] Health economists estimate that the annual cost of gonorrhea and its complications is more than $1.1 billion.[35] Caused by the bacterial pathogen *Neisseria gonorrhoeae,* this infection primarily infects the linings of the urethra, genital tract, pharynx, and rectum. It may spread to the eyes or other body regions via the hands or body fluids, typically during vaginal, oral, or anal sex. Most victims are males between the ages of 20 and 24; sexually active females between the ages of 15 and 19 are also at high risk.[36]

In males, a typical symptom is a white milky discharge from the penis accompanied by painful, burning urination two to nine days after contact. This is usually enough to send most men to the physician for treatment. However, about 20 percent of all males with gonorrhea are asymptomatic.

In females, the situation is just the opposite: only 20 percent experience any discharge, and few develop a burning sensation upon urinating until much later in the course of the infection (if ever). The organism can remain in the woman's vagina, cervix, uterus, or fallopian tubes for long periods with no apparent symptoms other than an occasional slight fever. Thus, a woman can be unaware that she has been infected and is infecting her sexual partners.

If the infection is detected early, antibiotic treatment is generally effective within a short period of time. If the infection goes undetected in a woman, it can spread throughout the genital–urinary tract to the fallopian tubes and ovaries, thus causing sterility or, at the very least, severe inflammation and PID. The bacteria can also spread up the reproductive tract or, more rarely, can spread through the blood and infect the joints, heart valves, or brain. If an infected woman becomes pregnant, the infection can cause conjunctivitis in her infant. To prevent this, physicians routinely administer silver nitrate or penicillin preparations to the eyes of newborn babies.

Untreated gonorrhea may spread to the prostate, testicles, urinary tract, kidney, and bladder. Blockage of the vasa deferentia due to scar tissue may cause sterility. In some cases, the penis develops a painful curvature during erection.

Syphilis

Syphilis is also caused by a bacterial organism, the *spirochete* known as *Treponema pallidum.* Because it is extremely delicate and dies readily upon exposure to air, dryness, or cold, the organism is generally transferred only through direct sexual contact. Typically, this means contact between sexual organs during intercourse, but in rare instances, the organism enters the body through a break in the skin, through deep kissing, or through some other transmission of body fluids.

Syphilis is called the "great imitator" because its symptoms resemble those of several other infections. Left untreated, syphilis generally progresses through distinct stages. It should be noted, however, that some people experience no symptoms at all.

Primary Syphilis   The first stage of syphilis, particularly for males, is often characterized by the development of a **chancre** (pronounced "shank-er"), a sore at the site of initial infection. This dime-sized chancre is painless, but it oozes with bacteria, ready to infect an unsuspecting partner. Usually the chancre appears three to four weeks after contact.

In males, the site of the chancre tends to be the penis or scrotum because this is the site where the organism first enters the body. But if the infection was contracted through oral sex, the sore can appear in the mouth, throat, or other "first contact" area. In females, the site of infection is often internal, on the vaginal wall or high on the cervix. Because the chancre is not readily apparent, the likelihood of detection is not great. In both males and females, the chancre will completely disappear in three to six weeks.

Secondary Syphilis   From a month to a year after the chancre disappears, secondary symptoms may appear, including a rash or white patches on the skin or on the mucous membranes of the mouth, throat, or genitals. Hair loss may occur, lymph nodes may enlarge, and the victim may develop a slight fever or a headache. In rare cases, sores develop around the mouth or genitals. As during the active chancre phase, these sores contain infectious bacteria, and contact with them can spread the infection. In a few cases, there may be arthritic pain in the joints. Because symptoms vary so much and appear so much later than the sexual contact that caused them, the victim seldom connects the two. The infection thus often goes undetected even at this second stage. Symptoms may persist for a few weeks or

---

Gonorrhea   Second most common STD in the United States; if untreated, may cause sterility.

Syphilis   One of the most widespread STDs; characterized by distinct phases and potentially serious results.

Chancre   Sore often found at the site of syphilis infection.

---

months and then disappear, thus leaving the victim thinking that all is well.

Latent Syphilis   After the secondary stage, the syphilis spirochetes begin to invade body organs. Symptoms, including infectious lesions, may reappear periodically for two to four years after the secondary period. After this period, the infection is rarely transmitted to others, except during pregnancy, when it can be passed to the fetus. The child will then be born with *congenital syphilis,* which can cause death or severe birth defects such as blindness, deafness, or disfigurement. Because in most cases the fetus does not become infected until after the first trimester, treatment of the mother during this period will usually prevent infection of the fetus.

In some instances, a child born to an infected mother will show no apparent signs of the infection at birth but within several weeks will develop body rashes, a runny nose, and symptoms of paralysis. Congenital syphilis is usually detected before it progresses much further. But sometimes the child's immune system will ward off the invading organism, and further symptoms may not surface until the teenage years. Fortunately, most states protect against congenital syphilis by requiring prospective marriage partners to be tested for syphilis prior to obtaining a marriage license.

If untreated, latent syphilis will progress and infect more and more organs.

Late Syphilis   Years after syphilis has entered the body, its effects become all too evident. Late-stage syphilis indications include heart damage, central nervous system damage, blindness, deafness, paralysis, premature senility, and, ultimately, insanity.

Treatment for Syphilis   Because the organism is bacterial, it is treated with antibiotics. The major obstacle to treatment is misdiagnosis of this "imitator" infection.

Pubic Lice

Pubic lice, often called "crabs," are small parasites that are usually transmitted during sexual contact. More annoying than dangerous, they move easily from partner to partner during sex. They have an affinity for pubic hair and attach themselves to the base of these hairs, where they deposit their eggs (nits). One to two weeks later, these nits develop into adults that lay eggs and migrate to other body parts, thus perpetuating the cycle.

Treatment includes washing clothing, furniture, and linens that may harbor the eggs. It usually takes two to three weeks to kill all larval forms. Although sexual contact is the most common mode of transmission, you can "catch" pubic lice from lying on sheets that an infected person has slept on. Sleeping in hotel and dormitory rooms in which sheets are not washed regularly, or sitting on toilet seats where the nits or larvae have been dropped and lie in wait for a new carrier, will put you at risk.

Genital HPV

Genital warts (also known as venereal warts or condylomas) are caused by a small group of viruses known as **human papillomaviruses (HPVs).** A person becomes infected when an HPV penetrates the skin and mucous membranes of the genitals or anus through sexual contact. HPV is among the most common forms of STI. The virus appears to be relatively easy to catch. The typical incubation period is from six to eight weeks after contact. Many people have no symptoms, particularly if the warts are located inside the reproductive tract. Others may develop a series of itchy bumps on the genitals that range in size from small pinheads to large cauliflowerlike growths. On dry skin (such as the shaft of the penis), the warts are commonly small, hard, and yellowish-gray, resembling warts that appear on other parts of the body. Genital warts are of two different types: (1) *full-blown genital warts* that are noticeable as tiny bumps or growths, and (2) the much more prevalent *flat warts* that are not usually visible to the naked eye.

Risks and Treatments of Genital Warts   Many genital warts eventually disappear on their own. Others grow and generate unsightly flaps of irregular flesh on the external genitalia. If they grow large enough to obstruct urinary flow or become irritated by clothing or sexual intercourse, they can cause significant problems.

The greatest threat from genital warts lies in the apparent relationship between them and a tendency for *dysplasia,* or changes in cells that may lead to a precancerous condition. It is known that within five years after infection, 30 percent of all HPV cases progress to the precancerous stage. If precancerous cases are left untreated, 70 percent of them will result in actual cancer. New research also implicates HPV as a possible risk factor for coronary artery disease, possibly because it causes an inflammatory response in artery walls. In addition, venereal warts pose a threat to a pregnant woman's fetus if it is exposed to the virus during birth. Cesarean deliveries may be considered in serious cases.

Genital warts can be treated with topical medications or removed by being frozen with liquid nitrogen. Large warts may require surgical removal.

Candidiasis (Moniliasis)

Unlike many STIs, which are caused by pathogens that come from outside the body, the yeastlike fungus caused by the *Candida albicans* organism normally inhabits the vaginal tract

---

Pubic lice   Parasites that can inhabit various body areas, especially the genitals; also called "crabs."

Genital warts   Warts that appear in the genital area or the anus; caused by the human papillomaviruses (HPVs).

Human papillomaviruses (HPV)   A small group of viruses that cause genital warts.

in most women. Only under certain conditions, in which the normal chemical balance of the vagina is disturbed, will these organisms multiply and cause problems.

The likelihood of **candidiasis** (also known as moniliasis or a *yeast infection*) increases if a woman has diabetes; if her immune system is overtaxed or malfunctioning; if she is taking birth control pills, other hormones, or broad-spectrum antibiotics; or if she uses douches or spermicides. All of these factors decrease the acidity of the vagina and create favorable conditions for a yeastlike infection.

Symptoms of candidiasis include severe itching and burning of the vagina and vulva, swelling of the vulva, and a white, cheesy vaginal discharge. These symptoms are collectively called **vaginitis**, or inflammation of the vagina. When this microbe infects the mouth, whitish patches form, and the condition is referred to as *thrush*. This monilial infection also occurs in males and is easily transmitted between sexual partners.

Candidiasis strikes at least half a million American women a year. Antifungal drugs applied on the surface or by suppository usually cure it in just a few days. For approximately one out of ten women, however, nothing seems to work, and the infection returns again and again. Symptoms can be aggravated by contact of the vagina with soaps, douches, perfumed toilet paper, chlorinated water, and spermicides. Tight-fitting jeans and pantyhose can provide the combination of moisture and irritant the organism thrives on.

Trichomoniasis

Unlike many STIs, **trichomoniasis** is caused by a protozoan. Although as many as half of the men and women in the United States may carry this organism, most remain free of symptoms until their bodily defenses are weakened. Both men and women may transmit the infection, but women are the more likely candidates for infection. Symptoms include a foamy, yellowish, unpleasant-smelling discharge accompanied by a burning sensation, itching, and painful urination. These symptoms are most likely to occur during or shortly after menstruation, but they can appear at any time or be absent altogether. Although usually transmitted by sexual contact, the "trich" organism can also be spread by toilet seats, wet towels, or other items that have discharged fluids

on them. You can also contract trichomoniasis by sitting naked on the locker room bench at your local gym. Treatment includes oral metronidazole, usually given to both sexual partners to avoid the possible "ping-pong" effect of repeated cross-infection so typical of STIs.

General Urinary Tract Infections

Although *general urinary tract infections (UTIs)* can be caused by various factors, some forms are sexually transmitted. Anytime invading organisms enter the genital area, they can travel up the urethra and enter the bladder. Similarly, organisms normally living in the rectum, urethra, or bladder may travel to the sexual organs and eventually be transmitted to another person.

You can also get a UTI through autoinoculation, often during the simple task of wiping yourself after defecating. Wiping from the anus forward can transmit organisms found in feces to the vaginal opening or the urethra. Contact between the hands and the urethra and between the urethra and other objects are also common means of autoinoculation. Women, with their shorter urethras, are more likely to contract UTIs. Hand washing with soap and water prior to sexual intimacy, foreplay, and so on, is recommended. Treatment depends on the nature and type of pathogen.

Herpes

Herpes is a general term for a family of infections characterized by sores or eruptions on the skin. Herpes infections range from mildly uncomfortable to extremely serious. **Genital herpes** is an infection caused by the herpes simplex virus (HSV).

There are two types of HSV. Historically, the herpes simplex type 2 virus was considered the primary culprit in genital herpes, and herpes simplex virus type 1 was thought to affect the area of the lips and other body areas.[37] We now know that both type 1 and type 2 can infect any area of the body and produce lesions (sores) in and around the vaginal area, on the penis, around the anal opening, on the buttocks or thighs, and occasionally on other parts of the body. HSV remains in certain nerve cells for life and can flare up, or cause symptoms, when the body's ability to maintain itself is weakened.

The prodromal (precursor) phase of the infection is characterized by a burning sensation and redness at the site of infection. During this time, prescription medicines will often keep the disease from spreading. However, this phase of the disease is quickly followed by the second phase, in which a blister filled with a clear fluid containing the virus forms. If you pick at this blister or otherwise touch the site and spread this fluid with fingers, lipstick, lip balm, or other products, you can autoinoculate other body parts. Particularly dangerous is the possibility of spreading the infection to your eyes, for a herpes lesion on the eye can cause blindness.

Over a period of days, the unsightly blister will dry up and disappear, and the virus will travel to the base of an

---

Candidiasis   Yeastlike fungal disease often transmitted sexually.

Vaginitis   Set of symptoms characterized by vaginal itching, swelling, and burning.

Trichomoniasis   Protozoan infection characterized by foamy, yellowish discharge and unpleasant odor.

Genital herpes   STI caused by the herpes simplex virus.

---

affected nerve supplying the area and become dormant. Only when the victim becomes overly stressed, when diet and sleep are inadequate, when the immune system is overworked, or when excessive exposure to sunlight or other stressors occurs will the virus become reactivated (at the same site every time) and begin the blistering cycle all over again. These sores cast off (shed) viruses that can be highly infectious. However, it is important to note that a herpes site can shed the virus even when no overt sore is present, particularly during the prodromal stages (the interval between the earliest symptoms and blistering). People may get genital herpes by having sexual contact with others who don't know they are infected or who are having outbreaks of herpes without any sores. A person with genital herpes can also infect a sexual partner during oral sex. The virus is spread only rarely, if at all, by touching objects such as a toilet seat or hot tub seat.[38]

Genital herpes is especially serious in pregnant women because the baby could be infected as it passes through the vagina during birth. Many physicians recommend cesarean deliveries for infected women. Additionally, women who have a history of genital herpes appear to have a greater risk of cervical cancer.

Although there is no cure for herpes at present, certain drugs can reduce symptoms. Unfortunately, they seem to work only if the infection is confirmed during the first few hours after contact. As you may guess, this is rather rare. The effectiveness of other treatments, such as L-lysine, is largely unsubstantiated. Newer over-the-counter medications seem to be moderately effective in reducing the severity of symptoms. Although lip balms and cold-sore medications may provide temporary relief, remember that rubbing anything on a herpes blister can spread herpes-laden fluids to other body parts.

Preventing Herpes You can take precautions to reduce your risk of herpes.

- Avoid any form of kissing if you notice a sore or blister on your partner's mouth. Kiss no one, not even a peck on the cheek, if you know that you have a herpes lesion. Allow time after the sores go away before you start kissing again.
- Be extremely cautious if you have casual sexual affairs. Not every partner will feel obligated to tell you that he or she has a problem. It's up to you to protect yourself.
- Wash your hands immediately with soap and water after any form of sexual contact.
- If you have questionable sores or lesions, seek medical help at once. Do not be afraid to name your contacts.
- If you have herpes, be responsible in your sexual contacts with others. If you have any suspicious lesions that might put your partner at risk, say so. Find an appropriate time and place, and hold a candid discussion.
- Reduce your risk of herpes outbreaks by avoiding excessive stress, sunlight, or whatever else appears to trigger an episode.

HIV/AIDS

Acquired immune deficiency syndrome (AIDS) is a significant global health threat. Since 1981, when AIDS was first recognized, more than 60 million people in the world have become infected with **human immunodeficiency virus (HIV),** the virus that causes AIDS. Today, more than 42 million people are estimated to be living with HIV or AIDS, and an estimated 5 million new cases were diagnosed worldwide in 2002.[39] Women are becoming increasingly affected by the virus and account for approximately 50 percent of cases.[40] In the United States, as of 2002, more than 886,575 men, women, and children with AIDS have been reported to the CDC, and at least 501,669 have died.[41] The CDC estimates that at least 40,000 new infections occur each year in the United States. See the Health in a Diverse World box on page 382 for more on the global impact of HIV/AIDS.

A Shifting Epidemic

Under old definitions, people with HIV were diagnosed as having AIDS only when they developed blood infections, the cancer known as Kaposi's sarcoma, or any of 21 other indicator diseases, most of which were common in males. The CDC has expanded the indicator list to include pulmonary tuberculosis, recurrent pneumonia, and invasive cervical cancer. Perhaps the most significant new indicator is a drop in the level of the body's master immune cells, called CD4s, to 200 per cubic millimeter (one-fifth the level in a healthy person).

AIDS cases have been reported state by state throughout the United States since the early 1980s as a means of tracking the disease. While the numbers of actual reported cases have always been suspect, improved reporting and surveillance methods have helped increase accuracy. Today, the CDC recommends that all states report HIV infections as well as AIDS. Because of medical advances in treatment and increasing numbers of HIV-infected persons who do not progress to AIDS, it is believed that AIDS incidence statistics may not provide a true picture of the epidemic, the long-term costs of treating HIV-infected individuals, and other key information. HIV incidence data also provide a better picture of infection trends. Currently, most states mandate that those who test positive for the HIV antibody be reported.

Acquired immune deficiency syndrome (AIDS) Extremely virulent sexually transmitted disease that renders the immune system inoperative.

Human immunodeficiency virus (HIV) The slow-acting virus that causes AIDS.

The Staggering Toll of HIV/AIDS in the Global Community

Although the rates of HIV/AIDS may be slowing in the United States, the disease has had an increasingly devastating impact on other regions of the world. By the year 2003, an estimated 34 to 46 million people from all regions of the world were infected with HIV, which translates to nearly 1 out of every 100 men, women, and children. Every day in 2003, an estimated 14,000 people were newly infected with HIV. Here are some facts about this global epidemic.

AFRICA

- In southern Africa, one in every five people is now infected. Almost 39% of the population in Botswana and Swaziland is living with HIV.

- About 30% of people living with HIV worldwide live in southern Africa, an area that is home to just 2% of the world's population.
- South Africa is home to an estimated 5.3 million people with HIV, more than any other country in the world.

LATIN AMERICA AND THE CARIBBEAN

- In 2003, an estimated 2 million people in this region were living with the HIV virus. The epidemic was mainly spread through heterosexual intercourse, injecting drug use, and men who have sex with men.
- Haiti was worst hit, with 6% of adults infected.

EASTERN EUROPE AND CENTRAL ASIA

- In eastern Europe and central Asia combined, an estimated 1.5 million people were living with the AIDS virus at the end of 2003.
- Rates of infection are increasing among drug users sharing needles in eastern Europe and Russia.

ASIA

- An estimated 7.4 million people in the region were living with the AIDS virus in 2003.
- Thailand has an infection rate of 2%. This country and Cambodia seem to have controlled the once-rampant spread of HIV by promoting condom use, especially among sex workers.
- An estimated 3.82 to 4.58 million people in India live with the virus, the second highest national total behind South Africa, with an infection rate of 0.7%.

Source: Joint United Nations Programme on HIV/AIDS (UNAIDS), "AIDS Epidemic Update 2003," December 2003. www.unaids.org/wad/2003/press/epiupdate.html

---

What do you think?

Do you favor mandatory reporting of HIV and AIDS cases? ☀ *If you knew that your name and vital statistics would be "on file" if you tested positive for HIV, would you be less likely to take the HIV test?* ☀ *On the other hand, do people who carry this contagious fatal disease have a responsibility to inform the general public and the health professionals who will provide their care? Explain your answer.*

Women and AIDS

HIV is an equal-opportunity pathogen that can attack anyone who engages in high-risk behaviors. This is true regardless of race, gender, sexual orientation, or socioeconomic status. Consider the following facts:[42]

- Women are four to ten times more likely than men to contract HIV through unprotected sexual intercourse with an infected partner.[43]
- By 2002, women accounted for more than 50 percent of all AIDS cases in the United States.[44]

- HIV/AIDS due to heterosexual sexual transmission is increasing faster in rural America than in any other part of the country. Women most at risk are ethnic minorities and the economically disadvantaged. Among sexually active heterosexual teenagers, college students, and health care workers, nearly 60 percent of HIV cases are women.
- Most women with AIDS were infected through heterosexual exposure to HIV, followed by injection drug use (sharing needles).
- Women of color are disproportionately affected by HIV; African American and Hispanic women together account for 76 percent of AIDS cases among women in the United States, though they comprise less than 25 percent of all U.S. women.
- Of all AIDS cases among women, 61 percent were reported from five states: New York (26 percent), Florida (13 percent), New Jersey (10 percent), California (7 percent), and Texas (5 percent).
- AIDS is the leading cause of death among African American women age 25 to 44, and the fourth leading cause of death among all American women in this age group.
- AIDS is one of the top ten causes of death for people age 15 to 64 in the United States.

Compounding the problems are serious deficiencies in our health and social service systems, including inadequate treatment for women addicts and lack of access to child care, health care, and social services for families headed by single women. Women with HIV/AIDS are of special interest because they are the major source of infection in infants. Virtually all new HIV infections among children in the United States are attributable to perinatal transmission of HIV.[45]

Although contracting HIV is a serious problem for both males and females, women often have an even more difficult time protecting themselves from infection and taking care of themselves once they become ill. Irrefutable evidence indicates that HIV/AIDS disproportionately affects women. This discrepancy can be traced to biological and socioeconomic factors.

Biological factors include:

- HIV can enter through mucous membrane surfaces of the genital tract; the vagina has a greater exposed mucous membrane than does the urethra of the penis.
- The vaginal area is more likely to incur micro-tears during sexual intercourse, which facilitates entry of HIV.
- During intercourse, a woman is exposed to more semen than is the male to vaginal fluids.
- Semen is more likely to enter the vagina with force, whereas vaginal fluids do not enter the penis with force.
- Women who have STIs are more likely to be asymptomatic and therefore unaware they have an STI; STIs increase the risk of HIV transmission.

Socioeconomic factors include:

- There are more HIV-infected men than HIV-infected women in the United States; thus, it is more likely for a woman to have an HIV-infected male partner.
- Women have been underrepresented in clinical trials for HIV treatment and prevention.
- Many cultural norms place women in subordination to men, especially in developing nations. This reduces women's decision-making power and ability to negotiate safer sex.
- Women are more vulnerable to sexual abuse from their male partners.
- Women are more likely to be economically dependent on men.
- Women may be less likely to seek medical treatment because of lack of money, caregiving burdens, and transportation problems.
- In the United States, HIV-positive women are more likely than are HIV-positive men to be younger and less educated.

What do you think?

Why do you think HIV/AIDS is increasing among women and minority groups in America? ✻ *Why are some women particularly vulnerable?* ✻ *What actions can we take as a nation to reduce the spread of HIV/AIDS among women and among minority groups?* ✻ *Should Americans be concerned about the global HIV/AIDS epidemic? Why or why not?*

How HIV Is Transmitted

HIV typically enters one person's body when another person's infected body fluids (semen, vaginal secretions, blood, etc.) gain entry through a breach in body defenses. Mucous membranes of the genital organs and the anus provide the easiest route of entry. If there is a break in the mucous membranes (as can occur during sexual intercourse, particularly anal intercourse), the virus enters and begins to multiply. After initial infection, HIV multiplies rapidly, invading the bloodstream and cerebrospinal fluid. It progressively destroys helper T-lymphocytes, thus weakening the body's resistance to disease. The virus also changes the genetic structure of the cells it attacks. In response to this invasion, the body quickly begins to produce antibodies.

Despite some myths, HIV is not a highly contagious virus. Studies of people living in households with a person with HIV/AIDS have turned up no documented cases of HIV infection due to casual contact. Other investigations provide overwhelming evidence that insect bites do not transmit HIV.

Engaging in High-Risk Behaviors   AIDS is not a disease of gay people or minority groups. If you engage in high-risk behaviors, you increase your risk for the disease. If you do not practice these behaviors, your risk is minimal. Anyone who engages in unprotected sex is at risk, especially sex with a partner who has engaged in other high-risk behaviors. Sex with multiple partners is the greatest threat.

Exchange of Body Fluids   The greatest risk factor is the exchange of HIV-infected body fluids during vaginal and anal intercourse. Substantial research evidence indicates that blood, semen, and vaginal secretions are the major fluids of concern. Most health officials state that saliva is not a high-risk body fluid unless blood is present. But the fact that the virus has been found in isolated samples of saliva does provide a good rationale for using caution when engaging in deep, wet kissing.[46]

Initially, public health officials also included breast milk in the list of high-risk fluids because a few infants apparently contracted HIV while breast-feeding. Subsequent research has indicated that HIV transmission could have been caused by bleeding nipples as well as by actual consumption of breast milk and other fluids. Infection through contact with feces and urine is believed to be highly unlikely though technically possible.

Receiving a Blood Transfusion Prior to 1985   A small group of people became infected with HIV after receiving blood transfusions. In 1985, the Red Cross and other blood donation programs implemented a stringent testing program for all donated blood. Today, because of these massive screening efforts, the risk of receiving HIV-infected blood is almost nonexistent.

Injecting Drugs   A significant percentage of AIDS cases in the United States are believed to result from sharing or using

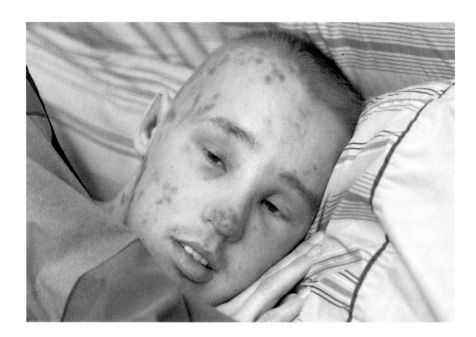

The effects of HIV/AIDS can be seen here in the form of Kaposi's sarcoma and wasting syndrome.

HIV-contaminated needles and syringes. Though users of illegal drugs are commonly considered the only members of this category, others may also share needles—for example, people with diabetes who inject insulin or athletes who inject steroids. People who share needles and also engage in sexual activities with members of high-risk groups, such as those who exchange sex for drugs, increase their risks dramatically.

Mother-to-Infant Transmission (Perinatal) Approximately one in three of the children who has contracted AIDS received the virus from an infected mother while in the womb or while passing through the vaginal tract during delivery.

Symptoms of HIV Disease

A person may go for months or years after infection by HIV before any significant symptoms appear. The incubation time varies greatly from person to person. Children have shorter incubation periods than do adults. Newborns and infants are particularly vulnerable to AIDS because human beings do not become fully immunocompetent (that is, their immune system is not fully developed) until they are 6 to 15 months old. New information suggests that some very young children show the "adult" progression of AIDS.[47]

For adults who receive no medical treatment, it takes an average of eight to ten years for the virus to cause the

slow, degenerative changes in the immune system that are characteristic of AIDS. During this time, the person may experience a large number of opportunistic infections (infections that gain a foothold when the immune system is not functioning effectively). Colds, sore throats, fever, tiredness, nausea, night sweats, and other generally non–life-threatening conditions commonly appear, and are described as pre-AIDS symptoms.

Testing for HIV Antibodies

Once antibodies have formed in reaction to HIV, a blood test known as the **ELISA** test may detect their presence. If sufficient antibodies are present, the ELISA test will be positive. When a person who previously tested *negative* (no HIV antibodies present) has a subsequent test that is *positive,* seroconversion is said to have occurred. In such a situation, the person would typically take another ELISA test, followed by a more expensive, precise test known as the **Western blot,** to confirm the presence of HIV antibodies.

It should be noted that these tests are not AIDS tests per se. Rather, they detect antibodies for the disease that would indicate the presence of HIV in the person's body. Whether the person will develop AIDS depends to some extent on the strength of the immune system. However, the vast majority of all infected people develop some form of the disease.

As testing for HIV antibodies has been perfected, scientists have explored various ways of making it easier for individuals to be tested. Health officials distinguish between *reported* and *actual* cases of HIV infection because it is believed that many HIV-positive people avoid being tested. One reason may be fear of knowing the truth. Another is the

---

ELISA Blood test that detects presence of antibodies to HIV virus.

Western blot A test more accurate than the ELISA to confirm presence of HIV antibodies.

---

fear of discrimination from employers, insurance companies, and medical staff if a positive test becomes known to others. However, early detection and reporting are important, because immediate treatment for someone in the early stages of HIV disease is critical.

New Hope and Treatments

New drugs have slowed the progression from HIV to AIDS and have prolonged life expectancies for many AIDS patients. While these new therapies offered the promise of life for many, they may have inadvertently led to increases in risky behaviors. This may have led to a noteworthy rise in cases by 2 percent in 2002.[48] Although the death rate from AIDS has declined each year since 1995, many fear that we are taking steps backward. Advocates for AIDS patients believe the medications still cost too much money and cause too many side effects. Multidrug treatment for AIDS for one person now exceeds $20,000 per year.

Current treatments combine selected drugs, especially protease inhibitors and reverse transcriptase inhibitors. Protease inhibitors (for example, Amprenavir, Ritonavir, and Saquinavir) resemble pieces of the protein chain that the HIV protease normally cuts. They block the HIV protease enzyme from cutting the protein chains needed to produce new viruses. Older AIDS drugs work by preventing the virus from infecting new cells.

Although protease inhibitors show promise, they have proved difficult to manufacture, and some have failed while others have been successful. Side effects vary, and getting the right dose is critical for effectiveness. All of the protease drugs seem to work best in combination with other therapies. These combination treatments are still quite experimental, and no combination has proved to be absolute for all people as yet. Also, as with other antiviral treatments, resistance to the drugs can develop. Individuals who already show resistance to AZT may not be able to use a protease-AZT combination. This can pose a problem for many people who have been taking the common drugs and then find their options for combination therapy limited.

Although these drugs provide new hope and longer survival for people living with HIV, we are still a long way from a cure. In addition, the number of people becoming HIV-infected each year has not declined which means that we are still a long way from beating this disease.

Preventing HIV Infection

Although scientists have been searching for an HIV vaccine since 1983, they have had no success so far. The only way to prevent HIV infection is to avoid risky behaviors. HIV infection and AIDS are not uncontrollable conditions. You can reduce your risk by the choices you make in sexual behaviors and by taking responsibility for your health and the health of your loved ones. The Skills for Behavior Change box on page 386 presents ways to reduce your risk for contracting HIV.

Noninfectious Diseases

Typically, when we think of major noninfectious ailments, we think of "killer" diseases such as cancer and heart disease. Clearly, these diseases make up the major portion of life-threatening diseases—accounting for nearly two-thirds of all deaths. Yet, although these diseases capture much media attention, other chronic conditions can also cause pain, suffering, and disability. Fortunately, most of them can be prevented or their symptoms relieved.

Generally, noninfectious diseases are not transmitted by a pathogen or by any form of personal contact. Lifestyle and personal health habits are often implicated as underlying causes. Healthy changes in lifestyle and public health efforts aimed at research, prevention, and control can minimize the effects of these diseases.

Chronic Lung Disease

Chronic lung diseases pose a serious and significant threat to Americans today. Collectively, they have become the fourth leading cause of death, with most sufferers living with a condition known as chronic **dyspnea,** or chronic breathlessness. Depending on the situation, dyspnea may limit the ability to climb stairs, walk unassisted, or even sleep. Chronic lung disease can result in major disability and lack of function as the lungs fill with mucous, become susceptible to bacterial or viral infections, or cause acute stress on the heart as they struggle to get valuable oxygen. Chronic cough, excessive phlegm, wheezing, or coughing up blood are frequent symptoms. Over time, many of these underlying conditions lead to hospitalization and possible death.

Among the more deadly chronic lung diseases are the **chronic obstructive pulmonary diseases (COPDs):** asthma, emphysema, and chronic bronchitis. Other chronic lung diseases also cause significant health risks, the most common of which are allergy-induced problems and hay fever. Each of these may exacerbate or contribute to the development of COPD.

Allergy-Induced Respiratory Problems

An **allergy** occurs as a part of the body's attempt to defend itself against a specific *antigen* or *allergen* by producing

---

Dyspnea   Chronic breathlessness.

Chronic obstructive pulmonary diseases (COPDs) A collection of chronic lung diseases including asthma, emphysema, and chronic bronchitis.

Allergy   Hypersensitive reaction to a specific antigen or allergen in the environment in which the body produces excessive antibodies to that antigen or allergen.

Staying Safe in an Unsafe Sexual World

HIV transmission depends on specific behaviors; this is true of other STIs as well. The following will help you protect yourself and reduce your risk.

- Avoid casual sexual partners. Ideally, have sex only if you are in a long-term, mutually monogamous relationship with someone who is equally committed to the relationship and whose HIV status is negative.
- Avoid unprotected sexual activity involving the exchange of blood, semen, or vaginal secretions with people whose present or past behaviors put them at risk for infection. Do not be afraid to ask intimate questions about your partner's sexual past. Remember, whenever you choose to have sexual relations, you expose yourself to your partner's history. Postpone sexual involvement until you are assured that he or she is not infected.
- All sexually active adults who are not in a lifelong monogamous relationship should practice safer sex by using latex condoms. Remember, however, that condoms still do not provide 100% safety.
- Never share injecting needles with anyone for any reason.
- Never share any devices through which the exchange of blood could occur, including needles, razors, tattoo instruments, body-piercing instruments, and any other sharp objects.
- Avoid injury to body tissue during sexual activity. HIV can enter the bloodstream through microscopic tears in anal or vaginal tissues.
- Avoid unprotected oral sex or any sexual activity in which semen, blood, or vaginal secretions could penetrate mucous membranes through breaks in the membrane. Always use a condom or a dental dam during oral sex.
- Avoid using drugs that may dull your senses and affect your ability to make decisions about responsible precautions with potential sex partners.
- Wash your hands before and after sexual encounters. Urinate after sexual relations and, if possible, wash your genitals.
- Although total abstinence is the only absolute means of preventing the sexual transmission of HIV, abstinence can be a difficult choice to make. If you have any doubt about the potential risks of having sex, consider other means of intimacy, at least until you can assure your safety. Try massage, dry kissing, hugging, holding and touching, and masturbation (alone or with a partner).
- Be sure medical professionals take appropriate precautions to prevent potential transmission, including washing their hands and wearing gloves and masks. All equipment used for treatment should be properly sterilized.
- If you are worried about your own HIV status, have yourself tested. Don't risk infecting others inadvertently.
- If you are a woman and HIV positive, you should take the steps necessary to ensure that you do not become pregnant.
- If you suspect that you may be infected or if you test positive for HIV antibodies, do not donate blood, semen, or body organs.

At no time in your life is it more important to communicate openly than when you are considering an intimate relationship. Ask questions, so you can then make an informed decision about whether to get involved. Remember that you can't tell if someone has an STI. Anyone who has ever had sex with anyone else or has injected drugs is at risk, and they may not even know it. The following will help you to communicate about potential risks.

- Remember that you have a responsibility to your partner to disclose your own status. You also have a responsibility to yourself to stay healthy. Ask about your partner's HIV status. Suggest going through the testing together as a means of sharing something important.
- Be direct, honest, and determined in talking about sex before you become involved. Do not act silly or evasive. Get to the point, ask clear questions, and do not be put off in receiving a response. A person who does not care enough to talk about sex probably does not care enough to take responsibility for his or her actions.
- Discuss the issues without sounding defensive or accusatory. Develop a personal comfort level with the subject prior to raising the issue with your partner. Be prepared with complete information, and articulate your feelings clearly. Reassure your partner that your reasons for desiring abstinence or safer sex arise from respect and not distrust. Sharing feelings is easier in a calm, suspicion-free environment in which both people feel comfortable.
- Encourage your partner to be honest and to share feelings. This will not happen overnight. If you have never had a serious conversation with this person before you get into an intimate situation, you cannot expect honesty and openness when the lights go out.
- Analyze your own beliefs and values ahead of time. Know where you will draw the line on certain actions, and be very clear with your partner about what you expect. If you believe that using a condom is necessary, make sure you communicate this.
- Decide what you will do if your partner does not agree with you. Anticipate potential objections or excuses, and prepare your responses accordingly.
- Ask about your partner's history. Although it may seem as though you are prying into another person's business, your own health future depends upon knowing basic information about your partner's past sexual practices and use of injectable drugs.
- Discuss the significance of monogamy in your partner's relationships. Ask, "How important is a committed relationship to you?" Decide early how important this relationship is to you and how much you are willing to work at arriving at an acceptable compromise on lifestyle.

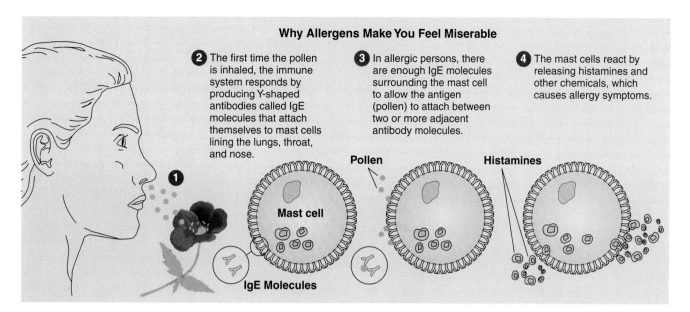

Why Allergens Make You Feel Miserable

2 The first time the pollen is inhaled, the immune system responds by producing Y-shaped antibodies called IgE molecules that attach themselves to mast cells lining the lungs, throat, and nose.

3 In allergic persons, there are enough IgE molecules surrounding the mast cell to allow the antigen (pollen) to attach between two or more adjacent antibody molecules.

4 The mast cells react by releasing histamines and other chemicals, which causes allergy symptoms.

1

Mast cell

Pollen

Histamines

IgE Molecules

Figure 14.4
Steps of an Allergy Response

specific *antibodies.* When foreign pathogens such as bacteria or viruses invade the body, the body responds by producing antibodies to destroy these invading antigens. Under normal conditions, the production of antibodies is a positive element in the body's defense system. However, for unknown reasons, in some people the body overreacts by developing an overly elaborate protective mechanism against relatively harmless substances. The resultant *hypersensitivity reaction* to specific allergens or antigens in the environment is fairly common, as anyone who has awakened with a runny nose or itchy eyes will testify. Most commonly, these hypersensitivity, or allergic, responses occur as a reaction to environmental antigens such as molds, animal dander (hair and dead skin), pollen, ragweed, or dust. Once excessive antibodies to these antigens are produced, they trigger the release of **histamines,** chemical substances that dilate blood vessels, increase mucous secretions, cause tissues to swell, and produce other allergy-like symptoms, particularly in the respiratory system (Figure 14.4).

Although many people think of allergies as childhood diseases, in reality allergies tend to become progressively worse with time and with increased exposure to allergens. In these circumstances, allergic responses become chronic in nature, and treatment becomes difficult. Many people take allergy shots to reduce the severity of their symptoms, with some success. In most cases, once the offending antigen has disappeared, allergy-prone people suffer few symptoms. Although allergies can cause numerous problems, one of the most significant effects is on the immune system.

Hay Fever

Perhaps the best example of a chronic respiratory disease is **hay fever.** Usually considered a seasonally related disease (most prevalent when ragweed and flowers are blooming),

hay fever is common throughout the world. Hay fever attacks, which are characterized by sneezing and itchy, watery eyes and nose, make countless people miserable. The disorder appears to run in families, and research indicates that lifestyle is not as great a factor in developing hay fever as it is in other chronic diseases. Instead, an overzealous immune system and exposure to environmental allergens including pet dander, dust, pollen from various plants, and other substances appear to be the critical factors that determine vulnerability. For those people who are unable to get away from the cause of their hay fever response, medical assistance in the form of injections or antihistamines may provide the only relief.

Asthma

Unfortunately, for many persons who suffer from allergies such as hay fever, their condition often becomes complicated by the development of one of the major COPDs: asthma, emphysema, or bronchitis. **Asthma** is a long-term, chronic inflammatory disorder that blocks air flow in and out of the lungs. Asthma causes tiny airways in the lung to overreact

---

Histamines Chemical substances that dilate blood vessels, increase mucous secretions, and produce other symptoms of allergies.

Hay fever A chronic respiratory disorder that is most prevalent when ragweed and flowers bloom.

Asthma A chronic respiratory disease characterized by attacks of wheezing, shortness of breath, and coughing spasms.

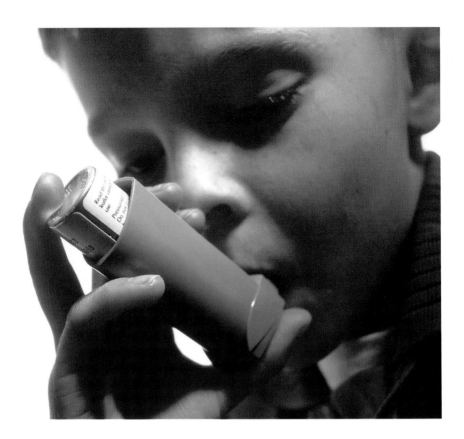

Although a number of new medications are available to relieve the symptoms of asthma, the marked increase of this problem among young children concerns health officials.

with spasms in response to certain triggers. Symptoms include wheezing, difficulty breathing, shortness of breath, and coughing spasms. Although most asthma attacks are mild and non–life-threatening, they can trigger bronchospasms (contractions of the bronchial tubes in the lungs) that are so severe that without rapid treatment, death may occur. Between attacks, most people have few symptoms.

A number of things can trigger an asthma attack, including air pollutants; particulate matter, such as wood dust; indoor air pollutants, such as sidestream smoke from tobacco; and allergens, such as dust mites, cockroach saliva, and pet dander. Stress is also believed to trigger attacks in some individuals.[49]

Asthma can occur at any age, but it is most likely in children between infancy and age 5 and in adults before age 40. In childhood, asthma strikes more boys than girls; in adulthood, it strikes more women than men. Also, the asthma rate is 50 percent higher among African Americans than whites, and four times as many African Americans die of asthma than do whites. Midwesterners appear to be more prone to asthma than people from other areas of the country. In recent years, concern over the rise in incidence of asthma has grown considerably. Consider these points:[50]

- Asthma has become the most common chronic disease of childhood and accounts for one-fourth of all school absences.
- Asthma is the number one cause of hospitalization and absenteeism.
- Asthma affects more than 17 million Americans, including 5 million children; 13 percent of all students age 5 to 19 have it.

- The number of asthma sufferers has increased by more than 65 percent since the 1980s; one in ten new asthma cases is diagnosed in people over age 65.
- The death toll from asthma has nearly doubled since 1980 to more than 5,000 persons per year.

People with asthma have one of two distinctly different types. The most common type, known as *extrinsic* (or *slow onset*) *asthma,* is most commonly associated with allergic triggers. This form tends to run in families and begins to develop in childhood. Often, by adulthood, a person has few episodes, or the disorder completely goes away. *Intrinsic asthma* also may have allergic triggers, but the main difference is that any unpleasant event or stimulant may trigger an attack. A common form of extrinsic asthma is *exercise-induced asthma (EIA),* which may or may not have an allergic connection. Some athletes have no allergies yet live with asthma. Cold, dry air is believed to exacerbate EIA; thus, keeping the lungs moist and warming up prior to working out may reduce risk. The warm, moist air around a swimming pool is one of the best environments for people with asthma.

Relaxation techniques appear to help some asthma sufferers. Drugs may be necessary for serious cases. Determining whether a specific allergen provokes asthma attacks, taking steps to reduce exposure, avoiding triggers such as certain types of exercise or stress, and finding the most effective medications are big steps in asthma prevention and control. Numerous new drugs are available that cause fewer side effects than do older medications. Finding a doctor who specializes in asthma treatment and stays up-to-date on possible options is critical.

Emphysema

Emphysema involves the gradual destruction of the **alveoli** (tiny air sacs) of the lungs. As the alveoli are destroyed, the affected person finds it more and more difficult to exhale. The victim typically struggles to take in a fresh supply of air before the air held in the lungs has been expended. The chest cavity gradually begins to expand, thus producing the barrel-shaped chest characteristic of the chronic emphysema victim.

The cause of emphysema is uncertain. There is, however, a strong relationship between emphysema and long-term cigarette smoking and exposure to air pollution. Victims of emphysema often suffer discomfort over a period of many years. In fact, studies have shown that lung function decline may begin well before age 50 and the early morning "smoker's cough" may signal that damage has already begun.[51] What most of us take for granted—the easy, rhythmic flow of air in and out of the lungs—becomes a continuous struggle for people with emphysema. Inadequate oxygen supply, combined with the stress of overexertion on the heart, eventually takes its toll on the cardiovascular system and leads to premature death.

Bronchitis

Bronchitis refers to an inflammation of the lining of the bronchial tubes. These tubes, the bronchi, connect the windpipe with the lungs. When the bronchi become inflamed or infected, less air is able to flow from the lungs, and heavy mucous begins to form. *Acute bronchitis* is the most common of the bronchial diseases and results in millions of visits to the doctor every year at a cost of more than $300 million per year.[52] More than 95 percent of these acute cases are caused by viruses; however, they are often misdiagnosed and treated with antibiotics, even though little evidence supports this treatment. Typically, misdiagnosis occurs when a cluster of symptoms is labeled as bronchitis, despite the fact that there is no true laboratory diagnosis. *Chronic bronchitis,* in contrast, is defined by the presence of a productive (mucous-laden) cough most days of the month, more than three months of a year for two successive years without underlying disease to explain the cough. Typically, cigarette smoking causes chronic bronchitis, and once bronchitis begins, secondary bacterial or viral infections often make the condition worse. Air pollution and industrial dusts and fumes are also risk factors.

Sleep Apnea

Sleep apnea, although not as life threatening as asthma and other COPDs, affects about 5 percent of the general population. This condition is characterized by periodic episodes when breathing stops completely for ten seconds or longer. Each time it occurs, the sleeper awakens and breathing resumes, but the pattern causes a restless night's sleep. Over time, sleep apnea can lead to high blood pressure and subse-

quent risk of CVD. Reducing alcohol use, changing sleeping position and schedules, and other medical interventions are common treatments.

> ### What do you think?
> *Which of the respiratory diseases described in this section do you or your family have problems with?* ✳ *How many of your college friends have these COPDs?* ✳ *What difficulties do they have in controlling their diseases?* ✳ *Why do you think the incidence of COPDs, as a group, is increasing?* ✳ *What actions can you or your community take to reduce risks and problems from these diseases?*

Neurological Disorders

Headaches

Almost all of us have experienced at least one major headache. In fact, more than 80 percent of women and 65 percent of men experience headaches on a regular basis.[53] Common types of headaches and their treatments are described below.

Tension Headache Tension headaches, also referred to as muscular contraction headaches, are generally caused by muscle contractions or tension in the neck or head. This tension may be caused by actual strain placed on neck or head muscles due to overuse, static positions held for long periods of time, or tension triggered by stress. Recent research indicates that tension headaches may be a product of a more "generic mechanism" in which chemicals deep inside the brain may cause the muscular tension, pain, and suffering often associated with an attack. Possible triggers include red wine, lack of sleep, fasting, menstruation, or other factors, and the same symptoms (sensitivity to light and sound, nausea, and/or throbbing pain) may characterize different types of headaches. Relaxation, hot water treatment, and massage have surfaced as the new holistic treatments, while aspirin, Tylenol, Aleve, and Advil remain the old standby forms of pain relief. Although such painkillers may bring temporary relief of symptoms, it is believed that, over time, the drugs

> **Emphysema** A respiratory disease in which the alveoli become distended or ruptured and are no longer functional.
>
> **Alveoli** Tiny air sacs of the lungs.
>
> **Bronchitis** An inflammation of the lining of the bronchial tubes.
>
> **Sleep apnea** Disorder in which a person has numerous episodes of breathing stoppage during a night's sleep.

may dull the brain's own pain-killing weapons and result in more rather than fewer headaches.

Migraine Headache   Migraine is not just a name for an unusually bad headache; it is a specific diagnosis, involving pain that begins on one side of the head, often accompanied by nausea and sensitivity to light and sounds. Many migraine sufferers experience the sensation of an "aura" in their visual field, typically some form of disturbance such as flashing lights or blind spots, along with numbness or weakness on one side of the body or slurred speech,[54] all signals of an ensuing bad headache. Most people report pain behind or around one eye and always on the same side of the head—a pain that can last for hours or days and then disappear. A migraine can strike at any time, although the hormonal changes around menstruation and ovulation often seem to set off migraines in women, who are three times more likely to get them than men.[55]

Patients report that migraines can be triggered by emotional stress, weather, certain foods, lack of sleep, and a litany of other causes. When tested under laboratory settings, however, much of this evidence is inconclusive. What is known is that migraines occur when blood vessels dilate in the membrane that surrounds the brain. Historically, treatments have centered on reversing or preventing this dilation, with the most common treatment derived from the rye fungus *ergot*. Today, many fast-acting ergot compounds are available by nasal spray, thus vastly increasing the speed of relief. However, ergot drugs have many side effects, the least of which may be that they are habit forming, which causes users to wake up with "rebound" headaches each morning after use.[56]

Critics of the blood vessel dilation theory question why only blood vessels of the head dilate in these situations. Furthermore, why aren't people who exercise or take hot baths more prone to migraine attacks? They suggest that migraines originate in the cortex of the brain, where certain pain sensors are stimulated.

When true migraines occur, relaxation is only minimally effective. Often, strong pain-relieving drugs prescribed by a physician are necessary. Imitrex, a drug tailor-made for migraines, works for about 80 percent of those who try it. Recently, treatment with lidocaine has also shown promising results, and newer drugs called triptans, such as Zomig, Amerge, and Maxalt, are now available.[57]

Secondary Headaches   Secondary headaches arise as a result of some other underlying condition. Hypertension, blocked sinuses, allergies, low blood sugar, diseases of the spine, the common cold, poorly fitted dentures, problems with eyesight, and other problems can trigger this condition. Relaxation and pain relievers such as aspirin are of little help in treating secondary headaches. Rather, medications or other therapies designed to relieve the underlying organic cause of the headache must be included in the treatment regimen.

Seizure Disorders

The word **epilepsy** is derived from the Greek *epilepsia,* meaning "seizure." Approximately 1 percent of all Americans suffer from some form of seizure-related disorder. These disorders are generally caused by abnormal electrical activity in the brain and are characterized by loss of control of muscular activity and unconsciousness. Symptoms vary widely from person to person. Common forms of epilepsy include the following.

- *Grand mal, or major motor seizure.* These seizures are often preceded by a shrill cry or a seizure aura (body sensations such as ringing in the ears or a specific smell or taste). Convulsions and loss of consciousness generally occur and may last from 30 seconds to several minutes or more. Keeping track of the length of time elapsed is one aspect of first aid.
- *Petit mal, or minor seizure.* These seizures involve no convulsions. Rather, a minor loss of consciousness that may go unnoticed occurs. Minor twitching of muscles may take place, usually for a shorter time than for grand mal convulsions.
- *Psychomotor seizure.* These seizures involve both mental processes and muscular activity. Symptoms may include mental confusion and a listless state characterized by activities such as lip smacking, chewing, and repetitive movements.
- *Jacksonian seizure.* This is a progressive seizure that often begins in one part of the body, such as the fingers, and moves to other parts, such as the hand or arm. Usually only one side of the body is affected.

In most cases, people afflicted with seizure disorders can lead normal, seizure-free lives when under medical supervision. Public ignorance about these disorders is one of the most serious obstacles confronting them. Improvements in medication and surgical intervention to reduce some causes of seizures are among the most promising treatments today.

> **What do you think?**
> *Do you suffer from recurrent headaches or other neurological problems?* ✳ *What might cause your problems?* ✳ *What actions could you take to reduce your risks and symptoms?*

Other Neurological Disorders

Parkinson's disease and multiple sclerosis are two other conditions related to the nervous system. Parkinson's has come to public attention due to actor Michael J. Fox's

---

Migraine   A condition characterized by localized headaches that possibly result from alternating dilation and constriction of blood vessels.

Epilepsy   A neurological disorder caused by abnormal electrical brain activity; can be accompanied by altered consciousness or convulsions.

announcement that he suffers from it. **Parkinson's disease** is a chronic, slowly progressive condition that typically strikes after age 50. The symptom most commonly associated with the disease is a tremor. These tremors can become so severe that simple daily tasks can become difficult or impossible. The most common theories for the causes of the disease are familial disposition, acceleration of age-related changes, and exposure to environmental toxins. Although the disease is progressive and incurable, drug therapies can keep the symptoms under control, possibly for years.

Multiple sclerosis (MS) is a degenerative disease in which myelin, a material composed of fats that serves as an insulator and conduit for transmission of nerve impulses, breaks down and causes nerve malfunction. MS typically appears between ages 15 and 50 and is characterized by a periods of relapse, when symptoms flare up, and remissions, when symptoms are not present. Symptoms can range in severity from fatigue and episodic numbness to severe weakness. Most MS patients have few flare ups and can lead fairly normal lives. Theories for the cause of MS are inconclusive.

Gender-Related Disorders

Menstrual Problems

Premenstrual syndrome (PMS) comprises the mood changes and physical symptoms that occur in some women a week to ten days preceding the menstrual period. Symptoms include depression, tension, irritability, headaches, tender breasts, bloated abdomen, backache, abdominal cramps, acne, fluid retention, diarrhea, and fatigue. About 80 percent of all women have some negative symptoms associated with their menstrual cycle; about 3 to 5 percent have more severe symptoms, which are known collectively as **premenstrual dysphoric disorder (PMDD).** Unlike PMS, PMDD symptoms are severe and difficult to manage. They include severe mood disturbances in addition to the physical symptoms associated with PMS.

Strategies for managing PMS include decreasing caffeine and salt intake, increasing intake of complex carbohydrates, practicing stress reduction techniques, and getting exercise. These strategies can also help PMDD. The use of SSRI antidepressants has shown significant promise in the treatment of the mood disturbances associated with PMDD.

Dysmenorrhea, a condition that causes pain in the lower abdomen just before or after menstruation, and toxic shock syndrome (discussed elsewhere in this chapter) are other problems associated with menstruation.

Endometriosis

Whether the incidence of **endometriosis** is on the rise in the United States or whether the disorder is simply attracting more attention is difficult to determine. Victims of endometriosis tend to be women between the ages of 20 and 40. Symptoms include severe cramping during and between menstrual cycles, irregular periods, unusually heavy or light menstrual flow, abdominal bloating, fatigue, painful bowel movements with periods, painful intercourse, constipation, diarrhea, menstrual pain, infertility, and low back pain.

Endometriosis is characterized by the abnormal growth and development of endometrial tissue (the tissue lining the uterus) in regions of the body other than the uterus. Among the most widely accepted theories concerning its causes are the transmission of endometrial tissue to other body regions during surgery or birth; backward flow of menstrual fluid through the fallopian tubes during menstruation; and abnormal cell migration through the movement of body fluids. Women with cycles shorter than 27 days and those with flows lasting over a week are at increased risk. The more aerobic exercise a woman engages in and the earlier she starts it, the less likely she is to develop endometriosis.

Treatment ranges from bed rest and stress reduction to **hysterectomy** (the removal of the uterus) and/or the removal of one or both ovaries and fallopian tubes. Recently, physicians have been criticized by some segments of the public for being too quick to select hysterectomy as the treatment of choice. More conservative treatments that involve dilation and curettage, surgically scraping endometrial tissue off the fallopian tubes and other reproductive organs, and combinations of hormone therapy have become more acceptable. Hormonal treatments include gonadotropin-releasing hormone (GnRH) analogs, various synthetic progesterone-like drugs (Provera), and oral contraceptives.

Digestion-Related Disorders

Diabetes

Diabetes is a serious, widespread, and costly chronic disease, affecting not just the more than 18 million Americans who must live with it, but their families and communities.

Parkinson's disease   A chronic, progressive neurological condition that causes tremors and other symptoms.

Multiple sclerosis (MS)   A degenerative neurological disease in which myelin, an insulator of nerves, breaks down.

Premenstrual syndrome (PMS)   The mood changes and physical symptoms that occur in many women prior to menstruation.

Premenstrual dysphoric disorder (PMDD)   A group of symptoms similar to but more severe than PMS; especially involves mood disturbances.

Endometriosis   Abnormal development of endometrial tissue outside the uterus; results in serious side effects.

Hysterectomy   Surgical removal of the uterus.

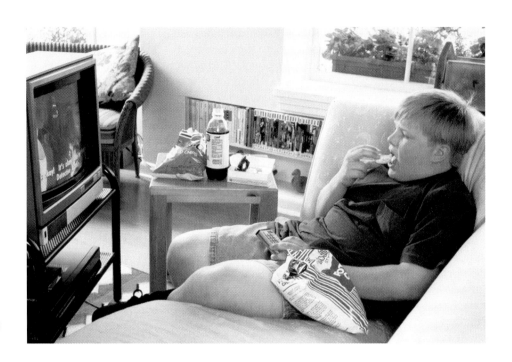

Unhealthy eating habits and a sedentary lifestyle can lead to type 2 diabetes even among children.

Between 1990 and 2000, diagnosed diabetes increased 49 percent among U.S. adults, which gives it the dubious distinction of being the fastest growing chronic disease in American history.[58] A recent CDC study indicated that diabetes seems to be increasing even more dramatically among younger adults—up by almost 70 percent among those in their thirties.[59] More than 2,200 people are diagnosed with diabetes each day in America, and more than 200,000 die each year of related complications, thus making diabetes the sixth leading cause of death in America today.[60]

What causes this serious disease? In healthy people, the *pancreas,* a powerful enzyme-producing organ, secretes the hormone **insulin** in sufficient quantities to allow the body to use or store glucose (blood sugar). When the pancreas fails to produce enough insulin to regulate sugar metabolism or when the body fails to use insulin effectively, a disease known as **diabetes mellitus** occurs. Diabetics exhibit **hyperglycemia,** or elevated blood sugar levels, and high glucose levels in their urine. Other symptoms include excessive thirst, frequent urination, hunger, tendency to tire easily, wounds that heal slowly, numbness or tingling in the extremities, changes in vision, skin eruptions, and, in women, a tendency toward vaginal yeast infections.

The most serious form, known as type 1 (insulin-dependent) diabetes, is an autoimmune disease in which the immune system destroys the insulin-making beta cells.[61] Type 1 diabetics typically must depend on insulin injections or oral medications for the rest of their lives because insulin is not present in their bodies. Type 2 (non–insulin-dependent) diabetes, in which insulin production is deficient or the body resists or is unable to utilize available insulin, tends to develop in later life. People with Type 2 diabetes can often control their symptoms with a healthy diet, weight control, and regular exercise. They may be able to avoid oral medications or insulin indefinitely. A third type of diabetes, *gestational diabetes,* can develop in a woman during pregnancy. The condition usually disappears after childbirth, but it does leave the woman at greater risk of developing type 2 diabetes at some point.

Understanding Risk Factors Diabetes tends to run in families. Being overweight, coupled with inactivity, dramatically increases the risk of type 2 diabetes. Older persons and mothers of babies weighing more than 9 pounds also run an increased risk. Approximately 80 percent of all type 2 patients are overweight at the time of diagnosis. Weight loss and exercise are important factors in lowering blood sugar and improving the efficiency of cellular use of insulin. Both can help to prevent overwork of the pancreas and the development of diabetes. In fact, recent findings show that modest, consistent physical activity and a healthy diet can cut a person's risk of developing type 2 diabetes by nearly 60 percent.[62] African Americans, Hispanics, and Native Americans have the highest rates of type 2 diabetes in the world—much higher than that of Caucasians. The reasons for this increased risk are not clear.[63]

Controlling Diabetes Most physicians attempt to control diabetes with a variety of insulin-related drugs. Most of these

---

Insulin   A hormone produced by the pancreas; required by the body for the metabolism of carbohydrates.

Diabetes mellitus   A disease in which the pancreas fails to produce enough insulin or the body fails to use insulin effectively.

Hyperglycemia   Elevated blood sugar levels.

---

drugs are taken orally, although self-administered hypodermic injections are prescribed when other treatments are inadequate. Recent breakthroughs in individual monitoring and implantable insulin monitors and insulin infusion pumps that regulate insulin intake "on demand" have provided many diabetics with the opportunity to lead normal lives. Newer forms of insulin that last longer in the body and have fewer side effects are now available. An insulin inhaler is being tested and may soon be available.

Lactose Intolerance

As many as 50 million Americans are unable to eat dairy products such as milk, cheese, ice cream, and other foods that the rest of us take for granted. These people suffer from **lactose intolerance,** which means that they have lost the ability to produce the digestive enzyme lactase, which is necessary for the body to convert milk sugar (lactose) into glucose. That glass of milk becomes a source of stomach cramping, diarrhea, nausea, gas, and related symptoms. Once diagnosed, however, lactose intolerance can be treated by introducing low-lactose or lactose-free foods into the diet. Through trial and error, people usually find that they can tolerate one type of low-lactose food better than others. As an alternative to eating foods without lactose, some purchase special products that contain the missing lactase and thus eat dairy foods without serious side effects. Most large grocery chains, food cooperatives, and drug stores have these products available in liquid or tablet form. It should be noted, however, that these products do not work for everyone. Someone who is lactose intolerant may need to experiment before settling into a diet that works.

Colitis and Irritable Bowel Syndrome

Ulcerative colitis is a disease of the large intestine in which the mucous membranes of the intestinal walls become inflamed. Victims with severe cases may have as many as 20 bouts of bloody diarrhea a day. Colitis can also produce severe stomach cramps, weight loss, nausea, sweating, and fever. Although some experts believe that colitis occurs more frequently in people with high stress levels, this theory is controversial. Hypersensitivity reactions, particularly to milk and certain foods, have also been considered as a cause. It is difficult to determine the cause of colitis because the disease goes into unexplained remission and then recurs without apparent reason. This pattern often continues over periods of years and may be related to the later development of colorectal cancer. Since the cause of colitis remains unknown, treatment focuses on relieving the symptoms. Increasing fiber intake and taking anti-inflammatory drugs, steroids, and other medications designed to reduce inflammation and soothe irritated intestinal walls can relieve symptoms.

Many people develop a related condition known as **irritable bowel syndrome (IBS),** characterized by nausea, pain, gas, diarrhea attacks, or cramps that occur after eating certain foods or when a person is under unusual stress. IBS symptoms commonly begin in early adulthood. Symptoms may vary from week to week and can fade for long periods of time, only to return. The cause is unknown, but researchers suspect that people with IBS have digestive systems that are overly sensitive to food and drink, stress, and certain hormonal changes. They may also be more sensitive to pain signals from the stomach. Stress management, relaxation techniques, regular activity, and diet can bring IBS under control in the vast majority of cases. Problems with diarrhea can be reduced by cutting down on fat and avoiding caffeine and excessive amounts of sorbitol, a sweetener found in dietetic foods and chewing gum.

Peptic Ulcers

An ulcer is a lesion or wound that forms in body tissue as a result of some irritant. A **peptic ulcer** is a chronic ulcer that occurs in the lining of the stomach or the section of the small intestine known as the *duodenum.* The lining of these organs becomes irritated, the protective covering of mucous is reduced, and the gastric acid begins to digest the dying tissue, just as it would a piece of food. Typically, this irritation causes pain that disappears when the person eats, but it returns about an hour later.

Research indicates that most peptic ulcers result from infection by a common bacterium, *Helicobacter pylori.* The disorder, which affects more than 4 million Americans every year, generally responds to antibiotics. Peptic ulcers caused by excess stomach acid or overuse of stomach-irritating drugs such as aspirin and ibuprofen can be treated with acid-reducing medications.

> ### What do you think?
> *What role can a healthy diet play in reducing risks for and symptoms of the diseases discussed here?* * *Are you or any of your family members at risk for these problems?* * *What actions can you take today that will cut your risk?*

Lactose intolerance   The inability to produce lactase, an enzyme needed to convert milk sugar into glucose.

Ulcerative colitis   An inflammatory disorder that affects the mucous membranes of the large intestine, producing bloody diarrhea.

Irritable bowel syndrome (IBS)   Nausea, pain, gas, or diarrhea caused by certain foods or stress.

Peptic ulcer   Damage to the stomach or intestinal lining, usually caused by digestive juices.

Musculoskeletal Diseases

Arthritis

Called the "nation's primary crippler," **arthritis** strikes one in seven Americans, or more than 38 million people. Symptoms range from the occasional tendinitis of the weekend athlete to the severe pain of rheumatoid arthritis. There are more than 100 types of arthritis diagnosed today. Together, they cost the U.S. economy over $65 billion per year in lost wages and productivity and untold amounts in hospital and nursing home services, prescriptions, and over-the-counter pain relief.[64]

Osteoarthritis, also known as degenerative joint disease, is a progressive deterioration of bones and joints that has been associated with the wear-and-tear theory of aging. More recent research indicates that as joints are used, they release enzymes that digest cartilage while other cells in the cartilage try to repair the damage. When the enzymatic breakdown overpowers cellular repair, the cartilage is destroyed, thus causing bones to rub against each other. Weather extremes, excessive strain, and injury often lead to osteoarthritis flare-ups, but a specific precipitating event does not seem to be necessary. Obesity, joint trauma, and repetitive joint usage all contribute to increased risk, and thus are important targets for prevention.

Of the 20.7 million Americans with osteoarthritis, the majority of them are women.[65] Although age and injury are undoubtedly factors, heredity, abnormal use of the joint, diet, abnormalities in joint structure, and impaired blood supply to the joint may also contribute. Joint replacement and bone fusion are common surgical repair techniques. For most people, anti-inflammatory drugs and pain relievers such as aspirin and cortisone-related agents ease discomfort. Heat, mild exercise, and massage may also relieve the pain.

Rheumatoid arthritis is an autoimmune disease involving chronic inflammation that can appear at any age, but most commonly between ages 20 and 45. Rheumatoid arthritis is three times more common among women than among men during early adulthood but equally common among men and women in the over-70 age group. Symptoms include stiffness, pain, and swelling of multiple joints, often including the joints of the hands and wrists; they can be gradually progressive or sporadic, with occasional unexplained remissions.

Treatment for rheumatoid arthritis is similar to that for osteoarthritis. Emphasis is placed on pain relief and attempts to improve the functional mobility of the patient. Sometimes immunosuppressant drugs can reduce the inflammatory response.

Fibromyalgia

Fibromyalgia is a chronic, painful, rheumatoidlike disorder that affects as many as 5 to 6 percent of the general population. Persons with fibromyalgia experience an array of symptoms, including headaches, dizziness, numbness and tingling, itching, fluid retention, chronic joint pain, abdominal or pelvic pain, and even occasional diarrhea. Suspected causes include sleep disturbances, stress, emotional distress, viruses, and autoimmune disorders; however, none has been proved in clinical trials. Because of fibromyalgia's multiple symptoms, it is usually diagnosed only after myriad tests have ruled out other disorders. The American College of Rheumatology identifies these major diagnostic criteria:[66]

- History of widespread pain of at least three months' duration in the axial skeleton as well as in all four quadrants of the body
- Pain in at least 11 of 18 paired tender points on digital palpation of about 4 kilograms of pressure

Fibromyalgia primarily affects women in their 30s and 40s. It can be extremely debilitating, causing feelings of unrelieved pain, bloating or swelling, and fatigue. Many people with fibromyalgia also become depressed and report chronic fatigue-like symptoms. Treatment varies based on the severity of symptoms. Typically, adequate rest, stress management, relaxation techniques, dietary supplements and selected herbal remedies, and pain medications are prescribed.

Systemic Lupus Erythematosus

Systemic lupus erythematosus (SLE), or **lupus,** is an autoimmune disease in which antibodies destroy or injure organs such as the kidneys, brain, and heart. The symptoms vary from mild to severe and may disappear for periods of time. A butterfly-shaped rash covering the bridge of the nose and both cheeks is common. Nearly all SLE sufferers have aching joints and muscles, and 60 percent of them develop redness and swelling that move from joint to joint. The disease affects 1 in 700 Caucasians but 1 in 250 African Americans; 90 percent of all victims are females. Extensive research has not yet found a cure for this sometimes fatal disease.

Arthritis   Painful inflammatory disease of the joints.

Osteoarthritis   A progressive deterioration of bones and joints that has been associated with the "wear and tear" theory of aging.

Rheumatoid arthritis   A serious inflammatory joint disease.

Fibromyalgia   A chronic rheumatoidlike disorder that can be highly painful and difficult to diagnose.

Lupus   A disease in which the immune system attacks the body and produces antibodies that destroy or injure organs such as the kidneys, brain, and heart.

Table 14.2
Other Modern Afflictions

Disease	Description	Treatment
Cystic fibrosis	Inherited disease occurring in 1 out of every 1,600 births. Characterized by pooling of large amounts of mucus in lungs, digestive disturbances, and excessive sodium excretion. Results in premature death.	Most treatments are geared toward relief of symptoms. Antibiotics are administered for infection. Recent strides in genetic research suggest better treatments and potential cure in the near future.
Sickle-cell anemia	Inherited disease affecting 8–10% of all African Americans. Disease affects hemoglobin, forming sickle-shaped red blood cells that interfere with oxygenation. Results in severe pain, anemia, and premature death.	Reduce stress, and attend to minor infections immediately. Seek genetic counseling.
Cerebral palsy	Disorder characterized by the loss of voluntary control over motor functioning. Believed to be caused by a lack of oxygen to the brain at birth, brain disorders or an accident before or after birth, poisoning, or brain infections.	Follow preventive actions to reduce accident risks; improved neonatal and birthing techniques show promise.
Graves' disease	A thyroid disorder characterized by swelling of the eyes, staring gaze, and retraction of the eyelid. Can result in loss of sight. The cause is unknown, and the disease can occur at any age.	Medication may help control symptoms. Radioactive iodine supplements also may be administered.

Low Back Pain

Approximately 80 percent of all Americans will experience low back pain (LBP) at some point. Some LBP episodes result from muscular damage and may be short-lived and acute. Other episodes may involve dislocations, fractures, or other problems with spinal vertebrae or discs, thus resulting in chronic pain or requiring surgery. Low back pain is epidemic throughout the world. It is the major cause of disability for people age 20 to 45 in the United States, who suffer more frequently and severely from this problem than older people do.[67] LBP causes more lost work time in the United States than any other illness except upper respiratory infections. In fact, costs associated with back injury exceeded those associated with all other industrial injuries combined.[68]

Almost 90 percent of all back problems occur in the lumbar spine region (lower back). You can avoid many problems by consciously maintaining good posture. Other preventive hints include:

- Purchase a firm mattress, and avoid sleeping on your stomach.
- Avoid high-heeled shoes, which often tilt the pelvis forward.
- Control your weight.
- Lift objects with your legs, not your back.
- Buy a good chair for doing your work, preferably one with lumbar support.
- Move your car seat forward so your knees are elevated slightly.
- Warm up before exercising.

- Engage in regular exercise, particularly exercises that strengthen the abdominal muscles and stretch the back muscles.

Other Maladies

During the past 20 years, several afflictions have surfaced that seem to be products of our time. Some of these health problems relate to specific groups of people; some are due to technological advances; and others have not been explained (Table 14.2).

Chronic Fatigue Syndrome

Fatigue is a subjective condition in which people feel tired before they begin activities, lack the energy to accomplish tasks that require sustained effort and attention, or become abnormally exhausted after normal activities. In the late 1980s, several U.S. clinics noted a characteristic set of symptoms including chronic fatigue, headaches, fever, sore throat, enlarged lymph nodes, depression, poor memory, general weakness, nausea, and symptoms remarkably similar to mononucleosis.

Despite extensive testing, No viral cause has been found.[69] In the absence of a known pathogen, many researchers believe that the illness, commonly referred to as *chronic fatigue syndrome (CFS)*, may have strong psychosocial roots. Our heightened awareness of health makes some of us scrutinize our bodies so carefully that the slightest deviation becomes amplified. In addition, people who suffer from depression seem to be good candidates for CFS. Experts worry, however, that too many people approach CFS as something that is "in the person's head" and that such an attitude may prevent scientists from doing the serious research needed to find a cure.

The diagnosis of CFS depends on two major criteria and eight or more minor criteria. The major criteria are debilitating fatigue that persists for at least six months and the absence of other illnesses that could cause the symptoms. Minor criteria include headaches, fever, sore throat, painful lymph nodes, weakness, fatigue after exercise, sleep problems, and rapid onset of these symptoms. Treatment focuses on improved

---

Repetitive stress injury (RSI) An injury to nerves, soft tissue, or joints due to the physical stress of repeated motions.

Carpal tunnel syndrome A common occupational injury in which the median nerve in the wrist becomes irritated, thus causing numbness, tingling, and pain in the fingers and hands.

---

nutrition, rest, counseling for depression, judicious exercise, and development of a strong support network.

Repetitive Stress Injuries

The Bureau of Labor Statistics estimates that 25 percent of all injuries in the labor force that result in lost work time are due to a **repetitive stress injury (RSI).** These are injuries to nerves, soft tissue, or joints that result from the physical stress of repeated motions. They are estimated to cost employers more than $22 billion a year in workers' compensation and an additional $85 billion in related costs, such as absenteeism.

One of the most common RSIs is **carpal tunnel syndrome.** Hours spent typing at the computer, flipping groceries through computerized scanners, or other jobs made simpler by technology can irritate the median nerve in the wrist, thus causing numbness, tingling, and pain in the fingers and hands. Although carpal tunnel syndrome risk can be reduced by proper placement of the keyboard, mouse, wrist pads, and other techniques, RSIs are often overlooked until significant damage has been done. Better education and ergonomic workplace designs can eliminate many injuries of this nature.

Taking Charge

Make It Happen!

Assessment: The Assess Yourself box on page 376 gave you the chance to consider your beliefs and attitudes about STIs, and possible risks you may be facing. Now that you have considered these results, you can begin to take steps toward changing certain behaviors that may be putting you at risk.

Making a Change: In order to change your behavior, you need to develop a plan. Follow these steps.

1. Evaluate your behavior, and identify patterns and specific things you are doing. What can you change now? What can you change in the near future?
2. Select one pattern of behavior that you want to change.
3. Fill out a Behavior Change Contract. It should include your long-term goal for change, your short-term goals,

the rewards you'll give yourself for reaching these goals, potential obstacles along the way, and strategies for overcoming these obstacles. For each goal, list the small steps and specific actions that you will take.

4. Chart your progress in a journal. At the end of a week, consider how successful you were in following your plan. What helped you be successful? What made change more difficult? What will you do differently next week?
5. Revise your plan as needed. Are the short-term goals attainable? Are the rewards satisfying?

Example: Carlos had never thought that he was at risk for an STI. He only dated one woman at a time, and he had never had an STI himself. After he reviewed his answers to the self-assessment, however, he saw that there were several ways in which he was putting himself at risk.

He had thought that he would be able to tell whether someone was infected with an STI but the answer to question #1 described how, especially among women, there are few if any obvious signs or symptoms of some STIs. Carlos also believed that he was not at risk because he dated only one woman at a time, but the answer to question #8 pointed out that a person can pass on an STI that he or she contracted from a previous sex partner. Carlos decided it was time to take responsibility for his sexual activity. He had been on three dates with Sherry, and felt things were progressing to a more intimate stage soon. He wanted to be sure that they took the time to discuss STIs before they put themselves at risk.

Carlos was nervous when he thought about talking to Sherry about STIs, so he wrote out a few ideas of ways to bring up the subject. This made him more confident that he would be able to talk honestly with Sherry before they became more intimate. He also made sure that he had a supply of condoms, so there wouldn't be any reason not to practice safe sex. At the end of their next date, Carlos asked Sherry if they could have a serious conversation about the next step. When he told her that he wanted to talk about STIs, she told him that she was relieved that he had brought up the subject. She knew that she was healthy, and hadn't been sure how to find out his status. Carlos was relieved that Sherry was as concerned about the issue as he was, and they were both glad that embarrassment had not prevented them from having this conversation.

Summary

✳ The major uncontrollable risk factors for contracting infectious diseases are heredity, age, environmental conditions, and organism resistance. The major controllable risk factors are stress, nutrition, fitness level, sleep, hygiene, avoidance of high-risk behaviors, and drug use.

✳ The major pathogens are bacteria, viruses, fungi, protozoa, prions, and parasitic worms. Bacterial infections include staphylococcal infections, streptococcal infections, pneumonia, Legionnaire's disease, tuberculosis, and periodontal diseases. Major viruses include the common cold, influenza, mononucleosis, hepatitis, and measles.

✳ Your body uses a number of defense systems to keep pathogens from invading. The skin is the body's major protection, helped by enzymes. The immune system creates antibodies to destroy antigens. In addition, fever and pain play a role in defending the body. Vaccines bolster the body's immune system against specific diseases.

✳ Emerging and resurgent diseases pose significant threats for future generations. Many factors contribute to these risks. Possible solutions focus on a public health approach to prevention.

✳ Sexually transmitted infections (STIs) are spread through intercourse, oral sex, anal sex, hand–genital contact, and sometimes through mouth-to-mouth contact. Major STIs include chlamydia, pelvic inflammatory disease (PID), gonorrhea, syphilis, pubic lice, genital warts, candidiasis, trichomoniasis, and herpes. Sexual transmission may also be involved in some general urinary tract infections.

✳ Acquired immune deficiency syndrome (AIDS) is caused by the human immunodeficiency virus (HIV). HIV is not confined to certain high-risk groups. Globally, HIV/AIDS has become a major threat to the world's population. Anyone can get HIV by engaging in high-risk sexual activities that include exchange of body fluids, by having received a blood transfusion before 1985, and by injecting drugs (or having sex with someone who does). Women appear to be particularly susceptible to infection. You can cut your risk for AIDS by deciding not to engage in risky sexual activities.

✳ Chronic lung diseases include allergies, hay fever, asthma, emphysema, and chronic bronchitis. Allergies are part of the body's natural defense system. Chronic obstructive pulmonary diseases are the fifth leading cause of death in the United States.

✳ Neurological conditions include headaches, seizure disorders, Parkinson's disease, and multiple sclerosis. Headaches may be caused by a variety of factors, the most common of which are tension, dilation and/or rapid contraction of blood vessels in the brain, chemical influences on muscles and vessels that cause inflammation and pain, and underlying physiological and psychological disorders.

✳ Premenstrual syndrome (PMS) and premenstrual dysphoric disorder (PMDD) are conditions related to the menstrual cycle. Endometriosis is the buildup of endometrial tissue in regions of the body other than the uterus.

✳ Diabetes occurs when the pancreas fails to produce enough insulin to regulate sugar metabolism. Other conditions, such as colitis, irritable bowel syndrome (IBS), and peptic ulcers, are the direct result of functional problems in various digestion-related organs or systems.

✳ Musculoskeletal diseases such as arthritis, lower back pain, repetitive stress injuries, and other problems cause significant pain and disability in millions of people. Chronic fatigue syndrome (CFS) and repetitive stress injuries (RSIs, such as carpal tunnel syndrome) have emerged in the past decade as major chronic maladies. CFS is associated with depression. Repetitive stress injuries are preventable by proper equipment placement and usage.

Questions for Discussion and Reflection

1. What are the major controllable risk factors for contracting infectious diseases? Using this knowledge, how would you change your current lifestyle to prevent such infection?

2. What is a pathogen? What are the similarities and differences between pathogens and antigens? Discuss uncontrollable and controllable risk factors that can threaten your health.

3. What are the six types of pathogens? What are the various means by which they can be transmitted? How have social conditions among the poor and homeless increased the risks for certain diseases, such as tuberculosis,

influenza, and hepatitis? Why are these conditions a challenge to the efforts of public health officials?

4. Identify possible reasons for the spread of emerging and resurgent diseases. Indicate public policies and programs that might reduce this trend.

5. Identify five STIs. What are their symptoms? How do they develop? What are their potential long-term effects?

6. Should Americans be concerned about soaring HIV/AIDS rates elsewhere in the world? Explain your answer.

7. What are some of the major noninfectious chronic diseases affecting Americans today? Do you think there is a pattern in the types of diseases that we get? What are the common risk factors?

8. List common respiratory diseases affecting Americans. Which of these diseases has a genetic basis? An environmental basis? An individual basis? What, if anything, is being done to prevent, treat, and control each of these conditions?

9. Describe the symptoms and treatment of diabetes. What is the difference between type 1 diabetes and type 2 diabetes?

10. What are the major disorders of the musculoskeletal system? Why do you think there aren't any cures? Describe the difference between osteoarthritis and rheumatoid arthritis.

Accessing Your Health on the Internet

Visit the following Internet sites to explore further topics and issues related to personal health. To visit an organization's website, go to the Companion Website for *Health: The Basics, Sixth Edition* at www.aw-bc.com/donatelle, click on the book image, and select "Accessing Your Health on the Internet" from the navigation menu on the left.

1. *American Academy of Allergy, Asthma, and Immunology.* Provides an overview of asthma and allergies. Offers interactive quizzes to test your knowledge and an "ask an expert" section.

2. *American Diabetes Association.* Excellent resource for diabetes information.

3. *Centers for Disease Control and Prevention (CDC).* Home page for the government agency dedicated to disease intervention and prevention, with links to all the latest data and publications put out by the CDC, including the *Morbidity and Mortality Weekly Report, HIV/AIDS Surveillance Report,* and the *Journal of Emerging Infectious Diseases,* and access to the CDC research database, Wonder.

4. *National Center for Chronic Disease Prevention and Health Promotion.* Provides access to a wide range of information from this CDC-affiliated organization dedicated to chronic diseases and health promotion.

5. *World Health Organization (WHO).* Provides access to the latest information on world health issues, including infectious disease, as put out by WHO. Provides direct access to publications and fact sheets, with keywords to help users find topics of interest.

Further Reading

Champeau, D., and R. Donatelle. *AIDS and STIS: A Global Perspective.* Englewood Cliffs, NJ: Prentice Hall, 2002.

An overview of issues, trends, and ethics surrounding the global pandemic of HIV/AIDS and STIs.

Chin, J., ed. *Control of Communicable Diseases Manual, 17th ed.* Washington, D.C.: American Public Health Association, 2003.

Outstanding pocket reference for information on infectious diseases. Updated every three to five years to cover emerging diseases.

National Center for Health Statistics. *Monthly Vital Statistics Report and Advance Data from Vital and Health Statistics.* Hyattsville, MD: Public Health Service.

Detailed government reports, usually published monthly, concerning mortality and morbidity data for the United States. Includes changes occurring in the rates of particular diseases and in health practices so patterns and trends can be analyzed.

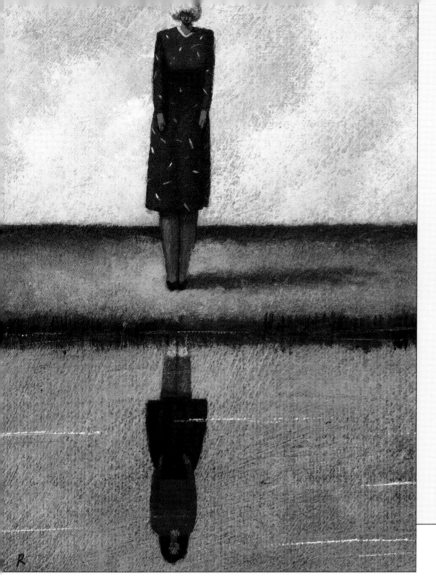

Life's Transitions
The Aging Process

Objectives

* Define aging, and explain the related concepts of biological, psychological, social, legal, and functional age.

* Explain how the growing population of older adults will impact society.

* Discuss the unique health challenges faced by older adults, such as alcohol abuse, use of prescription and over-the-counter drugs, osteoporosis, urinary incontinence, depression, senility, and Alzheimer's disease.

* Discuss strategies for healthy aging that can begin during young adulthood.

* Define *death* and analyze why people deny death in Western culture.

* Discuss the stages of the grieving process and describe strategies for coping more effectively with death.

* Describe the ethical concerns that arise from the concepts of the right to die and rational suicide.

* Review the decisions that need to be made when someone is dying or has died, including hospice care, funeral arrangements, wills, and organ donations.

Exercise and Setting Ease Alzheimer's Effects

By Anahad O'Connor

For many, a diagnosis of Alzheimer's disease can mean life in a dreary nursing home and a treatment centered on powerful anti-psychotics to combat the onset of memory loss, dementia and other signs of a mind that is slowly unraveling.

But now, some scientists say the best way to treat Alzheimer's is with a broader approach, one that emphasizes regular exercise and a healthy environment. Even encouraging participation in an activity as simple as gardening, one researcher noted, can reduce depression and ease anxiety in some Alzheimer's patients.

The findings were detailed in two studies released last month.

One, published in the October 15 issue of *The Journal of the American Medical Association,* looked at 153 Alzheimer's patients living in the Seattle area over several years. Some of the patients, whose symptoms of the disease varied in their severity, were randomly assigned to an exercise program that focused on strength, balance and flexibility training.

For about 30 minutes a day, the patients went for walks, stretched or used light hand weights for quick exercises that they could do at home.

Read the complete article online in the eThemes section of this book's website: www.aw-bc.com/donatelle.

Original article published November 4, 2003. Copyright © 2003 The New York Times. Reprinted with permission.

Grow old along with me!
The best is yet to be,
The last of life, for which the first was made. . . .

  Robert Browning, *Rabbi Ben Ezra*

In a society that seems to worship youth, researchers have begun to offer good—even revolutionary—news about the aging process. Growing old doesn't have to mean a slow slide to declining physical and mental health. Health promotion, disease prevention, and wellness-oriented activities can prolong vigor and productivity, even among those who haven't always led model lifestyles or made healthful habits a priority. In fact, getting older can mean getting better in many ways—particularly socially, psychologically, and intellectually.

The manner in which you view aging (either as a natural part of living or an inevitable decline toward disease and death) is a crucial factor in how successfully you will adapt to life's transitions. If you view these transitions as periods of growth in your development as a human being, your journey through even the most difficult times will be easier. Explore your own notions about aging in the Assess Yourself box.

Aging   The patterns of life changes that occur in members of all species as they grow older.

Ageism   Discrimination based on age.

Gerontology   The study of individual and collective aging processes.

Aging has traditionally been described as the patterns of life changes that occur in members of all species as they grow older. Some people believe that aging begins at the moment of conception. Others contend that it starts at birth. Still others believe that true aging does not begin until we reach our forties. Typically, experts and laypersons alike have used chronological age to assign a person to a particular life-cycle stage.

Redefining Aging

Discrimination against people based on age is known as **ageism.** When directed against the elderly, this discrimination carries with it social ostracism and negative portrayals of older people.

The study of individual and collective aging processes, known as **gerontology,** explores the reasons for aging and the ways in which people cope with and adapt to this process. Gerontologists have identified several age-related characterstics that define where a person is in terms of biological, psychological, social, legal, and functional life-stage development:[1]

- *Biological age* refers to the relative age or condition of the person's organs and body systems. There are 70-year-old runners who have the cardiovascular system of a 40-year-old, and 40-year-olds who have less energy than their parents do. Arthritis and other chronic conditions can accelerate the aging process.
- *Psychological age* refers to a person's adaptive capacities, such as coping abilities and intelligence, and to the person's

Where Do You Want to Be?

When we are young, aging most likely is the furthest thing from our minds. However, thinking about aging and what we expect from life are important elements of a satisfying adult develop-ment process. Take a few minutes to answer the following questions. Your answers may tell you a great deal about yourself.

1. At this point in your life, what do you value most?
2. What do you think will be most important to you when you reach your forties? fifties? sixties? What similarities and differences do you notice, and what causes these similarities and differences?
3. Do you think your parents are happy and content with the way their lives have turned out? If they could change anything, what do you think they might do differently?
4. What about your own direction so far in life is similar to that of your parents? What have you done differently? Are the similarities and differences good? Why or why not?
5. What do you think are the keys to a happy and satisfying life?
6. What do you want to accomplish by the time you are 40? By the time you are 50? By the time you are 60?
7. Have you ever thought of retirement? Describe your retirement.
8. Describe the "you" that you would like to be at the age of 70. How is that person similar to or different from the "you" of today? What actions will you need to take to be that "you" in the future?

awareness of his or her individual capabilities, self-efficacy, and general ability to adapt to situations. Although chronic illness may render people physically handicapped, they may possess tremendous psychological reserves and remain alert and fully capable of making decisions.

- *Social age* refers to a person's habits and roles relative to society's expectations. People in a particular life stage usually share similar tastes in music, television shows, and politics.
- *Legal age* is probably the most common definition of age in the United States. Based on chronological years, legal age is used as a factor in determining voting rights, driving privileges, drinking age, eligibility for Social Security payments, and a host of other rights and obligations.
- *Functional age* refers to the ways—heart rate, hearing, etc.—in which people compare to others of a similar age. It is difficult to separate functional aging from other types of aging, particularly chronological and biological aging.

What Is Successful Aging?

Many of today's older individuals lead active, productive lives. For instance, 49,000 Americans age 65 and older are currently enrolled in college, and 14 percent are employed. Seventy-two percent of U.S. citizens age 65 to 74 voted in the last presidential election—a higher percentage than any other age group.[2]

Typically, people who have aged successfully have the following characteristics.

- In general, they have managed to avoid serious, debilitating diseases and disability.

- They maintain a high level of physical functioning, live independently, and engage in most normal activities of daily living.
- They have maintained cognitive functioning and are actively engaged in mentally challenging and stimulating activities.
- They are actively engaged in social and productive activities.
- They are resilient and able to cope reasonably well with physical, social, and emotional changes.

Though the process of aging has often been viewed with dread due to physical changes that inevitably occur, only in the past decade have we begun to fully appreciate the gains and positive aspects of normal adult development throughout the lifespan. According to gerontologist Dr. Karen Hooker, older adults as a population display much more differentiation in personalities, coping styles, and "possible selves" than any other age group. She states that "successful aging and development as individuals can be viewed as dynamic processes of adaptation between the self and the environment. Throughout our lives we make choices and respond to changes in vastly different ways. Each person is born with certain traits that stay reasonably stable throughout life, but character is deeply affected by personal action constructs that change with time and life history."[3]

Aging is not a static process, but one in which we change and become someone uniquely fashioned by our life's story. Gerontologists have devised several categories for specific age-related characteristics. People age 65 to 74 are viewed as the **young-old;** those aged 75 to 84 are the **middle-old** group; those 85 and over are classified as **old-old.**

Older Adults: A Growing Population

There are more than 35 million people age 65 or older in the United States, nearly 13 percent of the total population. The number of older Americans has increased more than tenfold since 1900, when there were only about 3 million people age 65 or older, 4 percent of the total population[4] (Figure 15.1). According to researchers at the National Institute on Aging, "the aging of the 75 million–strong baby boomer generation could have an impact on our society of equal magnitude to that of immigration at the turn of the last century."[5] Life expectancy for a person born in 2000 is 76.9 years, about 29 years longer than for a child born in 1900.[6]

Health Issues for an Aging Society

Health Care Costs

Today, older adults account for approximately 38 percent of total national health care costs, with estimated costs in excess of $6,800 per person. Out-of-pocket health expenses for them have risen by 33 percent since 1990.[7] As people live longer, the chances of developing a costly chronic disease increase. In 2000, 26.3 percent of older persons assessed their health as fair or poor, compared to 9.2 percent of all age groups taken together. Nearly 29 percent of older people also reported activity limitations.[8] As our technology improves, chronic illnesses that once were quickly fatal may now be treated successfully for years. Projected future costs from these two trends are staggering.

Will working Americans be willing to pay an increased share of the health care costs for people on fixed incomes who cannot pay for themselves? If not, what will become of older Americans? Perhaps most important, who ultimately will pay?

Young-old   People age 65 to 74.

Middle-old   People age 75 to 84.

Old-old   People age 85 and over.

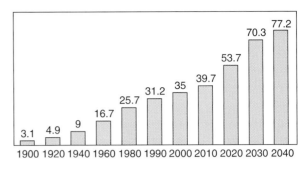

Figure 15.1
Number of Americans 65 and Older (in Millions)
Sources: U.S. Bureau of the Census, "Projections of the Total Resident Population by 5 Year Age Groups, Race, and Hispanic Origin with Special Age Categories: Middle Series, 1999 to 2000," 2000. www.census.gov; U.S. Bureau of the Census "Population Projections of the United States by Age, Sex, Race, and Hispanic Origin: 1995–2050," *Current Population Reports,* 25–1130. Data for 2000 are from the 2000 Census.

Housing and Living Arrangements   Contrary to popular opinion, most older people (more than 95 percent) never live in a nursing home. Community living, assisted living, skilled nursing care, and other options are new possibilities for those who have financial means or who have purchased some form of long-term care insurance.[9] However, housing problems for low-income individuals remain. Who will provide the necessary social services, and who will pay the bill? Will the family of the future be forced to coexist with several generations under one roof?

Ethical and Moral Considerations   Difficult ethical questions arise when we consider the implications for an already overburdened health care system. Given the shortage of donor organs, will we be forced to decide whether a 50-year-old should receive a heart transplant instead of a 75-year-old? Questions have already surfaced regarding the efficacy of hooking up a terminally ill older person to costly machines that prolong life for a few weeks or months but overtax health care resources. Is the prolongation of life at all costs a moral imperative, or will future generations be forced to devise a set of criteria for deciding who will be helped and who will not? Understanding the process of aging and knowing what actions you can take to prolong your own healthy years are part of our collective responsibility.

Theories of Aging

Biological Theories

Explanations for the biological causes of aging include the following.

- The *wear-and-tear theory* states that, like everything else in the universe, the human body wears out. Inherent in this theory is the idea that the more you abuse your body, the faster it will wear out. Fortunately, today's older adults can achieve high levels of fitness without having to be marathon runners. Strength training, walking, gardening, and other activities allow even the most out of shape to improve.
- The *cellular theory* states that at birth we have only a certain number of usable cells, which are genetically programmed to divide or reproduce a limited number of times. Once these cells reach the end of their reproductive cycle, they die, and the organs they make up begin to deteriorate. The rate of deterioration varies from person to person, and its impact depends on the system involved.
- The *autoimmune theory* attributes aging to the decline of the body's immunological system. Studies indicate that as we age, our immune systems become less effective in fighting disease. Eventually, bodies that are subjected to too much stress, lack of sleep, and so on, show signs of disease and infirmity, especially if these factors are coupled with poor nutrition. In some instances, the immune system appears to lose control, turn its protective mechanisms inward, and actually attack a person's own body. Although autoimmune disorders occur in all age groups, some gerontologists believe that they increase in frequency and severity with age.
- The *genetic mutation theory* proposes that the number of cells exhibiting unusual or different characteristics increases with age. Proponents of this theory believe that aging is related to the amount of mutational damage within the genes. The greater the mutation, the greater the chance that cells will not function properly, which leads to eventual dysfunction of body organs and systems.

Psychosocial Impacts on Aging

Numerous psychological and sociological factors also influence the manner in which people age. Psychologists Erik Erikson and Robert Peck have formulated theories of personality development that emphasize adaptation and adjustment. In his developmental model, Erikson states that people must progress through eight critical stages during a lifetime. If a person does not receive the proper stimulus or develop effective methods of coping with life's turmoil from infancy onward, problems are likely to develop later in life. According to this theory, maladjustments in old age are often a result of problems encountered in earlier stages of life.

Peck argues that during middle age and old age, people face a series of increasingly stressful tasks. Those who are poorly adjusted psychologically or who have not developed appropriate coping skills are likely to undergo a painful aging process.

Both Erikson and Peck suggest that a combination of psychosocial and biological factors and environmental trigger mechanisms causes each of us to age in a unique manner. But what is normal and what is unique in aging? How much change is inevitable, and how much can we avoid?

Changes in the Body and Mind

Typical Physical Changes

Although the physiological consequences of aging can differ in severity and timing, certain standard changes occur as a result of the aging process.

The Skin   As a normal consequence of aging, the skin becomes thinner and loses elasticity, particularly in the outer surfaces. Fat deposits, which add to the soft lines and shape of the skin, diminish. Starting at about age 30, lines develop on the forehead as a result of smiling, squinting, and other facial expressions. These lines become more pronounced, with added "crow's feet" around the eyes, during the forties. During a person's fifties and sixties, the skin begins to sag and lose color, which leads to pallor in the seventies. Body fat in underlying layers of skin continues to be redistributed away from the limbs and extremities into the trunk region of the body. Age spots become more numerous because of excessive pigment accumulation under the skin, particularly in those areas of the skin exposed to heavy sun.

Bones and Joints   Throughout the life span, bones are continually changing because of the accumulation and loss of minerals. By the third or fourth decade of life, mineral loss from bones becomes more prevalent than does mineral accumulation, which results in a weakening and porosity (diminishing density) of bony tissue. This loss of minerals (particularly calcium) occurs in both sexes, although it is more common in females. Loss of calcium can contribute to **osteoporosis,** a disease characterized by low bone density and structural deterioration of bone tissue. These porous, fragile bones are susceptible to fracture.

However, osteoporosis can occur at any age and develops over the course of many years.[10] There are several risk factors for osteoporosis, some of which cannot be controlled (gender, age, body size, ethnicity, and family history). However, there are factors that can be controlled starting from adolescence. Young women who have eating disorders

---

Osteoporosis   A degenerative bone disorder characterized by increasingly porous bones.

(anorexia or bulimia) are not getting adequate nutrients, particularly calcium and vitamin D, and are at high risk. Other factors among young adults that can contribute to a propensity to osteoporosis later in life are cigarette smoking and a lack of exercise. Weight-bearing exercise such as walking, jogging, weight training, and tennis all strengthen bone and improve bone density. Often overlooked in the discussion of osteoporosis are young men, who are at risk for developing the disease as well. Just as for women, preventive measures include eating a nutritious diet with plenty of calcium and vitamin D, engaging in regular exercise, and avoiding tobacco use.[11]

Two of the most important preventive measures are adequate calcium intake and regular weight-bearing exercise throughout your life. Diets low in calcium and vitamin D (such as those among young adults who substitute sodas and energy drinks for milk) increase the risk of osteoporosis. Doing weight-bearing exercise, which strengthens bones and improves bone density, is another measure that can delay or prevent the onset of this condition.

The Head   With age, features of the head enlarge and become more noticeable. Increased cartilage and fatty tissue cause the nose to grow a half-inch wider and another half-inch longer. Earlobes get fatter and grow longer, while overall head circumference increases one-quarter of an inch per decade, even though the brain itself shrinks. The skull becomes thicker with age.

The Urinary Tract   At age 70, the kidneys can filter waste from the blood only half as fast as they could at age 30. The need to urinate more frequently occurs because the bladder's capacity declines from 2 cups of urine at age 30 to 1 cup at age 70.

One problem often associated with aging is **urinary incontinence,** which ranges from passing a few drops of urine while laughing or sneezing to having no control over urination. As many as 19 percent of older men and 38 percent of older women have some degree of urinary incontinence.[12]

Urinary incontinence   The inability to control urination.

Cataracts   Clouding of the lens that interrupts the focusing of light on the retina, which results in blurred vision or eventual blindness. This condition is correctable with surgery.

Glaucoma   Elevation of pressure within the eyeball, which leads to hardening of the eyeball, impaired vision, and possible blindness.

Macular degeneration   Disease that breaks down the macula, the light-sensitive part of the retina responsible for sharp, direct vision.

Incontinence can pose major social, physical, and emotional problems. Embarrassment and fear of wetting oneself may cause an older person to become isolated and avoid social functions. Caregivers may become frustrated with incontinent patients. Prolonged wetness and the inability to properly care for oneself can lead to irritation, infections, and other problems.

However, incontinence is not an inevitable part of aging. Most cases are caused by medications, highly treatable neurological problems that affect the central nervous system, infections of the pelvic muscles, weakness in the pelvic wall, or other problems. When the problem is treated, the incontinence usually vanishes.[13]

The Heart and Lungs   Resting heart rate stays about the same over the course of a person's life, but the stroke volume (the amount of blood the muscle pushes out per beat) diminishes as heart muscles deteriorate. Vital capacity, or the amount of air that moves when you inhale and exhale at maximum effort, also declines with age. Exercise can do a great deal to preserve heart and lung function.

Eyesight   By age 30, the lens of the eye begins to harden, which causes problems by the early forties. The lens begins to yellow and loses transparency, while the pupil of the eye shrinks, which allows less light to penetrate. Activities such as reading become more difficult, particularly in dim light. By age 60, depth perception declines, and farsightedness often develops. A need for glasses usually develops in the forties, and this evolves into a need for bifocals in the fifties and trifocals in the sixties. **Cataracts** (clouding of the lens) and **glaucoma** (elevated pressure within the eyeball) become more likely. Eventually, a tendency toward color blindness may develop, especially for shades of blue and green. **Macular degeneration** is the breakdown of the light-sensitive part of the retina responsible for the sharp, direct vision needed to read or drive. Its effects can be devastating to independent older adults; the causes are still being investigated.

Hearing   The ability to hear high-frequency consonants (for example, *s, t,* and *z*) diminishes with age. Much of the actual hearing loss lies in the inability to distinguish extreme ranges of sound rather than in the inability to distinguish normal conversational tones.

Sexual Changes   As men age, they experience notable changes in sexual functioning. Whereas the degree and rate of change vary greatly from person to person, the following changes generally occur.

- The ability to obtain an erection is slowed.
- The ability to maintain an erection is diminished.
- The length of the refractory period between orgasms increases.
- The angle of the erection declines with age.
- The orgasm itself grows shorter in duration.

Women also experience several changes.

- Menopause usually occurs between the ages of 45 and 55. Women may experience symptoms such as hot flashes, mood swings, weight gain, development of facial hair, or other hormone-related problems.
- The walls of the vagina become less elastic and the epithelium thins, which possibly make intercourse painful.
- Vaginal secretions, particularly during sexual activity, diminish.
- The breasts become less firm. Loss of fat in various areas leads to fewer curves, with a decrease in the soft lines of the body contours.

While these physiological changes may seem somewhat discouraging, a recent study by the National Council on Aging indicates that older Americans continue to be sexually active. This study refutes long-held beliefs that sexual desire decreases as we age. Results indicate that nearly half of Americans over age 60 engage in sexual activity at least once a month, and four out of ten would like to have sex more frequently than they currently do.[14] With the advent of drugs designed to treat sexual dysfunction, such as Viagra, many older adults may get their wish.

Body Comfort   Because of the loss of body fat, thinning of the epithelium, and diminished glandular activity, older people experience greater difficulty in regulating body temperature. This limits their ability to withstand extreme cold or heat, which increases the risks of hypothermia, heatstroke, and heat exhaustion.

> **What do you think?**
>
> *Of the health conditions discussed in this section, which ones can you prevent? Which ones can you delay?* ✳ *What actions can you take now to protect yourself from these problems?*

Typical Mental Changes

Intelligence   Recent research demonstrates that many of our previous beliefs about intelligence later in life were based on inappropriate testing procedures. Given an appropriate length of time, older people learn and develop skills in a similar manner to younger people. Researchers have also determined that what many older adults lack in speed of learning they make up for in practical knowledge—that is, they have the wisdom of age.

Memory   Have you ever wondered why your grandfather seems unable to remember what he did last weekend even though he can graphically describe an event that occurred 40 years ago? This phenomenon is not unusual. Although short-term memory may fluctuate on a daily basis, the ability to remember events from past decades seems to remain largely unchanged.

Flexibility versus Rigidity   Although it is widely believed that people become more like one another as they age, nothing could be further from the truth. Having lived through a multitude of experiences and faced diverse joys, sorrows, and obstacles, the typical older person has developed unique methods of coping with life. These unique adaptive variations make for interesting differences in how we confront the many changes brought on by the aging process. As a group, older adults are extremely heterogeneous. They adapt and "make do" in ways that younger adults may not be able to duplicate. Labeling this highly flexible and resilient group as rigid is inaccurate and misleading.

Depression   Most adults continue to lead healthy, fulfilling lives. However, some older people do suffer from mental and emotional disturbances. Some research indicates that depression may be the most common psychological problem facing older adults.[15] However, the rate of major depression is actually lower among older people than it is among younger adults.

Regardless of age, people who have a poor perception of their health, who have multiple chronic illnesses, who take a lot of medications, and who do not exercise have greater rates of depression. Strong coping skills and support systems often will lessen the duration and severity of the depression.

Senility: Getting Rid of Ageist Attitudes   Over the years, older adults have often suffered from ageist attitudes. People who were chronologically old were often labeled "senile" whenever they displayed memory failure, errors in judgment, disorientation, or erratic behaviors. Today scientists recognize that these same symptoms can occur at any age and for various reasons, including disease or the use of over-the-counter and prescription drugs. When the underlying problems are corrected, the memory loss and disorientation also improve. Currently, the term **senility** is seldom used except to describe a very small group of organic disorders.

Alzheimer's Disease   **Dementias** are progressive brain impairments that interfere with memory and normal intellectual functioning. Although there are many types of dementia, one of the most common forms is **Alzheimer's disease (AD)**. Attacking more than 4 million Americans and killing more than 100,000 of them every year, this disease is one of the most

---

Senility   A term associated with loss of memory and judgment and orientation problems occurring in a small percentage of the elderly.

Dementias   Progressive brain impairments that interfere with memory and normal intellectual functioning.

Alzheimer's disease (AD)   A chronic condition involving changes in nerve fibers of the brain that results in mental deterioration.

painful and devastating conditions that families can endure. It kills its victims twice: first through a slow loss of personhood (memory loss, disorientation, personality changes, and eventual loss of the ability to function independently), and then through the deterioration of bodily systems as they gradually succumb to the powerful impact of neurological problems. On average, patients with AD live for 8 to 10 years after diagnosis, though the disease can last for up to 20 years.[16]

Currently, Alzheimer's afflicts an estimated one in ten people over age 65 and one in five people over age 85, including actor Charlton Heston and former president Ronald Reagan. These numbers are certain to increase. It currently is estimated to cost society more than $100 billion a year. With the U.S. population gradually aging, the economic burden of the future seems even more dismal. While most people associate Alzheimer's with the aged, it has been diagnosed in people in their late forties. In fact, about 5 percent of all cases occur before age 65.

Contrary to what many people think, Alzheimer's is not a new disease. Named after Alois Alzheimer, a German neuropathologist who recorded it as early as 1906, Alzheimer's disease refers to a degenerative disease of the brain in which nerve cells stop communicating with one another. Ordinarily, brain cells communicate by releasing chemicals that allow the cells to receive and transmit messages for various types of behavior. In Alzheimer's patients, the brain doesn't produce enough of these chemicals, cells can't communicate, and eventually the cells die. This degeneration occurs in the sections of the brain that affect memory, speech, and personality; the regions that control other bodily functions, such as heartbeat and breathing, function at near normal levels. Thus, the mind begins to go as the body lives on. It all happens in a slow, progressive manner, and it may take 20 years before symptoms are noticed.

Alzheimer's generally is detected first by families, who note changes, particularly memory lapses and personality changes, in their loved ones. Medical tests rule out underlying causes, and certain neurological tests help confirm the diagnosis.

Alzheimer's disease characteristically progresses in three stages. During the *first stage,* symptoms include forgetfulness, memory loss, impaired judgment, increasing inability to handle routine tasks, disorientation, lack of interest in one's surroundings, and depression. These symptoms accelerate in the *second stage,* which also includes agitation and restlessness (especially at night), loss of sensory perceptions, muscle twitching, and repetitive actions. Many patients become depressed, combative, and aggressive. In the *final stage,* disorientation is often complete. The person becomes completely dependent on others for eating, dressing, and other activities. Identity loss and speech problems are common. Eventually, control of bodily functions may be lost.

Once Alzheimer's disease strikes, the victim's life expectancy is cut in half. Tragically, little can be done at present to treat the disorder, although scientists are experimenting with various drug regimens. Researchers are investigating a number of possible causes, including genetic predisposition, malfunction of the immune system, a slow-acting virus, chromosomal or genetic defects, oxidative stress, chronic inflammation, and neurotransmitter imbalance.[17] A 2003 study indicates that being overweight or obese may predispose individuals to Alzheimer's.[18] Obesity increases the incidence of high blood pressure, high cholesterol, and high blood sugar, all of which have been implicated as risk factors in Alzheimer's disease. However, more research with greater numbers of participants and sufficient controls will be needed to validate these initial findings.

Health Challenges of Older Adults

Some health problems common in the elderly are brought on by failing health, others by society or a perceived loss of control over life's events. Developing life skills and a network of social support during earlier years can reduce problems in old age significantly.

Alcohol Use and Abuse

Early studies reported that 2 to 10 percent of older Americans were alcoholics, but the exact percentages are controversial today. However, a person who is prone to alcoholism during the younger and middle years is more likely to continue during later years. The elderly alcoholic is probably no more common in American society than is the young alcoholic, despite the stereotype of the old, lost soul, drowning his or her sorrows in a bottle. Often, when many people think they see a drunken older person, they are really seeing a confused individual who has taken too many different prescription medications and is experiencing a form of drug interaction.

Men tend to have a higher risk for alcoholism at all ages. Alcohol abuse is five times more common among older men than it is among older women. Yet, as many as half of all older men and an even higher proportion of older women don't drink at all.[19] Those who do drink do so less than younger persons and consume only five to six drinks weekly. It is important to note that most older adults who consume alcohol are neither alcoholics nor people who drink to cope with their losses. Most of their drinking is social and, in fact, may be less of a problem than previously thought.[20]

Prescription Drug Use

It is extremely rare for older people to use illicit drugs, but some do overuse and grow dependent upon prescription drugs. Anyone who combines different drugs runs the risk of dangerous drug interactions. The risks of adverse effects are even greater for people with impaired circulation and declining kidney and liver function. Older adults displaying symptoms of these drug-induced effects, which may include bizarre behavior patterns or disorientation, are all-too-often misdiagnosed as senile rather than examined for underlying

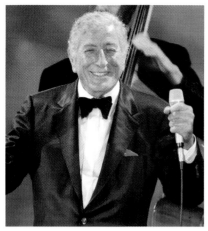
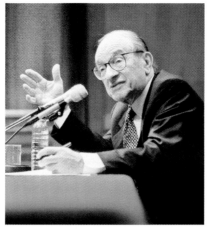
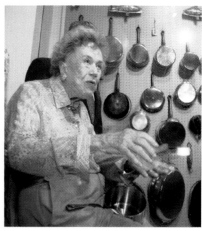

Singer Tony Bennett, economist Alan Greenspan, and chef Julia Child are examples of people who stay vigorous and active in their professions well into their seventies, eighties, and even nineties.

causes and treated. Doctors often have difficulty medicating older individuals, particularly when the patient is taking several drugs at the same time.

Over-the-Counter Remedies

A substantial segment of the over-60 population avoids orthodox medical treatment and views it as a last resort. This is becoming increasingly true as Medicare coverage becomes less adequate and older adults are forced to pay larger medical bills out of their own resources. The poor are particularly prone to turn to folk medicine and over-the-counter preparations as cheaper, less intimidating alternatives.

Preventive Actions for Healthy Aging

As you know from reading this book, you can do many things to prolong and improve the quality of your life. Some factors, however, are especially important. To provide for healthy older years, make each of the following part of your younger years.

Develop and Maintain Healthy Relationships

Social bonds lend vigor and energy to life. Be willing to give to others, and seek variety in your relationships rather than befriending only people who agree with you. By experiencing diverse people and interacting with different points of view, we gain a new perspective on life.

Enrich the Spiritual Side of Life

Although we often take this for granted, cultivating a relationship with nature, the environment, a higher being, and yourself is a key factor in personal growth and development. Take time for thought and quiet contemplation, and enjoy the sunsets, sounds, and energy of life. These moments spent in time prioritized for you will leave you invigorated and fresh—better able to cope with the ups and downs of life. If you don't take time for yourself now, it may be that you won't have time in the later years.

Improve Fitness

If you're basically sedentary, just about any moderate-intensity exercise that gets your heart beating faster and increases strength and/or flexibility will maximize your physical health and functional years. One of the inevitable physical changes that the body undergoes is **sarcopenia,** age-associated loss of muscle mass. The less muscle you have, the less energy you will burn even while resting. The lower your metabolic rate, the more likely you will gain weight. With regular strength training, you can increase your muscle mass, boost your metabolism, strengthen your bones, prevent osteoporosis, and, in general, feel better and function more efficiently.

Eat for Health

Although other chapters in this text provide detailed information about nutrition and weight control, certain nutrients are especially essential to healthy aging.

- *Calcium.* Bone loss tends to increase in women, particularly in the hip region, shortly before menopause. During perimenopause and menopause, bone loss accelerates rapidly, with an average of 3 percent of skeletal mass lost per year over a five-year period. The result is an increased risk for fracture and disability. Few women

---

Sarcopenia Age-related loss of muscle mass.

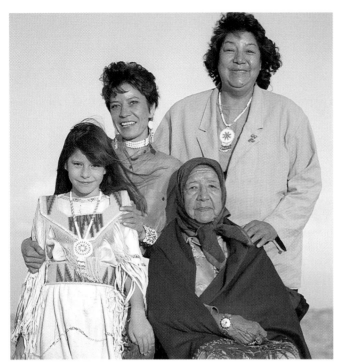

In most cases, you need look no further than your family tree to get an idea of the effects that aging will have on you.

actually consume the 1,000 milligrams (mg) of calcium recommended during the younger years, or the 1,500 mg recommended during and after menopause.

- *Vitamin D.* Vitamin D is necessary for adequate calcium absorption. Yet, as people age, particularly in their fifties and sixties, they do not absorb vitamin D from foods as readily as they did when they were younger. If vitamin D is unavailable, calcium levels are also likely to be lower.
- *Protein.* As older adults become more concerned about cholesterol and fatty foods, as their budgets shrink, one nutrient that often takes the "hit" is protein. Many cut back on protein to a point that is below the recommended daily amount. Because protein is necessary for muscle mass, protein insufficiencies can spell trouble.

Other nutrients, including vitamin E, folic acid (folate), iron, potassium, and vitamin B_{12}, are also important to the aging process. Most of these are readily available in any diet that follows Food Guide Pyramid recommendations.

Comorbidity The presence of a number of diseases at the same time.

Respite care The care provided by substitute caregivers to relieve the principal caregiver from his or her continuous responsibility.

Dying The process of decline in body functions, resulting in the death of an organism.

Death The permanent ending of all vital functions.

Caring for Older Adults

Elderly women far outnumber elderly men in American society, and the discrepancy increases with age. Because women live seven years longer than men do on average, older women are more likely to be living alone. Further, they are more likely to experience poverty and multiple chronic health problems, a situation referred to as **comorbidity.** Consequently, more women than men are likely to need assistance from children, other relatives, friends, and neighbors.

Women usually have been the primary caregivers for older Americans, often for their ailing husbands. Research also indicates that women spend more hours than men do (38 hours versus 27 hours per week) in caregiving activities and perform a wider range of services. Regardless of the time spent, caregiving is a difficult and stressful experience for both women and men. **Respite care,** or care that is given by someone who relieves the primary caregiver, should be available to ease the burden.

What do you think?
Why are women often the primary caregivers for aging spouses and other family members?
❋ *What problems can such caregiving cause?*
❋ *How can caregivers learn to cope with the stresses and strains of their situation?*

Understanding Death

Death eventually comes to everyone, but if you live life to the fullest and learn as much about end-of-life issues as you can, you will be better able to accept the inevitable. To cope effectively with dying, we must address the individual needs of those who are facing life's final transition. Let's begin by investigating what death means, at least in medical terms.

Defining Death

Dying is the process of decline in body functions that results in the death of an organism. **Death** can be defined as the "final cessation of the vital functions" and also refers to a state in which these functions are "incapable of being restored."[21] This definition has become more significant as medical advances make it increasingly possible to postpone death.

Legal and ethical issues led to the Uniform Determination of Death Act in 1981, which has been endorsed by the American Medical Association, the American Bar Association, and the National Conference for Commissioners on Uniform State Laws. This act, which has been adopted by several states, reads as follows: "An individual who has sustained either (1) irreversible cessation of circulatory and respiratory functions, or (2) irreversible cessation of all functions of the entire brain, including the brain stem, is dead. A determination of death must be made in accordance with accepted medical standards."[22]

The concept of **brain death,** defined as the irreversible cessation of all functions of the entire brain stem, has gained increasing credence. As defined by the Ad Hoc Committee of the Harvard Medical School, brain death occurs when the following criteria are met:

- Unreceptivity and unresponsiveness—that is, no response even to painful stimuli
- No movement for a continuous hour after observation by a physician and no breathing after three minutes off a respirator
- No reflexes, including brain stem reflexes; fixed and dilated pupils
- A "flat" electroencephalogram (EEG) for at least ten minutes
- All of these tests repeated at least 24 hours later with no change
- Certainty that hypothermia (extreme loss of body heat) and depression of the central nervous system caused by use of drugs such as barbiturates are not responsible for these conditions[23]

The Harvard report provides useful guidelines; however, the definition of *death* and all its ramifications continue to concern us.

> **What do you think?**
>
> *Why is there so much concern over the definition of* death? ✻ *How does modern technology complicate the understanding of when death occurs?*

Denying Death

Attitudes toward death tend to fall on a continuum. At one end of the continuum, death is viewed as the mortal enemy of humankind. Both medical science and certain religions have promoted this idea. At the other end of the continuum, death is accepted and even welcomed by some religious groups and segments of the population.[24] For people whose attitudes fall at this end, death is a passage to a better state of being. But most of us perceive ourselves to be in the middle of this continuum. From this perspective, death is a bewildering mystery that elicits fear and apprehension while profoundly influencing beliefs and actions throughout life.

In the United States, a high level of discomfort is associated with death and dying. We may avoid speaking about death to limit our own discomfort. Those who deny death tend to:

- Avoid people who are grieving after the death of a loved one so they won't have to talk about it

- Fail to validate a dying person's frightening situation by talking to the person as if nothing were wrong
- Substitute euphemisms for the word *death* (for example, "passing away," "kicking the bucket," "no longer with us," "going to heaven," or "going to a better place")
- Give false reassurances to dying people by saying things like "everything is going to be okay"
- Shut off conversation about death by silencing people who are trying to talk about it
- Avoid touching people who are dying

Recent years have shown a greater effort on the part of the American public to mourn openly, as is indicated by roadside memorials placed at the sites of violent or unexpected deaths. Although these are fairly new additions to the American landscape, these memorials have long been popular in other parts of the world, particularly in predominantly Catholic countries.[25]

> **What do you think?**
>
> *"The art of living well and the art of dying well are one."* ✻ *What do you think this quote from the Greek philosopher Epicurus means? Do you agree?*

The Process of Dying

Dying is a complex process that includes physical, intellectual, social, spiritual, and emotional dimensions. Now that we have examined the physical indicators of death, we must consider the emotional aspects of dying and "social death."

Coping Emotionally with Death

Although emotional reactions to dying vary, many people share similar experiences during this process. Much of our knowledge about reactions to dying stems from the work of Elisabeth Kübler-Ross, a major figure in modern **thanatology,** the study of death and dying. In 1969, Kübler-Ross published *On Death and Dying,* a sensitive analysis of the reactions of terminally ill patients. This pioneering work encouraged the development of death education as a discipline and prompted efforts to improve the care of dying patients. Kübler-Ross identified five psychological stages that terminally ill patients often experience as they approach death.

1. *Denial.* ("Not me, there must be a mistake.") This is usually the first stage, experienced as a sensation of shock

---

Brain death The irreversible cessation of all functions of the entire brain stem.

Thanatology The study of death and dying.

Funeral and Mourning Customs around the World

Traditions associated with death vary around the world and reflect differing cultures and religious practices. However, every culture recognizes death as a significant rite of passage. Here is a global sampling of funeral customs.

BUDDHISM

In several Japanese Buddhist traditions, a funeral ceremony resembles a Christian ceremony with a eulogy and prayers at a funeral home. Cambodian, Thai, and Sri Lankan traditions may have up to three ceremonies. In the first, which is held two days after the death, monks conduct a ceremony at the home of the bereaved. In the second, two to five days after the death, monks hold a service at a funeral home. The third, seven days after burial or cremation, is a monk-led ceremony at a temple or the home of the bereaved. This last ceremony, called a "merit transference," seeks to generate good energy for the deceased in his or her new incarnation. There is always an open casket, with the sight of the body reminding guests of the impermanence of life.

GREEK ORTHODOX CHURCH

Mourners bow in front of the open casket and kiss an icon or cross placed on the chest of the deceased. The traditional words said to the bereaved are "May you have an abundant life" and "May their memory be eternal." At the graveside, there is a five-minute prayer ceremony, and each person present places one flower on the casket. A memorial service is held on the Sunday closest to the fortieth day after the death.

HINDUISM

The body remains at the home until it is taken to the place of cremation, usually 24 hours after death. It is customary to wear white at the funeral. The major officiants at the service are Hindu priests or senior, male members of the family. Special books containing mantras for funeral services are used, but only by the priests. At the cremation, a last food offering is symbolically made to the deceased, and then the body is cremated. An additional ceremony at home, performed 10 days after death for the Brahmin caste and 30 days after death for other castes, liberates the soul of the deceased for its ascent to heaven.

ISLAM

Mourners wash the body of the deceased, perfume it, and wrap it in white cloth. Mourners face Mecca and recite prayers, and then a silent procession carries the body to its burial place. All the mourners participate in filling the grave with soil.

JUDAISM

A Jewish funeral is a time of intense mourning and public grieving. Traditional Jewish law forbids cremation, but it is allowed among Reform Jews. Flowers are never appropriate for Orthodox or Conservative funerals but are sometimes appropriate for Reform funerals. There is never an open casket. The officiants include a rabbi who delivers a eulogy, a cantor who sings, and family members or friends who may also deliver a eulogy or memorial. At the simplest graveside service, the rabbi recites prayers and leads the family in the mourner's *kaddish,* the prayer for the deceased. At a traditional service, there is a slow procession to the grave itself with several pauses along the way. After prayers and *kaddish* have been recited, each person puts one spade of earth into the grave.

The family sits in mourning for seven days after the funeral, which is called the *shiva* period. To symbolize the mourners' lack of interest in their comfort or how they appear to others, family members may cover mirrors in the home, wear a black ribbon that has been cut and slippers or socks rather than shoes; men may refrain from shaving. A special memorial candle may be burned for seven days.

NATIVE AMERICAN RELIGIONS

Funeral and mourning rituals are linked to the belief that this is the beginning of a journey into the next world. Strict rules govern the behavior of the living relatives to ensure the deceased a good start on his or her journey. Some Potawatomi, for instance, set a place for the deceased at a funeral feast so the spirit can partake of the food. Among the Yuchi, personal items such as a hunting rifle, blanket, and tobacco may be placed in an adult male's coffin, which reflects the belief that needs in the next life do not differ significantly from needs in this one.

While Native American beliefs assert that death is not necessarily the termination of life, the bereaved still mourn the absence of the one who has died. Many tribes restrict what bereaved relatives can eat or the activities they can engage in. This represents a sacrifice by the living for those who have moved on.

SOCIETY OF FRIENDS (QUAKERS)

There are two types of Quaker funerals. An unprogrammed meeting is held in silence in the traditional manner of Friends. Worshippers sit and wait for divine guidance; if so moved, they speak to the group. Programmed meetings are planned in advance and usually include singing, prayers, Bible reading, silent worship, and a sermon.

Source: Adapted from Arthur J. Magida and Stuart M. Matlins, eds, *How to Be a Perfect Stranger* (Woodstock, VT: SkyLight Paths Publishing, 2003). www.skylightpaths.com

and disbelief. A person intellectually accepts the impending death but rejects it emotionally. The patient is too confused and stunned to comprehend "not being" and thus rejects the idea. Within a relatively short time, the anxiety level may diminish, which enables the patient to sort through the powerful web of emotions.

2. *Anger.* ("Why me?") Anger is another common reaction. The person becomes angry at having to face death when others, including loved ones, are healthy and not threatened. The dying person perceives the situation as unfair or senseless and may be hostile to friends, family, physicians, or the world in general.

3. *Bargaining.* ("If I'm allowed to live, I promise . . .") This stage generally occurs at about the middle of the progression. The dying person may resolve to be a better person in return for an extension of life or may secretly pray for a short reprieve from death in order to experience a special event, such as a family wedding or birth.

4. *Depression.* ("It's really going to happen to me, and I can't do anything about it.") Depression eventually sets in as vitality diminishes, and the person begins to experience distressing symptoms with increasing frequency. The person's deteriorating condition becomes impossible for him or her to deny, and feelings of doom and tremendous loss may become pervasive. Feelings of worthlessness and guilt are also common because the dying person may feel responsible for the emotional suffering of loved ones and the arduous but seemingly futile efforts of caregivers.

5. *Acceptance.* ("I'm ready.") This is often the final stage. The patient stops battling with emotions and becomes tired and weak. The need to sleep increases, and wakeful periods become shorter and less frequent. With acceptance, the person does not give up and become sullen or resentfully resigned to death but rather becomes passive. According to one dying person, the acceptance stage is "almost void of feelings . . . as if the pain had gone, the struggle is over, and there comes a time for the final rest before the long journey."[26] As he or she lets go, the dying person may no longer welcome visitors and may not wish to engage in conversation. Death usually occurs quietly and painlessly while the person is unconscious.

Some of Kübler-Ross's peers consider her theory too neat and orderly. The experiences of dying people do not always fit easily into specific stages, and patterns vary from person to person. Even if it is not accurate in all particulars, however, Kübler-Ross's theory offers valuable insights for those seeking to understand or deal with the process of dying.

> **What do you think?**
>
> * *Do you agree with Elisabeth Kübler-Ross's stages of dying?* * *Do you think it is important to help a person get through all the stages that Kübler-Ross has identified? Why or why not?*

Social Death

The need for recognition and appreciation within a social group is nearly universal. Although the size and nature of the social group may vary widely, the need to belong exists in all of us. Loss of being valued or appreciated by others can lead to **social death,** a seemingly irreversible situation in which a person is not treated like an active member of society. Dramatic examples of social death include the exile of nonconformists from their native countries or the excommunication of dissident members of religious groups. More often, however, social death is inflicted by denying a person normal social interaction. Numerous studies indicate that people are treated differently when they are dying. The following common behaviors contribute to the social death that often isolates people who are terminally ill:

- The dying person is referred to as if he or she were already dead.
- The dying person may be inadvertently excluded from conversations.
- Dying patients often are moved to terminal wards and given minimal care.
- Bereaved family members are avoided, often for extended periods, because friends and neighbors feel uncomfortable in the presence of grief.
- Medical personnel may make degrading comments about patients in their presence.[27]

This decrease in meaningful social interaction often strips dying and bereaved people of their identity as valued members of society at a time when belonging is critical. Some dying people choose not to speak of their inevitable fate in an attempt to make others feel more comfortable and thus preserve vital relationships.

Coping with Loss

The losses resulting from the death of a loved one are extremely difficult to cope with. The dying person, as well as close family and friends, frequently suffers emotionally and physically from the impending loss of critical relationships and roles. Words used to describe feelings and behavior related to losses resulting from death include *bereavement, grief, grief work,* and *mourning.* These terms are related but not identical in meaning. Understanding them may help in comprehending the emotional processes associated with loss and the cultural constraints that often inhibit normal coping behavior. Figure 15.2 on page 412 depicts the stages of grief that many people commonly experience.

> **Social death** A seemingly irreversible situation in which a person is not treated like an active member of society.

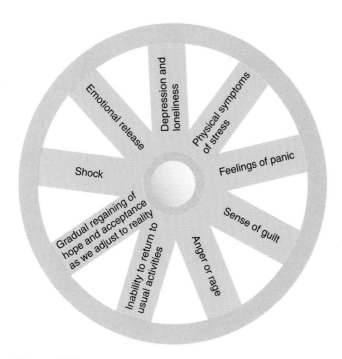

Figure 15.2
The Stages of Grief
People react differently to losses, but most eventually adjust. Generally, the stronger the social support system, the smoother the progression through the stages of grief.

Bereavement generally is defined as the loss or deprivation experienced by a survivor when a loved one dies. Because relationships vary in type and intensity, reactions to loss also vary. In the lives of the bereaved or of close survivors, the loss of loved ones leaves "holes." We can think of bereavement as the awareness of these holes. Time and courage are necessary to fill these spaces.

A special case of bereavement occurs in old age. Loss is an intrinsic part of growing old. The longer we live, the more losses we are likely to experience. They include physical, social, and emotional losses as our bodies deteriorate and more and more of our loved ones die. The theory of *bereavement overload* has been proposed to explain the effects of multiple losses and the accumulation of sorrow in the lives of some older people. This theory suggests that the gloomy outlook,

---

Bereavement The loss or deprivation experienced by a survivor when a loved one dies.

Grief The state of mental distress that occurs in reaction to significant loss, including one's own impending death, the death of a loved one, or a quasi-death experience.

Disenfranchised grief Grief concerning a loss that cannot be openly acknowledged, publicly mourned, or socially supported.

Mourning The culturally prescribed behavior patterns for the expression of grief.

---

disturbing behavior patterns, and apparent apathy that characterize these people may be related more to bereavement overload than to intrinsic physiological degeneration in old age.[28]

Grief is a state of mental distress that occurs in reaction to significant loss, including one's own impending death, the death of a loved one, or a quasi-death experience (a loss, such as the end of a relationship or job, that resembles death because it involves separation, grief, or change in personal identity). Grief reactions include any adjustments needed for one to make it through the day and may include changes in patterns of eating, sleeping, working, and even thinking.

When a person experiences a loss that cannot be openly acknowledged, publicly mourned, or socially supported, coping may be much more difficult. This type of grief is referred to as **disenfranchised grief**.[29] It may occur among those who miscarry, are developmentally disabled, or are close friends rather than relatives of the deceased. It may also include those relationships that are not socially approved, such as those between extramarital lovers or homosexual couples. When society does not assign significance to a high-grief death, grieving becomes more difficult.

The term **mourning** is often incorrectly equated with the term *grief*. As we have noted, *grief* refers to a wide variety of feelings and actions that occur in response to bereavement. *Mourning,* in contrast, refers to culturally prescribed and accepted time periods and behavior patterns for the expression of grief. In Judaism, for example, *"sitting shiva"* is a designated mourning period of seven days that involves prescribed rituals and prayers. Depending on a person's relationship with the deceased, various other rituals may continue for up to a year.

Symptoms of grief vary in severity and duration, depending on the situation and the individual. However, the bereaved person can benefit from emotional and social support from family, friends, clergy, employers, and the traditional support organizations, including the medical community and the funeral industry. The larger and stronger the support system, the easier readjustment is likely to be.

What Is "Normal" Grief?

Grief responses vary widely from person to person, but frequently include the following symptoms:

- Periodic waves of physical distress lasting from 20 minutes to an hour
- A feeling of tightness in the throat
- Choking and shortness of breath
- A frequent need to sigh
- Feelings of emptiness and muscular weakness
- Intense anxiety that is described as actually painful

Other common symptoms of grief include insomnia, memory lapse, loss of appetite, difficulty concentrating, a tendency to engage in repetitive or purposeless behavior, an "observer" sensation or feeling of unreality, difficulty in making decisions, lack of organization, excessive speech, social withdrawal or hostility, guilt feelings, and preoccupation with the image of the deceased. Susceptibility to disease increases with grief and may even be life threatening in severe and enduring cases.

A bereaved person may suffer emotional pain and exhibit a variety of grief responses for many months after the death. The rate of the healing process depends on the amount and quality of grief work that a person does. **Grief work** is the process of integrating the reality of the loss into everyday life and learning to feel better. Often, the bereaved person must deliberately and systematically work at reducing denial and coping with the pain that results from memories of the deceased. This process takes time and requires emotional effort.

> **What do you think?**
> *Do you think men grieve differently from women?*
> ✳ *What have you personally observed about these differences, if any?*

Life-and-Death Decision Making

Many complex, and often expensive, life-and-death decisions must be made during a highly distressing period in people's lives. We will not attempt to present definitive answers to moral and philosophical questions about death; instead, we offer these topics for your consideration. We hope that this discussion of the needs of the dying person and the bereaved will help you negotiate these difficult decisions in the future.

The Right to Die

Few people would object to a proposal for the right to a dignified death. Going beyond that concept, however, many people today believe that they should be allowed to die if their condition is terminal and their existence depends on mechanical life support devices or artificial feeding or hydration systems. Artificial life support techniques that may be legally refused by competent patients in some states include:

- Electrical or mechanical heart resuscitation
- Mechanical respiration by machine
- Nasogastric tube feedings
- Intravenous nutrition
- Gastrostomy (tube feeding directly into the stomach)
- Medications to treat life-threatening infections

As long as a person is conscious and competent, he or she has the legal right to refuse treatment, even if this decision will hasten death. However, when a person is in a coma or otherwise incapable of speaking on his or her own behalf, medical personnel and administrative policy will dictate treatment. This issue has evolved into a battle involving personal freedom, legal rulings, health care policy, and physician responsibility. The living will was developed to assist in solving these conflicts.

Cases have been reported in which the wishes of people who have signed a living will (also called an advanced directive) indicating their desire not to receive artificial life support were not honored by their physician or medical institution. This problem can be avoided by choosing a physician and a hospital that will carry out the directives of a living will. Taking this precaution and discussing your wishes with your family should eliminate anxiety about how you will be treated at the end of your life. Many legal experts suggest that you take the following steps to ensure that your wishes are carried out.

1. *Be specific.* Rather than signing an advanced directive (which speaks only in generalities), complete a directive that permits you to make specific choices about a variety of procedures under different circumstances. Attach this document to a completed copy of the standard advance directive for your state.
2. *Get an agent.* Even the most detailed directive cannot anticipate every situation that may arise. You may also want to appoint a family member or friend to act as your agent, or *proxy,* by making out a form known as either a *durable power of attorney for health care* or a *health care proxy.*
3. *Discuss your wishes.* Discuss your wishes with your proxy and your doctor. Going over the situations described in the form will give them a clear idea of just how much you are willing to endure to preserve your life.
4. *Deliver the directive.* Distribute several copies, not only to your doctor and your agent but also to your lawyer and to immediate family members or a close friend. Make sure *someone* knows to bring a copy to the hospital in the event you are hospitalized.[30]

Rational Suicide

We have discussed suicide in earlier chapters. The concept of **rational suicide** as an alternative to an extended dying process, however, deserves mention here. Although exact numbers are not known, medical ethicists and specialists in forensic medicine (the study of legal issues in medicine) estimate that thousands of terminally ill people every year decide to kill themselves rather than endure constant pain and slow decay. To these people, the prospect of an undignified death is unacceptable. This issue has been complicated by advances in death prevention techniques that allow terminally ill patients to exist in an irreversible disease state for extended periods of time. Medical personnel, clergy, lawyers, and patients all must struggle with this ethical dilemma.

> **Grief work**   The process of accepting the reality of a person's death and coping with memories of the deceased.
>
> **Rational suicide**   The decision to kill oneself rather than endure constant pain and slow decay.

Preparing to Support a Dying Person

Whether we have months to prepare for death or it comes suddenly, most people have difficulty knowing what to do. We push death from our consciousness, which leads to problems before and after the moment of death comes for loved ones. Although you can never be fully prepared for the loss of a loved one, you can learn skills that will help you through the trauma of loss. The following suggestions will help you, particularly in situations where you have time to prepare.

1. *Follow the wishes of the patient.* Make sure that a copy of his or her advance directive is available and accepted as the wishes of the patient. Most people, particularly in hospice, want a natural death. Think of comfort, not cure. Whenever possible, talk to the patient and allow choices to be made about the dying process. For example, if the patient wants to stay at home but being in a hospital bed would be easier for caregivers, talk this out with the patient.

2. *Help with comfort and rest.* Don't be afraid to ask for medications to help the patient deal with pain, sleeplessness, or anxiety.

3. *Prepare a list of people to call near the time of death, including family, friends, and religious support.* Talk about who the patient wants present, if anyone. Make a list of people to notify once death occurs. Keep a list of home health nurses, hospice staff, and physicians nearby so they can be contacted quickly.

4. *Call for professional help if any of the following occur:*
   - If the patient is in extreme pain or discomfort
   - If the patient has difficulty breathing. Oxygen can calm the patient and make the last hours more comfortable.
   - If the patient has trouble urinating or passing stool. Usually the urine will be dark and in small quantity. Medications can help ease discomfort.
   - If your emotions are getting the best of you. Thoughts of impending loss can prevent you from being supportive to the dying person.

5. *Touch is often comforting for the dying person.* Give back, hand, or foot rubs. Do not stand back and avoid contact. Help the patient adjust his or her position in bed if at all possible. Usually an extra sheet placed under the patient and the help of a second person will make this easier.

6. *Moisten the eyes and lips with warm, damp cloths and apply skin lotions to insure comfort.* Apply warm or cool compresses if the person wants them.

7. *Know what to expect.* Be ready to say goodbye. Talk to the person. In some cases soft, relaxing music may be comforting. During the last moments of life, the body begins to slow down, breathing rates slow, sometimes there are long pauses between breaths. Sometimes the person will appear to wake up but will be unable to speak or recognize you. Usually this means patients are in or near coma state, and they may progress to longer and longer periods of sleep. The skin may be cool, especially around the feet and hands, and may become blue- or gray-tinged. In the last stages as death nears, the person may become incontinent or lose bowel control. Finally, the chest will stop rising, the eyes may appear glassy, and there is no more pulse.

8. *You may choose to assist with preparing the body for transport to the funeral home or other facility, or you may choose to let others take over.* Try to think about this in advance and make decisions based on your own preferences and needs.

A form of mercy killing in which someone plays a passive role in the death of a terminally ill person is **dyathanasia.** This passive role may include withholding life-prolonging treatments or withdrawing life-sustaining medical support, which thereby allows the person to die. Euthanasia often is referred to as mercy killing. The term **active euthanasia** refers to ending the life of a person (or animal) that is suffering greatly and has no chance of recovery. An example might be a physician-prescribed lethal injection. **Passive euthanasia** refers to the intentional withholding of treatment that would prolong life. Deciding not to place a person with massive brain trauma on life support is an example of passive euthanasia.

Dr. Jack Kevorkian, a physician in Michigan, started a one-person campaign to force the medical profession to change its position regarding physician-assisted death. Kevorkian has assisted many terminally ill patients in dying and, until recently, had escaped conviction despite being taken into court several times for his actions. Kevorkian has argued that the Hippocratic oath, an ancient ethical pledge still taken by medical students, is not binding. He believes that the present situation in our society demands a shift in

Dyathanasia   The passive form of mercy killing in which life-prolonging treatments or interventions are not offered or are withheld which thereby allows a terminally ill person to die naturally.

Active euthanasia   Mercy killing in which a person or organization knowingly acts to hasten the death of a terminally ill person.

Passive euthanasia   The intentional withholding of treatment that would prolong life.

the practice of medicine and the acceptance of euthanasia, specifically in the practice of physician-assisted death. In 1998, Kevorkian took his argument to prime time, as the CBS News program *60 Minutes* broadcast his latest case of assisting a terminally ill patient with ending his life. This time, however, the courts determined that Kevorkian had gone too far. He was convicted of murder and sentenced to prison, where he remains.

Kevorkian's actions have focused a great deal of attention on the issue and have caused many to speculate on the merits of physician-assisted suicide. A study in Michigan revealed that a greater number of physicians were in favor of legalizing assisted suicide than were against it.[31] A similar study in Oregon found that physicians have a more favorable attitude toward legalized physician-assisted suicide, are more willing to participate, and currently are participating in greater numbers than other surveyed groups in the United States.[32] In both studies, however, a sizable minority of physicians still had reservations about the practical applications of the proposed law.

> ### What do you think?
> *Are there any end-of-life situations in which you would ask a physician to help you die? Explain your answer.* ✳ *Do you believe people should have the right to ask a physician to help them die? Why or why not?*

Planning for Death and After

Caring for dying people and dealing with the practical and legal questions surrounding death can be difficult and painful. The problems of the dying person and the bereaved loved ones involve a wide variety of psychological, legal, social, spiritual, economic, and interpersonal issues.

Hospice Care: Positive Alternatives

Since the mid-1970s, **hospice** programs have grown from a mere handful to more than 2,500 and are available in nearly every community. Unlike even ten years ago, families facing terminal illness often are expected to make difficult medical decisions, including where their loved ones will die. Improving quality of care at the end of life is a top priority of the American Medical Association.

The primary goals of hospice programs are to relieve the dying person's pain; offer emotional support to the dying person and loved ones; and restore a sense of control to the dying person, family, and friends. Although home care with maximum involvement by loved ones is emphasized, hospice programs are directed by cooperating physicians; coordinated by specially trained nurses; and fortified with the skills of counselors, clergy, and trained volunteers. Hospital

inpatient beds are available if necessary. Hospice programs usually include the following characteristics.

1. The patient and family constitute the unit of care, because the physical, psychological, social, and spiritual problems of dying confront the family as well as the patient.
2. Emphasis is placed on symptom control, primarily the alleviation of pain. Curative treatments are curtailed as requested by the patient, but sound judgment must be applied to avoid a feeling of abandonment.
3. There is overall medical direction of the program, with all health care being provided under the direction of a qualified physician.
4. Services are provided by an interdisciplinary team because no one person can provide all the needed care.
5. Coverage is provided 24 hours a day, seven days a week, with emphasis on the availability of medical and nursing skills.
6. Carefully selected and extensively trained volunteers who augment but do not replace staff service are an integral part of the health care team.
7. Care of the family extends through the bereavement period.
8. Patients are accepted on the basis of their health needs, not on their ability to pay.

Despite the growing number of people considering the hospice option, many people prefer to go to a hospital to die. Others choose to die at home, without the intervention of medical staff or life-prolonging equipment. Each dying person and his or her family should decide as early as possible what type of terminal care is most desirable and feasible. This will allow time for necessary emotional, physical, and financial preparations. Hospice care also may help the survivors cope better with the death experience.

Making Funeral Arrangements

Anthropological evidence indicates that all cultures throughout history have developed some sort of funeral ritual. For this reason, social scientists agree that funerals assist survivors of the deceased in coping with their loss.

In the United States, with its diversity of religious, regional, and ethnic customs, funeral patterns vary. In some faiths, the deceased may be displayed to formalize last respects and increase social support for the bereaved. This part of the funeral ritual is referred to as a *wake* or *viewing*. The funeral service may be held in a church, in a funeral chapel, or at the burial site. Some people choose to replace the funeral service with a simple memorial service held within a few days of the burial. Social interaction associated with funeral and memorial services is valuable in helping survivors cope with their loss.

> **Hospice** A concept of care for terminally ill patients designed to maximize quality of life.

Common methods of body disposal include burial in the ground, entombment above ground in a mausoleum, cremation, and anatomical donation. Expenses vary according to the method chosen and the available options. It should be noted that if burial is selected, an additional charge may be assessed for a burial vault. Burial vaults—concrete or metal containers that hold the casket—are required by most cemeteries to limit settling of the gravesite as the casket disintegrates and collapses. The actual container for the remains is only one of many choices that must be dealt with when a person dies.

Pressures on Survivors

There are many other decisions concerning the funeral ritual that can be burdensome for survivors. Many have to be made within 24 hours. These decisions relate to the method and details of body disposal, the type of memorial service, display of the body, the site of burial or body disposition, the cost of funeral options, organ donation, ordering floral displays, contacting friends and relatives, planning for guests, choosing markers, gathering and submitting obituary information to newspapers, printing memorial folders, and many other details. In our society, people who make their own funeral arrangements can save their loved ones from having to deal with unnecessary problems. Even making the decision regarding the method of body disposal can reduce the stress on survivors greatly.

Wills

The issue of inheritance is controversial in some families and should be resolved before the person dies to reduce conflict and needless expense. Unfortunately, many people are so

---

Intestate   Not having made a will.

Holographic will   A will written in the testator's own handwriting and unwitnessed.

Testator   A person who leaves a will or testament at death.

---

intimidated by the thought of making a will that they never do so and die **intestate** (without a will). This is tragic, especially because the procedure for establishing a legal will is relatively simple and inexpensive. In addition, if you don't make up a will before you die, the courts (as directed by state laws) will make up a will for you. Legal issues, rather than your wishes, will preside. Clearly, we all need wills that are updated regularly.

In some cases, other types of wills may substitute for the traditional legal will. One alternative is the **holographic will,** which is written in the handwriting of the **testator** (person who leaves a will) and unwitnessed. Caution should be taken concerning holographic wills and other alternatives to legally written and witnessed wills because they are not honored in all states. For example, holographic wills are contestable in court. Think of the parents who never approved of the fact that their child lived with someone outside marriage; they could challenge the holographic will in court successfully.

Organ Donation

Another decision concerns organ donation. Organ transplant techniques have become so refined, and the demand for transplant tissues and organs is so great, that many people are being encouraged to donate these gifts of life upon death. Uniform donor cards are available through the National Kidney Foundation; donor information is printed on the backs of drivers' licenses; and many hospitals include the opportunity for organ donor registration in their admission procedures. Although some people are opposed to organ transplants and tissue donation, others experience personal fulfillment from knowing that their organs may extend and improve someone else's life after their own deaths.

What do you think?
* *What can you do to ensure that your wishes will be carried out at the time of your death?*

Make It Happen!

Assessment: The Assess Yourself box on page 401 encouraged you to consider some of the deepest questions in life: What are your values? How do you want your life to compare with that of your parents? How would you like to be described at age 70? Now that you have considered your answers, perhaps there are actions you can take that will help you create the life that you want.

Making a Change: In order to change your behavior, you need to develop a plan. Follow these steps.

1. Evaluate your behavior, and identify patterns and specific things you are doing. What can you change now? What can you change in the near future?

2. Select one pattern of behavior that you want to change.
3. Fill out a Behavior Change Contract. It should include your long-term goal for change, your short-term goals, the rewards you'll give yourself for reaching these goals, potential obstacles along the way, and strategies for overcoming these obstacles. For each goal, list the small steps and specific actions that you will take.
4. Chart your progress in a journal. At the end of a week, consider how successful you were in following your plan. What helped you be successful? What made change more difficult? What will you do differently next week?
5. Revise your plan as needed: Are the short-term goals attainable? Are the rewards satisfying?

Example: When Eric answered the Assess Yourself questions, he realized he had not thought deeply about where he wanted to be at various stages in his life. In particular, he wanted to take more time to look at his parent's lives and careers, as well as those of older adults around him in the community. He set a goal of asking his parents and grandparents some of these same questions about their goals and lives in order to see where he might agree and disagree with them and how he might develop his own values and priorities. As he began thinking more seriously about the types of careers that he thought might be fulfilling, he arranged to meet with adults who had gone into professions that he was considering. He also decided to take a philosophy class as one of his electives in the next year, in which he could actually get school credit for thinking about these big questions.

Summary

* Aging can be defined in terms of biological age, which refers to a person's physical condition; psychological age, which refers to a person's coping abilities and intelligence; social age, which refers to a person's habits and roles relative to society's expectations; legal age, based on chronological years; or functional age, which is relative to how other people function at varied ages.
* The growing numbers of older adults (people age 65 and older) will have a growing impact on society in terms of economy, health care, housing, and ethical considerations.
* Two broad groups of theories—biological and psychosocial—purport to explain the physiological and psychological changes that occur with aging. Biological explanations include the wear-and-tear theory, the cellular theory, the autoimmune theory, and the genetic mutation theory. Psychosocial theories center on adaptation and adjustments related to self-development.
* Aging changes the body and mind in many ways. Physical changes occur in the skin, bones and joints, head, urinary tract, heart and lungs, senses, sexual functioning, and temperature regulation. Major physical concerns are osteoporosis and urinary incontinence. Most older people maintain a high level of intelligence and memory. Potential mental problems include depression and Alzheimer's disease.

* Special challenges for older adults include alcohol abuse, prescription and over-the-counter drug interactions, questions about vitamin and mineral supplementation, and issues regarding caregiving.
* Lifestyle choices we make today will affect health status later in life. Choosing to exercise, eat a healthy diet, and foster lasting relationships will contribute to healthy aging. Decisions about caring for older adults and stresses related to caregiving are ongoing concerns as the United States population ages.
* *Death* can be defined biologically in terms of brain death and/or the final cessation of vital functions. Denial of death results in limited communication about death, which can lead to further denial.
* Death is a multifaceted process, and individuals may experience emotional stages of dying, which include denial, anger, bargaining, depression, and acceptance. Social death results when a person is no longer treated as living. Grief is the state of distress felt after loss.
* The right to die by rational suicide involves ethical, moral, and legal issues. Dyathanasia involves passive help in suicide for a terminally ill patient; euthanasia involves direct help.

✳ Practical and legal issues surround dying and death. Choices of care for the terminally ill include hospice care. After death, funeral arrangements must be made almost immediately, which adds to pressures on survivors. Decisions should be made in advance of death through wills and organ donation cards.

Questions for Discussion and Reflection

1. Discuss the various definitions of aging. At what age would you place your parents for each category?
2. As the older population grows, how will it affect your life? Would you be willing to pay higher taxes to support government social programs for the elderly? For example, do you believe that Social Security should continue its yearly increases in payments, which are pegged to inflation? Why or why not?
3. Which of the biological theories of aging do you think is most correct? Why?
4. List the major physiological changes that occur with aging. Which of these, if any, can you change?
5. Explain the major health challenges that older adults may face. What advice would you give to your grandparents before they took a prescription or over-the-counter drug?
6. Discuss actions you can start taking now to ensure a healthier aging process.
7. Discuss why so many of us deny death. How could death become a more acceptable topic to discuss?
8. Debate whether rational suicide should be legalized for the terminally ill. What restrictions would you include in a law?
9. Compare and contrast the hospital experience with hospice care. What must one consider before arranging for hospice care?
10. Discuss the legal matters surrounding death, including wills, physician directives, organ donations, and funeral arrangements.

Accessing Your Health on the Internet

Visit the following Internet sites to explore further topics and issues related to personal health. To visit an organization's website, go to the Companion Website for *Health: The Basics, Sixth Edition* at www.aw-bc.com/donatelle, click on the book image, and select "Accessing Your Health on the Internet" from the navigation menu on the left.

1. *Administration on Aging.* A link to the Health and Human Services agency dedicated to addressing the health needs of older adults.
2. *Alzheimer's Association.* Includes media releases, position statements, fact sheets, and research on Alzheimer's disease.
3. *Funerals: A Consumer Guide.* Guides the consumer through the thinking process of planning for a funeral, including preplanning, types of funerals, costs, choosing a casket, burial, and many other aspects of funeral preparation.
4. *Hospice Web.* Includes information and links about hospice, including frequently asked questions.
5. *Loss, Grief, and Bereavement.* This site from the National Cancer Institute covers a variety of topics related to loss, grief, and bereavement. Includes a summary written by cancer experts.
6. *SeniorCom.* Home page links to numerous resources for senior citizens, including chatrooms, databases, and services dedicated to assisting the aging.
7. *Social Security Online.* Provides information about Social Security benefits and entitlements. Also offers links to related sites.
8. *Terminal Illness and Hospice.* Addresses all aspects of dealing with terminal illness, including loss, ALS (Lou Gehrig's disease), Alzheimer's disease, legal issues, and funeral planning.

Further Reading

The Johns Hopkins Medical Letter—Health After 50. www.hopkinsafter50.com

Monthly newsletter providing comprehensive, accurate overviews of health topics relevant to older adults.

Jacobs Altman, L. *Death: An Introduction to Medical–Ethical Dilemmas.* Berkeley Heights, NJ: Enslow, 2000.

A multifaceted exploration of death that gives the reader much to consider.

Muth, A. S., ed. *Death and Dying Sourcebook: Basic Consumer Health Information for the Layperson About End-of-Life Care and Related Ethical and Legal Issues.* Detroit, MI: Omnigraphics, 2000.

Provides up-to-date information on the issues of nursing care, living wills, pain management, and counseling.

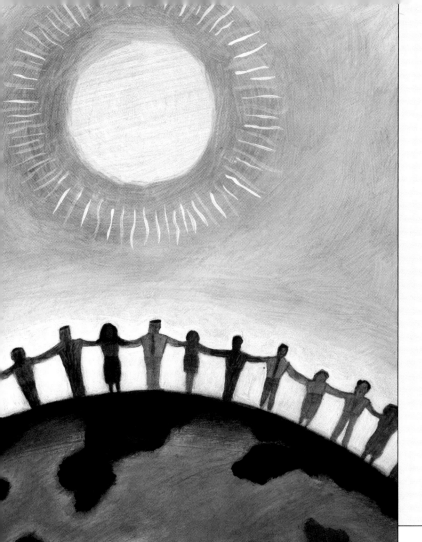

Environmental Health

Thinking Globally, Acting Locally

Objectives

✸ Explain problems and ethical issues associated with current levels of global population growth.

✸ Discuss major causes of air pollution, including photochemical smog and acid rain, and the global consequences of the accumulation of greenhouse gases and of ozone depletion.

✸ Identify sources of water pollution and the chemical contaminants often found in water.

✸ Describe the physiological consequences of noise pollution.

✸ Distinguish between municipal solid waste and hazardous waste.

✸ Discuss the health concerns associated with ionizing and non-ionizing radiation.

Subways Are Noisy, Study Finds, to the Point of Being Harmful

By Winnie Hu

Everyone who rides the subways knows they can be irritating during rush hours and sweltering in the summer. But a new report by the City Council says they can also be hazardous to hearing.

Screeching trains at the Union Square and Queens Plaza stations are noisier than airplanes taking off at La Guardia and Kennedy International Airports, and decibel levels are high enough to cause hearing damage, according to the report released yesterday at City Hall.

"It is the most pervasive and common noise problem that most New Yorkers cannot avoid being exposed to," the Council speaker, Gifford Miller, said at a news conference.

Investigators for the Council conducted the study during the summer, monitoring noise at 14 subway stations and street locations. The highest decibels were registered in and around subway stations; four stations and one street corner, at Brooklyn Borough Hall, were noisier than an intersection near Kennedy Airport. In the sampling, the noisiest station, Union Square, was measured at 98.3 decibels, compared with 84.5 at Kennedy.

Read the complete article online in the eThemes section of this book's website: www.aw-bc.com/donatelle.

Original article published November 1, 2003. Copyright © 2003 The New York Times. Reprinted with permission.

Since 1950, the world population has doubled which has increased the demand for water, food, firewood, and fossil fuel. Pro-growth advocates argue that these scarcities drive efforts to discover new sources of raw materials and new technologies to extract and process them, and they suggest that consumption is thus actually beneficial. However, supporters of sustainable resources maintain that in many parts of the world, resources are being depleted faster than they can be replenished, and they point to shrinking forests, falling water tables, eroding soils, disappearing wetlands, rising temperatures, and disappearing species as examples of such depletion.

Which view do you agree with? What are the arguments for and against population growth? How long might current social structures survive if population growth is unchecked? What steps could be taken worldwide to prevent population growth from depleting resources and polluting the environment? What would you propose as components of a global program to decrease consumption and pollution?

Human health, well-being, and the survival of all living things depend on the health and integrity of our planet. Today the natural world is under siege from the pressures of a burgeoning population that requires massive use of natural resources to survive. In response to public and political concerns, there has been a surge in federal and state regulations, along with a multibillion-dollar national infrastructure—but doubt remains regarding the effectiveness of that infrastructure in reducing environmental health risks.[1] An informed citizenry with a strong commitment to be responsible for the planet and maintain it for future generations is essential to the survival of the earth and all living things. With the many environmental challenges the planet faces, sometimes these problems can seem overwhelming. See the Assess Yourself box on page 422 for some ideas of individual actions you can take to be more environmentally healthy.

Overpopulation

Anthropologist Margaret Mead wrote, "Every human society is faced with not one population problem but two: how to beget and rear enough children and how not to beget and rear too many."[2] The United Nations projects that the world population will grow from its present total of more than 6.3 billion to 9.4 billion in 2050.[3] Though the population is expanding, the earth's resources are not. Population experts believe that many areas of the world are already struggling with "demographic fatigue" and that the most critical environmental challenge today is to slow global population growth.[4]

The population explosion is not distributed equally. The United States and western Europe have the lowest birth rates. At the same time, these two regions produce more grain and other foodstuffs than their populations consume. Countries that can least afford a high birth rate in economic, social, health, and nutritional terms are the ones with the most rapidly expanding populations.

The bulk of population growth in developing countries is occurring in urban areas. Populations in the cities within developing countries are doubling every 10 to 15 years and are overwhelming their governments' attempts to provide clean water, sewage facilities, adequate transportation, and other basic services. Every week, the population of the world's urban centers grows by more than 1 million.[5] In 1800, London was the only city in the world with 1 million people; today, 14 cities each have populations of more than 10 million.[6]

As the global population expands, so does competition for the earth's resources. Environmental degradation caused by loss of topsoil, pesticides, toxic residues, deforestation, global warming, air pollution, acid rain, a rapidly expanding population, and increasing poverty is exerting heavy pressure on natural resources and the capacity of natural resources to support human life and world health.[7]

Overpopulation threats are most evident in Latin America, Africa, and Asia. The country projected to have the largest increase in population is India, which could add another 600 million people by 2050 and surpass China as the most populous country in the world.[8]

These projections could change, however, if governments are not able to cope with the increased resource and economic demands. For example, the AIDS epidemic has stabilized in industrial countries to an adult infection rate of under 1 percent, but countries such as Zimbabwe, Botswana,

Table 16.1
Oil Consumption (Thousands of Barrels per Day) in Selected Countries

Country	1992	2002	Percentage of World Consumption
United States	17,033	19,708	25.4
Japan	5,521	5,337	6.9
China	2,662	5,362	7.0
India	1,296	2,090	2.8
Canada	1,708	1,988	2.5
Brazil	1,328	1,849	2.4
Saudi Arabia	1,095	1,363	1.8
Iran	1,017	1,115	1.5
Australia	679	846	1.1
Egypt	457	550	0.7
South Africa	369	501	0.7

Source: British Petroleum. "BP Statistical Review of World Energy, 2003." 2003. www.bp.com/centres/energy/oil/consumption.asp

and Zambia may lose one-fifth or more of their adult population within the next decade to AIDS.[9] The loss of a significant part of the workforce would have devastating economic as well as health consequences. Diseases such as AIDS are not the only threats to countries with unstable population growth. As governments strain to support growing numbers of people, the infrastructure designed to protect health (such as sewer systems and water purification) may not be sufficient to meet demands. Left unsolved, these problems grow and can result in increased rates of infectious diseases, especially among the poor, children, the elderly, and other groups at the margins of society.

We can do our part by recognizing that the United States consumes more energy and raw materials per person than does any other nation on earth (see Table 16.1). Many of these resources come from other countries, and our consumption is depleting the resource balances of those countries.

Perhaps the simplest course of action is to control our own reproductivity. The concept of zero population growth (ZPG) was born in the 1960s. Proponents of this idea believed that each couple should produce only two offspring. When the parents die, the two offspring are their replacements, and the population stabilizes. Globally, we are moving slowly toward this goal. In 1970, the worldwide total fertility rate peaked at an estimated 5 births per woman; at present it averages 2.7 births. However, although population growth is slowing, we have yet to achieve ZPG.[10]

The continued preference for large families in many developing nations is related to several factors: high infant mortality rates; the traditional view of children as social security (they work from a young age to assist the family, and

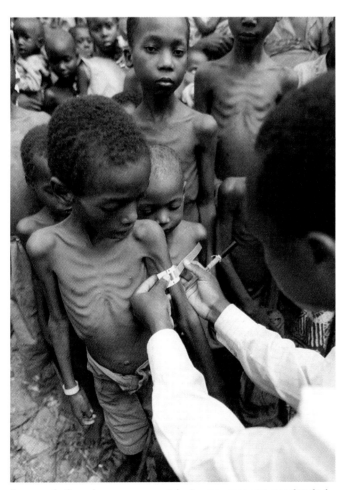

As populations increase, countries' resources are overloaded. In many parts of the world, governments cannot meet the needs of their most vulnerable citizens, and outside organizations must get involved.

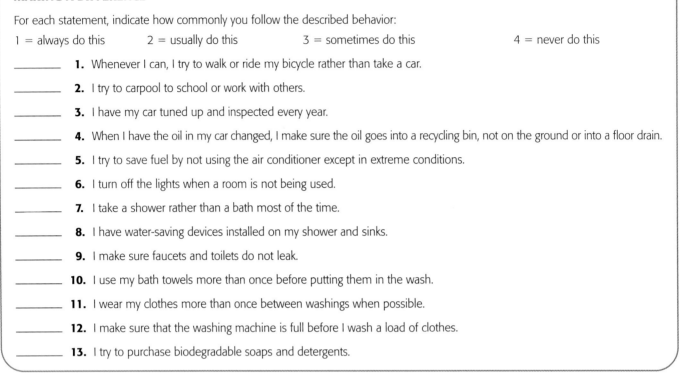

What Can I Do to Preserve the Environment?

Environmental problems often seem overwhelming and too big for an individual to make a difference. Each day, though, there are things you can do that contribute to the health of the planet.

MAKING A DIFFERENCE

For each statement, indicate how commonly you follow the described behavior:

1 = always do this   2 = usually do this   3 = sometimes do this   4 = never do this

_____ **1.** Whenever I can, I try to walk or ride my bicycle rather than take a car.

_____ **2.** I try to carpool to school or work with others.

_____ **3.** I have my car tuned up and inspected every year.

_____ **4.** When I have the oil in my car changed, I make sure the oil goes into a recycling bin, not on the ground or into a floor drain.

_____ **5.** I try to save fuel by not using the air conditioner except in extreme conditions.

_____ **6.** I turn off the lights when a room is not being used.

_____ **7.** I take a shower rather than a bath most of the time.

_____ **8.** I have water-saving devices installed on my shower and sinks.

_____ **9.** I make sure faucets and toilets do not leak.

_____ **10.** I use my bath towels more than once before putting them in the wash.

_____ **11.** I wear my clothes more than once between washings when possible.

_____ **12.** I make sure that the washing machine is full before I wash a load of clothes.

_____ **13.** I try to purchase biodegradable soaps and detergents.

they support parents when the parents grow too old to work); the low educational and economic status of women; and the traditional desire for sons, which keeps parents of daughters reproducing until they have male offspring.

Air Pollution

The daily impact of a growing population makes clean air more difficult to find. Concern about air quality prompted Congress to pass the Clean Air Act in 1970 and to amend it in 1977 and again in 1990. The object was to develop standards for six of the most widespread air pollutants that seriously affect health: sulfur dioxide, particulates, carbon monoxide, nitrogen dioxide, ozone, and lead.

Sulfur dioxide   A yellowish brown gaseous by-product of the burning of fossil fuels.

Particulates   Nongaseous air pollutants.

Sources of Air Pollution

Sulfur Dioxide   A yellowish brown gas, **sulfur dioxide** is a by-product of burning fossil fuels. Electricity-generating stations, smelters, refineries, and industrial boilers are the main source points. In humans, sulfur dioxide aggravates symptoms of heart and lung disease; obstructs breathing passages; and increases the incidence of respiratory diseases such as colds, asthma, bronchitis, and emphysema. Sulfur dioxide is toxic to plants, destroys some paint pigments, corrodes metals, impairs visibility, and is a precursor to acid rain, which we discuss later in this chapter.

Particulates   **Particulates** are tiny solid particles or liquid droplets that are suspended in the air. Cigarette smoke, for example, releases particulates. They are also by-products of industrial processes and the internal combustion engine. Particulates irritate the lungs and can carry heavy metals and carcinogenic agents deep into the lungs. When combined with sulfur dioxide, they exacerbate respiratory diseases. Particulates also can corrode metals and obscure visibility. Numerous scientific studies have found significant

_____ **14.** I try to use biodegradable trash bags.

_____ **15.** At home, I use dishes and silverware rather than Styrofoam or plastic.

_____ **16.** When I buy pre-packaged foods, I choose the ones with the least packaging.

_____ **17.** I try not to subscribe to newspapers and magazines when I can view them online.

_____ **18.** I try not to use a hair dryer.

_____ **19.** I recycle plastic bags that I get when I bring something home from the store.

_____ **20.** I don't run water continuously when washing the dishes, shaving, or brushing my teeth.

_____ **21.** I prefer to use unbleached or recycled paper.

_____ **22.** I use both sides of printer paper and other paper when possible.

_____ **23.** If I have items I do not want to use anymore, I donate them to charity so someone else can use them.

_____ **24.** I try not to buy drinks in cans with plastic rings attached to them.

_____ **25.** I try not to buy bottled water in small plastic containers.

_____ **26.** I clean up after myself while enjoying the outdoors (picnicking, camping, etc.).

_____ **27.** I volunteer for clean-up days in the community in which I live.

_____ **28.** I consider candidates' positions on environmental issues before casting my vote.

FOR FURTHER THOUGHT

Review your scores. Are your responses mostly 1s and 2s? If not, what actions you can take to become more environmentally responsible? Are there some ways to help the environment on the list that you had not thought of before? Are there some behaviors not on the list that you are already doing?

---

links between exposure to air particulate concentrations at or below current standards and adverse health effects, including premature death.[11]

Carbon Monoxide   An odorless, colorless gas, **carbon monoxide** originates primarily from motor vehicle emissions. Carbon monoxide interferes with the blood's ability to absorb and carry oxygen and can impair thinking; slow reflexes; and cause drowsiness, unconsciousness, and death. Many people have purchased home monitors to test for carbon monoxide.

Ozone   Ground-level **ozone** is a form of oxygen that is produced when nitrogen dioxide reacts with hydrogen chloride. These gases release oxygen, which is altered by sunlight to produce ozone. In the lower atmosphere, ozone irritates the mucous membranes of the respiratory system, which causes coughing and choking. It can impair lung functioning; reduce resistance to colds and pneumonia; and aggravate heart disease, asthma, bronchitis, and pneumonia. One of the irritants found in smog, this ozone corrodes rubber and paint and can injure or kill vegetation. The natural ozone found in the upper atmosphere (sometimes called "good" ozone), however, serves as a protective membrane against heat and radiation from the sun. We will discuss atmospheric ozone later in the chapter.

Nitrogen Dioxide   Coal-powered electrical utility boilers and motor vehicles emit **nitrogen dioxide,** an amber-colored gas. High concentrations can be fatal. Lower concentrations increase susceptibility to colds and flu, bronchitis, and pneumonia. Nitrogen dioxide is also toxic to plant life and causes a brown discoloration of the atmosphere. It is a precursor of ozone and, along with sulfur dioxide, of acid rain.

Carbon monoxide   An odorless, colorless gas that originates primarily from motor vehicle emissions.

Ozone   A gas formed when nitrogen dioxide interacts with hydrogen chloride.

Nitrogen dioxide   An amber-colored gas found in smog; can cause eye and respiratory irritations.

Lead Lead is a metal pollutant found in paint, batteries, drinking water, pipes, and dishes with lead-glazed bases. It affects the circulatory, reproductive, urinary, and nervous systems and can accumulate in bone and other tissues. Lead is particularly detrimental to children and fetuses. It can cause birth defects, behavioral abnormalities, and decreased learning abilities. Lead pollution has fallen significantly since lead was eliminated from gasoline and paint. However, an estimated 300,000 children in the United States still have unsafe blood lead levels.[12]

Hydrocarbons Although not listed specifically in the Clean Air Act, hydrocarbons encompass a wide variety of pollutants in the air. Sometimes known as volatile organic compounds, **hydrocarbons** are chemical compounds containing different combinations of carbon and hydrogen. Their principal source is the internal combustion engine. Most automobile engines emit hundreds of different hydrocarbon compounds. By themselves, hydrocarbons seem to cause few problems, but when they combine with sunlight and other pollutants, they form such poisons as formaldehyde, ketones, and peroxyacetylnitrate, all of which are respiratory irritants. Hydrocarbon combinations such as benzene and benzo(a)pyrene are carcinogenic. In addition, hydrocarbons play a major part in the formation of smog.

> **What do you think?**
> *Should automakers be responsible for developing cars with low emissions?* ☀ *As a motorist, how can you help eliminate carbon monoxide emissions?*

Photochemical Smog

When oxygen-containing compounds of nitrogen and hydrocarbons react in the presence of sunlight, **photochemical smog,** a brown, hazy mix of particulates and gases, forms.

Lead A metal found in the exhaust of motor vehicles powered by fuel containing lead and in emissions from lead smelters and processing plants.

Hydrocarbons Chemical compounds that contain carbon and hydrogen.

Photochemical smog The brownish-yellow haze resulting from the combination of hydrocarbons and nitrogen oxides.

Temperature inversion A weather condition occurring when a layer of cool air is trapped under a layer of warmer air.

Acid rain Precipitation contaminated with acidic pollutants.

It is sometimes called *ozone pollution* because ozone is created when vehicle exhaust reacts with sunlight. In most cases, smog forms in areas that experience a **temperature inversion,** a weather condition in which a cool layer of air is trapped under a layer of warmer air, which prevents the air from circulating. When gases such as hydrocarbons and nitrogen oxides are released into the cool air layer, they remain suspended until winds move away the warmer air layer. Sunlight filtering through the air causes chemical changes in the hydrocarbons and nitrogen oxides, which results in smog. Smog is more likely to be produced in valley regions blocked by hills or mountains—for example, Tokyo, Los Angeles, and Denver.

The most noticeable adverse effects of exposure to smog are difficulty breathing, burning eyes, headaches, and nausea. Long-term exposure poses serious health risks, particularly for children, older adults, pregnant women, and people with chronic respiratory disorders such as asthma and emphysema.

Acid Rain

Acid rain is precipitation in the form of rain, snow, or fog that has fallen through acidic air pollutants, particularly those containing sulfur dioxides and nitrogen dioxides. When introduced into lakes and ponds, acid rain gradually acidifies the water. When the acid content of the water reaches a certain level, plant and animal life cannot survive. Ironically, acidified lakes and ponds become a crystal-clear deep blue, which gives the illusion of beauty and health.

Sources of Acid Rain More than 95 percent of acid rain originates in human actions, chiefly in the burning of fossil fuels. The greatest sources of acid rain in the United States are coal-fired power plants, ore smelters, and steel mills.

When these and other industries burn fuels, the sulfur and nitrogen in the emissions combine with atmospheric oxygen and sunlight to become sulfur dioxide and nitrogen oxides (precursors of sulfuric acid and nitric acids, respectively). Small acid particles then are carried by the wind and combine with moisture to produce acidic rain or snow. Rain is more acidic in the summertime because of higher concentrations of sunlight. The ability of a lake to cleanse itself and neutralize its acidity depends on several factors, the most critical of which is bedrock geology.

Effects of Acid Rain In addition to damaging lakes and ponds, every year acid rain destroys millions of trees in Europe and North America. Scientists have concluded that 75 percent of Europe's forests now are experiencing damaging levels of sulfur deposition by acid rain. Forests in every country on the continent are affected.[13]

Doctors believe that acid rain aggravates and may cause bronchitis, asthma, and other respiratory problems. People with emphysema and those with a history of heart disease also may suffer from exposure to acid rain. In addition, it may be hazardous to a pregnant woman's unborn child.

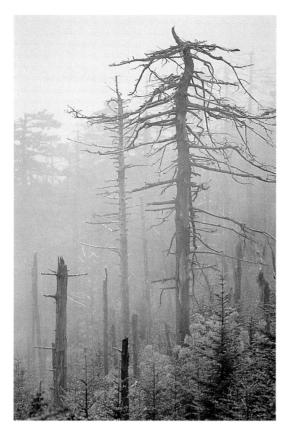

Acid rain has many harmful effects on the environment. Because its toxins seep into groundwater and enter the food chain, it also poses health hazards to humans.

Acidic precipitation can cause metals such as aluminum, cadmium, lead, and mercury to **leach** (dissolve and filter) out of the soil. If these metals make their way into water or food supplies (particularly fish), they can cause cancer in humans who consume them. Acid rain also damages crops; laboratory experiments show that it can reduce seed yield by up to 23 percent. Actual crop losses are being reported with increasing frequency. A final consequence of acid rain is the destruction of public monuments and structures, with billions of dollars in projected building damage each year.

Indoor Air Pollution

In the last several years, a growing body of scientific evidence has indicated that the air within homes and other buildings can be polluted more seriously than the outdoor air in even the most industrialized cities. Some of the most vulnerable people, particularly the young, elderly, and those who are already sick, spend more than 90 percent of their time indoors.[14]

Most indoor air pollution comes from sources that release gases or particles into the air. Table 16.2 on page 426 describes major sources of indoor air pollution and possible health effects. Inadequate ventilation, particularly in heavily insulated buildings with air-tight windows, may increase pollution by not allowing in outside air.

Prevention focuses on three main areas: source control (eliminating or reducing individual contaminants), ventilation improvements (increasing the amount of outdoor air coming indoors), and air cleaners (removing particulates from the air).[15]

Indoor air can be 10 to 40 times more hazardous than outdoor air. There are between 20 and 100 potentially dangerous chemical compounds in the average American home. An emerging source of indoor air pollution is mold (see the Reality Check box on page 427). It is not yet clear how widespread the effects of mold are.

Woodstove Smoke Woodstoves emit significant levels of particulates and carbon monoxide in addition to other pollutants, such as sulfur dioxide. If you rely on wood for heating, make sure that your stove is properly installed, vented, and maintained. Burning properly seasoned wood reduces particulates.

Furnace Emissions People who rely on oil- or gas-fired furnaces also need to make sure that these appliances are installed, ventilated, and maintained properly. Inadequate cleaning and maintenance can allow deadly carbon monoxide to build up in the home.

Asbestos Asbestos is a mineral that was commonly used in insulation materials in buildings constructed before 1970. When bonded to other materials, asbestos is relatively harmless. But if its tiny fibers become loosened and airborne, they can embed themselves in the lungs. Their presence leads to cancer of the lungs, stomach, and chest lining and is the cause of a fatal lung disease called mesothelioma.

Formaldehyde Formaldehyde is a colorless, strong-smelling gas present in some carpets, draperies, furniture, particle board, plywood, wood paneling, countertops, and many adhesives. It is released into the air in a process called *outgassing*. Outgassing is highest in new products, but the process can continue for many years.

Exposure to formaldehyde can cause respiratory problems, dizziness, fatigue, nausea, and rashes. Long-term exposure can lead to central nervous system disorders and cancer. Ask about the formaldehyde content of products you purchase, and avoid those that contain this gas. Some houseplants, such as philodendrons and spider plants, help clean

---

Leach   To dissolve and filter through soil.

Asbestos   A mineral that separates into stringy fibers and lodges in the lungs, where it can cause various diseases.

Formaldehyde   A colorless, strong-smelling gas released through outgassing; causes respiratory and other health problems.

Table 16.2
Health Effects of Indoor Air Pollution

Type of Pollutant	Sources	Health Effects
Radon	Uranium in the soil or rock on which homes are built; well water also can be a source	Lung cancer from exposure in air, other health risks from swallowing in water
Environmental tobacco smoke	Smoke that comes from burning end of cigarette, pipe, or cigar	Complex mixture of more than 4,000 compounds, over 40 of which cause cancer
Biological contaminants (molds, mildew, viruses, animal dander and cat saliva, dust mites, cockroaches, and pollen)	Improper ventilation and moisture buildup, lack of cleanliness/sanitation, contaminated heating systems, household pets, rodents, insects, damp carpets, etc.	Allergic reactions, including hypersensitivity, rhinitis, asthma, infectious illnesses, sneezing, watering eyes, coughing, shortness of breath, dizziness, lethargy, fever, digestive problems
Stoves, heaters, fireplaces, chimneys	Unvented kerosene heaters, woodstoves, fireplaces, gas stoves	Carbon monoxide causes headaches, dizziness, weakness, nausea, confusion and disorientation, chest pain, death. Nitrogen dioxide causes irritation of nose, eyes, respiratory distress. Particles cause lung damage and irritation.
Household chemicals (see partial list below)	Paints, varnishes; cleaning products, solvents, degreasers, and hobby products, etc.	Variable symptoms dependent on exposure level, including eye and respiratory tract problems, headaches, dizziness, visual disorders, and memory impairment
• Benzene	Paint, new carpet, new drapes, upholstery, fast-drying glues, caulks	Headaches, eye/skin irritation, fatigue, cancer
• Formaldehyde	Tobacco smoke, plywood, cabinets, furniture, particle board, new carpet and drapes, wallpaper, ceiling tile, paneling	Headaches, eye/skin irritation, drowsiness, fatigue, respiratory problems, memory loss, depression, gynecological problems, cancer
• Chloroform	Paint, new drapes, new carpet, upholstery	Headaches, asthma attacks, dizziness, eye/skin irritations
• Toluene	All paper products, most finished wood products	Headaches, eye/skin irritation, sinus problems, dizziness, cancer
• Hydrocarbons	Tobacco smoke, gas burners and furnaces	Headaches, fatigue, nausea, dizziness, breathing difficulty
• Ammonia	Tobacco smoke, cleaning supplies, animal urine	Eye/skin irritation, headaches, nosebleeds, sinus problems
• Trichlorethylene	Paints, glues, caulking, vinyl coatings, wallpaper	Headaches, eye/skin irritation, upper respiratory irritation

Source: U.S. Environmental Protection Agency, "The Inside Story: A Guide to Indoor Air Quality" (EPA Document #402-K-93-007), 1995. http://epa.gov/iaq/pubs/insidest.html

formaldehyde from the air. If you experience symptoms of formaldehyde exposure, have your home tested by a city, county, or state health agency.

Radon Radon, an odorless, colorless gas, is the natural by-product of the decay of uranium and radium in the soil. Radon penetrates homes through cracks, pipes, sump pits,

Radon A naturally occurring radioactive gas resulting from the decay of certain radioactive elements.

and other openings in the foundation. An estimated 15,000 cancer deaths per year are attributed to radon, which makes it second only to smoking as a leading cause of lung cancer.[16]

The EPA estimates that 1 in 15 American homes has an elevated radon level.[17] You can buy a kit from a hardware store to test your home yourself. "Alpha track" detectors are commonly used for this type of short-term testing. They must remain in your home for 2 to 90 days, depending on the device.

Household Chemicals Use cleansers and other cleaning products in a well-ventilated room, and be conservative in

Growing Concerns about Mold

WHAT IS MOLD?

Molds produce tiny spores in order to reproduce. Mold spores waft through the indoor and outdoor air continually. When they land on a damp spot indoors, they may begin growing and digesting whatever they are growing on, including wood, paper, carpet, and food. Potential health effects and symptoms associated with mold exposure include allergic reactions, asthma, and other respiratory complaints

CONTROLLING MOLD

Wherever excessive moisture accumulates, mold often will grow. There is no practical way to eliminate all mold and mold spores in the indoor environment, so the key to mold control is moisture control.

To prevent mold, dry water-damaged areas and items within 24–48 hours. If mold is already a problem, clean up the mold and get rid of the excess moisture. Fix leaky plumbing or other sources of water. Wash mold off hard surfaces with detergent and water, and dry completely. Absorbent materials (such as ceiling tiles and carpet) that become moldy may have to be replaced.

Reduce indoor humidity (to 30–60%) to decrease mold growth by venting bathrooms, dryers, and other moisture-generating sources to the outside. Use air conditioners and de-humidifiers; increase ventilation; and run exhaust fans whenever cooking, dishwashing, and cleaning.

Reduce the potential for condensation on cold surfaces (i.e., windows, piping, exterior walls, roof, or floors) by adding insulation. Do not install carpeting in areas where there is a perpetual moisture problem, such as near drinking fountains and sinks, or on concrete floors with leaks or frequent condensation.

Source: Environmental Protection Agency, "Mold Resources," 2003. www.epa.gov/iaq/molds/moldresources.html

---

their use. Those caustic chemicals that zap mildew and grease also pose a major risk to water and the environment. Regular cleanings will reduce the need to use potentially harmful substances. Cut down on dry cleaning; the chemicals used by many cleaners can cause cancer. If your newly cleaned clothes smell of chemicals, return them to the cleaner or hang them in the open air until the smell is gone. Avoid household air freshener products containing the carcinogenic agent *dichlorobenzene.*

Indoor air pollution is also a concern in the classroom and workplace. Studies show that one in five U.S. schools has problems with indoor air quality, which affect an estimated 8.4 million students.[18] Poor quality in classrooms may lead to drowsiness, headaches, and lack of concentration. It also may affect physical growth and development. Children with asthma are particularly at risk. Many people who work indoors complain of maladies that tend to lessen or vanish when they leave the building. **Sick building syndrome (SBS)** is said to exist when 80 percent of a building's occupants report problems. One of the primary causes of SBS is poor ventilation. Symptoms include eye irritation, sore throat, queasiness, and worsened asthma.[19]

Ozone Layer Depletion

As mentioned earlier, the ozone layer in the atmosphere protects our planet and its inhabitants from ultraviolet B (UVB) radiation, a primary cause of skin cancer. UVB radiation may also damage DNA and weaken immune systems in both humans and animals. Thus, the ozone layer is crucial to life on the planet's surface.

In the 1970s, scientists began to warn of a breakdown in the earth's ozone layer. Instruments developed to test atmospheric contents indicated that chemicals used on earth, **chlorofluorocarbons (CFCs),** were contributing to its rapid depletion.

CFCs were used as refrigerants (Freon); as aerosol propellants in products such as hairsprays and deodorants; as cleaning solvents; and in medical sterilizers, rigid foam insulation, and Styrofoam. Along with halons (found in many fire extinguishers), methyl chloroform, and carbon tetrachloride (found in cleaning solvents), CFCs eventually were found to be a major cause of ozone depletion. When released into the air through spraying or outgassing, CFCs migrate upward toward the ozone layer, where they decompose and release chlorine atoms. These atoms cause ozone molecules to break apart (Figure 16.1 on page 428).

In the 1970s, the U.S. government banned the use of aerosol sprays containing CFCs. The discovery of an "ozone hole" over Antarctica led to the 1987 Montreal Protocol treaty, whereby the United States and other nations agreed to reduce the use of CFCs and other ozone-depleting chemicals. The treaty was amended in 1995 to ban CFC production in developed countries. Today, more than 160 countries have signed the treaty.[20]

Sick building syndrome (SBS)   Problem that exists when 80 percent of a building's occupants report maladies that tend to lessen or vanish when they leave the building.

Chlorofluorocarbons (CFCs)   Chemicals that contribute to the depletion of the ozone layer.

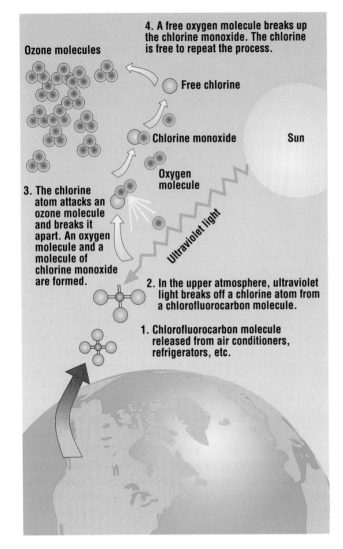

4. A free oxygen molecule breaks up the chlorine monoxide. The chlorine is free to repeat the process.

Ozone molecules

Free chlorine

Chlorine monoxide

Sun

Oxygen molecule

3. The chlorine atom attacks an ozone molecule and breaks it apart. An oxygen molecule and a molecule of chlorine monoxide are formed.

Ultraviolet light

2. In the upper atmosphere, ultraviolet light breaks off a chlorine atom from a chlorofluorocarbon molecule.

1. Chlorofluorocarbon molecule released from air conditioners, refrigerators, etc.

Figure 16.1
How the Ozone Layer Is Being Depleted

Global Warming

More than 100 years ago, scientists theorized that carbon dioxide emissions from burning of fossil fuels would create a buildup of *greenhouse gases* in the earth's atmosphere that could have a warming effect on the earth's surface. The predictions now seem to be coming true, with alarming results. According to the National Academy of Sciences, the earth's surface temperature has risen 1 degree Fahrenheit in the past century, with accelerated warming in the past two decades.[21] There is new and strong evidence that most of the warming over the last 50 years is due to human activities.[22]

Climate researchers predict that the buildup of greenhouse gases could produce life-threatening natural phenom-

---

Greenhouse gases   Gases that contribute to global warming by trapping heat near the earth's surface.

---

ena around the globe, including drought, more frequent forest fires, massive flooding, extended heat waves, and killer hurricanes. Recently, the planet has experienced all five of these phenomena, although whether they are connected to global warming remains a matter of debate.

Greenhouse gases include carbon dioxide, CFCs, ground-level ozone, nitrous oxide, and methane. They become part of a gaseous layer that encircles the earth, which allows solar heat to pass through and then traps it close to the earth's surface. The most predominant is carbon dioxide, which accounts for 49 percent of all greenhouse gases. Eastern Europe and North America are responsible for approximately half of all carbon dioxide emissions. Since the late nineteenth century, carbon dioxide concentrations in the atmosphere have increased by 30 percent, with half of this increase occurring since the 1950s. Carbon emissions from the burning of fossil fuels, oil, coal, and gas continue to climb. The United States emits about one-fifth of total global greenhouse gases.[23]

Rapid deforestation of the tropical rain forests of Central and South America, Africa, and Southeast Asia is also contributing to the rapid rise in greenhouse gases. Trees take in carbon dioxide, transform it, store the carbon for food, and then release oxygen into the air. As we lose forests at the rate of hundreds of acres per hour, we lose the capacity to dissipate carbon dioxide.[24]

Reducing Air Pollution

Air pollution problems are rooted in our energy, transportation, and industrial practices. We must develop comprehensive national and global strategies to clean our air for the future. We must support policies that encourage the use of renewable resources such as solar, wind, and water power to provide most of the world's energy.

Most experts agree that shifting away from automobiles as the primary source of transportation is the only way to reduce air pollution significantly. Many cities have taken steps in this direction by setting high parking fees, imposing bans on city driving, and establishing high road usage tolls. Governments should be encouraged to provide convenient, inexpensive, and accessible public transportation.

Although laws restricting carbon emissions and new hybrid cars that operate on electricity and gas are promising, we have a long way to go to reduce fossil fuel consumption. One promising initiative is bicycle power. Bicycles are gaining popularity. Currently, China leads the world in bicycle use, followed by India. In Germany, bicycle use has increased by 50 percent, and England has a plan to quadruple bicycle use by 2012.[25]

Water Pollution

Seventy-five percent of the earth is covered with water in the form of oceans, seas, lakes, rivers, streams, and wetlands. Beneath the landmass are reservoirs of groundwater. We draw our drinking water from either this underground source or from surface freshwater. The status of our water supply reflects the pollution level of our communities and, ultimately, of the entire earth.

Water Contamination

Any substance that gets into the soil can potentially enter the water supply. Industrial pollutants, acid rain, and pesticides eventually work their way into the soil, then into the groundwater. Oil spills such as the one off the coast of Spain in 2002 contaminate coastal waterways and spill into local rivers, along with hazardous farming and industrial wastes. Today more than 1.1 billion people (one-sixth of the world's population) do not have access to safe drinking water.[26]

Congress has coined two terms, *point source* and *nonpoint source,* to refer to the two general sources of water pollution. **Point source pollutants** enter a waterway at a specific point through a pipe, ditch, culvert, or other conduit. The two major sources of this type of pollution are sewage treatment plants and industrial facilities. **Nonpoint source pollutants**—commonly known as *runoff* and *sedimentation*— run off or seep into waterways from broad areas of land rather than through a discrete conduit. It is estimated that 99 percent of the sediment in our waterways, 98 percent of the bacterial contaminants, 84 percent of the phosphorus, and 82 percent of the nitrogen come from nonpoint sources.[27] Nonpoint pollution results from a variety of human land use practices, including soil erosion and sedimentation, construction wastes, pesticide and fertilizer runoff, urban street runoff, wastes from engineering projects, acid mine drainage, leakage from septic tanks, and sewage sludge.[28] (See Figure 16.2 on page 430.)

Septic Systems   Bacteria from human waste can leach into the water supply from improperly installed septic systems. Toxic chemicals that are dumped into septic systems also can enter groundwater.

Landfills   Landfills and dumps generate a liquid called **leachate,** a mixture of soluble chemicals from household garbage, office waste, biological waste, and industrial waste. If a landfill has not been lined properly, leachate trickles through its layers of garbage and eventually enters the water supply as acid and the atmosphere as methane gas.

Gasoline and Petroleum Products   In the United States, there are more than 2 million underground storage tanks for gasoline and petroleum products, most of which are located at gasoline filling stations. One-quarter of them are thought to be leaking.[29]

Most of these tanks were installed 25 to 30 years ago. They were made of fabricated steel that was unprotected from corrosion. Over time, pinpoint holes develop in the steel, and the petroleum products leak into groundwater. The most common way to detect the presence of petroleum products in water is to test for benzene, a component of oil and gasoline. Benzene is highly toxic and associated with the development of cancer.

Chemical Contaminants

Chemicals designed to dissolve grease and oil are called *organic solvents.* These extremely toxic substances, such as carbon tetrachloride, tetrachloroethylene, and trichloroethylene, are used to clean clothing, painting equipment, plastics, and metal parts. Many household products, such as stain and spot removers, degreasers, drain cleaners, septic system cleaners, and paint removers, also contain these toxic chemicals.

Organic solvents work their way into the water supply in different ways. Consumers often dump leftover products into the toilet or into street drains. Industries pour leftovers into large barrels, which are then buried. After a while, the chemicals eat through the barrels and leach into the groundwater system.

One related group of toxic substances contains chlorinated hydrocarbons. The most notorious are the **polychlorinated biphenyls (PCBs),** their cousins the *polybromated biphenyls,* and the *dioxins.* Pesticides and lead are also sources of chemical contamination.

PCBs   Fire resistant and stable at high temperatures, PCBs were used for many years as insulating materials in high-voltage electrical equipment such as transformers. PCBs bioaccumulate, which means that the body does not excrete them but stores them in fatty tissues and the liver. PCBs are associated with birth defects, and exposure to them is known to cause cancer. The manufacture of PCBs was discontinued in the United States in 1977, but approximately 500 million pounds of them have been dumped into landfills and waterways, where they continue to pose an environmental threat.[30] Western European countries phased out the use of many of these chemicals in the 1970s, but elevated levels still can be detected at the mouths of major rivers. Over three tons of PCBs flow into the North Sea every year, mainly from the Rhine River.[31]

Point source pollutants   Pollutants that enter waterways at a specific point.

Nonpoint source pollutants   Pollutants that run off or seep into waterways from broad areas of land.

Leachate   A liquid consisting of soluble chemicals that come from garbage and industrial waste that seeps into the water supply from landfills and dumps.

Polychlorinated biphenyls (PCBs)   Toxic chemicals that were once used as insulating materials in high-voltage electrical equipment.

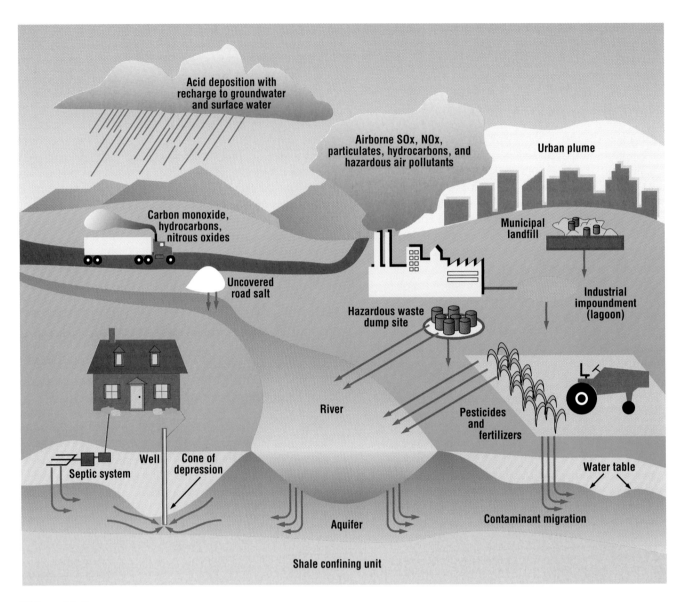

Figure 16.2
Sources of Groundwater Contamination

Dioxins Dioxins are chlorinated hydrocarbons found in herbicides (chemicals that are used to kill vegetation) and produced during certain industrial processes. Dioxins have the ability to bioaccumulate and are much more toxic than PCBs.

The long-term effects of bioaccumulation of these toxic substances include possible damage to the immune system and increased risk of infections and cancer. Exposure to high concentrations of PCBs or dioxins for a short period of time also can have severe consequences, including nausea, vomiting, diarrhea, painful rashes and sores, and chloracne, an ailment in which the skin develops hard, black, painful pimples that may never go away.

Pesticides Pesticides are chemicals that are designed to kill insects, rodents, plants, and fungi. Americans use more than 1.2 billion pounds of pesticides each year, but only 10 percent actually reach the targeted organisms. The remaining 1.1 billion pounds of pesticides settle on the land and in air and water.

Pesticides are volatile and evaporate readily, often to be dispersed by winds over a large area or carried to the sea. This is particularly true in tropical regions, where many

Dioxins Highly toxic chlorinated hydrocarbons contained in herbicides and produced during certain industrial processes.

Pesticides Chemicals that kill pests.

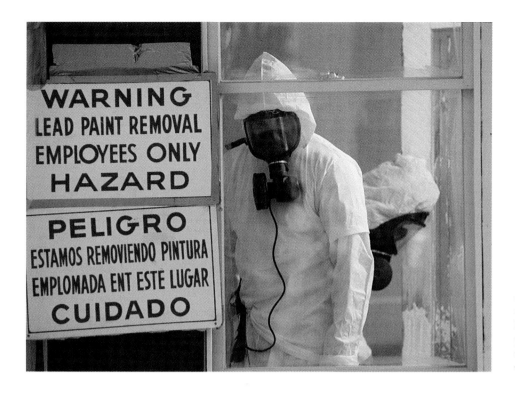

Although an expensive and cumbersome project, deleading a house is now one of the most important considerations of prospective homeowners, especially those with children.

farmers use pesticides heavily and the climate promotes their rapid release into the atmosphere. In Nigeria, for example, 98 percent of the insecticide DDT applied to a cowpea crop evaporated within four years.[32]

Pesticide residues cling to fresh fruits and vegetables and can accumulate in the body when people eat these items. A recent study found a correlation between breast cancer and Dieldrin, a popular pesticide used until the 1970s.[33] Women who had the highest traces of Dieldrin in their blood were twice as likely as women with the lowest levels to develop breast cancer. Other potential hazards associated with exposure to pesticides include birth defects, cancer, liver and kidney damage, and nervous system disorders.

Lead The Environmental Protection Agency (EPA) has issued new standards to reduce dramatically the levels of lead in U.S. drinking water. These standards are already in place in many municipalities and will eventually reduce lead exposure for approximately 130 million people. The new rules stipulate that tap water lead values must not exceed 15 parts per billion (the previous standard allowed an average lead level of 50 parts per billion). When water suppliers identify problem areas, they will have to lower the water's acidity with chemical treatment (because acidity increases water's ability to leach lead from the pipes through which it passes), or they will have to replace old lead plumbing in the service lines.

If lead does exist in your home's water, you can reduce your risk by running tap water for several minutes before taking a drink or cooking with it. This flushes out water that has been standing overnight in lead-contaminated lines. Although leaded paints and ceramic glazes used to pose health risks, particularly for small children who put painted toys in their mouths, the use of lead in such products has effectively been reduced in recent years.

> **What do you think?**
> *Who should bear the financial responsibility for cleaning up hazardous waste leaks?*
> ✳ *What can you do to avoid contributing to water contamination?*

Noise Pollution

Our bodies have definite physiological responses to noise, and it can become a source of physical or mental distress. Short-term exposure to loud noise reduces productivity, concentration level, and attention span and may affect mental and emotional health. Symptoms of noise-related distress include disturbed sleep patterns, headaches, and tension. Physically, our bodies respond to noise in a variety of ways. Blood pressure increases, blood vessels in the brain dilate, and vessels in other parts of the body constrict. The pupils of the eye dilate. Cholesterol levels in the blood rise, and some endocrine glands secrete additional stimulating hormones, such as adrenaline, into the bloodstream.

Sounds are measured in decibels. A jet takeoff from 200 feet has a noise level of approximately 140 decibels, while voice in normal conversation has a level of about 60 decibels. Hearing can be damaged by varying lengths of exposure to sound. If the duration of allowable daily exposure to different decibel levels is exceeded, hearing loss will result.

Unfortunately, despite increasing awareness that noise pollution is more than just a nuisance, noise control programs have been given a low budgetary priority in the United States. The European Union has been more active in combating certain forms of noise pollution, such as aircraft noise.[34] Still, the European Environment Agency estimates that more than 120 million people in the European Union are exposed daily to noise levels greater than 55 decibels on the front facade of their homes.[35] Clearly, to protect your hearing, you must take it upon yourself to avoid voluntary and involuntary exposure to excessive noise.

> **What do you think?**
> *What do you currently do that places your hearing at risk?* ✳ *What changes can you make in your lifestyle to protect your hearing?*

Land Pollution

Solid Waste

Each day, every person in the United States generates more than four pounds of **municipal solid waste**—containers and packaging, discarded food, yard debris, and refuse from residential, commercial, institutional, and industrial sources. This translates to more than 220 million tons per day. Approximately 73 percent of this waste is buried in landfills. Cities and smaller communities throughout the country are in danger of exhausting their landfill space.

As communities run out of landfill space, it is becoming more common to haul garbage out to sea to dump it or ship it to landfills in developing countries. Although experts believe that up to 90 percent of our trash is recyclable, only 26 percent of it is currently recycled. In today's throwaway

> **Municipal solid waste** Solid wastes such as durable goods, nondurable goods, containers and packaging, food wastes, yard wastes, and miscellaneous wastes from residential, commercial, institutional, and industrial sources.
>
> **Hazardous waste** Solid waste that, because of its toxic properties, poses a hazard to humans or to the environment.
>
> **Superfund** Fund established under the Comprehensive Environmental Response Compensation and Liability Act to be used for cleaning up toxic waste dumps.

society, we need to become aware of the amount of waste we generate every day and to look for ways to recycle, reuse, and—most desirable of all—reduce what we use.

Hazardous Waste

The community of Love Canal, New York, has come to symbolize **hazardous waste** dump sites. The Hooker Chemical Company used Love Canal as a chemical dump site for nearly 30 years, starting in the 1920s. Then the area was filled in by land developers and built up with homes and schools.

In 1976, homeowners began noticing strange seepage in their basements and strong chemical odors. Babies were born with abnormal hearts and kidneys, two sets of teeth, mental handicaps, epilepsy, liver disease, and abnormal rectal bleeding. The rate of cancer and miscarriages was far above normal.

The New York State Department of Health investigation found high concentrations of PCBs in the storm sewers near the old canal, but it took the department another two years to order the evacuation of Love Canal homes. More than 900 families were evacuated, and the state purchased their homes. Finally, in 1978, the expensive process of cleaning up the waste dump began. Many lawsuits for damages are still being litigated.

In 1980, the Comprehensive Environmental Response Compensation and Liability Act **(Superfund)** was enacted to provide funds for cleaning up chemical dump sites that endanger public health and land. This fund is financed through taxes on the chemical and petroleum industries (87 percent) and through general federal tax revenues (13 percent). Clean-up cost estimates from the year 1990 through 2020 range from $106 billion to $500 billion.[36]

To date, 32,500 potentially hazardous waste sites have been identified across the nation. After investigation, 17,800 of them were determined to require no further action, but more than 1,200 are still listed on the National Priorities List as a hazard to human health.[37]

The large number of hazardous waste dump sites in the United States indicates the severity of our toxic chemical problem. American manufacturers generate more than 1 ton of chemical waste per person per year (approximately 275 million tons). The *Agency for Toxic Substances and Disease Registry* and the EPA evaluate and rank the chemicals that are considered hazardous substances. The EPA and the states have undertaken a "cradle-to-grave" program to manage hazardous wastes by monitoring their generation, transportation, storage, treatment, and final disposal.[38]

> **What do you think?**
> *What items do you currently recycle?* ✳ *What are some of the reasons you do not recycle?* ✳ *What might encourage you to recycle more than you do?* ✳ *What concerns would you have about living near a landfill or hazardous waste disposal site?*

Speaking Out on the Environment

Here are eight ways to get involved in the crusade against pollution.

- Monitor legislation. All of the key environmental organizations keep tabs on state and national laws being considered in order to offer testimony and to generate letter-writing campaigns on behalf of (or against) proposed laws.
- Write letters or send emails. They may not seem like potent weapons, but letters to state and federal legislators on pending bills do influence their opinions. When writing to any public official, keep your letter simple. Focus on one subject and identify a particular piece of legislation, request a specific action, and state your reasons for taking your position. If you live or work in the legislator's district, make sure to say so. Keep the letter to one or two paragraphs, and never write more than one page. Send your letters to:

Hon. _____
House Office Building
Washington, D.C. 20515

Senator _____
Senate Office Building
Washington, D.C. 20510

You can find contact information for your Senators and Representative online at the websites listed at the end of this box.

- Complete customer comment cards, and call the toll-free phone numbers on packages. Let companies know your concerns.
- Educate others. You can do this in a variety of ways, from talking to your friends, coworkers, and neighbors, to organizing an educational activity.
- Campaign for environmental candidates. Consider the environmental positions of candidates at all levels of government.
- Launch a campaign at school or work. At Rutgers University, for example, members of the law association decided to target the use of plastic foam in the cafeterias. The students spoke with the director of food services, who readily agreed to stop using foam cups and foam food containers. Sometimes all you have to do is ask.

- Invite speakers to your organization. Most environmental organizations offer speakers on a wide range of topics who will speak at no charge to your civic, school, religious, or social organization. For maximum impact, consider scheduling a debate or panel discussion among representatives of environmental groups, government agencies, and industry.
- Get involved with government. Most communities offer a variety of boards, commissions, and committees that deal with environmental issues: planning, zoning and land use, parks and recreation, public transit, and so on. Play a role in setting policies that affect the quality of life in your area.

Sources: Except for the first paragraph, from *The Green Consumer Supermarket Guide,* 260–264, by J. Makower, J. Elkington, and J. Hailes. Copyright © 1991 by J. Elkington, J. Hailes, and Viking Penguin. Used by permission of Viking Penguin, a division of Penguin Group (USA) Inc. and Victor Gollancz Ltd., a division of the Orion Publishing Group Ltd. United States Senate, "Find Your Senators." www.senate.gov; United States House of Representatives, "Write Your Representatives." www.house.gov

Radiation

A substance is said to be radioactive when it emits high-energy particles from the nuclei of its atoms. There are three types of radiation: alpha particles, beta particles, and gamma rays. *Alpha* particles are relatively massive and are not capable of penetrating human skin. They pose health hazards only when inhaled or ingested. *Beta* particles can penetrate the skin slightly and are harmful if ingested or inhaled. *Gamma* rays are the most dangerous because they can pass straight through the skin, which causes serious damage to organs and other vital structures.

Ionizing Radiation

Exposure to ionizing radiation is an inescapable part of life on this planet. **Ionizing radiation** is caused by the release of particles and electromagnetic rays from atomic nuclei during the normal process of disintegration. Some naturally occur-

ring elements, such as uranium, emit radiation. Radiation can wreak havoc on human cells, which leads to mutations, cancer, miscarriages, and other problems.

Reactions to radiation differ from person to person. Exposure is measured in **radiation absorbed doses,** or **rads** (also called roentgens). Recommended maximum safe dosages range from 0.5 rad to 5 rads per year. Approximately 50 percent of the radiation to which we are exposed comes from natural sources, such as building materials. Another 45 percent comes from medical and dental X rays. The remaining 5 percent comes from computer display screens, microwave ovens, television sets, luminous watch dials, and

Ionizing radiation Radiation produced by photons having energy high enough to ionize atoms.

Radiation absorbed doses (rads) Units that measure exposure to radioactivity.

Wireless Worries

In less than a decade, cell phones have become a household staple. The number of subscribers has skyrocketed from 16 million in 1994 to more than 110 million today, and is still rising by 1 million per month.

Although cell phones have become commonplace, their use continues to spur controversy, particularly regarding questions of potential health risk. The cell phone industry assures consumers that phones are completely safe. But a former industry research director, Dr. George Carlo, argues that past studies have not provided conclusive evidence of safety, and we do not know the effects of cell phone usage on future generations. He observed, "This is the first generation that has put relatively high-powered transmitters against the head, hour after hour, day after day." Depending on how close the cell phone antenna is to the head, as much as 60 percent of microwave radiation may be absorbed by and actually penetrate the area around the head; some of this radiation may reach an inch to an inch-and-a half into the brain.

Are increases in the incidence and prevalence of brain tumors and other neurological conditions in the last decade related to cell phone use? At high power levels, radiofrequency energy, which is the energy used in cell phones, can heat biological tissue rapidly and cause damage, such as burns. However, cell phones operate at power levels well below the level at which such heating effects occur. Many countries, including the U.S. and most of Europe, use standards set by the Federal Communication Commission (FCC) for radiofrequency energy based on research by several scientific groups. These groups identified a whole-body *Specific Absorption Rate (SAR)* value for exposure to radiofrequency energy. Four watts per kilogram was identified as a threshold level of exposure at which harmful biological effects may occur. The FCC requires wireless phones to comply with a safety limit of 1.6 watts per kilogram. To find the SAR for your phone, see this website: www.fda.gov/cellphones/qa.html.

The Food and Drug Administration, the World Health Organization, and other major health agencies agree that the research to date has not shown radiofrequency energy emitted from cell phones to be harmful. However, they also point to the need for more research and caution that there is not enough information to say cell phones are risk-free. Three recently published large, case-control studies and one large cohort study have compared cell phone use among brain cancer patients and individuals free of brain cancer. Key findings from these studies indicate the following.

- Brain cancer patients did not report more cellular phone use overall than did the controls. In fact, for unclear reasons, most of the studies showed a lower risk of brain cancer among cell phone users.
- None of the studies showed a clear link between the side of the head on which the cancer occurred and the side on which the phone was used.
- There was no correlation between brain tumor risk and dose of exposure, as assessed by duration of use, date since first subscription, age at first subscription, or type of phone used.

However, these studies are not conclusive, and preliminary results from smaller, well-designed studies have continued to raise questions. At the moment, the biggest risk from cell phones appears to come from using them while driving, with a corresponding increase in crashes. However, if you prefer to err on the side of caution, follow these hints to lower your risk.

- Use lighter- or dash-mounted phones or headphones/ear buds when driving. This not only helps keep your hands free, helping to avoid accidents, but, if subsequent studies indicate potential health risk, you will also have minimized your exposure to radiofrequency energy.
- Limit cell phone usage. Use land-based phones whenever possible.
- Check the SAR level of your phone. Purchase one with a lower level if yours is near the FCC limit.
- Digital phones have lower radiofrequencies than do analog phones. An upgrade might be in order.

Sources: U.S. General Accounting Office (GAO), *Research and Regulatory Efforts on Mobile Cell Phone Health Issues* (GAO-01-545) (Washington, D.C. USGAO, 2001); H. Frumkin and M. Thun, "Environmental Carcinogens—Cellular Phones and Risk of Brain Tumors," *California Cancer Journal for Clinicians* 51 (2001): 137–141; Brian Ross, "Wireless Worries?" December 8, 2002. http://abcnews.go.com/onair/2020/2020_991020cellphones.html; Food and Drug Administration, "Cell Phone Facts: Consumer Information on Wireless Phones," July 29, 2003. www.fda.gov/cellphones/qa.html#4

---

radar screens and waves. Most of us are exposed to far less radiation than the safe maximum dosage per year.

Radiation can cause damage at dosages as low as 100 to 200 rads. At this level, signs of radiation sickness include nausea, diarrhea, fatigue, anemia, sore throat, and hair loss, but death is unlikely. At 350 to 500 rads, these symptoms become more severe, and death may result because the radiation hinders bone marrow production of the white blood cells we need to protect us from disease. Dosages above 600 to 700 rads are invariably fatal. The effects of long-term exposure to relatively low levels of radiation are unknown. Some scientists believe that such exposure can cause lung cancer, leukemia, skin cancer, bone cancer, and skeletal deformities. Researchers are also investigating the effects of long-term exposure to the radio frequency waves generated by cell phones (see the Consumer Health box).

Electric and Magnetic Fields: Emerging Risks?

If you believe what you hear on TV or read in the papers, electric and magnetic fields (EMFs) generated by electric power delivery systems are responsible for risks for cancer (particularly among children), reproductive dysfunction, birth defects, neurological disorders, Alzheimer's disease, and other ailments. But does research support these claims about EMFs? A six-year study by the National Institute of Environmental Health Sciences (NIEHS) found that the evidence for a link between cancer and EMFs is "weak," although the director of NIEHS warned that efforts to reduce exposure should continue.

The study did indicate a slight increase in risk for childhood leukemia, as well as chronic lymphocytic leukemia in occupationally exposed adults such as utility workers, machinists, and welders.[39] Since then, numerous studies in the United States, Canada, Sweden, Taiwan, New Zealand, and other regions have found only a small association or none at all between cancer and EMFs. Although rates of brain tumors and other cancers are on the increase, a clear link to EMFs has not been established. NIEHS suggests that the lack of consistent, positive findings weakens the contention that EMFs cause cancer.[40]

Nuclear Power Plants

Nuclear power plants account for less than 1 percent of the total radiation to which we are exposed. Other producers of radioactive waste include medical facilities that use radioactive materials as treatment and diagnostic tools and nuclear weapons production facilities.

Proponents of nuclear energy believe that it is a safe and efficient way to generate electricity. Initial costs of building nuclear power plants are high, but actual power generation is relatively inexpensive. A 1,000-megawatt reactor produces enough energy for 650,000 homes and saves 420 million gallons of fossil fuels each year. In some areas where nuclear power plants were decommissioned, electricity bills tripled when power companies turned to hydroelectric or fossil fuel sources to generate electricity.

Nuclear reactors also discharge fewer carbon oxides into the air than do fossil-fuel-powered generators. Advocates believe that conversion to nuclear power could help slow the global warming trend. Over the past 15 years, carbon emissions were reduced by 298 million tons, or 5 percent.

All these advantages of nuclear energy must be weighed against the disadvantages. First, disposal of nuclear wastes is extremely problematic for the entire world. Additionally, a reactor core meltdown could pose serious threats to a plant's immediate environment and to the world in general.

A **meltdown** occurs when the temperature in the core of a nuclear reactor increases enough to melt both the nuclear fuel and the containment vessel that holds it. Most modern facilities seal their reactors and containment vessels in concrete buildings that have pools of cold water on the bottom. If a meltdown occurs, the building and the pool are supposed to prevent the escape of radioactivity.

Two serious nuclear accidents within seven years of each other caused a steep decline in public support for nuclear energy. The first occurred in 1979 at Three Mile Island near Harrisburg, Pennsylvania, when a mechanical failure caused a partial meltdown of one reactor core, and small amounts of radioactive steam were released into the atmosphere. No loss of human life was reported, although residents in the area were evacuated. Miscarriages, birth defects, and cancer rates in the area are reported to have increased, but no public health statistics have been released.

Human error and mechanical failure were the reported causes of the 1986 reactor core fire and explosion at the Chernobyl nuclear power plant in the former Soviet Union. In just 4.5 seconds, the temperature in the reactor rose to 120 times normal, which caused the explosion. Eighteen people were killed immediately, 30 workers died later from radiation sickness, and 200 other workers were hospitalized for severe radiation sickness. Soviet officials evacuated towns and villages near the plant. Some medical workers estimate that the eventual death toll from radiation-induced cancers related to the Chernobyl incident topped 100,000.

Radioactive fallout from the Chernobyl disaster spread over most of the northern hemisphere. Milk, meat, and vegetables in Scandinavian countries were contaminated with radioactive iodine and cesium and were declared unfit for human consumption. Thousands of reindeer in Lapland were contaminated and had to be destroyed. In Great Britain, thousands of sheep had to be destroyed, and three years later sheep in the northern regions of the country were still found to be contaminated. Direct costs of the disaster totaled more than $13 billion, including lost agricultural output and the cost of replacing the power plant. Nuclear accidents continue to pose risks to human health, even in well-controlled settings.

> **What do you think?**
> *How much exposure do you have to ionizing and non-ionizing radiation in a year?* ∗ *What measures could you take to reduce your exposure?* ∗ *Do you feel the advantages outweigh the disadvantages of nuclear power? Explain why or why not.*

Meltdown   An accident that results when the temperature in the core of a nuclear reactor increases enough to melt the nuclear fuel and the containment vessel housing it.

Make It Happen!

Assessment: The Assess Yourself box on page 422 gave you the chance to look at your behavior and consider ways of saving water, reducing waste, and protecting the planet in other ways. Now that you have considered these results, you can begin to take steps to become more environmentally responsible.

Making a Change: In order to change your behavior, you need to develop a plan. Follow these steps:

1. Evaluate your behavior, and identify patterns and specific things you are doing. What can you change now? What can you change in the near future?
2. Select one pattern of behavior that you want to change.
3. Fill out a Behavior Change Contract. It should include your long-term goal for change, your short-term goals, the rewards you'll give yourself for reaching these goals, potential obstacles along the way, and strategies for overcoming these obstacles. For each goal, list the small steps and specific actions that you will take.
4. Chart your progress in a journal. At the end of a week, consider how successful you were in following your plan. What helped you be successful? What made change more difficult? What will you do differently next week?
5. Revise your plan as needed. Are the short-term goals attainable? Are the rewards satisfying?

Example: Marta saw that she was already doing several of the items recommended in the self-assessment. However, she had not considered several of the ideas regarding excess packaging of her food, drinks, and so on, although she knew that extra plastic wraps and other excess packaging contribute to the need for more landfills and other environmental problems. She decided that for a week she would try to pay more attention to the packaging of her favorite foods, and to buy large sizes of the food whenever possible instead of individually packed products. This meant spending more time in the grocery store to be sure she found items with the least packaging (although she also didn't have to make as many trips to the store that week). The next week, Marta looked at how many plastic bottles she used for her water each day. She bought a durable, dishwasher-safe plastic bottle and started filling it with water each day before she left the house. After a week she was happy to discover that her garbage was not full of plastic water bottles, and she had actually saved herself some money.

Summary

✳ Population growth is the single largest factor affecting the demands on the environment. Demand for more food, products, and energy—as well as places to dispose of waste, particularly in the industrialized world—places great strain on the earth's resources.

✳ The primary constituents of air pollution are sulfur dioxide, particulate matter, carbon monoxide, nitrogen dioxide, ozone, lead, and hydrocarbons. Air pollution takes the forms of photochemical smog and acid rain, among others. Indoor air pollution is caused primarily by woodstove smoke, furnace emissions, asbestos, passive smoke, formaldehyde, radon, and household chemicals. Pollution is depleting the earth's protective ozone layer, which causes global warming.

✳ Water pollution can be caused by either point (direct entry through a pipeline, ditch, etc.) or nonpoint (runoff or seepage from a broad area of land) sources. Major contributors to water pollution include dioxins, pesticides, and lead.

✳ Noise pollution affects our hearing and produces other symptoms such as reduced productivity, reduced concentration, headaches, and tension.

✳ Solid waste pollution includes household trash, plastics, glass, metal products, and paper. Limited landfill space creates problems. Hazardous waste is toxic; improper disposal creates health hazards for those in surrounding communities.

✳ Ionizing radiation results from the natural erosion of atomic nuclei. Non-ionizing radiation is caused by the electric and magnetic fields around power lines and household appliances, among other sources. The disposal and storage of radioactive wastes from nuclear power and weapons production plants pose serious potential problems for public health.

Questions for Discussion and Reflection

1. How are the rapidly increasing global population and consumption of resources related? Is population control the best solution? Why or why not?
2. What are the primary sources of air pollution? What can be done to reduce air pollution?
3. What causes poor indoor air quality? How does indoor air pollution affect schoolchildren?
4. What are the causes and consequences of global warming?
5. What are point and nonpoint sources of water pollution? What can be done to reduce or prevent water pollution?
6. What are the physiological consequences of noise pollution? What can you do to lessen your exposure to it?
7. Why do you think so little recycling occurs in the United States?
8. Would you feel comfortable living near a nuclear power plant? Do you think nuclear power is an important source of energy in the future? Why or why not?

Accessing Your Health on the Internet

Visit the following Internet sites to explore further topics and issues related to personal health. To visit an organization's website, go to the Companion Website for *Health: The Basics, Sixth Edition* at www.aw-bc.com/donatelle, click on the book image, and select "Accessing Your Health on the Internet" from the navigation menu on the left.

1. *Environmental Protection Agency (EPA).* Government agency responsible for overseeing environmental regulation and protection issues in the United States.

2. *National Center for Environmental Health (NCEH).* A section of the Centers for Disease Control and Prevention website, this site provides information on a wide variety of environmental health issues, including a series of helpful fact sheets.

3. *National Environmental Health Association (NEHA).* This organization provides educational resources and opportunities for environmental health professionals. The NEHA website lists conferences, trainings, and publications and offers informational position papers.

Further Reading

Cayne, B., and J. Tesar. *Food and Water: Threats, Shortages, and Solutions.* New York: Facts on File, 2002.

A basic introduction that discusses the vital importance of an adequate supply of food and water and the need for alternative water storage and agricultural strategies.

Godish, T. *Indoor Environmental Quality.* Boca Raton, FL: Lewis Publishers, 2000.

Explores the scope of the indoor environment, both in the home and workplace, and major indoor contaminants.

Nadakavukaren, N. *Our Global Environment: A Health Perspective.* Prospect Heights, IL: Waveland, 2000.

A survey of major global environmental issues and their ecological impact on personal and community health.

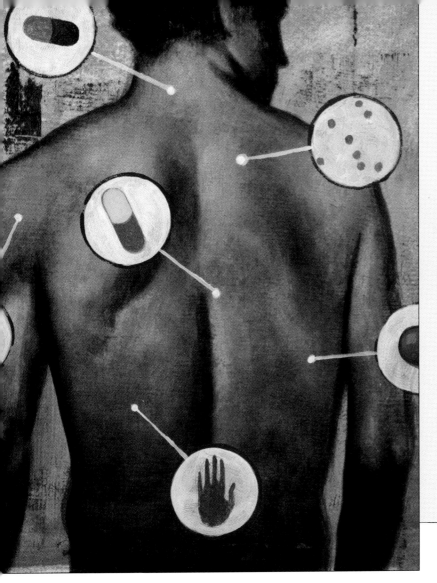

Consumerism

Selecting Health Care Products and Services

17 17 17 17 17 17 17

Objectives

* Explain why responsible consumerism is important to Americans and how to encourage consumers to take action.

* Explain why self-diagnosis, self-help, and self-care are becoming increasingly important in our quest for health and well-being.

* Discuss the choices available to Americans who seek health care through allopathic avenues, as well as factors that should be considered in making decisions about health care.

* Describe the U.S. health care system in terms of types of medical practice, provider groups, and the changing structures of managed care and other options.

* Discuss key issues in American health care services in terms of cost, quality, and access to services.

* Discuss the different types of health insurance available in the United States and the role insurers play in providing health care.

In Loco Parentis Doesn't Necessarily Pay the Doctor

By Sana Siwolop

Before heading off to college, students go through the rituals of packing, buying books and supplies and checking class schedules and living arrangements. Often low on the priority list, if it's there at all, is reviewing health insurance coverage.

Sure, college students are generally young and healthy, and many are already covered by employer-sponsored health plans, usually through their parents. But those plans are not foolproof:

some cover non-emergency expenses only if the school is within the plan's geographic area, while many others apply only to full-time students, and only until they are 23. Some policies may also require referrals for certain services or when patients go out of their network of physicians.

In some cases, health care experts say, students may be better off with their own policies, like those sponsored by the schools themselves or offered by private insurers.

Which type is best? Because so many plans are available with varying coverage, deductibles and restrictions the answer is not always clear.

Read the complete article online in the eThemes section of this book's website: www.aw-bc.com/donatelle.

There are many reasons for you to be an informed health care consumer. Most important, you have only one body, and if you don't treat it with care, you will pay a major price in terms of financial costs and health consequences. Doing everything you can to stay healthy and recover rapidly when you do get sick will enhance every other part of your life.

To obtain high-quality health care at an affordable cost, you need to be both informed and assertive. But, as you may already know, medical services are much harder to evaluate for need, availability, cost, and quality than are, say, clothing or vegetables. In addition, you may seek health care in circumstances of physical or emotional distress, when your decision-making powers are compromised.

This chapter will help you make better decisions that affect your health and health care. Our health care system is a maze of health care providers, payers (insurance, government, and individuals), and products. Many of us find it hard to thread our way through the maze. Health care is the fifth largest industry in our country. It accounts for more than 10 percent of our workforce. And many different companies aggressively market health products and services to the public. Increasingly, health care organizations are "for-profit" businesses that are sold and traded on the stock market. Medical professionals and consumers report that they feel overwhelmed, confused, and frustrated by the multitude of choices, seemingly divergent interests, and lack of coordination in our system.

Responsible Consumerism: Choices and Challenges

Perhaps the single greatest difficulty that we face as health care consumers is the sheer magnitude of choices available to us. If you try to select a general practitioner from the telephone book, you have to thumb through dozens of pages of specialists. When you want to purchase cough syrup, you are confronted with hundreds of options, each claiming to do more for you than the brand next to it. Even trained pharmacists find it difficult to keep up with the explosion of new drugs and health-related products. Because there are so many profit-seekers competing for a share of the lucrative health care market and because misinformation is so common, wise health care consumers use every means at their disposal to ensure that they are acting responsibly and economically. Answer the questions in the Assess Yourself box to see how you might become a better health care consumer.

Putting Cure into Perspective

People often fall victim to false health claims because they mistakenly believe that a product or provider has helped them. Frequently this belief arises from two conditions: spontaneous remission and the placebo effect.

Spontaneous Remission   It is commonly said that if you treat a cold, it will disappear in a week, but if you leave it alone, it will last seven days. A **spontaneous remission** from

Spontaneous remission   The disappearance of symptoms without any apparent cause or treatment.

Being a Better Health Care Consumer

Answer the following questions and determine what you might
do to become a better health care consumer.

1. Do you have a physician?
2. Do you have health insurance?
3. Have you determined which health care services are available free or at a reduced cost in your area? If so, what are they?
4. When you receive a prescription, do you ask the pharmacist if a generic brand could be substituted?
5. Do you ask the pharmacist for potential side effects before or after the prescription is filled?
6. Do you take medication as directed?
7. Do you report any unusual side effects to your doctor?
8. When you receive a diagnosis, do you seek more information about the diagnosis and treatment?
9. If surgery or an invasive type of treatment is indicated by your doctor, do you seek a second opinion?
10. Where do you find most health information?
11. How do you know this source of information is a reliable and credible source?
12. When you purchase an over-the-counter (OTC) medication, do you read the label?
13. What attracts you most to a new product? (check all that apply)

_____ price

_____ promises of a new lifestyle

_____ appears to meet a need

_____ positive testimonials

_____ savings or coupons

_____ spokesperson

_____ testing for product safety

14. How much of a role do you think advertising plays in your decision to purchase a new product?

an ailment refers to the disappearance of symptoms without any apparent cause or treatment. Many illnesses, like the common cold and even back strain, are self-limiting and will improve in time, with or without treatment. Other illnesses, such as multiple sclerosis and some cancers, are characterized by alternating periods of severe symptoms and sudden remissions. People experiencing spontaneous remissions can easily attribute their "cure" to a treatment that, in fact, had no real effect.

Placebo Effect   The **placebo effect** is an apparent cure or improved state of health brought about by a substance, product, or procedure that has no generally recognized therapeutic value. It is not uncommon for patients to report improvements based on what they expect, desire, or were told would happen after taking simple sugar pills that they believed were powerful drugs. About 10 percent of the population is believed to be exceptionally susceptible to the power

of suggestion and may be easy targets for such aggressive marketing. Although the placebo effect is generally harmless, it does account for the expenditure of millions of dollars on health products and services every year. Megadoses of vitamin C have never been proven to treat cancer. Mud baths do not smooth wrinkled skin, nor do electric shocks reduce muscle pain. People who mistakenly use placebos when medical treatment is urgently needed increase their risk for health problems.

> **Placebo effect**   An apparent cure or improved state of health brought about by a substance or product that has no medicinal value.

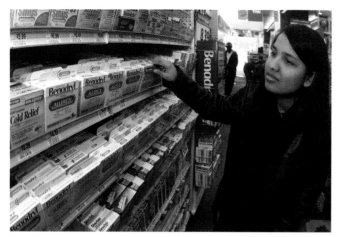

Deciding when to contact a physician can be difficult. Most people first try to diagnose and treat their condition themselves.

Taking Responsibility for Your Health Care

As the health care industry has become more sophisticated about seeking your business, so must you become more sophisticated about purchasing its products and services. Learn how, when, and where to enter the massive technological maze that is our health care system without incurring unnecessary risk and expense. Acting responsibly in times of illness can be difficult, but the person best able to act on your behalf is you.

If you are not feeling well, you must first decide whether you really need to seek medical advice. Not that long ago, as many as 70 percent of all trips to the doctor and nearly half of all hospital stays were believed to be unnecessary and potentially harmful.[1] These figures have decreased considerably, however, with the advent of managed care, which carries with it a degree of out-of-pocket shared costs. Theoretically, patients who have to pay for a portion of their care will not seek care unnecessarily. Managed care involves a number of measures designed to keep people out of hospitals and emergency rooms.[2] Although there are no exact figures, respected sources indicate that the number of emergency room visits has decreased dramatically, and the cost of emergency room care for nonemergencies has declined as well.[3]

Yet, critics of managed care point to cost savings as a part of the problem with quality and access. Not seeking treatment, whether because of high costs or limited coverage, or trying to medicate oneself when more rigorous methods of treatment are needed, is dangerous. Being knowledgeable about the benefits of and limits to self-care is critical for responsible consumerism.

Self-Help or Self-Care

A recent concept in health consumerism proposes that the patient is the primary health care provider or first line of defense. We can practice behaviors that promote health,

prevent disease, and minimize reliance on the formal medical system. We can also interpret basic changes in our own physical and emotional health and treat minor afflictions without seeking professional help. Self-care consists of knowing your body, paying attention to its signals, and taking appropriate action to stop the progression of illness or injury. Common forms of self-care include:

- Diagnosing symptoms or conditions that occur frequently but may not require physician visits (e.g., the common cold, minor abrasions)
- Performing breast and testicular self-examinations (monthly)
- Learning first aid for common, uncomplicated injuries and conditions
- Checking blood pressure, pulse, and temperature
- Using home pregnancy and ovulation kits and HIV test kits
- Doing periodic checks for blood cholesterol
- Using home stool test kits for blood and early colon cancer detection
- Using self-help books, tapes, software, websites, and videos
- Benefiting from relaxation techniques, including meditation, nutrition, rest, and exercise

When to Seek Help

Effective self-care also means understanding when to seek medical attention rather than treating a condition yourself. Deciding which conditions warrant professional advice is not always easy. Generally, you should consult a physician if you experience any of the following:

- A serious accident or injury
- Sudden or severe chest pains causing breathing difficulties
- Trauma to the head or spine accompanied by persistent headache, blurred vision, loss of consciousness, vomiting, convulsions, or paralysis
- Sudden high fever or recurring high temperature (over 102°F for adults and 103°F for children) and/or sweats
- Tingling sensation in the arm accompanied by slurred speech or impaired thought processes
- Adverse reactions to a drug or insect bite (shortness of breath, severe swelling, dizziness)
- Unexplained bleeding or loss of body fluid from any body opening
- Unexplained sudden weight loss
- Persistent or recurrent diarrhea or vomiting
- Blue-colored lips, eyelids, or nail beds
- Any lump, swelling, thickness, or sore that does not subside or that grows for over a month
- Any marked change or pain in bowel or bladder habits
- Yellowing of the skin or the whites of the eyes
- Any symptom that is unusual and recurs over time
- Pregnancy

With the vast array of home diagnostic devices currently available, it seems relatively easy for most people to take

Being Proactive in Your Own Health Care

Throughout this book, we have emphasized the importance of healthy preventive behaviors. Sometimes, however, regardless of the steps you take to care for yourself, you still get sick. At such times, it is important that you continue to be actively involved in your care. The more you know about your own body and the factors that can affect your health, the better you will be at communicating with your doctor. It also helps you make informed decisions and recognize when a certain treatment may not be right for you. The following points can help.

- Know your own and your family's medical history.
- Be knowledgeable about your condition—causes, physiological effects, possible treatments, prognosis. Don't rely on the doctor for this information. Do some research.
- Bring a friend or relative along for medical visits to help you review what the doctor says. If you go alone, take notes.
- Ask the practitioner to explain the problem and possible treatments, tests, and drugs in a clear and understandable way. If you don't understand something, ask for clarification.
- If the doctor prescribes any medications, ask whether you can take generic equivalents that cost less.
- Ask for a written summary of the results of your visit and any lab tests.

- If you have any doubt about the doctor's recommended treatment, seek a second opinion.
- If you will need to take a prescription medication for an extended time, ask for the maximum number of doses allowed by your plan if you have a small pharmacy copayment.

After seeing a health care professional, consider these ideas:

- Write down an accurate account of what happened and what was said. Be sure to include the names of the doctor and all other people involved in your care, the date, and the place.
- Shop around drugstores for the best prices in the same way that you would when shopping for clothes.
- When filling prescriptions, ask to see the pharmacist's package inserts that list medical considerations concerning the medicines. Request detailed information about potential drug and food interactions.
- Write clear instructions on the label to avoid risk to others who may take the drug in error.

Just like you, doctors are human. Their decisions are based on the best information they have available to them and may be influenced by a number of factors—workload, limited information, personal views. Therefore, in addition to following the practical steps listed above, being proactively involved in your health care also means that you should be aware of your rights as a patient. Your rights include the following.

1. The right of informed consent means that before receiving any care, you should be fully informed of what is being planned, the risks and potential benefits, and possible alternative forms of treatment, including the option of no treatment. Your consent must be voluntary and without any form of coercion. It is critical that you read any consent forms carefully and amend them as necessary before signing.
2. You are entitled to know whether the treatment you are receiving is standard or experimental. In experimental conditions, you have the legal and ethical right to know if the study is one in which some people receive treatment while others do not in order to compare the results, and if any drug is being used in the research project for a purpose not approved by the Food and Drug Administration (FDA).
3. You have the right to privacy, which includes the source of payment for treatment and care. It also includes protecting your right to make personal decisions concerning all reproductive matters.
4. You have the right to receive care. You also have the legal right to refuse treatment at any time and to cease treatment at any time.
5. You are entitled to access all your medical records and to have those records remain confidential.
6. You have the right to seek the opinions of other health care professionals regarding your condition.

---

care of themselves. But some caution is in order here: Although many of these devices are valuable for making an initial diagnosis, home health tests are no substitute for regular, complete examinations by a trained practitioner. See the Skills for Behavior Change box for information on taking an active role in your own health care.

Assessing Health Professionals

Suppose you decide that you do need medical help. You must then identify what type of help you need and where to obtain it. Initially, selecting a professional may seem a simple matter, yet many people have no idea how to assess the qualifications of a health care provider.

Knowledge of both traditional medical specialties and alternative, or complementary, medical treatment is critical to making an intelligent selection. You also need to be aware of your own criteria for evaluating a health professional. Several studies have pointed to bedside manner and positive interactions with doctors as key to patient satisfaction. In a survey of Health Maintenance Organization (HMO) members, it was shown that even in a setting of limited physician choice, the opportunity to select one's personal physician had a positive influence on patient satisfaction with that physician.[4] When selecting from a network of providers, make sure you fully understand your coverage options. Carefully consider the following factors about all prospective health care providers.

- What professional educational training have they had? What license or board certification do they hold? Note that there is a difference between "board eligible" and "board certified." *Board certified* indicates that they have passed the national board examination for their specialty (e.g., pediatrics) and have been certified as competent in that specialty. In contrast, *board eligible* merely means that they are eligible to take the specialty board's exam or even that they may have failed the exam.
- Are they affiliated with an accredited medical facility or institution? The Joint Commission on the Accreditation of Healthcare Organizations (JCAHO) requires these institutions to verify all education, licensing, and training claims of their affiliated practitioners. What other doctors are in their group, and who will assist in your treatment?
- Are they open to complementary or alternative strategies? Would they refer you for different treatment modalities, when appropriate?
- Do they indicate clearly how long a given treatment may last, what side effects you might expect, and what problems you should watch for?
- Do their diagnoses, treatments, and general statements appear to be consistent with established scientific theory and practice?
- Who will be responsible for your care when the doctor is on vacation or off call?
- Do they listen to you, respect you as an individual, and give you time to ask questions? Do they return your calls, and are they available to answer questions?
- How often has the doctor performed this test, surgery, or procedure, and with what proportion of successful outcome?

When a doctor orders a test, treatment, or medication, you might ask questions like these:

- What are the side effects, and can these side effects be treated or reduced?
- Does this procedure require an overnight stay at a hospital, or can it be performed in a doctor's office?
- Why has this test been ordered? What is the doctor trying to find or exclude?

Allopathic medicine   Traditional, Western medical practice; in theory, based on scientifically validated methods and procedures.

Primary care practitioner   A medical practitioner who treats routine ailments, advises on preventive care, gives general medical advice, and makes appropriate referrals when necessary.

Asking the right questions at the right time may save you personal suffering and expense. Many patients find that writing their questions down before an appointment helps them get answers to all their questions. You should not accept a defensive or hostile response; asking questions is your right as a patient.

A 2002 survey found that nearly two-thirds of Americans are confident that the medical information given to them by their doctor is accurate, while the remaining one-third opt for a second opinion on important issues or do independent research.[5]

Choices in Medical Care

How can you choose the right provider for your needs? You should understand the various health professions and sub-specialties. Many health professionals subscribe to allopathic medical procedures. Most people believe that **allopathic medicine,** or traditional Western medical practice, is based on scientifically validated methods. But remember that not all allopathic treatments have had the benefit of the extensive clinical trials and long-term studies of outcomes that would be necessary to conclusively prove effectiveness in different populations. Even when studies appear to support the health benefits of a particular treatment or product, other studies with equal or better scientific validity often refute these claims. Also, what is recommended treatment today may change dramatically in the future as new technology and medical advances replace older practices. Like other professionals, medical doctors are only as good as their training, continued knowledge acquisition, and resources allow them to be. A "consumer beware" attitude is always prudent, especially when making critical health care decisions.

Traditional Western (Allopathic) Medicine

Selecting a **primary care practitioner**—a medical practitioner whom you can go to for routine ailments, preventive care, general medical advice, and appropriate referrals—is not an easy task. The primary care practitioner for most people is a family practitioner, an internist, a pediatrician, or an obstetrician/gynecologist (OB/GYN). Many people routinely see nurse practitioners or physician assistants who work for an individual doctor or a medical group, and others use nontraditional providers as their primary source of care.

Active participation in your own treatment is the only sensible course in a health care environment that encourages "defensive medicine." That is, physicians will frequently order tests to rule out rare or unlikely diagnoses simply because they are worried about possible malpractice suits. Researchers have documented that this practice often leads to unnecessary tests and overtreatment. It has been well documented that most medical treatments carry risks and that there is no 100 percent guarantee of improved health outcomes. You may find that your condition worsens or that the treatment may create an iatrogenic disease (an illness caused by the medical treatment itself).

Informed consent refers to your right to have explained to you—in nontechnical language you can understand—all possible side effects, benefits, and consequences of a procedure as well as available alternatives to it. It also means that you have the right to refuse a treatment and to seek a second or even third opinion from unbiased, noninvolved providers.[6]

> ### What do you think?
> *Have you ever opted for a treatment other than what was recommended by your allopathic medical provider?* ✳ *What was the response?* ✳ *Did your health insurer cooperate fully and pay the bill?*

Other Allopathic Specialties

There are many types of health care professionals appropriate for certain medical issues other than medical doctors. **Osteopaths** are general practitioners who receive training similar to a medical doctor's but who put special emphasis on the skeletal and muscular systems. Their treatments may involve manipulation of the muscles and joints. Osteopaths receive the degree of doctor of osteopathy (D.O.) rather than doctor of medicine (M.D.).

Much confusion exists about the roles of optometrists and ophthalmologists. An **ophthalmologist** holds a medical degree and can perform surgery and prescribe medications. An **optometrist** typically evaluates visual problems and fits glasses but is not a trained physician. If you have an eye infection, glaucoma, or other eye condition needing diagnosis and treatment, you need to see an ophthalmologist.

Dentists are specialists who diagnose and treat diseases of the teeth, gums, and oral cavity. They attend dental school for four years and receive the title of doctor of dental surgery (D.D.S.) or doctor of medical dentistry (D.M.D.). They must also pass both state and national board examinations before receiving their licenses to practice. The field of dentistry includes many specialties. For example, **orthodontists** specialize in aligning teeth. **Oral surgeons** perform surgical procedures to correct problems of the mouth, face, and jaw.

Nurses are highly trained and strictly regulated health practitioners who provide a wide range of services for patients and their families, including patient education, counseling, community health and disease prevention information, and administration of medications. Nurses may today choose from several training options. There are more than 2.4 million licensed registered nurses (R.N.) in the United States who have completed either a four-year program leading to a bachelor of science in nursing (B.S.N.) degree or a two-year associate degree program. More than 0.5 million lower-level licensed practical or vocational nurses (L.P.N. or L.V.N.) have completed a one- to two-year training program, which may be community college–based or hospital-based.

Nurse practitioners (N.P.) are professional nurses with advanced training obtained through either a master's degree program or a specialized nurse practitioner program. Nurse practitioners have the training and authority to conduct diagnostic tests and prescribe medications (in some states). They work in a variety of settings, particularly in HMOs, clinics, and student health centers. Nurses may also earn the clinical doctor of nursing degree (N.D.) or a doctorate of nursing science (D.N.S. or D.N.Sc.), or a research-based Ph.D. in nursing.

More than 30,000 **physician assistants** (P.A.) currently practice in the United States. Most of these are in office-based practices, including school health centers, but approximately 40 percent practice in areas where physicians are in short supply. Studies have shown that this relatively new class of midlevel practitioners may competently care for the majority of patients seeking primary care. All physician assistants must work under the supervision of a licensed physician, but most states do allow physician assistants to prescribe drugs.[7]

Health Care Organizations, Programs, and Facilities

Today, managed care is the dominant health payer system in the United States. Because of this, many people are restricted in their choice of a health care provider. Selective contracting

---

Osteopath   General practitioner who receives training similar to a medical doctor's but with an emphasis on the skeletal and muscular systems; often uses spinal manipulation as part of treatment.

Ophthalmologist   Physician who specializes in the medical and surgical care of the eyes, including prescriptions for glasses.

Optometrist   Eye specialist whose practice is limited to prescribing and fitting lenses.

Dentist   Specialist who diagnoses and treats diseases of the teeth, gums, and oral cavity.

Orthodontist   Dentist who specializes in the alignment of teeth.

Oral surgeon   Dentist who performs surgical procedures to correct problems of the mouth, jaw, and face.

Nurse   Health practitioner who provides many services for patients and who may work in a variety of settings.

Physician assistant   A midlevel practitioner trained to handle most standard cases of care.

between insurers or employers and health providers has limited the freedom of choice that some Americans previously enjoyed under a fee-for-service system. Two critical decisions to make are (1) choosing an insurance carrier or type of plan, and then (2) choosing from among the health care providers who participate in that plan. This section lists the most common choices.

Types of Medical Practices

In the highly competitive market for patients, many health care providers have found it essential to combine resources into a **group practice,** which can be single- or multispecialty. Physicians share offices, equipment, utility bills, and staff costs. Besides sharing costs, they may also share profits. Proponents of group practice maintain that it provides better coordination of care, reduces unnecessary duplication of equipment, and improves the quality of health care through peer review. Critics argue that group practice may limit competition and patients' access to services.

Solo practitioners are medical providers who practice independently of other practitioners. It is hard for solo practitioners to survive in today's high-cost, high-technology health care market. Additionally, solo practitioners often have little time away from their offices and have to trade on-call hours with other doctors. For these reasons, there are far fewer solo practices today than in the past.

Integrated Health Care Organizations

Both hospitals and clinics provide a range of health care services, including emergency treatment, diagnostic tests, and inpatient and outpatient (ambulatory) care. The number of hospitals has decreased in recent years because of an oversupply of hospital beds, a decreasing need for inpatient care, an increase in competition, and the growing number of hospital-based outpatient clinics. These integrated health care organizations range from groups of loosely affiliated health care service organizations and hospitals, to HMOs that control their own very tightly joined hospitals, clinics, pharmacies, and even home health care agencies.

There are several ways to classify hospitals: by profit status (nonprofit or for-profit), ownership (private, city, county, state, federal), specialty (children's, maternity, chronic care, psychiatric, general acute), teaching status (teaching-affiliated or not), size, and whether they are part of a chain of hospitals. **Nonprofit (voluntary) hospitals** have traditionally been run by religious or other humanitarian groups. Earnings have generally been reinvested in the hospital to improve health care. These hospitals have often provided care regardless of a patient's ability to pay.

The number of **for-profit (proprietary) hospitals** has multiplied over the past two decades. Today they constitute more than 20 percent of nongovernmental acute-care hospitals. For-profit hospitals, which do not receive tax breaks, are not compelled to operate as a charity and typically provide fewer free services to the community than do nonprofit hospitals. Historically, some for-profit hospitals have quickly transferred indigent (poor) or uninsured patients to public hospitals or to nonprofit hospitals.[8] This practice, known as *patient dumping,* was prohibited by federal law in 1986. Today, all hospital emergency rooms are required to perform a screening medical exam on all patients, regardless of their ability to pay. Patients must be determined to be "medically stable" before they can be transferred to another facility or discharged from the emergency room.

More treatments or services, including surgery, are delivered on an **outpatient (ambulatory) care** basis (care that does not involve an overnight stay) by hospitals, traditional clinics, student health clinics, and nontraditional clinical centers. One type of ambulatory facility that is becoming common is the *surgicenter*—a place where minor, low-risk procedures such as vasectomies, tubal ligations, tissue biopsies, cosmetic surgery, abortions, and minor eye operations are performed. In 1982, nearly 85 percent of all surgeries in the United States involved an overnight hospital stay; by 2000, fewer than 30 percent of surgeries did so.

Many hospitals and group practices are affiliated with freestanding imaging and diagnostic laboratory centers through either direct ownership or other profit-sharing arrangements. Significant debate surrounds this practice. Critics argue that when doctors own the diagnostic and laboratory services to which they refer patients, they may order an excessive number of tests. Today, such practices amount to "conflict of interest situations" and are largely prohibited by anti-kickback legislation.

Once located within hospitals, most health clinics today are likely to be independent facilities run by medical practitioners. Other health clinics are run by county health departments; these offer low-cost diagnosis and treatment for financially needy patients. Additionally, some 1,500 college campuses have student health centers that, along with county, city, or community clinics, supply low-cost family planning, tests and services related to sexually transmitted infection, gynecological services, and vaccination services.

Group practice   A group of physicians who combine resources, sharing offices, equipment, and staff costs to render care to patients.

Solo practitioner   Physician who renders care to patients independently of other practitioners.

Nonprofit (voluntary) hospitals   Hospitals run by religious or other humanitarian groups that reinvest their earnings in the hospital to improve health care.

For-profit (proprietary) hospitals   Hospitals that provide a return on earnings to the investors who own them.

Outpatient (ambulatory) care   Treatment that does not involve an overnight stay in a hospital.

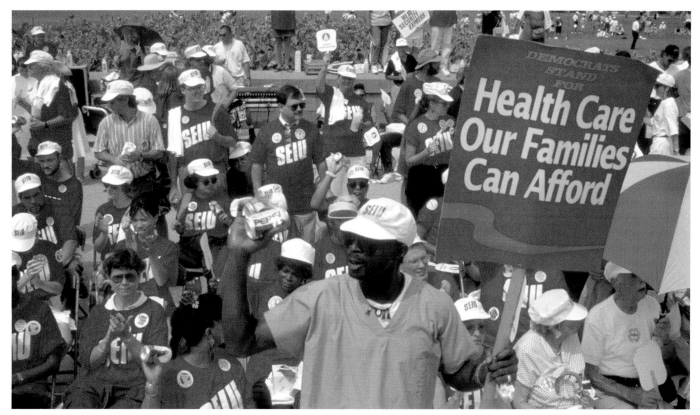
Increasing heath care costs have mobilized people to take political action. Debate continues over the proper role of government, the insurance industry, and other parties.

Consumers who consider using a hospital or clinic should scrutinize the facility's accreditation. Accredited hospitals have met rigorous standards set by the JCAHO. If you choose an institution having this form of accreditation, you have a high likelihood of obtaining quality care.

With the growth of managed care organizations, concerns have arisen about the quality of care offered under this type of payment system. These concerns compelled consumer groups and public health organizations to require managed care insurers to compile quality care "report cards," known as HEDIS Reports (Health Employer Data Information Set), so that health outcomes could be compared across different plans. The quality measures include preventive services (childhood immunizations, Pap smears, mammograms), disease indicators (eye exams and glucose control tests for diabetics), and screening exams (routine physical exams, including gynecological exams).

Consumers can obtain additional information regarding providers' malpractice insurance or sanctions from state licensure boards and the National Practitioner Data Bank, on request. It is the responsibility of every health care consumer to report concerns about their health care providers to local or state medical societies or licensing agencies for investigation. Report concerns about billing-related fraud or abuse directly to the Health Care Finance Administration (HCFA).

> **What do you think?**
>
> *If you had access to a HEDIS health care report card for the hospitals in your area, would you try to switch your upcoming surgery to the hospital having the lowest complication and mortality rate? ✳ Have you ever checked on a doctor's or health care facility's credentials, or do you take it for granted that they are licensed, certified, or accredited?*

Issues Facing Today's Health Care System

Many Americans believe that our health care system needs fundamental reform. What are the problems that have brought us to this point? Cost, access, malpractice, restriction in choice of provider and treatment modality, unnecessary procedures, complicated and cumbersome insurance rules, and dramatic ranges in quality are among the issues of concern. One of the most frequently voiced criticisms concerns lack of access to adequate health insurance, as many Americans have had increasing difficulty obtaining comprehensive coverage from their employers. Until recently, insurance benefits were often

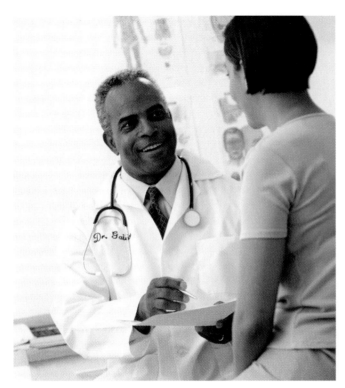

It is important to have an open and honest relationship with your health care provider. Asking questions and providing accurate information will help you make the best decisions about your medical treatment.

lost when employees changed jobs, which caused many to remain in undesirable positions to avoid losing health benefits. This phenomenon, known as *job lock,* led the federal government to pass legislation mandating the "portability" of health insurance benefits from one job to the next, thereby guaranteeing coverage during the transition. Today, individuals who leave their jobs have the option of continued group health insurance benefits under the Consolidated Omnibus Budget Reconciliation Act (COBRA) law. COBRA gives former employees, retirees, spouses, and dependents the right to temporary continuation of insurance at group rates. COBRA beneficiaries pay for their benefits, but they usually have better coverage than they can receive as individuals.

More than 90 million people in the United States suffer from chronic health conditions that should be at least monitored by medical practitioners.[9] Their access to care is largely determined by whether they have health insurance. Catastrophic or chronic illness among only 10 percent of the population accounts for 75 percent of all health expenditures.[10] Since we cannot perfectly predict who will fall into that 10 percent, every American is potentially vulnerable to the high cost and devastating effects of such illnesses.

Cost

Both per capita and as a percentage of gross domestic product (GDP), we spend more on health care than any other nation. Yet, unlike the rest of the industrialized world, we do not provide access for our entire population. In 2001, we spent more than $1.4 trillion on health care; this averages more than $5,035 for every man, woman, and child. This translates into nearly 13 percent of our GDP, up from 5 percent of the GDP in 1960. Health care expenditures are projected to reach $3.1 trillion annually by 2012, growing at a rate of 7.3 percent between 2002 and 2012. Amazingly, by 2012 health care costs will make up nearly 18 percent of our GDP.[11] Why do health care costs continue to spiral upward? There are many factors involved: excess administrative costs, duplication of services, an aging population, demand for new diagnostic and treatment technologies, an emphasis on crisis-oriented care instead of prevention, inappropriate utilization of services by consumers, and related factors.

Our system has more than 2,000 health insurance companies, each with different coverage structures and administrative requirements. This lack of uniformity prevents our system from achieving *economies of scale* (bulk purchasing at a reduced cost) and administrative efficiency realized in countries where there is a single-payer delivery system. According to the Health Insurance Association of America (HIAA), commercial insurance companies commonly experience administrative costs greater than 10 percent of the total health care insurance premium, whereas the administrative cost of the government's Medicare program is less than 4 percent. Administrative expenses in the private sector contribute to the high cost of health care and force companies to require employees to share more of the costs, cut back on benefits, and drop some benefits altogether. These costs are largely passed on to consumers in the form of higher prices.

The declining availability of health insurance coverage means more Americans are uninsured or underinsured. These people are unable to access preventive care and seek treatment only in the event of an emergency or crisis. Because emergency care is extraordinarily expensive, they often are unable to pay, and the cost is absorbed by those who *can* pay—the insured or taxpayers. This process is known as *cost shifting.*

Access

Access to health care is determined by numerous factors, including the supply of providers and facilities, proximity to care, ability to maneuver in the system, health status, and insurance coverage. Although there are approximately 700,000 physicians in the United States, many Americans do not have adequate access to health care or other health services because of insurance barriers or maldistribution of providers. There is an oversupply of higher-paid specialists and a shortage of lower-paid primary care physicians (family practitioners, pediatricians, internists, OB/GYNs, geriatricians, and gerontologists). Inner cities and some rural areas face constant shortages of physicians.

Managed-care health plans determine access on the basis of participating providers, health plan benefits, and administrative rules. Often this means that consumers do not have the freedom to choose specialists, facilities, or treatment options beyond those contracted with the health plan and recommended by their primary care provider (also known as *gatekeeper*). In the United States, consumer demand has led to an expansion of benefits to include nonallopathic therapies, such as chiropractic and acupuncture (see Chapter 18). However, many nonallopathic treatments remain unavailable through current health plans.

Quality and Malpractice

The U.S. health care system employs several mechanisms for ensuring quality services: education, licensure, certification/registration, accreditation, peer review, and, as a last resort, the legal system of malpractice litigation. Some of these mechanisms are mandatory before a professional or organization may provide care, whereas others are purely voluntary. (Be aware that licensure, although state mandated for some practitioners and facilities, is only a minimum guarantee of quality.) Insurance companies and government payers may also require a higher level of quality by linking payment to whether a practitioner is board certified or a facility is accredited by the appropriate agency. In addition, most insurance plans now require prior authorization and/or second opinions not only to reduce costs but also to improve quality of care.

Quality is now measured using "outcome" as the primary indicator. This involves assessing not only what is done to the patient, but what subsequently happens to the patient's health status.

Of course, medical errors and mistakes do happen. An Institute of Medicine report indicates that as many as 44,000 to 98,000 people die in U.S. hospitals each year as the result of medical errors—more than the number who die from motor vehicle accidents, breast cancer, or AIDS.[12] Clearly, we must be as proactive as possible in our health care.

> ### What do you think?
> *Do you believe prospective patients should have access to information about practitioners' and facilities' malpractice records? ✳ About their success and failure rates or outcomes of various procedures?*

Third-Party Payers

The fundamental principle of insurance underwriting is that the cost of health care can be predicted for large populations. This is how health care premiums (payments) are determined. Policyholders pay premiums into a pool, which is held in reserve until needed. When you are sick or injured, the insurance company pays out of the pool, regardless of your total amount of contribution. Depending on circumstances, you may never pay for what your medical care

costs, or you may pay much more for insurance than your medical bills ever total. The idea is that you pay in affordable premiums so that you never have to face catastrophic bills. In today's profit-oriented system, insurers prefer to have healthy people in their plans who pour money into risk pools without taking money out.

Unfortunately, not everyone has health insurance. Almost 40 million Americans are uninsured at any given point in time—that is, they have no private health insurance and are not eligible for Medicare, Medicaid, or other health programs. The number of the uninsured has been growing since the late 1970s. Lack of health insurance has been associated with delayed health care and increased mortality. *Underinsurance* (i.e., the inability to pay out-of-pocket expenses despite having insurance) also may result in adverse health consequences. Findings from the most recent Agency for Healthcare Research and Quality survey indicate that a large proportion of all adults are either uninsured or underinsured. In 2001, 25.9 percent of the nonelderly population was uninsured at some point during the year, and 13.1 percent was uninsured for the entire year.[13] Another 41 million Americans are estimated to be underinsured (at risk for spending more than 10 percent of their income on medical care because their insurance is inadequate).[14]

Contrary to the common belief that the uninsured are unemployed, 75 percent of them are either workers or the dependents of workers. Twenty-five percent are children under age 16. College students are one of the largest groups of the uninsured who are not in the labor force. This presents a difficult dilemma for both universities and students when they must seek care because most university insurance plans are designed as short-term, noncatastrophic plans having low upper limits of benefits. As a full-time student, you should consider purchasing a higher level catastrophic plan to protect yourself in the event of a rare, but very costly, illness or accident.

Private Health Insurance

Health insurance, as it originally developed in the past century, consisted solely of coverage for hospital costs (it was called *major medical*), but gradually it was extended to cover routine physicians' treatment and other areas such as dental services and pharmaceuticals. Payment mechanisms used until recently laid the groundwork for today's steadily rising health care costs. Hospitals were reimbursed for the costs of providing care plus an amount for profit. This system provided no incentive to contain costs, limit the number of procedures, or curtail capital investment in redundant equipment and facilities. Physicians were reimbursed on a fee-for-service (indemnity) basis determined by "usual, customary, and reasonable" fees. This system encouraged physicians to charge high fees, raise them often, and perform as many procedures as possible. At the same time, because most insurance did not cover routine or preventive services, consumers were encouraged to use hospitals whenever possible (the coverage was better) and to wait until illness developed to seek care instead of seeking preventive care. Consumers were also free to choose any provider or service they wished, including even inappropriate—and often very expensive—levels of care.

Private insurance companies have increasingly employed several mechanisms to limit potential losses: cost-sharing (in the form of deductibles, copayments, and coinsurance), exclusions, "preexisting condition" clauses, waiting periods, and upper limits on payments. *Deductibles* are front-end payments (commonly $250 to $1,000) that you must make to your provider before your insurance company will start paying for any services you use. *Copayments* are set amounts that you pay per service received, regardless of the cost of the service (e.g., $10 per doctor visit or per prescription). *Coinsurance* is the percentage of the bill that you must pay throughout the course of treatment (e.g., 20 percent of the total bill). *Preexisting condition clauses* limit the insurance company's liability for medical conditions that a consumer had before obtaining coverage (i.e., if a woman takes out coverage while she is pregnant, the insurance company may cover pregnancy complications and infant care but may not cover charges related to "normal pregnancy"). Because many insurance companies use a combination of these mechanisms, keeping track of the costs you are responsible for can become very difficult.

Group plans of large employers (government agencies, school districts, and corporations, for example) generally do not have preexisting condition clauses in their plans. But smaller group plans (a group may be as small as two people) often do. Some plans never cover preexisting conditions, whereas others specify a *waiting period* (such as six months) before they will provide coverage. All insurers set some limits on the types of services they will cover (e.g., most exclude cosmetic surgery, private rooms, and experimental procedures). Some insurance plans may also include an *upper* or *lifetime limit,* after which coverage will end. Although $250,000 may seem like an enormous sum, medical bills for a sick child or chronic disease can easily run this high within a few years.

Medicare and Medicaid

After years of debate about whether we should have a national health program like those of most industrialized countries, the U.S. government directed the system toward a mixed private and public approach in the 1960s. Most Americans obtained their health insurance through their employers. But this left out two groups—the nonworking poor and the aged. In 1965, amendments to the 1935 Social Security Act established Medicare and Medicaid. Although enacted simultaneously, these programs were vastly different.

Medicare—basically federal social insurance covering 99 percent of the elderly over 65 years of age, all totally and permanently disabled people (after a waiting period), and all people with end-stage renal failure—is a universal program that covers a broad range of services except long-term care. In 2003, coverage was expanded to include prescription drugs, subject to restrictions. It currently covers 36 million people. Medicare is widely accepted by physicians and hospitals and has relatively low administrative costs.

In contrast, **Medicaid,** which covers approximately 35 million people, is a federal–state matching funds welfare program for people who are defined as poor. Because each state determines income eligibility levels and payments to providers, there are vast differences in the way Medicaid operates from state to state.

To control hospital costs, in 1983 the federal government set up a prospective payment system based on **diagnosis related groups (DRGs)** for Medicare. Based on a complicated formula, nearly 500 groupings of diagnoses were created to establish how much a hospital would be reimbursed for a particular patient. If a hospital can treat the patient for less than that amount, it can keep the difference. However, if a patient's care costs more than the set amount, the hospital must absorb the difference (with a few exceptions that must be reviewed by a panel). This system gives hospitals the incentive to discharge patients quickly after doing as little as possible for them, provide more ambulatory care, and admit only patients with favorable (profitable) DRGs.

In its continued efforts to control rising costs, HCFA has encouraged the growth of prepaid HMO senior plans for Medicare-eligible persons. Under this system, commercial managed care insurance plans receive a fixed per-capita premium from HCFA and then offer more preventive services with lower out-of-pocket copayments. These managed care plans encourage providers and patients to utilize health care resources under administrative rules similar to commercial HMO plans. Similarly, states have encouraged the growth of managed Medicaid programs.

Managed Care

Managed care describes a health care delivery system composed of the following elements:

1. A budget based on an estimate of the annual cost of delivering health care for a given population
2. A network of physicians, hospitals, and other providers and facilities linked contractually to deliver comprehensive health benefits within that predetermined budget, thus sharing economic risk for any budget deficit or surplus

---

Medicare   Federal health insurance program for the elderly and the permanently disabled.

Medicaid   Federal–state health insurance program for the poor.

Diagnosis related groups (DRGs)   Diagnostic categories established by the federal government to determine in advance how much hospitals will be reimbursed for the care of a particular Medicare patient.

Managed care   Cost-control procedures used by health insurers to coordinate treatment.

---

3. An established set of administrative rules requiring patients to follow the advice of participating health care providers in order to have their health care paid under the terms of the health plan

Many such plans pay their contracted health care providers through **capitation,** that is, prepayment of a fixed monthly amount for each patient without regard of the type or number of health services provided. Some plans pay health care providers' salaries, and some are still fee-for-service plans. As with other insurance plans, enrollees are members of a risk pool, and it is expected that some persons will use no services, some will use a modest amount, and others will have high-cost utilization over a given year. Doctors have the incentive to keep their patient pool healthy and avoid catastrophic ailments that are preventable; usually such incentives come back in terms of increased salaries, bonuses, and other benefits. As such, prevention and health education to reduce risk and intervene early to avoid major problems should be capstone components of such plans.

Managed care plans are commonplace, with more than 60 million Americans enrolled in one type, the HMO, and another 90 million in other forms of managed care. Four million beneficiaries are in Medicare HMOs, with enrollment growing by about 80,000 people a month.[15] Types of managed care plans include HMOs, point of service (POS) plans, and preferred provider organizations (PPOs).

Health Maintenance Organizations

HMOs provide a wide range of covered health benefits, such as checkups, surgery, doctor visits, and lab tests, for a fixed amount prepaid by you, your employer, Medicaid, or Medicare.[16] Usually, HMO premiums are the least expensive form of managed care (saving between 10 and 40 percent more than other plans), but also the most restrictive. There are low or no deductibles or coinsurance payments, and copayments are $5 to $10 per office visit. HMOs contract with providers to supply health services for enrollees through various systems,[17] such as the following:

- *The staff model.* You receive care from salaried staff doctors at the HMO's facility.
- *The group network model.* The HMO contracts with one or several groups of doctors who provide care for a fixed amount per plan member. Groups often practice in one facility.
- *The independent practice association (IPA).* Doctors in private practice form an IPA that contracts with HMOs. The physicians generally work in their own offices.

The downside of HMOs is that patients are typically required to use the plan's doctors and hospitals and to get approval from a "gatekeeper" or primary care physician for treatment and referrals. Although more and more people have opted for HMOs, criticisms of the plans are mounting. Currently, a class action suit is pending against a major HMO over "denial of service" that plaintiffs say endangered their lives. If such cases succeed, HMOs may need to change their business practices or face significant financial risk.

Other concerns leveled against HMOs include issues such as the following.

- Do highly paid administrators and stockholders ration care, thus allocating more care to those who are better able to pay and enjoy better health?
- Does the huge administrative structure imposed by the HMO make it virtually impossible for patients to sue in the event of clear violations?
- Are patients denied costly diagnostic tests because such tests cut into bottom-line profits? Are some tests given too late because of cost concerns?
- Are HMOs really focused on prevention or intervention? Evidence exists that the fee structure of many HMOs actually discourages basic preventive services, such as immunizations.
- Are doctors allowed to use their best judgment and skills to treat patients, or do policies and profit-motivated concerns interfere with the doctors' roles as advocates for their patients?
- Are the obstacles imposed by HMOs too daunting for patients in need of urgent care?
- Do HMO cost-saving policies force patients out of hospitals and treatment centers too early?

Point of Service

The POS option often provides a more acceptable form of managed care for those used to the traditional indemnity plan of insurance; this probably explains why POS is among the fastest growing of the managed care plans. Under POS, patients can go to providers outside their HMO for care but must pay for the extra cost. Usually this is a reasonable alternative for middle-class or wealthy Americans who are willing to pay extra for choices in care.[18]

Preferred Provider Organizations

PPOs are networks of independent doctors and hospitals that contract to provide care at discounted rates. Although they offer greater choices in doctors than HMOs do, they are less likely to coordinate a patient's care. In addition, although members have a choice of seeing doctors who are not on the preferred list, this choice may come at considerable cost (such as having to pay 30 percent of the charges out of pocket, rather than 10 to 20 percent for PPO doctors and services).[19]

> **What do you think?**
>
> *Why is it important for private insurance to cover preventive or lower-level care as well as hospitalization and high-technology interventions?*
> * *What kinds of incentives would cause you to seek help early rather than to delay care?*

> **Capitation** Prepayment of a fixed monthly amount without regard to the type or number of services provided.

Make It Happen!

Assessment: The Assess Yourself box on page 441 asks you to look at your behavior as a health care consumer. Once you have considered your responses, you may want to change or improve certain behaviors in order to get the best treatment from your health care provider and the heath care system.

Making a Change: In order to change your behavior, you need to develop a plan. Follow these steps.

1. Evaluate your behavior, and identify patterns and specific things you are doing. What can you change now? What can you change in the near future?
2. Select one pattern of behavior that you want to change.
3. Fill out a Behavior Change Contract. It should include your long-term goal for change, your short-term goals, the rewards you'll give yourself for reaching these goals, potential obstacles along the way, and strategies for overcoming these obstacles. For each goal, list the small steps and specific actions that you will take.

4. Chart your progress in a journal. At the end of a week, consider how successful you were in following your plan. What helped you be successful? What made change more difficult? What will you do differently next week?
5. Revise your plan as needed. Are the short-term goals attainable? Are the rewards satisfying?

Example: When Theo reviewed his answers in the self-assessment, it was clear to him that he needed to pay more attention to the medication he took for his asthma. Although he was supposed to take the same dose every day, when he was feeling healthy he would take only half of the prescribed dosage in order to save money. Theo also wasn't sure what side effects were considered normal with his medication and had not mentioned any of them to his doctor, Dr. Higuchi. He also had recently started taking an herbal supplement that his roommate had recommended to help his weight-lifting, but he hadn't mentioned the supplement to his doctor either.

Theo's first step was to make an appointment with Dr. Higuchi to discuss some of his questions and concerns about his medication. He made a list

ahead of time of what he wanted to talk about to be sure he didn't forget any of his questions. He also started keeping track of the side effects he was experiencing, so he could give the doctor a clear picture of his health. Finally, he made a note of the name and ingredients of the supplement and decided not to take it until he could ask about any potential interaction it might have with his asthma medication.

Theo's meeting with Dr. Higuchi went well. When Theo explained that he was trying to save money by using less of the medication than prescribed, Dr. Higuchi found a generic equivalent that cost much less. He reminded Theo about the importance of taking the correct dose and explained that some of the side effects that he reported were caused by the variation in the amount of medication he was taking. He also told Theo that the herbal supplement would make the asthma medication much less effective, an interaction not disclosed on the supplement's label. Theo agreed that now he could afford to take the medication exactly as prescribed, and scheduled a follow-up appointment in six months to report on any further concerns he might have.

Summary

* Advertisers of health care products and services use sophisticated tactics to attract attention and get business. Advertising claims sometimes appear to be supported by spontaneous remission (symptoms disappearing without any apparent cause) or the placebo effect (symptoms disappearing because you think they should), rather than the efficacy of the product or service.
* Self-care and individual responsibility are key factors in reducing rising health care costs and improving health status. Advance planning can help you navigate health care treatment in unfamiliar situations or emergencies. Assess health professionals by considering their qualifications, their record of treating problems like yours, and their ability to work with you.

* In theory, allopathic (traditional Western) medicine is based on scientifically validated methods and procedures. Medical doctors, specialists of various kinds, nurses, physician assistants, and other health care professionals practice allopathic medicine.
* Health care providers may provide services as solo practitioners or in group practices that share overhead cost. Hospitals and clinics are classified by profit status, ownership, specialty, and teaching status.
* Concerns about the U.S. health care system include cost, access, choice of treatment modality, quality and malpractice, and fraud and abuse.
* Health insurance is based on the concept of spreading risk. Insurance is provided by private insurance companies

(which charge premiums) and the government Medicare and Medicaid programs (funded by taxes). Managed care (in the form of HMOs, POS plans, and PPOs) attempts to control costs by streamlining administrative procedures and stressing preventive care (among other initiatives).

Questions for Discussion and Reflection

1. What claims do marketers use to get people to try their health-related products? Why are consumers susceptible to such ploys? What could be done to increase the accuracy of messages related to health care?
2. List several conditions (resulting from illness or accident) for which you wouldn't need to seek medical help. When would you consider each condition to be bad enough to require medical attention? How would you decide to whom and where to go for treatment?
3. What are the pros and cons of group practices? Of non-profit and for-profit hospitals? If you had health insurance, where do you believe you would get the best care? On what do you base your choice?
4. What are the inherent benefits and risks of managed care organizations?
5. Explain the differences between traditional indemnity insurance and managed health care. Which would you feel more comfortable with? Should insurance companies dictate rates for various medical tests and procedures in an attempt to keep prices down?

Accessing Your Health on the Internet

Visit the following Internet sites to explore further topics and issues related to personal health. To visit an organization's website, go to the Companion Website for *Health: The Basics, Sixth Edition* at www.aw-bc.com/donatelle, click on the book image, and select "Accessing Your Health on the Internet" from the navigation menu on the left.

1. *Agency for Health Care Research and Quality (AHRQ).* A gateway to consumer health information. Provides links to sites that can address health care concerns and provide information on what questions to ask, what to look for, and what you should know when making critical decisions about personal care.

2. *Food and Drug Administration (FDA).* News on the latest government-approved home health tests and other health-related products.
3. *National Committee for Quality Assurance (NCQA).* The NCQA assesses and reports on the quality of managed care plans, including HMOs.
4. *National Library of Medicine—General Information Center for Health-Related Research.* Supports Medline/Pubmed information retrieval systems in addition to providing public health information for consumers.

Further Reading

Birenbaum, Arnold. *Wounded Profession: American Medicine Enters the Age of Managed Care.* Westport, CT: Praeger Publishers, 2002.

Birenbaum describes the rise of HMOs in the nineties and the increasing backlash against them, and presents ideas for reform of the health care system.

Geyman, John. *Health Care in America: Can Our Ailing System Be Healed?* London: Butterworth-Heinemann, 2001.

Written from the perspective of a physician, this book focuses on the challenges—escalating costs, limitations of access, and a wide range of quality—facing the health care system.

Lee, Philip, and Carroll Estes. *The Nation's Health, 7th ed.* Sudbury, MA: Jones and Bartlett, 2003.

Presents an overview of factors affecting the health of Americans and the roles of public health, medical care, and the community in ensuring the nation's health. Special emphasis on health determinants, women's health, long-term care, and the uncertainties of tomorrow's health care system.

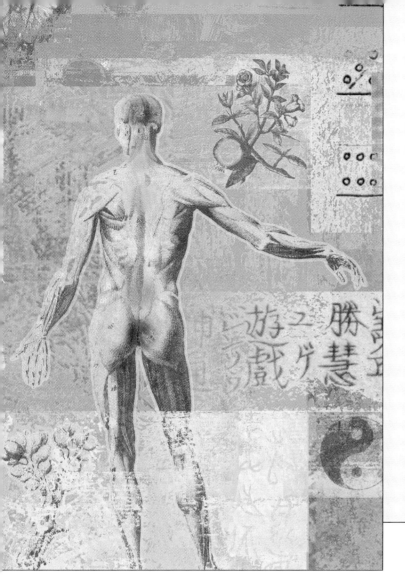

Complementary and Alternative Medicine

New Choices and Responsibilities for Healthwise Consumers

Objectives

* Describe complementary and alternative medicine and identify its typical domains. Explain why it is growing in popularity in the United States and throughout the world, and who is most likely to use it.

* Describe major types of complementary and alternative medicine providers and common treatments they offer.

* Discuss the various types of complementary and alternative medicines being used in America today, their patterns of use, and their potential benefits and risks.

* Explain how to evaluate testimonials and claims related to complementary and alternative products and services, and how to ensure that you are getting accurate information and sound treatment.

* Discuss the challenges and opportunities related to complementary and alternative medicine in ensuring our health and wellness.

At Bronx Botanical Garden, Mainstream Doctors Meet Kava and Cohosh

By Leslie Berger

It's hard to imagine a doctor more solidly mainstream than Frederick Small, a gynecologist from suburban Tenafly, NJ, with an old-school practitioner's reassuring manner, a grandfather's head of clipped white hair and not much experience with alternative medicine.

Yet there he was last week at the New York Botanical Garden, with his laminated name tag and neatly pressed summer shirt, participating in a conference called "Botanical Medicine in Modern Clinical Practice," immersed in the world of roots and decoctions and admiring live specimens like a kava tree.

"This is actually my first conference of this kind," Dr. Small said during lunch in the garden's Terrace Room.

Read the complete article online in the eThemes section of this book's website: www.aw-bc.com/donatelle.

Consumers today face an amazing array of choices when they consider taking action to improve their health. One of the newest movements toward self-care and health promotion focuses on *complementary and alternative medicine (CAM)*. Various foods, products, and services offer us a new range of health options and an opportunity for greater control over our own health care.

Complementary and Alternative Medicine: What Is It and Who Uses It?

If you think that alternative medicine is just a fad, you are in for a surprise. Today, Americans and people from most other cultures of the world are much more likely to try therapies once considered exotic and strange. This is particularly true as America becomes a composite of people from different regions and cultures of the world. Many of these cultures are contributing their unique beliefs about remedies to restore health and treat afflictions. Referred to as **complementary and alternative medicine (CAM),** these therapies are defined as "neither being taught widely in U.S. medical schools nor generally available in U.S. hospitals during the previous year."[1] Although often used interchangeably, there is a distinction between *complementary* and *alternative* medicine. **Complementary medicine** is used *with* conventional medicine, as part of the modern integrative medical approach (an aromatherapist might work with an oncologist to reduce a patient's nausea during chemotherapy, for example). **Alternative medicine** is used *in place of* conventional medicine; for example, following a special diet to treat cancer instead of using surgery or other traditional treatments.

Therapies vary widely in terms of nature of treatment, extent of therapy, and types of problems for which they offer help. Typically, CAM therapies are compared with the more familiar allopathic (traditional Western) treatments offered by individuals who graduate from schools of medicine accredited in the United States or are licensed medical practitioners recognized by the American Medical Association (AMA) and its governing board.[2] The list of practices that are considered CAM changes continually as CAM therapies that are proven safe and effective become accepted as "mainstream."[3] CAM therapies, in general, serve as alternatives to an allopathic system that some people regard as too invasive, high tech, and toxic in terms of laboratory-produced medications. Explore your opinions about CAM in the Assess Yourself box.

Complementary and alternative medicine (CAM)
Forms of treatment distinct from traditional allopathic medicine that until recently were neither taught widely in U.S. medical schools nor generally available in U.S. hospitals.

Complementary medicine Treatment used in conjunction with conventional medicine.

Alternative medicine Treatment used in place of conventional medicine.

Evaluating Complementary and Alternative Medicine

You may have a range of opinions about CAM, depending on the therapies described. Use the questions below to explore your assumptions about CAM.

1. What types of medical professionals do you think should call themselves a *holistic health practitioner*?
2. What is meant by the term *mind–body medicine*?
3. What type of person do you think is most likely to seek alternative or complementary medical treatment?
4. Would you tell your doctor you were taking herbal supplements?
5. Would you tell your doctor if you were consulting an alternative medicine practitioner?
6. Would you try hypnosis to quit smoking or lose weight? Why or why not?
7. Do you consider yoga or tai chi forms of alternative medicine?
8. If a person with severe pain claimed that wearing a magnetic bracelet worked, would you try it or recommend it to someone else?
9. Should health insurance cover complementary or alternative medical treatments?
10. Should herbal supplements be tested and regulated by the federal government?

CAM in the United States Today

In 1993, a landmark study showed that one in three Americans sought some form of alternative care.[4] A follow-up study five years later found that these numbers had jumped to 47 percent, reflecting an unprecedented explosion in use. By 2002, total out-of-pocket expenditures for alternative care were conservatively estimated at $307 billion, which is comparable to out-of-pocket expenditures for all U.S. physician services. Additionally, an estimated 15 million Americans took prescription medications concurrently with herbal remedies or high-dose vitamins and supplements, which are not considered in these estimates.[5]

Although it is widely assumed that increasing numbers of us are choosing alternative care, we have known little about the nature and extent of CAM use until fairly recently. According to the studies cited above, the most frequently used alternatives to conventional medicine are:

- Relaxation techniques (16.9 percent of respondents)
- Chiropractic (31 percent)
- Massage (18 percent)
- Self-help (13 percent)
- Energy healing (6 percent)
- Other therapies (16 percent)

Major Domains of CAM

The United States government not only has sanctioned the concept of CAM in prevention and treatment, but also has moved aggressively to create the National Center for Complementary and Alternative Medicine (NCCAM) within the National Institutes of Health (NIH). This center serves as a clearinghouse for CAM information and a focal point for re-search initiatives, policy development, and general recommendations for CAM use. NCCAM broadly groups CAM practices into five major domains: (1) alternative medical systems, (2) manipulative and body-based methods, (3) energy therapies, (4) mind–body interventions, and (5) biologically based treatments. Many of these alternatives are discussed in other parts of this book. In this chapter, we focus on alternatives that have become increasingly popular in recent years or that are of particular interest to college students.

Alternative Medical Systems

Alternative medical systems involve complete systems of theory and practice that have evolved independently of, and often prior to, the conventional biomedical approach that we tend to think of as "traditional." In the United States, the term *traditional* or *allopathic* has historically referred to a system that is directed by AMA guidelines for licensing and that most insurance plans cover as standard and acceptable procedure. In contrast, *nonallopathic* medicine has been dubbed as "alternative." This situation is changing. In the past decade, some specialists in nonallopathic medicine have been accepted by professional groups, and their inclusion in mainstream medicine is growing daily. Many traditional medical schools are now offering coursework in CAM, and many traditional doctors refer patients to alternative providers, who are, in turn, reimbursed by the patients' health insurance plans. Modalities that have received the greatest degree of acceptance include chiropractic medicine, acupuncture, herbal and homeopathic medicine, and naturopathy. However, it is important to realize that there are many other systems of medicine that have been practiced by various cultures throughout the world. Many come from venerable Asian approaches.[6]

Traditional Oriental Medicine and Ayurveda

Two major systems that are at the root of much of our CAM thinking today are the traditional oriental medicine system, and the Ayurvedic system, which is India's traditional system of medicine. **Traditional oriental medicine (TOM)** emphasizes the proper balance or disturbances of **qi** (pronounced "chi"), or vital energy in health and disease, respectively.[7] In TOM, diagnosis is based on history, on observation of the body (especially the tongue), on palpation, and on pulse diagnosis; this elaborate procedure requires considerable skill and experience by the practitioner. Techniques such as acupuncture, herbal medicine, oriental massage, and *qi gong* (a form of energy therapy described in more detail later in this chapter) are among the TOM approaches to health and healing.

Ayurveda (or **Ayurvedic medicine**) relates to the "science of life," which places equal emphasis on body, mind, and spirit and strives to restore the innate harmony of the individual. Ayurvedic practitioners diagnose mostly by observation and touch and assign patients to one of three major body types and a variety of subtypes. Once classified, patients are treated mostly through dietary modifications and herbal remedies that have been drawn from the vast botanical wealth of the Indian subcontinent. Treatments may also include animal and mineral ingredients, even powdered gemstones. Massage, steam baths, exposure to sunlight, and controlled breathing are among the more common Ayurvedic treatments.[8]

Homeopathy and Naturopathy

Other alternative systems of medicine include **homeopathy** and **naturopathy**. *Homeopathic medicine* is an unconventional Western system based on the principle that "like cures like." In other words, the same substance that in large doses produces the symptoms of an illness will in very small doses cure the illness.[9] Essentially, homeopathic physicians use herbal medicine, minerals, and chemicals in extremely diluted forms as natural agents to kill or ward off illnesses that are caused by more potent forms or doses of those agents.

Naturopathic medicine views disease as a manifestation of an alteration in the processes by which the body naturally heals itself. Disease results from the body's effort to ward off impurities and harmful substances from the environment. Naturopathic physicians emphasize restoring health rather than curing disease. They employ an array of healing practices, including diet and clinical nutrition; homeopathy; acupuncture; herbal medicine; hydrotherapy (the use of water in a range of temperatures and methods of applications); spinal and soft-tissue manipulation; physical therapies involving electric currents, ultrasound, and light therapy; therapeutic counseling; and pharmacology. Three major naturopathic schools in the United States and Canada provide thorough training, conferring the *naturopathic doctor (N.D.)* degree on students who have completed a four-year graduate program that emphasizes humanistically oriented family medicine.

While these medical philosophies and patterns of treatment have exerted great influence on populations worldwide, other, more regionally limited, traditional medical systems are also noteworthy. Native American, Aboriginal, African, Middle Eastern, Tibetan, and South American cultures also have their own unique alternative systems. International surveys of CAM outside the United States suggest that alternative therapies are popular throughout most of the world. Public opinion polls and consumer surveys in Europe and the United Kingdom suggest high CAM use in Italy, France, Denmark, Finland, and Australia, in addition to most Asian cultures.[10]

As the number of alternative therapists grows and systems become intertwined, so do the number of health care options available to consumers (see Table 18.1 for examples). Before considering any medical system, wise consumers will consult reliable resources to thoroughly evaluate risks, the scientific basis of claimed benefits, and any contraindications for using the CAM service or product. Avoid practitioners who promote their treatments as a cure-all for every health problem or who seem to promise remedies that have thus far defied the best scientific efforts of mainstream medicine. Wise consumers apply the same strategies to researching CAM as they do to choosing allopathic care (see Chapter 17).

Traditional oriental medicine (TOM) Comprehensive system of diagnosis and treatment in which dietary change, touch, massage, medicinal teas, and other herbal medicines are used extensively.

Qi Element of traditional oriental medicine that refers to the vital energy force that courses through the body. When qi is in balance, health is restored.

Ayurveda (Ayurvedic medicine) A method of treatment derived largely from ancient India, in which practitioners diagnose by observation and touch and then assign a largely dietary treatment laced with herbal medicines.

Homeopathy Unconventional Western system of medicine based on principle that "like cures like."

Naturopathy System of medicine that attempts to restore natural processes of body and promote healing through natural means.

Manipulative and Body-Based Methods

Another category of CAM includes methods that are based on manipulation and/or movement of the body. For example, chiropractors focus on the relationship between the body's structures (primarily the spine) and function and on how that relationship affects the preservation and restoration of health. Chiropractors use manipulation as a key therapy.[11]

Table 18.1
Popular Complementary Treatments

Aromatherapy	Aromatherapists use scented materials to evoke sensations through the smell centers of the body. Treatment focuses on odors regarded as pleasurable.
Energy healing	Different therapies are based on the philosophy that humans produce waves of energy that are disrupted during illness.
Food therapy	Treatment is based on the belief that many disorders are based on allergies and toxic synergism among food combinations. Naturopaths test for and treat food allergies and assign special diets designed to produce nutritional balance.
Hypnosis	The treatment of disease by suggestion while the patient is in a hypnotic trance.
Massage	Massage involves rubbing, stroking, kneading, or lightly pounding the body with the hands or other instruments.
Megavitamins	Treatment with megavitamins promotes the consumption of large doses of common essential vitamins and minerals to prevent disease and heal illness.
Relaxation techniques	The goal is to remove stress and promote healing. Techniques include yoga, meditation, breathing and posture exercises, and visualization.

Chiropractic Medicine

Chiropractic medicine has been practiced for more than 100 years. A century ago, allopathic medicine and chiropractic medicine were in direct competition.[12] Today, however, many managed care organizations work closely with chiropractors, and many insurance companies will pay for chiropractic treatment, particularly if it is recommended by a medical doctor. More than 20 million Americans now visit chiropractors each year.

Chiropractic medicine is based on the idea that a life-giving energy flows through the spine via the nervous system. If the spine is subluxated (partly misaligned or dislocated), that force is disrupted. Chiropractors use a variety of techniques to manipulate the spine back into proper alignment so the life-giving energy can flow unimpeded. It has been established that their treatment can be effective for back pain, neck pain, and headaches. The average chiropractic training program requires four years of intensive courses in biochemistry, anatomy, physiology, diagnostics, pathology, nutrition, and related topics, combined with hands-on clinical training. Like allopathic physicians, chiropractors are licensed and regulated by the states in which they practice. You should investigate and question a chiropractor as carefully as you would any licensed medical doctor. As with many health professionals, you may note vast differences in technique among specialists. It is recommended that you choose a chiropractor who follows standard chiropractic regimens for treating musculoskeletal conditions.

Other Manipulation Therapies

There are other specialties that involve manipulation of the body. Recall from Chapter 17 that *D.O.s*, or *doctors of osteopathy*, place particular emphasis on the musculoskeletal system. Osteopaths believe that all of the body's systems work together and that disturbances in one system may have an impact upon function elsewhere in the body.[13] As such, they specialize in body manipulation yet also have a more traditional form of medical school training.

Energy Therapies

Energy therapies focus either on energy fields originating within the body (biofields) or on fields from other sources (electromagnetic fields). Biofield therapies are intended to affect energy fields, whose existence is not experimentally proven, that surround and penetrate the human body. Some forms of energy therapy manipulate biofields by applying pressure and/or manipulating the body by placing the hands in, or through, these fields.[14]

Examples of biofield therapy include qi gong, reiki, and therapeutic touch. *Qi gong,* a component of traditional Chinese medicine, combines movement, meditation, and regulation of breathing to enhance the flow of vital energy (qi), improve blood circulation, and enhance immune function.[15] *Reiki,* whose name derives from the Japanese word representing "universal life energy," is based on the belief that by channeling spiritual energy through the practitioner, the spirit is healed, and it, in turn, heals the physical body.[16] *Therapeutic touch* is derived from the ancient technique of "laying on" of hands. It is based on the premise that the healing force of the therapist can bring about the patient's recovery and healing by promoting a balance in the body's

---

Chiropractic medicine Manipulation of the spine to allow proper energy flow.

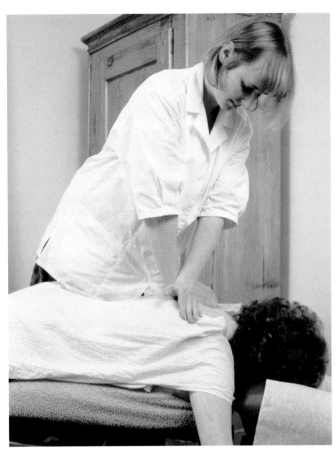

A chiropractor treats a patient using a variety of techniques to manipulate the spine into proper alignment.

energies. By passing the hands over the body, the healer identifies body imbalances.[17]

Bioelectromagnetic-based therapies involve the unconventional use of electromagnetic fields, such as pulsed fields, magnetic fields, or alternating current or direct current fields, to treat asthma, cancer, pain, migraines, and other conditions. At this point, the energy field techniques mentioned above have little scientific documentation to support their claims. However, there are two derivatives of energy therapy that have gained much wider acceptance in recent years: acupuncture and acupressure.

Acupuncture

Chinese medical treatments are growing in popularity and offer an important complement to Western biomedical care. **Acupuncture,** one of the more popular forms of Chinese medicine among Americans, is sought for a wide variety of health conditions, including musculoskeletal dysfunction, mood enhancement, and wellness promotion. Long, thin needles are inserted into the skin in specific locations to affect the qi, or

Acupuncture   The insertion of long, thin needles to affect the energy flow within the body.

energy pathways. Following acupuncture, most respondents report high satisfaction with the treatment, improved quality of life, improvement in or cure of the condition, and reduced reliance on prescription drugs and surgery.[18]

Acupuncturists in the United States are state licensed, and each state has specific requirements regarding training programs. Most acupuncturists have either completed a two- to three-year postgraduate program to obtain a master of traditional Oriental medicine (M.T.O.M.) degree or attended a shorter certification program in North America or Asia. They may be licensed in multiple areas—for example, the M.T.O.M. is also trained in the use of herbs and moxabustion (the application of a heated herbal moxa stick). Some licensed M.D.s and chiropractors have trained in acupuncture and obtained certification to use this treatment.

Acupressure

Acupressure is similar to acupuncture, but it does not use needles. Instead, the practitioner applies pressure to points critical to balancing yin and yang. Practitioners must have the same basic understanding of energy pathways as do acupuncturists. Acupressure should not be applied by an untrained person to pregnant women or to anyone with a chronic condition.

What do you think?

Why do you think more people are opting for complementary and alternative treatments? ✳ *What are the potential benefits of these treatments?* ✳ *What are the potential risks?* ✳ *What types of controls are reasonable to regulate the quality and consistency of foreign-trained health care providers?*

Mind-Body Interventions

Mind–body interventions employ a variety of techniques designed to facilitate the mind's capacity to affect bodily function and symptoms.[19] Many therapies might fall under this category, but some areas, such as biofeedback, patient education, and cognitive–behavioral techniques, have been so well investigated that they are no longer considered alternative. However, meditation, yoga, tai chi, certain uses of hypnosis, dance, music and art therapy, prayer and mental healing, and others are still categorized as complementary and alternative. (See Chapter 11 for more on yoga and tai chi.)

Body Work

Body work actually consists of several different forms of exercise. *Feldenkrais* work is a system of movements, floor exercises, and body work designed to retrain the central nervous system to find new pathways around areas of blockage or damage. It is gentle and effective in rehabilitating trauma victims. *Rolfing,* a more invasive form of body work, aims to restructure the musculoskeletal system by working on patterns of tension held in deep tissue. The therapist applies firm—sometimes painful—pressure to different areas of the body. Rolfing can release repressed emotions as well as dissipate muscle tension. *Shiatsu* is a traditional healing art from Japan that applies firm finger pressure to specified points on the body and is intended to increase the circulation of vital energy. The client lies on the floor, with the therapist seated alongside. *Trager work,* one of the least invasive forms of body work, employs gentle rocking and bouncing motions to induce states of deep, pleasant relaxation.[20]

> **What do you think?**
>
> *Have you ever tried any of these CAM therapies?* ✳ *Which of them are offered on your campus or in your community?* ✳ *What role does CAM have in your personal quest for physical fitness? Spiritual fitness?*

Biologically Based Therapies

Biologically based therapies use substances found in nature, such as herbs, foods, and vitamins. This is one of the most controversial domains of CAM practice, largely because of the sheer number of options available and the many claims that are made about their supposedly magic effects. Many of these claims have not been thoroughly investigated, and regulation of this aspect of CAM has been relatively slow in coming.

Herbs and plants have been part of medical practice for thousands of years. Today, an estimated 25 percent of all modern pharmaceutical drugs are derived from herbs, including aspirin (white willow bark), the heart medication digitalis (foxglove), and the cancer treatment taxol (Pacific yew tree). Practitioners who base their therapies primarily on the medicinal qualities of plants and herbs are referred to as *herbalists.*

Herbal remedies are not to be taken lightly. Just because something is natural does not necessarily mean that it is safe. For example, a recent Food and Drug Administration (FDA) Consumer Advisory warned that kava products may be associated with severe liver damage.[21] Many plants are poisonous, and others can be toxic if ingested in high doses. Still others are dangerous when combined with prescription or over-the-counter drugs, or they could disrupt the normal action of the drugs. Properly trained herbalists and homeopaths have received graduate-level training in special programs, such as herbal nutrition or traditional Chinese medicine. These practitioners have been trained in diagnosis; in mixing herbs, titrations, and dosages; and in the follow-up of patients.

Checking on the education and training of anyone who recommends or sells herbal medications is a part of intelligent consumerism as well as just plain good sense. Also, it is important to look at the research surrounding individual substances and remedies. The NCCAM website (http://nccam.nih.gov) is a good place to start, since it includes summaries of recent research. It is a good resource for information on the effectiveness and risks of any CAM therapy included in this chapter.

Herbal Remedies

Largely derived from Ayurvedic or traditional Chinese medicine, herbal medications are widely available in the United States. Fueled by mass advertising and promoted as part of multiple vitamin and mineral regimens by major drug manufacturers, herbal supplements represent the hottest trend in the health market.

Herbal remedies come in several different forms. **Tinctures** (extracts of fresh or dried plants) usually contain a high percentage of grain alcohol to prevent spoilage and are among the best herbal options. Freeze-dried extracts are stable and offer good value for your money. Standardized extracts are also among the more reliable forms of herbal preparations.

In general, herbal medicines tend to be milder than chemical drugs and produce their effects more slowly; they also are less likely to cause toxicity because they are diluted rather than concentrated forms of drugs.[22] But diluted or not, herbal products are still drugs. They should not be taken casually, any more than you would take over-the-counter or prescription medications without really needing them or knowing their side effects. No matter how natural they are, herbs still contain many of the same chemicals as synthetic prescription drugs. Too much of an herb can cause problems, particularly one from nonstandardized extracts. Some can interact with prescription drugs or cause unusual side effects. The following discussion gives an overview of some of the most common herbal supplements on the market.

Ginkgo Biloba Ginkgo biloba is an extract from the leaves of a deciduous tree that lives up to 1,000 years, thus making it the world's oldest living tree species that can be traced back more than 200 million years. The ginkgo was almost destroyed during the last Ice Age in all regions of the world except China, where it is considered a sacred tree with medicinal properties.[23] Today, ginkgo leaf extracts are among the leading prescription medicines in Germany and France,

---

Biologically based therapies Treatments that use substances found in nature, such as herbs, foods, and vitamins.

Tinctures Herbal extracts usually combined with grain alcohol to prevent spoilage.

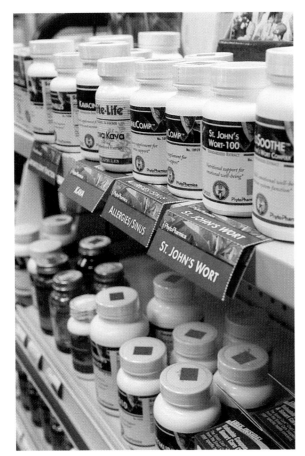

Buying herbal supplements can be confusing because so many brands exist and their manufacture is not strictly regulated for potency and quality.

where they account for nearly 2 percent of total prescription sales.[24]

Purported benefits are many, and ginkgo biloba is used to treat depression; impotence; premenstrual syndrome; diseases of the eye, such as retinopathy and macular degeneration; and general vascular disease. In particular, it has been shown to improve short-term memory and concentration for individuals with impaired blood flow to the brain due to narrowed blood vessels. A Harvard-based study of 202 men and women with mild to moderately severe dementia caused by stroke or Alzheimer's disease was among the first to promote ginkgo in the United States. After one year, the group receiving ginkgo experienced significant improvement in cognitive performance (memory, learning, reading) and social functioning (carrying on conversations, recognizing familiar faces) than those in the placebo group (those who did not receive ginkgo).[25] Much of this improvement was believed to be due to the antioxidant properties of the herb, as well as to its blood-thinning properties that seem to improve blood and oxygen flow through constricted blood vessels. Whether this herb will improve memory in people with normal blood flow remains largely unexplored.

Most nutritional experts and physicians recommend that people who are considering ginkgo take a 40-milligram tablet three times a day for a month or so. If there is no improvement, continuing to take this supplement is largely unwarranted. Also, remember that disturbing memory loss or difficulty thinking, regardless of age, should be checked by a doctor to determine underlying causes. Because the main action of ginkgo appears to be as a blood thinner, it should not be taken with other blood-thinning agents, such as aspirin, vitamin E, garlic, ginger, the prescription drug warfarin (trade name: Coumadin), or any other medications that list thinning of the blood as a potential side effect.[26] Doing so could increase the risk of hemorrhage.

St. John's Wort The bright yellow, star-shaped flowers of St. John's wort (SJW) have a long history of medical use in Europe, Asia, and Africa. Colonists to the United States brought SJW with them, only to find that Native Americans were already using it for everything from snake bite to a general health enhancer. In the United States, SJW grows in abundance in northern California and southern Oregon and is also referred to as *klammath weed*.[27]

Today, SJW enjoys global popularity. It is the favored therapy for depression in a number of countries, including Germany, and actually surpasses most standard antidepressants as the first mode of treatment for clinical depression. Research into the herb has yielded mixed results: some studies have indicated it is more effective than a placebo and has fewer side effects than prescription antidepressants, while others have found no effect on depression at all.[28] Proponents believe SJW acts as a positive mood enhancer by helping maintain levels of serotonin, a natural neurotransmitter that helps brain function and calms the body;[29] helps as a sleep enhancer for those having difficulty sleeping;[30] and supports immune functioning by suppressing the release of interleukin-6, a protein that controls certain aspects of the immune response.[31] As with most antidepressants, SJW's benefits are not felt for about four weeks.

Like other plants, SJW contains a number of different chemicals, many of which are not clearly understood. We do know that there seems to be more to SJW than myth and the simplistic explanations that many health food stores give their customers, and researchers are beginning to view SJW in a less favorable light.

The herb does have several side effects. Most are more bothersome than severe and range from slight gastrointestinal upset to fatigue, dry mouth, dizziness, skin rashes, and itching. Some people develop extreme sensitivity to sunlight. Most of these side effects are minor, however, when compared with those of major antidepressant medicines.

Due to conflicting news about SJW, consumers should proceed with caution. Since the herb is sold in the United States as a dietary supplement, not a drug, it is not regulated by the FDA and rigorous testing has not been done. Anyone suffering from clinical depression should be under a physician's and psychologist's care.

In addition, SJW should never be taken in combination with prescription antidepressants. When combined with other serotonin-enhancing drugs, such as Prozac, SJW may result in serotonin overload, leading to tremors, agitation, or convulsions. SJW also should not be used by pregnant women or women who are nursing, by young children, or by the frail elderly, because the safety margins have not been established.

Echinacea Echinacea, or the *purple coneflower,* is found primarily in the Midwest and the prairie regions of the United States. Two of the nine species of echinacea in the United States are now on the federal endangered species list, a cause of growing concern for many environmentalists as the herb's popularity has grown. In fact, echinacea is the best-selling herb in health and natural food stores in the United States and is widely used throughout most of the world. It is said to stimulate the immune system and increase the effectiveness of the white blood cells that attack bacteria and viruses. Many people believe it to be helpful in preventing and treating the symptoms of a cold or flu. However, echinacea remains controversial. Although many studies in Europe have provided preliminary evidence of its effectiveness, recent controlled trials in the United States indicate that echinacea is no more effective than a placebo in preventing a cold.[32]

As with many herbal treatments, little research has been conducted on the benefits and risks of echinacea. Because it can affect the immune system, people with autoimmune diseases such as arthritis should not take it. Other people who should avoid echinacea include pregnant women, people with diabetes or multiple sclerosis, and anyone allergic to the daisy family of plants.

Green Tea Several studies have shown promising links between green and white tea consumption and cancer prevention, although investigation continues. Now, new research from Japan suggests that drinking one or two cups of green tea per day may keep the heart attack doctor away.[33] Findings indicate that tea drinkers had lower rates of heart attack, thus indicating a possible protective effect. Some scientists suspect that green tea may boost heart health because it contains high levels of flavonoids. These plant compounds, which are also found in fruits, vegetables, and red wine, are thought to boost health by combating oxidation, a process in which cell-damaging free radicals accumulate. Oxidative damage can be caused by outside factors, such as cigarette smoking, or by factors on the cellular level. Oxidation is suspected of increasing the risk of heart disease, stroke, and several other diseases. Although promising, more research on the role of green tea in CVD risk must be conducted to determine whether the effect is actually due to the tea or to some other characteristic that tea drinkers have in common.

Ephedra An herbal ingredient in many weight loss and fitness supplements, ephedra's active ingredient is ephedrine,

which is similar to amphetamine. After years of controversy, a comprehensive study conducted for the FDA by the RAND Corporation released in 2003 indicated that there was limited evidence of an effect of ephedra on short-term weight loss and minimal evidence of an effect on performance enhancement in physical activity.[34] Furthermore, the study reviewed more than 16,000 reported adverse effects from ephedra and noted that heart attack, stroke, and death had occurred in the absence of other contributing factors. Other side effects such as heart palpitations, psychiatric problems, upper gastrointestinal effects, tremor, insomnia, and other problems had occurred at rates much greater than might be expected. In light of these risks, in December 2003 the FDA announced that it would ban the sale of all dietary supplements containing ephedra. The ban would become effective in spring 2004. These products are no longer legally available for sale.

Special Supplements

The FDA defines dietary supplements as "products (other than tobacco) that are intended to supplement or add to the diet and contain one or more of the following ingredients: vitamins, minerals, amino acids, herbs, or other substance that increases total dietary intake, and that is intended for ingestion in the form of a capsule, powder, soft gel, or gel-cap, and is not represented as a conventional food or as a sole item." Typically, people take these supplements to enhance health, prevent disease, or enhance mood. In recent years, we've heard increasing reports on the health benefits of a number of vitamins and minerals.

When taken to increase work output or the potential for it, dietary supplements are labeled as **ergogenic aids.** Examples include bee pollen, caffeine, glycine, carnitine, lecithin, brewer's yeast, and gelatin. In recent years, a new generation of performance-enhancing ergogenic aids has hit the market. Many of these claim to increase muscular strength and performance, boost energy, and enhance resistance to disease.

Muscle Enhancers In 1998, Mark McGwire made headline news not only for his home run record, but also for admitting that he took the diet supplement androstenedione. "Andro," a substance that is found naturally in meat and some plants and is also produced in the human body by the adrenal glands and gonads, is a precursor to the human hormone testosterone (see Chapter 7 for more on andro). In other words, the body converts andro directly into testosterone, which enables an athlete to train harder and recover more quickly. Ironically, although the NCAA, the NFL, and the International Olympic Committee have banned andro, it is readily available over the counter.

Ergogenic aids Special dietary supplements taken to increase strength, energy, and the ability to work.

News from the World of CAM Research

Research is being conducted on complementary and alternative therapies in all areas of health, with investigations into treatments for some conditions making headlines. Recently, experts from Harvard Medical School shared their insights about selected treatments for certain conditions.

CANCER

Although CAM therapies for cancer abound on the Internet and elsewhere, choosing a CAM therapy over conventional treatment is risky business. Promising new research focusing on diet, mind–body techniques, and even shark-cartilage supplements indicates that when CAM is coupled with traditional medicine, treatment may be more bearable and survival rates may improve. Interesting points include the following.

- "Natural" doesn't always mean "safe." High doses of vitamin E and ginkgo biloba have anticoagulant effects that could cause excessive bleeding during surgery, particularly in those already taking aspirin. Soy contains plant estrogens that have not been ruled out in breast or endometrial cancer.
- Some supplements, such as St. John's Wort (SJW), seem to counteract the effects of conventional cancer treatment drugs.
- Antioxidants may limit adverse effects of radiation and chemotherapy. However, recent studies suggest they may also sometimes make these treatments less effective.

- Mind–body therapies, acupuncture, massage, and other remedies may help comfort patients, relieve physical symptoms such as pain and insomnia, alleviate nausea, and improve recovery from treatment.

CARDIOVASCULAR DISEASE

Diet and exercise provide nearly indisputable benefits for reducing CVD risks. Research on other natural strategies is promising, although inconclusive at this time. Findings include the following.

- The Harvard's Nurses' Health Study and Health Professional's Follow-Up Study found reduced rates of CVD in people whose diets are rich in antioxidants such as vitamin E, vitamin A, and beta carotene. However, other studies have refuted these results.
- A large study of chelation therapy (a technique used to clear toxic metals from the bloodstream) may provide results within the next five years. Until this time, the jury is out on this one.
- Supplements to watch out for include ginkgo biloba (can cause excessive bleeding) and ephedra (ma huang), which has been banned by the FDA for its serious side effects, including high blood pressure and irregular heartbeat.

ARTHRITIS

Current treatment for arthritis sufferers has been primarily exercise and acetaminophen (Tylenol) plus non-steroidal anti-inflammatory drugs (NSAIDs) such as aspirin, ibuprofen (Advil), naproxen (Aleve), or celecoxib (Celebrex), and rofecoxib (Vioxx). Many of these, particularly Celebrex and Vioxx, have side effects that cause people to seek alter-

natives, including the following.

- Glucosamine. Although critics abound, many believe that glucosamine may help those suffering from arthritis pain while reducing the gastrointestinal irritation of NSAIDs. However, newer research also indicates that it can interfere with insulin, thus causing increases in blood sugar.
- Chondroitin. Often used with glucosamine, chondroitin may also elevate blood sugar levels and lead to excessive bleeding, particularly among those already on blood thinners and with other risks.
- Herbs and supplements. Although many are touted as arthritis treatments, scientific evidence of pain and symptom relief is lacking.

MEMORY LOSS

While Americans have been buying ginkgo biloba in search of supposed memory-aiding benefits, a 2002 study in *The Journal of the American Medical Association* suggests that the herb does not help healthy people. Another study has shown that it may slow the rate of decline among Alzheimer's patients. A six-year trial started in 1999 and due to be completed in 2005 may shed more light on this. Most research supports the idea that mental activities, such as playing brain teasers and working on puzzles, are the best remedy for slowed memory.

Sources: Adapted from W. Weiger and D. Eisenberg, "Health for Life: The New Science of Alternative Medicine. Cancer: Easing the Treatment," *Newsweek*, December 2, 2002, 49; W. Haskell and D. Eisenberg, "Health for Life: The New Science of Alternative Medicine. Cardiac Disease: Ways to Heal Your Heart," *Newsweek*, December 2, 2002, 52.

Creatine A naturally occurring compound found primarily in skeletal muscle that helps optimize the muscles' energy levels.

The McGwire controversy has encouraged new research into the compound. Results indicate that andro has a chemical structure that is very similar to anabolic steroids, which may result in long-term risks similar to those of the illegal androgens.[35]

Creatine is a naturally occurring compound found primarily in skeletal muscle that helps to optimize the muscles' energy levels. In recent years, the use of creatine supplements has increased dramatically because of claims that it increases muscle energy and allows a person to work harder with less muscle fatigue and build muscle mass with less effort. Reports of creatine's benefits, however, appear exaggerated. More than one-third of people taking creatine are unable to absorb it in the muscles and achieve no benefit. Side effects include muscle cramping, muscle strains, and possible liver and kidney damage.[36]

Ginseng   Grown commercially throughout many regions of the United States, ginseng is much prized for its reported sexual restorative value. It is believed that ginseng affects the pituitary gland, increasing resistance to stress, affecting metabolism, aiding skin and muscle tone, and providing the hormonal balance necessary for a healthy sex life. Other purported benefits include improved endurance, muscle strength, recovery from exercise, oxygen metabolism during exercise, auditory and visual reaction time, and mental concentration.[37] Studies of the effectiveness of ginseng, however, have raised questions about it: Primarily, what are appropriate dosages, and how long should it be taken to realize benefits? Because the potency of plants varies considerably, dosage is difficult to control, and side effects are fairly common. Noteworthy side effects of high doses of ginseng include nervousness, insomnia, high blood pressure, headaches, skin eruptions, chest pain, depression, and abnormal vaginal bleeding.[38]

Glucosamine   Glucosamine is a substance produced by the body that plays a key role in the growth and development of cartilage. When present in sufficient amounts, it stimulates the manufacture of substances necessary for proper joint function and joint repair. It is manufactured commercially and sold under a variety of different names, usually glucosamine sulfate. Glucosamine has been shown to be effective for treating osteoarthritis and related degenerative joint diseases and appears to relieve swelling and decrease pain. Unlike many other herbal supplements, glucosamine sulfate has an excellent safety record with few noteworthy side effects.[39]

Chromium Picolinate   A few years ago, chromium picolinate was believed to be the new miracle for anyone interested in weight loss. Since then, at least two major studies at the U.S. Department of Agriculture Human Nutrition Research Center have shown no benefit.[40]

SAMe   SAMe (pronounced "Sammy") is the nickname for S-adenosyl-methionine. This compound is produced biochemically in all humans to help perform some 40 functions in the body, ranging from bone preservation (hence its purported osteoarthritis benefits) to DNA replication.

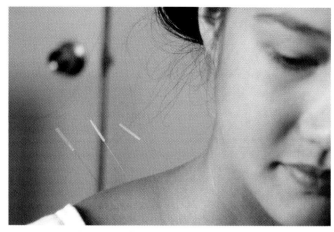

Acupuncture has been found to be effective in treating many problems, but should always be performed by a licensed practitioner.

SAMe has been reported to have a significant effect on mild to moderate depression without many of the typical side effects of prescription medications, such as sexual dysfunction, weight gain, and sleep disturbance. Scientists speculate that SAMe somehow affects brain levels of the neurotransmitters noradrenaline, serotonin, and, possibly, dopamine, all of which are related to the human stress response and the origins of depression in the body.[41] However, much of the hype has not been substantiated in large, randomized clinical trials, the type of research necessary to validate drug claims. Also, little is known about long-term side effects such as toxicity to the liver or carcinogenic properties. Anyone interested in SAMe should consider these factors:[42]

- While one large randomized trail showed modest pain relief in osteoarthritis patients using SAMe, results were not significantly better than results obtained using standard treatments.
- Many question the high cost of SAMe (between $15 and $35 or higher for 20 pills).
- Clinical depression requires more than self-treatment. Any depressed person should consult a physician to explore all options, including counseling as well as pharmaceutical and natural remedies.
- People with a family history of heart disease should not take SAMe, due to preliminary indications that it may trigger heart problems.

Under no circumstances should SAMe be taken by anyone on prescription antidepressants. The time lag between taking the prescription and beginning SAMe, and vice versa, should be carefully considered.[43]

Antioxidants   Although covered in depth in Chapter 9, it should be noted here that antioxidants are among the most sought-after supplements on the market. Primary antioxidants include beta-carotene, selenium, vitamin C, and vitamin E.

Who Seeks Alternative Medical Treatment?

People who decide to use complementary and alternative medicine tend not to make this decision on a whim. In fact, in many cases, they are more educated than people who rely solely on traditional health care. They are also more likely to be middle-aged and have a middle-class socioeconomic status. A randomized study of several thousand patients seeking care for low back pain, through traditional allopathic providers versus chiropractic providers, found that those opting for chiropractic help were more likely to question their providers about the nature and extent of recommended treatments. People who seek alternative care do so for one of three reasons.

1. *Dissatisfaction.* Patients may be unhappy with ineffective treatment or treatment that has resulted in adverse effects, may find traditional allopathic medicine too impersonal and technologically oriented, or may find it too costly. Also, it appears that managed care may have pushed some people out of the allopathic system. Many began to distrust it after watching family members experience problems.

2. *Need for personal control.* Patients view CAM therapies as less authoritarian and more empowering.

3. *Philosophical congruence.* For some people, CAM is just a better fit. Referred to as *cultural creatives,* these CAM users tend to be committed to the environment; to feminism; to involvement with esoteric forms of spirituality and personal growth psychology, including self-actualization and self-expression; and to exploring anything foreign and exotic. They also identify with cultural change and innovation and are among those most likely to adopt alternative treatments.

Research has also revealed the following:

✔ CAM users didn't have a particularly negative attitude toward traditional medicine.

✔ Racial or ethnic status didn't predict CAM usage.

✔ Men and women were equally likely to use CAM.

✔ Those with poorer health status were more likely to use CAM.

✔ Some conditions, particularly low back pain and other chronic pain conditions, predict higher CAM usage.

✔ Those who had gone through a transformational experience that had changed their world view were more likely to use CAM.

Sources: J. Astin, "Why Patients Use Alternative Medicine: Results of a National Study," *The Journal of the American Medical Association* 279 (1998): 1548–1552; D. Eisenberg et al., "Trends in Alternative Medicine Use in the United States, 1990–1997: Results of a Follow-up National Study," *The Journal of the American Medical Association* 280 (1998): 1569–1579; R. Donatelle, J. Nyiendo, and M. Haas, "Health Care Decision-Making among Those Seeking Care for Low Back Pain from Traditional Medical and Chiropractic Physicians" (paper presented at the American Public Health Association's annual meeting, 1998); P. H. Ray, "The Emerging Culture," *American Demographics,* February 1997.

Foods as Healing Agents

Many Americans rely on *functional foods*—foods or supplements designed to improve some aspect of physical or mental functioning. Sometimes referred to as **nutraceuticals** for their combined nutritional and pharmaceutical benefit, several are believed to actually work in much the same way as pharmaceutical drugs in making a person well or bolstering the immune system.

Foods contain many "nonnutrient" active ingredients that can affect us in different ways. For example, chili peppers contain ingredients that make your eyes water and clear your sinuses. Many of these active ingredients, or constituents, can promote good health. A number of foods, such as sweet potatoes, tangerines, and red peppers, are recognized as excellent sources of antioxidants. Onion and garlic contain allium compounds that reduce blood clotting. Other foods have natural anti-inflammatory properties or aid digestion. Some are known by the term *prebiotics,* foods that promote good bacteria in the body that may help fight off infection.[44]

Some of the most common healthful foods and their purported benefits include the following.

- *Plant stanol.* Can lower "bad" LDL cholesterol.
- *Oat fiber.* Can lower "bad" LDL cholesterol; serves as a natural soother of nerves; stabilizes blood sugar levels.
- *Sunflower.* Can lower risk of heart disease; may prevent angina.
- *Soy protein.* May lower heart disease risk; provides protective estrogen-like effect; may reduce risk from certain cancers.
- *Red meats and dark green, leafy vegetables.* Contain B vitamins (B_6, B_{12}, folate), which can lower levels of homocysteine, an amino acid associated with heart disease.
- *Garlic.* Is believed to lower cholesterol and reduce clotting tendency of blood; lowers blood pressure; may serve as form of antibiotic.
- *Ginger.* Fights motion sickness, stomach pain, and upset; discourages blood clots; may relieve rheumatism.
- *Yogurt.* Untreated, nonpasteurized yogurt contains active, friendly bacteria that can fight off infections.

Nutraceuticals Term often used interchangeably with *functional foods;* refers to the combined nutritional and pharmaceutical benefit derived through use of foods or food supplements.

Table 18.2
Common Herbal, Vitamin, and Mineral Supplements: Benefits vs. Risks

Supplement	Use	Claims of Benefits	Risks
Chaparral	Sold as teas and pills	Fights cancer and purifies blood	Linked to serious liver damage
Chondroitin (shark cartilage or sea cucumber)		Improves osteoporosis and arthritis by improving cartilage function	Fewer benefits than glucosamine; benefits still unproven
Comfrey	Originated as a poultice to reduce swelling, but later used internally	Wound healing, infection control	Contains alkaloids toxic to the liver, and animal studies suggest it is carcinogenic
DHEA	Hormone that turns into estrogen and testosterone in the body	Fights aging, boosts immunity, strengthens bones, and improves brain functioning	No anti-aging benefits proven; could increase cancer risk and lead to liver damage, even when taken briefly
Dieter's teas	Herbal blends containing senna, aloe, rhubarb root, buckthorn, cascara, and castor oil	Act as laxatives	Can disrupt potassium levels and cause heart arrhythmias; linked to diarrhea, vomiting, chronic constipation, fainting, and death
Flax seeds	Produce linseed oil	Omega-3 fatty acid benefits	Delay absorption of medicine
High-dose vitamin E	Antioxidants	Reduces risk of heart disease; better survivability after heart attack	Causes bleeding when taking blood thinners
L-Carnitine	Amino acid	Improves metabolism in heart muscle, purported to increase fat-burning enzymes	Heart palpitations, arrhythmias, sudden death; claims largely unsubstantiated
Licorice root		None proven	Speeds potassium loss
Melatonin	"Clock hormone"	Role in regulating circadian rhythms and sleep patterns	Anti-aging claims unfounded
Niacin (vitamin B_3)	Reduces serum lipids, vasodilation, and increased blood flow		Skin flushing, gastrointestinal distress, stomach pain, nausea and vomiting
Pennyroyal (member of the mint family)	Sold as tea	Helps digestive problems	Pregnancy-related complications, heart arrhythmias, death
Sassafras	Once a flavoring in root beer; used in tonics and teas	No real claims	Shown to cause liver cancer in animals
Vitamin C	Antioxidant, manufactures collagen, wound repair, nerve transmission	Improves blood vessel relaxation in people with CVD, diabetes, hypertension, and other problems; can relieve pain of angina pectoris	

Table 18.2 lists other foods and supplements with their risks and benefits.

Many people purchase foods labeled *organic*, because they expect these products to contain only health-promoting substances. See Chapter 9 for a complete discussion of what it means for a food to be labeled organic.

What do you think?

Why do you think the government has not acted more aggressively to regulate or control herbal and other dietary supplements? ✳ *Why are many CAM treatments not covered under typical insurance plans?*

Protecting Consumers and Regulating Claims

Although many CAM products appear promising, be aware that most of these products are not regulated in the United States as strictly as are foods and drugs. This is in sharp contrast to nations such as Germany, where the government holds companies to strict standards for ingredients and manufacturing. In the United States, nutritional supplements and genetically engineered and organic foods have had a long history of unregulated growth, including an abundance of claims and testimonials about their health-enhancing attributes. With few regulatory controls in place, many get-rich-quick charlatans have jumped into the health food and CAM market.

Strategies to Protect Consumers' Health

The burgeoning popularity of nutraceuticals and functional foods concerns many scientists. According to NIH nutritional biochemist Dr. Terry Krakower:

> NIH does have some concerns about them and we are looking into them, especially the potential for interaction with other medications. We advise anyone who uses them to talk to their physician. [Functional foods] are so new we don't know yet if they are good, bad, or indifferent. [Much] of the herb content in these food products is so small that it's probably ineffective, and if it were included in large amounts, it could be harmful. Anyone taking these supplements, whether in pill form or in foods, should do their homework and thoroughly research them rather than rely on health claims made by manufacturers.[45]

By legal definition, herbal supplements and functional foods are neither prescription drugs nor over-the-counter medications. Instead, classified as food supplements, they can be sold without FDA approval. Because they are not regulated by the FDA, these products are not subject to the strict guidelines that govern the research and development of medications.

Consumer groups, members of the scientific community, and government officials are calling for action. Pressure is mounting to establish consistent standards for herbal supplements and functional foods similar to those used in Germany and other countries. Many scientists advocate a more stringent FDA approval process for virtually all supplements sold in the United States.

The German Commission E

The German Commission E is among the most noteworthy of the international groups attempting to regulate alternative medicines and supplements. Consisting of an expert panel established in 1970, its mission was to conduct a formal evaluation of the hundreds of herbal remedies that have been part of traditional German medicine for centuries. Commission members carefully analyzed data from clinical trials, observational studies, biological experiments, and chemical analyses. Between 1983 and 1996, they evaluated 383 herbal remedies; they approved almost two-thirds of them for use but discounted nearly another third, some of which continue to be sold in the United States.[46]

Essentially, the German Commission E analyzed a growing list of **phytomedicines,** another name for medicinal herbs, many of which are sold over the counter in Europe. Typically, phytomedicines are integrated into conventional medical practice and are prepared in several different ways, usually as tablets or ground into powders.[47] Many are sold in much the same way as over-the-counter remedies in the United States.

Looking to Science for More Answers

Even as CAM treatments gain credibility, this credibility must be tempered with good science. Legislators have pushed for better science, increased funding, and an agency designed to help garner information useful to consumers—although all of these have been slow in coming.

The National Center for Complementary and Alternative Medicine (NCCAM) has established research centers at universities and other institutions throughout the United States, where many clinical trials are being conducted.[48] Studies into alternative treatments such as acupuncture, green tea, fish oil, flax seed, shark cartilage, and other treatments are taking place across the United States. To read about early test results and new initiatives, go to the NCCAM website (http://nccam.nih.gov).

Healthy Living in the New Millennium

Clearly, CAM is here to stay. It appears to serve a very real need for consumers. While consumers are making the adjustment to CAM in record numbers, members of the health care delivery system seem slow to act. Although progress has been noted, there is still a long way to go before CAM becomes fully accepted in mainstream medical practice.

Enlisting Support from Insurers and Providers

More and more insurers are hiring alternative practitioners as staff or covering alternative care as a routine benefit, at least to some degree. This is especially true as criticisms of managed care increase and government agencies get involved.

The changing nature of HMOs and health care insurers makes it impossible to determine exactly how many insurance companies currently cover CAM therapies. What is known is that the numbers are increasing despite a reimbursement system that is biased in favor of traditional treatments. While the

---

Phytomedicines   Another name for medicinal herbs, many of which are sold over the counter in Europe.

Selecting a CAM Provider

Selecting a CAM practitioner—indeed, any health care provider—can be difficult. Although these recommendations apply to CAM, you should also consider them when selecting any health care product or service. Before starting a CAM therapy or choosing a practitioner, talk with your primary health care provider(s) and others who are knowledgeable about CAM. If they dismiss the therapy, ask why. Check their explanations with other sources to see if their insights are confirmed.

FINDING A CAM PRACTITIONER

- Ask your doctor or other health professional to recommend or refer you to a CAM therapist.
- Ask people you trust who have used CAM practices if they have any recommendations based on experience.
- Contact a nearby hospital or medical school and ask if they could recommend CAM practitioners in your area. Some may actually have CAM providers on staff.
- If your therapy will be covered by insurance, ask your carrier for a list of approved CAM providers.
- Contact a professional organization for the type of practitioner you are seeking. Often they have standards of practice and websites or publications that list recommended providers. These resources will also answer common questions that you might have. If there is a regulatory or licensing board for this specialty, check to see that your practitioner has the proper credentials.

INTERVIEWING A CAM PRACTITIONER

- Make a list of your options, and gather information about each before making your first visit. Ask basic questions about providers' credentials and experience. Where did they obtain their training? What supporting degrees, licenses, or certifications do they have?
- Make a list of questions to ask at your first visit. You may want to bring a friend or family member who can help you ask questions and note answers.
- Bring medical information with you, including any tests you've had, information about your health history, surgical history, allergies, and any medications (including prescription, over-the-counter, and herbal or other supplements).
- Ask if there are diseases/health conditions in which the practitioner specializes and how frequently he or she treats patients with conditions like yours.
- Ask if there is any scientific research supporting the use of this treatment for your condition.

- Is the provider supportive of conventional as well as CAM treatments? Does he or she have a good relationship with conventional practitioners in order to give referrals to them?
- Were questions answered to your satisfaction?
- How many patients per day does the provider see, and how much time is spent with each one?
- Ask about charges and payment options. What percentage of the payment might you have to pay out of pocket?

After the visit, assess the interaction and how you felt about the practitioner.

UNDERSTANDING THE RECOMMENDED TREATMENT

- What benefits can I expect from this therapy?
- What are the risks and side effects associated with this therapy? Do the benefits outweigh the risks?
- Will I need to buy any special equipment or take any special supplements?
- Will this therapy interfere with any conventional medicine treatments?
- If there are problems, where would I be referred for further treatment?
- What is the history of success in treating this type of condition for someone of my age and health status?

---

nation's insurers spend more than $30 billion a year on bypass and angioplasty for CVD, only 40 companies cover the lifestyle-based program developed by Dr. Dean Ornish—despite repeated compelling research that demonstrates that the program is safe, effective, and much cheaper than surgery.[49] In some cases, consumers are offered an optional "extra-cost" rider on their insurance policy, through which they may choose to consult alternative practitioners for a higher premium and co-pay agreement. For many consumers, just knowing they have a choice seems to be worth the extra cost.

Support from professional organizations, such as the AMA, is also increasing as more physician training programs require or offer electives in alternative treatment modalities. In some cases, medical schools are educating a new generation of medical doctors to be better prepared to advise patients about the pros and cons of alternative treatments, and more comprehensive studies are underway to compare the efficacy of alternative strategies to traditional treatments.

What do you think?

What can you do as a consumer to obtain the greatest benefit from CAM? ✳ *How can you protect yourself from possible risks?*

Self-Care: Protecting Yourself

Like no other time in human history, today we are faced with an astounding array of possible health choices. Be aware that, with a few notable exceptions, much of what we read on the Internet about functional foods, herbal medicines, and CAM is unreliable at best—and strewn with potentially harmful and downright false information at worst.

When considering alternative treatments, do your homework and ask questions (see the Skills for Behavior Change box). Protect yourself by remembering the following points.

- Consult only reliable sources—texts, journals, periodicals, and government resources. Start with the websites listed at the end of this and every chapter.
- Remember that *natural* and *safe* are not necessarily synonyms. Many people have become seriously ill from seemingly harmless products. For example, some people have suffered serious liver damage from sipping teas brewed with comfrey, an herb used in poultices and ointments to treat sprains and bruises but that should not be taken internally. Pregnant women face special risks from herbs such as echinacea, senna, comfrey, and licorice.
- Realize that no one is closely monitoring the purity of herbal supplements. The FDA has verified industry reports that certain shipments of ginseng were contaminated with high levels of fungicides. Other problems with imported herbs have been noted.

- Recognize that dosage levels in many herbal products are not regulated. German manufacturers produce identical batches of herbal remedies as required by law. Look for reputable manufacturers.
- Tell your doctor if you are taking herbal medications. Several may interact with prescription (and over-the-counter) medications.
- Be cautious about combining herbal medications, just as you should be cautious about combining other drugs. Always remember that just because something is natural doesn't mean it is safe.
- Remember that no herbal medicine is likely to work miracles. Monitor your health, and seek help if you notice any unusual side effects from herbal products.
- Always look for the word *standardized* on any herbal product you buy.

As we enter a new era of medicine, more than ever, you are being called upon to take responsibility for what goes into your body. This means you must educate yourself. CAM can offer new avenues toward better health, but it is up to you to make sure that you are on the right path.

Taking Charge

18 18 18

Make It Happen!

Assessment: The Assess Yourself box on page 457 asks you to assess your opinions about CAM. Now that you have considered your results, you may want to take steps to explore your opinions further or discuss them with others.

Making a Change: In order to change your behavior, you need to develop a plan. Follow these steps.

1. Evaluate your behavior, and identify patterns and specific things you are doing. What can you change now? What can you change in the near future?
2. Select one pattern of behavior that you want to change.
3. Fill out a Behavior Change Contract. It should include your long-term

goal for change, your short-term goals, the rewards you'll give yourself for reaching these goals, potential obstacles along the way, and strategies for overcoming these obstacles. For each goal, list the small steps and specific actions that you will take.

4. Chart your progress in a journal. At the end of a week, consider how successful you were in following your plan. What helped you be successful? What made change more difficult? What will you do differently next week?
5. Revise your plan as needed. Are the short-term goals attainable? Are the rewards satisfying?

Example: When Melia answered the question about the type of person most likely to seek CAM treatment, she assumed that no one she knew would be

a user of anything but traditional treatment. She was surprised when she started asking her friends and family, and it turned out that several of them had tried various CAM therapies. Some had positive experiences: Her uncle Louis had developed back problems after a car accident, and a chiropractor had brought him relief. Also, her friend Tony had had acupuncture for his "tennis elbow" and reported that it had helped. On the other hand, Melia's mother had taken ginkgo biloba because she felt she needed help with her memory. However, she didn't tell her regular physician that she was taking it and, when she started taking a blood thinner he prescribed for her, the combination of the two caused dangerous bleeding. She had not experienced any memory enhancement from the ginkgo and was glad to stop it.

Melia had chronic knee pain, and her doctor had not discovered anything that could be treated with surgery or other conventional treatments. Now that she had thought more about CAM and saw how widely used some of the therapies are, Melia decided to investigate the most appropriate ones for knee pain and ask her doctor's opinion about pursuing one of them. Based on her mother's experience, she knew she would need to work together with her physician and any CAM provider to be sure that their treatments were compatible. She made an appointment with her doctor to discuss possible treatments and planned to research all of her options, including side effects and insurance coverage.

Summary

* The National Center for Complementary and Alternative Medicine (NCCAM) groups complementary and alternative medicine (CAM) practices into five major domains: (1) alternative medical systems; (2) manipulative and body-based methods; (3) energy therapies; (4) mind–body interventions; and (5) biologically based treatments.
* People throughout the world are choosing complementary and alternative medicine options, and these numbers are growing exponentially. Much of the influence of these CAM strategies may be traced to other cultures, particularly those with traditional oriental medicine (TOM) or ayurvedic roots.
* Major types of CAM providers and treatment modalities include chiropractic medicine, acupuncture, herbal remedies, homeopathy, and naturopathy.
* Herbal remedies, largely derived from traditional oriental medicine, include ginkgo biloba, St. John's wort, and echinacea. Other herbal remedies have also received widespread attention as potential miracle drugs without having harmful side effects. Special supplements include muscle enhancers, ginseng, glucosamine, chromium picolinate, SAMe, and antioxidants. A number of functional foods also serve as healing agents.
* Though many positive effects are associated with CAM, there are also many risks. The drive for profits and the lack of strict government regulation make the CAM market a free-for-all. As a consumer, you must be aware of the risks and check reputable sources to ensure that you are not being lured by false claims and promises.
* Health in the new millennium will provide an interesting assortment of choices for health care consumers. By enlisting the support of health care professionals and health care services, and by making informed decisions, you will reap positive rewards in your quest for health enhancement in the days ahead.

Questions for Discussion and Reflection

1. What are some of the potential benefits and risks of CAM? Why do you think these practices and products are becoming so popular?
2. What are the major domains of CAM treatments? Have you tried any of them? Would you feel comfortable trying any new ones? Why or why not?
3. What are the major herbal remedies? Special supplements? What are some of the risks and benefits associated with each?
4. What can you do to ensure that you are receiving accurate information regarding CAM treatments or medicines? Which federal agency oversees CAM in the United States?
5. What is being done in the United States to ensure continued growth of CAM?

Accessing Your Health on the Internet

Visit the following Internet sites to explore further topics and issues related to personal health. To visit an organization's website, go to the Companion Website for *Health: The Basics, Sixth Edition* at www.aw-bc.com/donatelle, click on the book image, and select "Accessing Your Health on the Internet" from the navigation menu on the left.

1. *Acupuncture.com.* Provides resources for consumers regarding traditional Asian therapies, geared to students and practitioners.

2. *Alternative Medicine Links.* Provides links to a number of the best alternative, complementary, and preventive health news pages.

3. *National Center for Complementary and Alternative Medicines (NCCAM).* A division of the National Institutes of Health dedicated to providing the latest information on complementary and alternative practices, including NCCAM-funded centers of research on alternative medicine.

4. *National Institutes of Health, Office of Dietary Supplements.* An excellent resource for information on dietary supplements.

Further Reading

Blumenthal, M., ed. *Complete German Commission E Monographs: Therapeutic Guide to Herbal Medicines.* Austin, TX: The American Botanical Council, 1998.

Overview of German E Commission findings and relevant information about supplement research for consumers. Provides an interesting perspective on international herbal research, policies, recommendations, and future directions.

Cassileth, B. R. *The Alternative Medicine Handbook: The Complete Reference Guide to Alternative and Complementary Therapies.* New York: W. W. Norton & Co., 1998.

A complete reference for patients and physicians alike on possible alternative treatments.

Pelletier, Ken. *The Best Alternative Medicine: What Works? What Does Not?* New York: Simon & Schuster, 2000.

Excellent overview of commonly used CAM techniques with scientific information for consumers.

Turchaninov, R., and C. A. Cox. *Medical Massage.* Scottsdale, AZ: Stress Less Publishing and Phoenix: Aesculapius Books, 1998.

An in-depth review of therapeutic practices from around the world.

Appendix

Injury Prevention and Emergency Care

Injury Prevention

Unintentional injuries are one of the major public health problems facing the United States today. On an average day, more than a million people will suffer a nonfatal injury; more than 100,000 people die each year as a result of unintentional injuries. Unintentional injuries are the leading cause of death for Americans under the age of 44. In the United States, unintentional injuries are the fifth leading cause of death, after heart disease, cancer, stroke, and lung disease.

Vehicle Safety

The risk of dying in an auto crash is related to age. Young drivers (ages 16 to 24) have the highest death rate, owing to their inexperience and immaturity. In 2002, 38,309 Americans died in automobile crashes. Each year another 1.9 million are disabled, 140,000 permanently. Most of these car crashes were avoidable. The best line of prevention against car crashes is to practice risk management driving and accident-avoidance techniques and to be aware of safety technology when purchasing a car.

Risk Management Driving   Practicing risk management driving techniques helps reduce chances of being involved in a collision. Techniques include the following.

- *Surround your car with a bubble space.* The rear bumper of the car ahead of you should be three seconds away. To measure your safety bubble, choose a roadside landmark such as a signpost or light pole as a reference point. When the car in front of you passes this point, count "one-one-thousand, two-one-thousand." Make sure you are not passing the reference point before you've finished saying "three-one-thousand."
- *Scan the road ahead of you and to both sides.*
- *Drive with your low-beam headlights on.* Having your low-beam headlights on, *day or night,* makes you more visible to other drivers.

- Other important strategies include anticipating other drivers' actions, driving refreshed and sober, obeying all traffic laws, and using safety belts.

Accident-Avoidance Techniques   Sometimes when driving, you need to react instantly to a situation. To avoid a more severe accident, you may need to steer into another, less severe collision. Here are AAA's rules for avoidance.

1. Generally, veer to the right.
2. Steer, don't skid, off the road.
3. If you have to hit a vehicle, hit one moving in the same direction as your own.
4. If you have to hit a stationary object, try to hit a soft one (bushes, small trees, etc.) rather than a hard one (boulders, brick walls, giant oaks).
5. If you have to hit a hard object, hit it with a glancing blow.
6. Avoid hitting pedestrians, motorcyclists, and bicyclists at all costs.

Safety Technology   The last line of defense against a collision is the car itself. How a car is equipped can mean the difference between life and death. When purchasing a car, the Insurance Institute for Highway Safety recommends that you look for the following features.

- Does the car have airbags? Remember, airbags do not eliminate the need for everyone to wear safety belts. Airbags inflate only in the case of frontal crashes.
- Does the car have antilock brakes? Antilock brakes help pump the brakes and prevent them from locking up and, hence, prevent the car from skidding.
- Does the car have impact-absorbing crumple zones?
- Are there strengthened passenger compartment side walls?
- Is there a strong roof support? (The center door post on four-door models gives you an extra roof pillar.)

In Case of Mechanical Breakdown

- Try to get off the road as far as possible.
- Turn on your car's emergency flashers, and raise the hood. Set out flares or reflective triangles.
- Stay in the car until a law enforcement officer arrives. If others stop to help, ask them to contact the authorities.
- If you must leave your car, leave a note with the car explaining the problem (as best you can), the time and date, your name, the direction in which you are walking, and what you are wearing. This information will help anyone who needs to look for you.
- Remove all valuables from the car if you must leave it.

Safe Refueling

Gasoline is a flammable substance. Follow these guidelines from the Petroleum Equipment Institute any time you are filling up a car, truck, or motorcycle.

- Turn off the engine while refueling.
- Do not reenter your vehicle during refueling. In the unlikely event of a static-caused fire, leave the nozzle in the tank and back away from the vehicle. Notify the attendant immediately.
- Avoid prolonged breathing of gasoline vapors. Keep gasoline away from your eyes and skin; it can cause irritation. Never use it to wash your hands or as a cleaning solvent.
- If you are dispensing gasoline into a container or storing it, be sure the container is approved for such use.
- Never siphon gasoline by mouth; it can be harmful or fatal if swallowed.

Pedestrian Safety

Each year, approximately 13 percent of all motor vehicle deaths involve pedestrians, and another 82,000 pedestrians are injured. The highest death rates involving pedestrians occur among the very young and elderly populations. Pedestrian injuries occur most frequently after dark, in urban settings, and primarily in intersections where pedestrians may walk or dart into traffic. It is not uncommon for alcohol to play a role in the death or injury of a pedestrian. AAA has the following safety suggestions for joggers and walkers.

- Carry or wear reflective material at night to help drivers see you.
- Cross only at crosswalks. Keep to the right in crosswalks.
- Before crossing, look both ways. Be sure the way is clear before you cross.
- Cross only on the proper signal.
- Watch for turning cars.
- Never go into the roadway from between parked cars.
- Where there is no sidewalk and it is necessary to walk in a roadway, walk on the left side, facing traffic.
- Don't wear headphones for a radio or CD player. These may interfere with your ability to hear sounds of motor vehicles.

Cycling Safety

Currently more than 63 million Americans of all ages ride bicycles for transportation, recreation, and fitness. The Consumer Product Safety Commission reports about 800 deaths per year from cycling accidents. The biggest risk factors are failure to wear a helmet, being male, and riding after dark. Children age 10 to 14 also are at higher risk for injury. Approximately 87 percent of fatal collisions were due to cyclists' errors, usually failure to yield at intersections. Alcohol also plays a significant role in bicycle deaths and injuries. Careful cyclists should do the following.

- Wear a helmet. It should be ANSI or Snell approved. This can reduce head injuries by 85 percent.
- Don't drink and ride.
- Respect traffic.
- Wear light reflective clothing that is easily seen at night and during the day.
- Avoid riding after dark.
- Ride with the flow of traffic.
- Know and use proper hand signals.
- Keep your bicycle in good working condition.
- Use bike paths whenever possible.
- Stop at stop signs and traffic lights.

Water Safety

Drowning is the third most common cause of accidental death in the United States, according to the National Safety Council. About 85 percent of drowning victims are teenage males. Many drowned swimmers are strong swimmers. Alcohol plays a significant role in many drowning cases. Most drownings occur in unorganized or unsupervised facilities, such as ponds or pools with no lifeguards present. Swimmers should take the following precautions.

- Don't drink alcohol before or while swimming.
- Don't enter the water unless you can swim at least 50 feet unassisted.
- Know your limitations; get out of the water as soon as you start to feel even slightly fatigued.
- Never swim alone, even if you are a skilled swimmer. You never know what might happen.
- Never leave a child unattended, even in extremely shallow water or wading pools.
- Before entering the water, check the depth. Most neck and back injuries result from diving into water that is too shallow.
- Never swim in muddy or dirty water that obstructs your view of the bottom.
- Never swim in a river with currents too swift for easy, relaxed swimming.

Emergency Care

In emergency situations, it may be necessary to administer first aid. Ideally, first-aid procedures should be performed by someone who has received formal training. If you do not have such training, contact a physician or call your local emergency medical service (EMS) by dialing 911 or your local emergency number. In life-threatening situations, however, you may not have time to call for assistance.

In cases of serious injury or sudden illness, you may need to begin first aid immediately and continue until help arrives. The remainder of this appendix contains basic information and general steps to follow for various emergency situations. Simply reading these directions, however, may not prepare you fully to handle these situations. For this reason, you may want to enroll in a first-aid course.

Calling for Emergency Assistance

When calling for emergency assistance, be prepared to give exact details. Be clear and thorough, and do not panic. Never hang up until the dispatcher has all the information needed. Be ready to answer the following questions.

1. Where are you and the victim located? This is the most important information the EMS will need.
2. What is your phone number and name?
3. What has happened? Was there an accident, or is the victim ill?
4. How many people need help?
5. What is the nature of the emergency? What is the victim's apparent condition?
6. Are there any life-threatening situations that the EMS should know about (for example, fires, explosions, or fallen electrical lines)?
7. Is the victim wearing a medic-alert tag (a tag indicating a specific medical problem such as diabetes)?

Are You Liable?

According to the laws in most states, you are not required to administer first aid unless you have a special obligation to the victim. For example, parents must provide first aid for their children, and a lifeguard must provide aid to a swimmer.

Before administering first aid, you should obtain the victim's consent. If the victim refuses aid, you must respect that person's rights. However, you should make every reasonable effort to persuade the victim to accept your help. In emergency situations, consent is *implied* if the victim is unconscious.

Once you begin to administer first aid, you are required by law to continue. You must remain with the victim until someone of equal or greater competence takes over.

Can you be held liable if you fail to provide adequate care or if the victim is further injured? To help protect people who render first aid, most states have "Good Samaritan"

laws. These laws grant immunity (protection from civil liability) if you act in good faith to provide care to the best of your ability, according to your level of training. Because these laws vary from state to state, you should become familiar with the Good Samaritan laws in your state.

When Someone Stops Breathing

If someone has stopped breathing, you should perform mouth-to-mouth resuscitation. This involves the following steps.

1. Check for responsiveness by gently tapping or shaking the victim. Ask loudly, "Are you OK?"
2. Call the local EMS for help (usually 911).
3. Gently roll the victim onto his or her back.
4. Open the airway by tilting the victim's head back, placing your hand nearest the victim's head on the victim's forehead, and applying backward pressure to tilt the head back and lift the chin.
5. Check for breathing (3 to 5 seconds): look, listen, and feel for breathing.
6. Give two slow breaths.
   - Keep the victim's head tilted back.
   - Pinch the victim's nose shut.
   - Seal your lips tightly around the victim's mouth.
   - Give two slow breaths, each lasting $1\frac{1}{2}$ to 2 seconds.
7. Check for pulse at side of neck; feel for pulse for 5 to 10 seconds.
8. Begin rescue breathing.
   - Keep the victim's head tilted back.
   - Pinch the victim's nose shut.
   - Give one breath every 5 to 6 seconds.
   - Look, listen, and feel for breathing between breaths.
9. Recheck pulse every minute.
   - Keep the victim's head tilted back.
   - Feel for pulse for 5 to 10 seconds.
   - If the victim has a pulse but is not breathing, continue rescue breathing. If there is no pulse, begin CPR.

There are some variations when performing this procedure on infants and children. For children ages one to eight, at step 8, give one slow breath every 4 seconds. For infants, you should not pinch the nose. Instead, seal your lips tightly around the infant's nose and mouth. Also, at step 8, you should give one slow breath every 3 seconds.

In cases in which the victim has no pulse, CPR should be performed. This technique involves a combination of artificial respiration and chest compressions. You should not perform CPR unless you have received training in it. You cannot learn CPR simply by reading directions, and without training, you could cause further injury to the victim. The American Red Cross offers courses in mouth-to-mouth resuscitation and CPR as well as general first aid. If you have taken a CPR course in the past, be aware that certain changes have been made in the procedure and you may need a refresher course.

When Someone Is Choking

Choking occurs when an object obstructs the trachea (windpipe), thus preventing normal breathing. Failure to expel the object and restore breathing can lead to death within 6 minutes. The universal signal of distress related to choking is the clasping of the throat with one or both hands. Other signs of choking include not being able to talk and/or noisy and difficult breathing. If a victim can cough or speak, do not interfere. The most effective method for assisting choking victims is the Heimlich maneuver, which involves the application of pressure to the victim's abdominal area to expel the foreign object. The maneuver involves these steps.

If the Victim Is Standing or Seated

1. Recognize that the victim is choking.
2. Wrap your arms around the victim's waist, making a fist with one hand.
3. Place the thumb side of the fist on the middle of the victim's abdomen, just above the navel and well below the tip of the sternum.
4. Cover your fist with your other hand.
5. Press fist into victim's abdomen, with up to five quick upward thrusts.
6. After every five abdominal thrusts, check the victim and your technique.
7. If the victim becomes unconscious, gently lower him or her to the ground.
8. Try to clear the airway by using your finger to sweep the object from the victim's mouth or throat.
9. Give two rescue breaths. If the passage is still blocked and air will not go in, proceed with the Heimlich maneuver.

If the Victim Is Lying Down

1. Facing the person, kneel with your legs astride the victim's hips. Place the heel of one hand against the abdomen, slightly above the navel and well below the tip of the sternum. Put the other hand on top of the first hand.
2. Press inward and upward using both hands with up to five quick abdominal thrusts.
3. Repeat the following steps in this sequence until the airway becomes clear or the EMS arrives:
   a. Finger sweep.
   b. Give two rescue breaths.
   c. Do up to five abdominal thrusts.

Alcohol Poisoning

Alcohol overdose is considered a medical emergency when one or both of the following occur: an irregular heartbeat or coma. The two immediate causes of death in such cases are cardiac arrhythmia and respiratory depression. If a person is seriously uncoordinated and has possibly also taken a depressant, the risk of respiratory failure is serious enough that a physician should be contacted. When dealing with someone who is drunk, remember these points.

1. Stay calm. Assess the situation.
2. Keep the person still and comfortable.
3. Stay with the person if she or he is vomiting. When lying him or her down, turn the head to the side to prevent it from falling back. This helps to keep the person from choking on vomit.
4. Monitor the person's breathing.
5. Keep your distance. Before approaching or touching the person, explain what you intend to do.
6. Speak in a clear, firm, reassuring manner.

When Someone Is Bleeding

External Bleeding   Control of external bleeding is an important part of emergency care. Survival is threatened by the loss of 1 quart of blood or more. There are three major procedures for the control of external bleeding.

1. *Direct pressure.* The best method is to apply firm pressure by covering the wound with a sterile dressing, bandage, or clean cloth. Wearing disposable latex gloves or an equally protective barrier, apply pressure for 5 to 10 minutes to stop bleeding.
2. *Elevation.* Elevate the wounded section of the body to slow bleeding. For example, a wounded arm or leg should be raised above the level of the victim's heart.
3. *Pressure points.* Pressure points are sites where an artery that is close to the body's surface lies directly over a bone. Pressing the artery against the bone can limit the flow of blood to the injury. This technique should be used only as a last resort when direct pressure and elevation have failed to stop bleeding.

Knowing where to apply pressure to stop bleeding is critical (Figure A.1). For serious wounds, seek medical attention immediately.

Internal Bleeding   Although internal bleeding may not be immediately obvious, you should be aware of the following signs and symptoms:

- Symptoms of shock (discussed later in this appendix)
- Coughing up or vomiting blood
- Bruises or contusions of the skin
- Bruises on chest or fractured ribs
- Black, tarlike stools
- Abdominal discomfort or pain (rigidity or spasms)

In some cases, a person who has suffered an injury (such as a blow to the head, chest, or abdomen) that does not cause external bleeding may experience internal bleeding. If you suspect that someone is suffering from internal bleeding, follow these steps.

1. Have the person lie on a flat surface with knees bent.
2. Treat for shock. Keep the victim warm. Cover the person with a blanket, if possible.
3. Expect vomiting. If it occurs, keep the victim on his or her side to prevent inhalation of vomit and to prevent expulsion of vomit from the stomach.
4. Do *not* give the victim any medications or fluids.
5. Send someone to call for emergency medical help immediately.

Nosebleeds To control a nosebleed, follow these steps:

1. Have the victim sit down and lean slightly forward to prevent blood from running into the throat. If you do not suspect a fracture, pinch the person's nose firmly closed using the thumb and forefinger. Keep the nose pinched for at least 5 minutes.
2. While the nose is pinched, apply a cold compress to the surrounding area.
3. If pinching does not work, gently pack the nostril with gauze or a clean strip of cloth. Do not use absorbent cotton, which will stick. Be sure that the ends of the gauze or cloth hang out so that it can be easily removed later. Once the nose is packed with gauze, pinch it closed again for another 5 minutes.
4. If the bleeding persists, seek medical attention.

Treatment for Burns

Minor Burns For minor burns caused by fire or scalding water, apply running cold water or cold compresses for 20 to 30 minutes. Never put butter, grease, salt water, aloe vera, or topical burn ointments or sprays on burned skin. If the burned area is dirty, gently wash it with soap and water and blot it dry with a sterile dressing.

Major Burns For major burn injuries, call for help immediately. Wrap the victim in a dry sheet. Do not clean the burns or try to remove any clothing attached to burned skin. Remove jewelry near the burned skin immediately, if possible. Keep the victim lying down and calm.

Chemical Burns Remove clothing surrounding the burn. Wash skin that has been burned by chemicals by flushing with water for at least 20 minutes. Seek medical assistance as soon as possible.

Shock

Shock is a condition in which the cardiovascular system fails to provide sufficient blood circulation to all parts of the body. Victims of shock display dilated pupils; cool, moist skin; weak, rapid pulse; vomiting; and/or delayed or unrelated responses to questions.

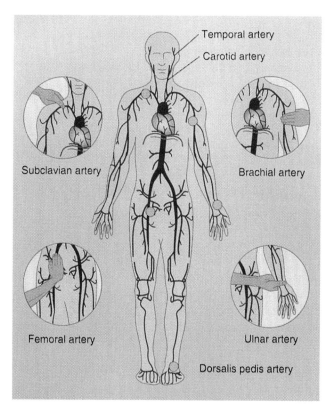

Figure A.1
Pressure Points
Pressure can be applied to these points to stop bleeding. However, unless absolutely necessary, avoid applying pressure to the carotid arteries, which supply blood to the brain. Also, never apply pressure to both carotid arteries at the same time.

All injuries result in some degree of shock. Therefore, treatment for shock should be given after every major injury. The following are basic steps for treating shock.

1. Have the victim lie flat with his or her feet elevated approximately 8 to 12 inches. (In the case of chest injuries, difficulty breathing, or severe pain, the victim's head should be slightly elevated if there is no sign of spinal injury.)
2. Keep the victim warm. If possible, wrap him or her in blankets or other material. Keep the victim calm and reassured.
3. Seek medical help.

Electrical Shock

Do not touch a victim of electrical shock until the power source has been turned off. Approach the scene carefully, avoiding any live wires or electrical power lines. Pay attention to the following.

1. If the victim is holding onto the live electrical wire, do not remove it unless the power has been shut off at the plug, circuit breaker, or fuse box.

2. Check the victim's breathing and pulse. Electrical current can paralyze the nerves and muscles that control breathing and heartbeat. If necessary, give mouth-to-mouth resuscitation. If there is no pulse, CPR might be necessary. (Remember that only trained people should perform CPR.)
3. Keep the victim warm and treat for shock. Once the person is breathing and stable, seek medical help or send someone else for help.

Poisoning

Of the 1 million cases of poisoning reported in the United States each year, about 75 percent occur in children under age five, and the majority are caused by household products. Most cases of poisoning involving adults are attempted suicides or attempted murders.

You should keep emergency telephone numbers for the poison control center and the local EMS close at hand. Many people keep these numbers on labels on their telephones. Check the front of your telephone book for these numbers. Be prepared to give the following information when calling for help.

- What was ingested. Have the container of the product and the remaining contents ready so you can describe it. Bring the container to the hospital with you.
- When the substance was taken.
- How much was taken.
- Whether vomiting has occurred. If the person has vomited, save a sample to take to the hospital.
- Other symptoms.
- How long it will take to get to the nearest emergency room.

When caring for a person who has ingested a poison, keep these basic principles in mind.

1. Maintain an open airway. Make sure the person is breathing.
2. Call the local poison control center. Follow their advice for neutralizing the poison.
3. If the poison control center or another medical authority advises you to induce vomiting, then do so.
4. If a corrosive or caustic (i.e., acid or alkali) substance was swallowed, immediately dilute it by having the victim drink at least one or two 8-ounce glasses of cold water or milk.
5. Place the victim on his or her left side. This position will delay advancement of the poison into the small intestine, where absorption into the victim's circulatory system is faster.

Injuries of Joints, Muscles, and Bones

Sprains   Sprains result when ligaments and other tissues around a joint are stretched or torn. The following steps should be taken to treat sprains.

1. Elevate the injured joint to a comfortable position.
2. Apply an ice pack or cold compress to reduce pain and swelling.
3. Wrap the joint firmly with a (roller) bandage.
4. Check the fingers or toes periodically to ensure that blood circulation has not been obstructed. If the bandage is too tight, loosen it.
5. Keep the injured area elevated, and continue ice treatment for 24 hours.
6. Apply heat to the injury after 48 hours if there is no further swelling.
7. If pain and swelling continue or if a fracture is suspected, seek medical attention.

Fractures   Any deformity of an injured body part usually indicates a fracture. A fracture is any break in a bone, including chips, cracks, splinters, and complete breaks. Minor fractures (such as hairline cracks) might be difficult to detect and might be confused with sprains. If there is doubt, treat the injury as a fracture until X rays have been taken.

Do not move the victim if a fracture of the neck or back is suspected because this could result in a spinal cord injury. If the victim must be moved, splints should be applied to immobilize the fracture, to prevent further damage, and to decrease pain. Following are some basic steps for treating fractures and applying splints to broken limbs.

1. If the person is bleeding, apply direct pressure above the site of the wound.
2. If a broken bone is exposed, do not try to move it back into the wound. This can cause contamination and further injury.
3. Do not try to straighten out a broken limb. Splint the limb as it lies.
4. The following materials are needed for splinting:
   - *Splint:* wooden board, pillow, or rolled-up magazines and newspapers
   - *Padding:* towels, blankets, socks, or cloth
   - *Ties:* cloth, rope, or tape
5. Place splints and padding above and below the joint. Never put padding directly over the break. Padding should protect bony areas and the soft tissue of the limb.
6. Tie splints and padding into place.
7. Check the tightness of the splints periodically. Pay attention to the skin color, temperature, and pulse below the fracture to make sure the blood flow is adequate.
8. Elevate the fracture, and apply ice packs to prevent swelling and reduce pain.

Head Injuries

Any head injury can potentially lead to brain damage from a cessation of breathing and pulse.

For Minor Head Injuries

1. For a minor bump on the head resulting in a bruise without bleeding, apply ice to decrease the swelling.

2. If there is bleeding, apply even, moderate pressure. Because there is always the danger that the skull may be fractured, excessive pressure should not be used.
3. Observe the victim for a change in consciousness. Observe the size of pupils, and note signs of inability to think clearly. Check for any signs of numbness or paralysis. Allow the victim to sleep, but wake him or her periodically to check for awareness.

For Severe Head Injuries

1. If the victim is unconscious, check the airway for breathing. If necessary, perform mouth-to-mouth resuscitation.
2. If the victim is breathing, check the pulse. If it is less than 55 or more than 125 beats per minute, the victim may be in danger.
3. Check for bleeding. If fluid is flowing from the ears or nose, do not stop it.
4. Do not remove any objects embedded in the victim's skull.
5. Cover the victim with blankets to maintain body temperature, but guard against overheating.
6. Seek medical help as soon as possible.

Temperature-Related Emergencies

Frostbite   Frostbite is damage to body tissues caused by intense cold, generally at temperatures below 32°F. The body parts most likely to suffer frostbite are the toes, ears, fingers, nose, and cheeks. When skin is exposed to the cold, ice crystals form beneath the skin. Avoid rubbing frostbitten tissue, because the ice crystals can scrape and break blood vessels. To treat frostbite, follow these steps.

1. Bring the victim to a health facility as soon as possible.
2. Cover and protect the frostbitten area. If possible, apply a steady source of external warmth, such as a warm compress. The victim should avoid walking if the feet are frostbitten.
3. If the victim cannot be transported, you must rewarm the body part by immersing it in warm water (100°F to 105°F). Continue to rewarm until the frostbitten area is warm to the touch when removed from the bath. Do not allow the body part to touch the sides or bottom of the water container. After rewarming, dry gently and wrap the body part in bandages to protect from refreezing.

Hypothermia   Hypothermia is a condition of generalized cooling of the body, resulting from exposure to cold temperatures or immersion in cold water. It can occur at any temperature below 65°F and can be made more severe by wind chill and moisture. The following are key symptoms of hypothermia:

- Shivering
- Vague, slow, slurred speech

- Poor judgment
- A cool abdomen
- Lethargy, or extreme exhaustion
- Slowed breathing and heartbeat
- Numbness and loss of feeling in extremities

After contacting the EMS, you should take the following steps to provide first aid to a victim of hypothermia.

1. Get the victim out of the cold.
2. Keep the victim in a flat position. Do not raise the legs.
3. Squeeze as much water from wet clothing, and layer dry clothing over wet clothing. Removal of clothing may jostle victim and lead to other problems.
4. Give the victim warm drinks only if he or she is able to swallow. Do not give the victim alcohol or caffeinated beverages, and do not allow the victim to smoke.
5. Do not allow the victim to exercise.

Heatstroke   Heatstroke, the most serious heat-related disorder, results from the failure of the brain's heat-regulating mechanism (the hypothalamus) to cool the body. The following are signs and symptoms of heatstroke.

- Rapid pulse
- Hot, dry, flushed skin (absence of sweating)
- Disorientation leading to unconsciousness
- High body temperature

As soon as these symptoms are noticed, the body temperature should be reduced as quickly as possible. The victim should be immersed in a cool bath, lake, or stream. If there is no water nearby, a fan should be used to help lower the victim's body temperature.

Heat Exhaustion   Heat exhaustion results from excessive loss of salt and water. The onset is gradual, with the following symptoms.

- Fatigue and weakness
- Anxiety
- Nausea
- Profuse sweating
- Clammy skin
- Normal body temperature

To treat heat exhaustion, move the victim to a cool place. Have the victim lie down flat, with feet elevated 8 to 12 inches. Replace lost fluids slowly and steadily. Sponge or fan victim.

Heat Cramps   Heat cramps result from excessive sweating, causing an excessive loss of salt and water. Although heat cramps are the least serious heat-related emergency, they are the most painful. The symptoms include muscle cramps, usually starting in the arms and legs. To relieve symptoms, the victim should drink electrolyte-rich beverages or a light saltwater solution or eat salty foods.

First-Aid Supplies

Every home, car, or boat should be supplied with a basic first-aid kit. In order to respond effectively to emergencies, you must have the basic equipment. This kit should be stored in a convenient place but out of reach of children. Supplies should include:

- Bandages, including triangular bandages (36 inches by 36 inches), butterfly bandages, a roller bandage, rolled white gauze bandages (2- and 3-inch widths), adhesive bandages
- Sterile gauze pads and absorbent pads
- Adhesive tape (2- and 3-inch widths)
- Cotton-tip applicators
- Scissors
- Thermometer
- Antibiotic ointment
- Aspirin
- Calamine lotion
- Antiseptic cream or petroleum jelly
- Safety pins
- Tweezers
- Flashlight
- Paper cups
- Blanket

You cannot be prepared for every medical emergency. Yet these essential tools and a knowledge of basic first aid will help you cope with many emergency situations.

References

CHAPTER 1

1. J. Rossouw and Writing Group for the Women's Health Initiative Investigators, "Risks and Benefits of Estrogen Plus Progestin in Health of Postmenopausal Women," *The Journal of the American Medical Association* 288, no. 3 (July 17, 2002); Million Women Study Collaborators, "Breast Cancer and Hormone-replacement Therapy in the Million Women Study," *The Lancet* 362 (August 9, 2003): 419–427.
2. World Health Organization, "Constitution of the World Health Organization," *Chronicles of the World Health Organization* (Geneva, Switzerland: WHO, 1947).
3. R. Dubos, *So Human the Animal* (New York: Scribners, 1968), 15.
4. D. Satcher, *Keynote Address* (Washington, DC: National Association of School Psychologists, Government and Professional Relations Committee, Public Policy Institute, February 2001), 10–12.
5. National Center for Health Statistics, "About Healthy People 2010." www.cdc.gov/nchs
6. Centers for Disease Control and Prevention, *Best Practices for Comprehensive Tobacco Control Programs, August 1999* (Atlanta: National Center for Chronic Disease Prevention and Health Promotion, Office on Smoking and Health, 1999). Reprinted with corrections.
7. R. Donatelle and S. Prows, *The Use of Financial Incentives and Social Support to Motivate Smoking Cessation among High-Risk Pregnant Smokers* (Birmingham, AL: R. W. Johnson Smoke-Free Families Office: 2000).
8. Adapted from "Ten Great Public Health Achievements—United States, 1900–1999," *Morbidity and Mortality Weekly Report* 48, no. 12 (April, 1999): 241–243; Centers for Disease Control and Prevention, "Poliomyelitis Prevention in the United States: Updated Recommendations of the Advisory Committee on Immunization Practices," *Morbidity and Mortality Weekly Report* (2000): 49 (RR-5).
9. L. Miller, "Medical Schools Put Women in Curricula," *The Wall Street Journal,* May 24, 1994, B1, B7.
10. E. Austin, "Women in Focus," *Shape,* September 1994, 46–47.
11. C. Tavris, *The Mismeasure of Woman* (New York: Touchstone, 1992), 99.
12. National Heart, Blood, and Lung Institute, "Facts about the Women's Health Initiative." www.nhlbi.nih.gov
13. K. Glanz, F. Lewis, and B. Rimer, *Health Behavior and Health-Education* (San Francisco: Jossey-Bass, 1997), Chapter 4.
14. E. P. Sarafino, *Health Psychology* (New York: Wiley, 1990), 189–191.
15. G. D. Bishop, *Health Psychology* (Boston: Allyn and Bacon, 1994), 84–86.
16. Glanz, Lewis, and Rimer, *Health Behavior and Health Education,* Chapters 8 and 9.
17. Ibid.
18. R. Donatelle et al., *Using Incentives to Motivate Behavior Change* (Middleton, WI: Society for Nicotine and Tobacco Research, 2004) (forthcoming); S. Higgins et al., "Participation of Significant Others in Outpatient Behavioral Treatment Predicts Greater Cocaine Abstinence," *American Journal of Drug and Alcohol Abuse* (1994): 2047.
19. A. Ellis and M. Bernard, *Clinical Application of Rational Emotive Therapy* (New York: Plenum, 1985).
20. P. Watson and R. Tharp, *Self-Directed Behavior: Self-Modification for Personal Adjustment* (Pacific Grove, CA: Brooks/Cole, 1993), 13.

CHAPTER 2

1. S. Benton, J. Robertson, T. Wen-Chih, F. Newton, and S. Benton, "Changes in Counseling Center Client Problems across 13 Years," *Professional Psychology: Research and Practice* 34, no. 1 (2003). www.apa.org/journals/pro/press_releases/february_32003/pro341666.html
2. National Mental Health Association, *Mental Health* (Alexandria, VA: National Mental Health Association, 1988), 3–4; W. Menninger, "Emotional Maturity," in *A Psychiatrist for a Troubled World: Selected Papers of William Menninger,* ed. B. H. Hall (New York: Viking, 1967), 789–807.
3. R. Lazarus, *Emotion and Adaptation* (New York: Oxford University Press, 1991).
4. C. Ritter, "Social Supports, Social Networks, and Health Behaviors," in *Health Behavior: Emerging Research Perspectives,* ed. D. Gochman (New York: Plenum, 1988); S. Kashubeck and S. Christensen, "Parental Alcohol Use, Family Relationships Quality, Self-Esteem, and Depression in College Students," *Journal of College Health* 36 (1995): 431–445; Linda K. George, *The Health-Promoting Effects of Social Bonds* (Durham, NC: Center for the Study of Aging and Human Development, Duke University, 2003. lkg@geri.duke.edu
5. S. Hawks, M. Hull, R. Thalman, and P. Richins, "Review of Spiritual Health: Definition, Role, and Intervention Strategies in Health Promotion," *American Journal of Health Promotion* 9, no. 5 (1995): 371–378.
6. A. Scandurra, "Everyday Spirituality: A Core Unit in Health Education and Lifetime Wellness," *Journal of Health Education* 30, no. 2 (1999): 104–109.
7. Ibid., 106.
8. L. Chapman, "Developing a Useful Perspective on Spiritual Health: Love, Joy, Peace and Fulfillment," *American Journal of Health Promotion* 2 (1987): 121–127.
9. Ibid., 122.
10. Ibid., 124.
11. R. Sloan, E. Bagiella, and T. Powell, "Religion, Spirituality, and Medicine," *The Lancet* (1999): 664–672.
12. D. Elkins, *Beyond Religion—A Personal Program for Building a Spiritual Life Outside the Walls of Traditional Religion* (Wheaton, IL: Quest Books, 1998).
13. Ibid.
14. D. Elkins, "Spirituality: It's What's Missing in Mental Health," *Psychology Today,* September/October, 1999, 48.

15. Patrick McGuire, "Seligman Touts the Art of Arguing with Yourself," *The APA Monitor Online* 29, no. 10 (October 1998).

16. M. Seligman, *Learned Optimism* (New York: Knopf, 1990).

17. Steve Proffit, "Pursuing Happiness with a Positive Outlook, Not a Pill." *Los Angeles Times,* January, 24, 1999. www.apa.org/releases/pursuing.html; APA HelpCenter: Mind/Body Connection,1996, "Learned Optimism Yields Health Benefits," http://helping.apa.org

18. P. Zimbardo, A. Weber, and R. Johnson, *Psychology* (Boston: Allyn and Bacon, 2000), 403.

19. G. Wilson, P. Nathan, K. O'Leary, and L. E. Clark, *Abnormal Psychology* (Boston: Allyn and Bacon, 1996), 137.

20. Excerpted by permission from the *University of California at Berkeley Wellness Letter* (July 1992): 3–4. © Health Letter Associates, 1992.

21. D. G. Myers and E. Diener, "Who Is Happy?" *Psychological Science* 6 (1995): 10–19.

22. Ibid.

23. Ibid.

24. B. Fredrickson, "Cultivating Positive Emotions to Optimize Health and Well-Being," *American Psychological Association: Prevention and Treatment* 3 (March 7, 2000), Article 0001a.

25. P. Doskoch, "Happily Ever Laughter," *Psychology Today* 29 (1996): 32–34.

26. B. Fredrickson, "Cultivating Positive Emotions."

27. D. Grady, "Think Right, Stay Well," *American Health* 11 (1992): 50–54.

28. B. Siegel, *Love, Medicine, and Miracles* (New York: HarperCollins, 1988).

29. MayoClinic.com, "Mental Health Definitions, March 12, 2003." www.mayoclinic.com/

30. World Health Organization, "GBD 2001 Estimates by Region," www.who.int/en; Burden of Disease Unit, *The Global Burden of Disease: A Comprehensive Assessment of Mortality and Disability from Diseases, Injuries, and Risk Factors in 1990 and Projected to 2020* (Cambridge, MA: Harvard University Press, 1996).

31. MayoClinic.com, "Lifting the Curtain on Mental Illness: Growing Awareness of a Common Problem," April 19, 2001. www.mayoclinic.com

32. L. A. Lefton, *Psychology,* 7th ed (Boston: Allyn and Bacon, 2000).

33. National Institute of Mental Health, "Depression, NIH Publication No. 02-3561," 2003. www.nimh.nih.gov

34. Lefton, *Psychology,* 540.

35. National Institute for Mental Health, 2000. www.nimh .nih.gov/; Lefton, *Psychology,* 541.

36. D. R. Rubinow, P. J. Schmidt, and C. A. Roca, "Estrogen–Serotonin Interactions: Implications for Affective Regulation," *Biological Psychiatry* 44, no. 9 (1998): 839–850; P. J. Schmidt, L. K. Neiman, M. A. Danaceau, L. F. Adams, and D. R. Rubinow, "Differential Behavioral Effects of Gonadal Steroids in Women with and in Those without Premenstrual Syndrome," *The Journal of the American Medical Association* 338 (1998): 209–216.

37. R. G. Gladstone and L. Koenig, "Sex Differences in Depression across the High School to College Transition," *Journal of Youth and Adolescence* 23 (1994): 643–669.

38. S. Scott, "Biology and Mental Health: Why Do Women Suffer More Depression and Anxiety?" *Maclean's,* January 12, 1998, 62–64.

39. National Institute of Mental Health, "Real Men. Real Depression," 2003, 6. www.menanddepression.nimh.nih.gov/

40. Ibid., 7.

41. A. K. Ferketick, J. A. Schwarzbaum, D. G. Frid, and M. L. Moeschberger, "Depression as an Antecedent to Heart Disease among Women and Men in the NHANES I Study. National Health and Nutrition Examination Survey," *Archives of Internal Medicine* 160, no. 9 (2002): 1261–1268.

42. I. Levav, R. Kohn, J. Golding, and M. Weissman, "Vulnerability of Jews to Affective Disorders," *American Journal of Psychiatry* 154 (1997): 941–947.

43. S. Wood and E. Wood, *The World of Psychology* (Boston: Allyn and Bacon, 1999), 513.

44. S. Banks and R. Kerns, "Explaining High Rates of Depression in Chronic Pain: A Diathesis–Stress Framework," *Psychological Bulletin* 119 (1996): 995–110.

45. Lefton, *Psychology,* 543.

46. Adapted by permission of the author from Kathryn Rose Gertz, "Mood Probe: Pinpointing the Crucial Differences between Emotional Lows and the Gridlock of Depression," *Self,* November 1990, 165–168, 204.

47. L. Rabasca, "Psychotherapy May Be as Useful as Drugs in Treating Depression, Study Suggests," *The APA Monitor Online* 30, no. 8 (September 1999). www.apa.org/monitor

48. MayoClinic.com, "Medical and Health Information for a Healthier Life," 2003. www.mayoclinic.com

49. MayoClinic.com, "Bipolar disorder," 2003. www.mayoclinic.com

50. National Institute of Mental Health, "Anxiety Disorders, NIH Publication No. 02-3879," 2002. www.nimh.nih.gov

51. "Anxiety Disorders," *USA Weekend,* October 12, 2000, 12.

52. Zimbardo, Weber, and Johnson, *Psychology,* 505.

53. MayoClinic.com, "Panic Attacks," July 2, 2002. www.mayoclinic.com

54. Ibid.

55. G. Wilson, P. Nathan, K. O'Leary, and L. Clark, *Abnormal Psychology* (Boston: Allyn and Bacon, 1996), 147.

56. Ibid., 147.

57. R. Saltus, "The PMS Debate," *Boston Globe Magazine,* July 25, 1999, 8–9.

58. U.S. Centers for Disease Control and Prevention, 2000. www.cdc.gov

59. K. Kendler and C. Gardner, "Boundaries of Major Depression: An Evaluation of DSM-IV Criteria," *The American Journal of Psychiatry* 155 (1998): 172–176.

60. Lefton, *Psychology,* 542.

CHAPTER 3

1. H. Selye, *Stress without Distress* (New York: Lippincott, 1974), 28–29.

2. W. Schafer, *Stress Management for Wellness, 2nd ed.* (New York: Harcourt Brace, Jovanovich, 1992).

3. R. Ader and S. Cohen, "Psychoneuroimmunology: Conditioning and Stress," *Annual Review of Psychology* 44 (1993): 53–85.

4. M. D. Jeremko, "Stress Inoculation Training: A Generic Approach for the Prevention of Stress-Related Disorders," *The Personal and Guidance Journal* 62 (1984): 544–550; H. S. Freidman and S. Booth-Kewley, "The Disease-Prone Personality: A Meta-Analytic View of the Construct," *American Psychologist* 42 (1987): 539–555.

5. G. E. Vaillant, *Adaptation to Life* (Boston: Little, Brown, 1977).

6. S. A. Lyness, "Predictions of Differences between Type A and B Individuals in Heart Rate and Blood Pressure Reactivity," *Psychological Bulletin* 114 (1993): 266–295; J. C. Barefoot and M. Schroll, "Symptoms of Depression, Acute Myocardial Infarction, and Total Mortality in a Community Sample, 1976–1980," *Circulation* 93 (1996): J. G. Schiraldi, T. Spalding, and C. Holford, "Expanding Health Educators' Roles to Meet Critical Needs in Stress Management and Mental Health," *Journal of Health Education* (1998): 70.

7. J. Chi and R. Kloner, "Stress and Myocardial Infarction," *Heart* 89, no. 5 (May 2003): 555–556.

8. F. Jones and J. Bright, *Stress: Myth, Theory and Research* (New York: Prentice Hall, 2001).

9. R. Glaser, B. Rabin, M. Chesney, S. Cohen, and B. Natelson, "Updates Linking Evidence and Experience: Stress-Induced

Immunomodulation," *The Journal of the American Medical Association* 281, no. 24 (1999): 2268–2270.

10. B. Rabin, *Stress, Immune Function, and Health: The Connection* (New York: Wiley-Liss, 1999).

11. J. Kiecolt-Glaser et al., "Chronic Stress and Age-Related Increases in the Proinflammatory Cytokine IL-6," *Proceedings of the National Academy of Sciences, USA* 100 (2003): 9090–9095.

12. D. Padgett et al., "Social Stress and the Reactivation of Latent Herpes Simplex Virus-Type 1," *Proceedings of the National Academy of Sciences, USA* 9 (1998): 7231–7235.

13. J. Kiecolt-Glaser et al., "Chronic Stress Alters the Immune Response to Influenza Virus Vaccines in Older Adults," *Proceedings of the National Academy of Sciences, USA* 93 (1996): 3043–3047.

14. R. Glaser et al., "The Influence of Psychological Stress on the Immune Response to Vaccines," *Annals of the New York Academy of Sciences* 840 (1998): 649–655.

15. A. Smith, "Breakfast, Stress, and Catching Colds," *Journal of Family Health Care* 13, no. 1 (2003): 2.

16. S. Cohen et al., "Types of Stressors That Increase Susceptibility to the Common Cold in Adults," *Health Psychology* 17 (1998): 214–223.

17. S. Cohen et al., "Social Ties and Susceptibility to the Common Cold," *The Journal of the American Medical Association* 277 (1997): 1940–1944.

18. R. Kessler, "The Effects of Stressful Life Events on Depression," *Annual Reviews of Psychology* 48 (1997): 191–214.

19. Schiraldi, Spalding, and Holford, "Expanding Health Educators' Roles," 69.

20. T. Holmes and R. Rahe, "The Social Readjustment Rating Scale," *Journal of Psychosocial Research* (1967): 213–217.

21. Ibid., 214.

22. R. Lazarus, "The Trivialization of Distress," in *Preventing Health Risk Behaviors and Promoting Coping with Illness,* eds. J. Rosen and L. Solomon (Hanover, NH: University Press of New England, 1985), 279–298.

23. L. Lefton, *Psychology* (Boston: Allyn and Bacon, 1994), 471.

24. M. Kenny and K. Rice, "Attachment to Parents and Adjustment in College Students: Current Status, Applications, and Future Considerations," *The Counseling Psychologist* 23 (1995): 433–456.

25. Kevin Nadal, "Ethnic Minority Students' Stressors: Their Impact on Campus Climate Perceptions and Academic Achievement," *R. E. McNair Fellowship Paper.* http://members.tripod.com/ ~knall/minoritystress.html

26. R. C. Kessler et al., "Social Support, Depressed Mood, and Adjustment to Stress: A Genetic Epidemiological Investigation," *Journal of Personality and Social Psychology* 62 (1992): 257–272.

27. M. Friedman and R. H. Rosenman, *Type A Behavior and Your Heart* (New York: Knopf, 1974).

28. R. Ragland and R. Brand, "Distrust, Rage May Be Toxic Cores That Put Type A Person at Risk," *The Journal of the American Medical Association* 261 (1989): 813, 814.

29. P. L. Rice, *Stress and Health* (Pacific Grove, CA: Brooks/Cole, 1992), 471.

30. Ibid.

31. American College Health Association. *National College Health Assessment: Reference Group Executive Summary* (Baltimore, MD: ACHA, 2001).

32. L. Reisberg. "Student Stress Is Rising, Especially among Women," *Chronicle of Higher Education* 46 (2000): A49–A50.

33. P. Jackson and M. Finney, "Negative Life Events and Psychological Distress among Young Adults," *Social Psychology Quarterly* (2003) (forthcoming). www.homepages.indiana.edu/101201/ ext/stress.html

34. L. Towbes and L. Cohen, "Chronic Stress in the Lives of College Students: Scale Development and Prospective Prediction of Distress," *Journal of Youth and Adolescence* 25 (1996): 206–217.

35. C. Crandell, J. Preisler, and J. Ausspring, "Measuring Life Event Stress in the Lives of College Students: The Undergraduate Stress Questionnaire (USQ)," *Journal of Behavioral Medicine* 15 (1992): 627–642.

36. S. Levine, D. M. Lyons, and A. F. Schatzberg, "Psychobiological Consequences of Social Relationships," *The Annals of the New York Academy of Science* 89, no. 7 (1999): 210–218; M. G. Marmot et al., "Contributions of Psychosocial Factors to Socioeconomic Difference in Health," *Milbank Quarterly* 76 (1998): 403–448; D. P. Phillips, T. E. Ruth, and L. M. Wagner, "Psychology and Survival," *The Lancet* 342 (1993): 1142–1145; D. Ornish et al., "Intensive Lifestyle Changes for Reversal of Coronary Heart Disease," *The Journal of the American Medical Association* 280 (1998): 2001–2007; D. Spiegel, "Healing Words: Emotional Expression and Disease Outcome," *The Journal of the American Medical Association* 281 (1999): 1328–1329.

37. G. R. Deckro et al., "The Evaluation of Mind/Body Intervention to Reduce Psychological Distress and Perceived Stress in College Students," *Journal of American College Health* 50, no. 6 (May 2002): 281–287.

CHAPTER 4

1. D. Zucchio, "Today's Violent Crime Is an Old Story with a New Twist," *San Jose Mercury News,* November 21, 1994.

2. U.S. Department of Justice, Office of Justice Programs, Bureau of Justice Statistics, "Expenditures and Employment Report: 1997," 1998. www.ojp.usdoj.gov/bjs

3. Bureau of Justice Statistics, "Key Facts at a Glance," 2000. www.ojp.usdoj.gov/bjs

4. L. Cohen and S. Swift, "A Public Health Approach to the Violence Epidemic in the United States," *Environment and Urbanization* (October 1993): 1–12; L. Lamberg, "Prediction of Violence Both Art and Science," *The Journal of the American Medical Association* 275 (1996): 1712–1715; D. P. Barash, *Understanding Violence* (Boston: Allyn and Bacon, 2001), 118–122.

5. Ibid.

6. M. Leeds, *Violence Prevention Conference* (Linnfield Community College, McMinnville, OR: 1996).

7. Ibid.

8. Ibid.

9. Lamberg, "Prediction of Violence," 1713.

10. Leeds, *Violence Prevention Conference.*

11. Ibid.

12. Ibid.

13. F. Rivera et al., "Alcohol and Illicit Drugs and the Risk of Violent Death in the Home," *The Journal of the American Medical Association* 278 (1997): 569–572.

14. "Substance Abuse: A Significant Characteristic in Domestic Violence Assailants," *Brown University Digest of Addiction Theory and Application* 16: 1–3.

15. M. Swartz et al., "Violence and Severe Mental Illness: The Effects of Substance Abuse and Non-Adherence to Medication," *The American Journal of Psychiatry* 155 (1998): 226.

16. Rivera et al., "Alcohol and Illicit Drugs," 571.

17. Bureau of Justice Statistics. "Homicide Trends in the United States," 2002. www.ojp.usdoj.gov/bjs/homicide/ homtrnd.htm

18. U.S. Center for Health Statistics, *Health: United States, 2001. Highlights: Health Status and Determinants—Disparities in Mortality* (Atlanta: Centers for Disease Control and Prevention, 2001), 6.

19. Ibid.

20. Ibid., 44.

21. Violence Policy Center, "A Deadly Myth: Women, Handguns, and Self-Defense," 2001. www.vpc.org/studies/myth.htm

22. U.S. Center for Health Statistics, *Health: United States, 2001. Highlights.*

23. R. Lacyo, "Still Under the Gun?" *Time,* July 6, 1998, 32–56.
24. Federal Bureau of Investigation, "Hate Crimes Statistics Report, 1999," 2000. www.fbi.gov/ucr/99hate.pdf
25. R. Fenske and L. Gordon, "Reducing Racial and Ethnic Hate Crimes on Campus: The Need for Community," in *Violence on Campus: Defining the Problems, Strategies for Action,* eds. A. Hoffman, J. Schuh, and R. Fenske (Gaithersburg, MD: Aspen, 1998).
26. Ibid.
27. Ibid.
28. Bureau of Justice Statistics. "2001 National Crime Victimization Survey," 2002. www.ojp.usdoj.gov/bjs
29. National Center for Domestic Violence and Abuse, Fact Sheet, 2000.
30. J. Barley et al., "Risk Factors for Violent Death in the Home," *Archives of Internal Medicine* 157 (1997): 786.
31. D. Brookkoff et al., "Characteristics of Participants in Domestic Violence: Assessment at the Scene of Domestic Violence," *The Journal of the American Medical Association* 277 (1997): 1369.
32. "Injury and Domestic Violence Prevention," *Nurse Practitioner* 22 (1997): 122.
33. F. Trevino, S. Walker, and G. Ramirez, "Violent Crime in American Society," in *Violence on Campus* (see note 25); Federal Bureau of Investigation, *Uniform Crime Report* (Washington, DC: U.S. Department of Justice, 1997).
34. A. Joerger and L. McClellan, "Why Men Batter: Why Women Stay," *Community Safety Quarterly* 5 (1992): 22–23.
35. N. West, "Crimes against Women" (see note 34): 3.
36. M. A. Straus and R. Gelles, eds., *Physical Violence in American Families: Risk Factors and Adaptations to Violence in 8,145 Families* (New Brunswick, NJ: Transaction, 1993), 101–201.
37. H. Pan, P. Neidig, and K. O'Leary, "Physical Aggression in Early Marriage: Pre-relationship and Relationship Effects," *Journal of Consulting and Clinical Psychology* 62 (1994): 975–981.
38. G. T. Wilson et al., *Abnormal Psychology* (Boston: Allyn and Bacon, 1996).
39. Ibid.
40. Ibid.
41. E. Newberger, "Child Sexual Abuse," in *Violence in America: A Public Health Approach,* ed. M. Rosenberg and M. Fenley (New York: Oxford University Press, 1991), 85.
42. National Criminal Justice Reference Service, "Family Violence Resources-Facts & Figures." www.ncjrs.org/family_violence/facts.html
43. M. Whittaker, "The Continuum of Violence against Women: Psychological and Physical Consequences," *Journal of American College Health* 40 (1992): 155. Reprinted with permission of the Helen Dwight Reid Education Foundation. Published by Heldref Publications, 1319 Eighteenth Street NW, Washington, DC 20036-1802. Copyright © 1992.
44. D. Finkelhor, "Child Sexual Abuse," in *Violence in America* (see note 41), 25.
45. N. West, "Children: The Invisible Victims of Domestic Violence," *Community Safety Quarterly* 5 (1992): 20.
46. Whittaker, "The Continuum of Violence against Women," 152.
47. K. Hunnicutt, "Women and Violence on Campus," in *Violence on Campus* (see note 25), 150.
48. Ibid., 149.
49. A. Berkowitz, "College Men as Perpetrators of Acquaintance Rape and Sexual Assault: A Review of Recent Literature," *Journal of American College Health* 40 (1992): 175.
50. J. Lenssen, *Update on Violence Statistics for Young Adults* (Corvallis, OR: Violence Prevention Summer Institute, 2000).
51. Bureau of Justice Statistics, "2001 National Crime Victimization Survey."
52. Hoffman, Schuh, and Fenske, *Violence on Campus,* 149–168.
53. D. Benson, C. Charlton, and F. Goohart, "Acquaintance Rape on Campus: A Literature Review," *Journal of American College Health* (1992): 157.
54. Raquel Kennedy Bergen, "Violence against Women Online Resources," 2003. www.vaw.umn.edu/Vawnet/mrape.htm.
55. Ibid.
56. Benson, Charlton, and Goohart, "Acquaintance Rape on Campus,"158.
57. M. W. Leidig, "The Continuum of Violence Against Women" (see note 43): 151.
58. Berkowitz, "College Men as Perpetrators of Acquaintance Rape," 177.
59. Ibid., 175.
60. Whittaker, "The Continuum of Violence against Women" (see note 43), 153–154.
61. Berkowitz, "College Men as Perpetrators of Acquaintance Rape," 718.
62. Ibid., 175.
63. Ibid., 176.
64. Hoffman, Schuh, and Fenske, *Violence on Campus,* 1–40.
65. Ibid., 175.
66. Ibid., 183.
67. J. Baier, M. Rosenzweig, and E. Shipple, "Patterns of Sexual Behavior, Coercion, and Victimization of University Students," *Journal of College Student Development* 32 (1991): 178.
68. M. Koss, "Rape: Scope, Impact, Interventions, and Public Policy Responses," *American Psychologist* 48 (1993): 1062–1069.
69. Hoffman, Schuh, and Fenske, *Violence on Campus,* 242.
70. E. Dersinger, C. Cychosz, and L. Jaeger, "Strategies for Dealing with Campus Violence," in *Violence on Campus* (see note 25).
71. American Association of University Professors, *Hostile Hallways: The AAUW Survey on Sexual Harassment in America's Schools* (1996); Hunnicutt, "Women and Violence on Campus" (see note 47), 160.
72. Ibid.
73. Ibid.
74. A. Matthews, "Campus Crime 101," *Eugene Register Guard* (March 1993): 4B.
75. Dersinger, Cychosz, and Jaeger, "Strategies for Dealing with Campus Violence" in *Violence on Campus* (see note 25), 248.
76. B. Moyers, "What Can We Do about Violence?" Public Broadcasting Service, January 1995.
77. U.S. Center for Health Statistics, *Health: United States 2001. U.S. Department of Labor, Bureau of Labor Statistics, Census of Fatal Occupational Injuries.* (Atlanta: Centers for Disease Control and Prevention, 2001).
78. Bureau of Labor Statistics, U.S. Department of Labor, "National Census of Fatal Occupational Injuries, 1999." www.bls.gov

CHAPTER 5

1. G. Goenthals, S. Worchel, and L. Heatherington, *Pathways to Personal Growth: Adjustments in Today's World* (Boston: Allyn and Bacon, 1999), 480.
2. MayoClinic.com, "Living Longer. Healthy Links: Invest in Relationships." Copyright 2001 Mayo Foundation for Medical Education and Research (MFMER). www.mayohealth.org
3. C. Snapp and M. Leary, "Hurt Feelings among New Acquaintances: Moderating Effects of Interpersonal Familiarity," *Journal of Social and Personal Relationships* 18, no. 3 (June 2001): 1344–1350.
4. V. Manusov and J. Harvey, eds., *Attribution, Communication Behavior and Close Relationships* (New York: Cambridge University Press, 2001).
5. S. S. Brehm, *Intimate Relationships* (New York: McGraw Hill, 1992), 4–5.
6. L. Lefton, *Psychology* (Boston: Allyn and Bacon, 2000), 480.
7. Ibid., 481.

8. C. Weiskopf, "Real Friends," *Current Health* 24 (1998): 16–18.
9. J. Turner and L. Rubinson, *Contemporary Human Sexuality* (Englewood Cliffs, NJ: Prentice Hall, 1993), 457.
10. Ibid., 457.
11. G. Levinger, "Can We Picture Love?" in *The Psychology of Love,* ed. R. J. Sternberg and M. Barnes (New Haven: Yale University Press, 1988), 139–159.
12. E. Hatfield, "Passionate and Companionate Love," in *The Psychology of Love* (see note 11), 191–217.
13. R. A. Baron and D. Byrne, *Social Psychology* (Boston: Allyn and Bacon, 1997), 290–295.
14. E. Hatfield and G. W. Walster, *A New Look at Love* (Reading, MA: Addison Wesley, 1981).
15. Sternberg, R. "Construct Validation of a Triangular Love Scale," *European Journal of Social Psychology* 27 (1997): 313–335.
16. A. Toufexis and P. Gray, "What Is Love? The Right Chemistry," *Time,* 1993, 47–52.
17. Ibid., 51.
18. Ibid., 49.
19. H. Fisher, *Anatomy of Love: The Natural History of Monogamy, Adultery, and Divorce* (New York: Norton, 1993).
20. E. Hatfield, *Love, Sex, and Intimacy: Their Psychology, Biology, and History* (Reading, MA: Addison-Wesley, 1993).
21. D. Tannen, *You Just Don't Understand: Women and Men in Conversation* (New York: William Morrow, 1990).
22. S. L. Michaud and R. M. Warner, "Gender Differences in Self-Reported Response in Troubles Talk," *Sex Roles: A Journal of Research* 37 (1997): 527–541; Kay Palsey, Jennifer Kerpelman, and Doug Guilbert, "Gender Conflict, Identity Disruption and Marital Instability. Expanding Gottman's Model," *Journal of Social and Personal Relationships* 18, no. 2 (February 2001): 1107–1114; Linda C. Gallo and Timothy W. Smith, "Attachment Style in Marriage: Adjustments and Responses to Interaction," *Journal of Social and Personal Relationships* 18, no. 2 (April 2001):1231–1237; Valerie Manusov and John Harvey, eds., *Attribution, Communication Behavior and Close Relationships.*
23. M. McGill, *The McGill Report on Male Intimacy* (New York: Holt, Rinehart and Winston, 1985), 87–88.
24. C. Morris, *Understanding Psychology* (Englewood Cliffs, NJ: Prentice Hall, 1993).
25. McGill, *The McGill Report,* 87–88.
26. M. Klausner and B. Hasselbring, *Aching for Love: The Sexual Drama of the Adult Child* (New York: Harper and Row, 1990).
27. Brehm, *Intimate Relationships,* 263.
28. B. Strong, C. DeVault, and B. Sayad, *Human Sexuality* (Mountain View, CA: Mayfield Publishing, 1999), 219.
29. U.S. Census Bureau, "Estimated Median Age at First Marriage, by Sex: 1890 to Present," June 12, 2003. www.census.gov/population/www/socdemo/hh-fam.html history
30. A. P. Greeff and H. L. Malherbe, "Intimacy and Marital Satisfaction in Spouses," *Journal of Sex and Marital Therapy* 27 (May–June 2001, Special Issue): 247–257; "Is Your Love Life Making You Sick?" *Ebony,* July 2001, 38–41; L. Waite and M. Gallagher, *The Case for Marriage: Why Married People Are Healthier, Happier, and Better Off Financially* (New York: Doubleday, 2000).
31. M. Young, M. Denny, T. Young, and R. Tuquis, "Sexual Satisfaction among Married Women," *American Journal of Health Studies* 16, no. 2 (2000): 73–78.
32. R. Alsop, "As Same-Sex Households Grow More Mainstream, Businesses Take Note," *The Wall Street Journal,* August 8, 2001, B1, B4.
33. Ibid.
34. Ibid.
35. U.S. Census Bureau, "Marital Status of People 15 Years and Older, March 2002," June 2003. www.census.gov/population/www/socdemo/hh-fam.html; Centers for Disease Control and Prevention, Advanced Data, *First Marriages Dissolution, Divorce, and Remarriage, United States,* May 31, 2001, 323.
36. Ibid.
37. Ibid.
38. Alsop, "Same-Sex Households," B1, B4.
39. Centers for Disease Control and Prevention, "National Vital Statistics Report," 49 no. 6 (August 2001).
40. USDA Center for Nutrition Policy and Promotion, "Expenditures on Children by Families, 2002," May 2003. www.cnpp.usda.gov.
41. National Center for Health Statistics and U.S. Census Bureau, "Divorce, Provisional 2001 Data." www.cdc.gov/nchs/fastats/divorce.htm
42. H. Markman, "Love Lessons: 6 New Moves to Improve Your Relationship," *Psychology Today,* March/April 1997, 42–49.
43. A. H. Slyper, "Childhood Obesity, Adipose Tissue Distribution, and the Pediatric Practitioner," *Pediatrics* 102 (1998): 4.
44. Mayo Foundation for Medical Education and Research, "HRT: A Risk/Benefit Analysis," 2000. www.mayohealth.org/mayo/0003/htm/hrt.htm
45. American Academy of Pediatrics, "Just the Facts: Circumcision," 2003. www.aap.org/mrt/factscir.htm
46. American Psychological Association, "Lesbian, Gay, and Bisexual Concerns Policy Statements," 2003. www.apa.org/pi/lgbc/policy/statements.html
47. D. J. Bem, "Exotic Becomes Erotic: A Developmental Theory of Sexual Orientation," *Psychological Review* 103, no. 2: 320–335; J. P. DeCecco and D. A. Parker, "The Biology of Homosexuality: Sexual Orientation or Sexual Preference?" *Journal of Homosexuality* 28. no. 1 (1995): 1–28; G. Haumann, "Homosexuality, Biology, and Ideology," *Journal of Homosexuality* 28. no. 1 (1995): 57–77; S. LeVay, *Queer Science: The Use and Abuse of Research into Homosexuality* (Cambridge, MA: MIT Press, 1996).
48. G. M. Herek, J. Roy Gillis, and J. C. Cogan, "Psychological Sequelae of Hate-Crime Victimization among Lesbian, Gay, and Bisexual Adults," *Journal of Consulting and Clinical Psychology* 67, no. 6: 945–951.
49. G. F. Kelly, *Sexuality Today: The Human Perspective* (Dubuque, IA: McGraw Hill, 1998), 203–206.
50. Ibid.
51. R. T. Michael, J. H. Gagnon, E. O. Laumann, and G. Kolata, *Sex in America: A Definitive Survey* (Boston: Little, Brown, 1994).
52. Ibid.
53. J. G. Beck, "Hypoactive Sexual Desire Disorder: An Overview," *Journal of Consulting and Clinical Psychology* 36, no. 6 (1995): 919–927.
54. B. Handy, "The Potency Pill," *Time,* May 4, 1998, 50–57.
55. Arnot Ogden Medical Center, "Frequently Asked Questions." 1998. www.aomc.org
56. S. A. Lyman, C. Hughes-McLain, and G. Thompson, "'Date-Rape Drugs: A Growing Concern," *Journal of Health Education* 29, no. 5 (1998): 271–274.

CHAPTER 6

1. Centers for Disease Control, *Contraceptive Options: Increasing Your Awareness* (Washington, D.C.: Nurses' Association of the American College of Obstetricians and Gynecologists, 1990).
2. World Health Organization, "Nonoxynol-9 Ineffective in Preventing HIV infection," June 28, 2002. www.who.int/mediacentre/notes/release55/en
3. University of Southern California School of Medicine, "Non-Contraceptive Health Benefits," *Dialogues in Contraception* 3 (1990): 2.
4. National Center for Health Statistics, "Fertility, Family Planning, and Women's Health," 23 (1997): 7.
5. K. N. Anderson, L. E. Anderson, and W. D. Glanze, eds., *Mosby's Medical, Nursing & Allied Health Dictionary* (Philadelphia: W.B. Saunders Co., 2002).
6. "FDA Approves Emergency Contraceptive Kit," *College Health Report* 1 (1998): 8.

7. Boston Women's Health Collective, *Our Bodies Ourselves for the New Century: A Book by Women and for Women* (New York: Simon and Schuster, 1998).

8. P. Gober, "The Role of Access in Explaining State Abortion Rates," *Social Science and Medicine* 44 (1997): 7.

9. The Allan Guttmacher Institute, "Facts in Brief: Induced Abortion" (2000). www.agi-usa.org

10. J. Gans Epner, H. Jonas, and D. Seckinger, "Late Term Abortion," *The Journal of the American Medical Association* 280 (1998): 726.

11. D. A. Grimes and R. J. Cook, "Mifepristone (RU-486)—An Abortifacient to Prevent Abortion?" *The New England Journal of Medicine* 327, no. 15 (1992): 1041–1044.

12. C. O. Byer, L. W. Shainberg, and G. Galliano, *Dimensions of Human Sexuality* (Boston: McGraw-Hill College, 1999), 489.

13. K. Schmidt, "The Dark Legacy of Fatherhood," *U.S. News and World Report* (December 14, 1992): 94–95.

14. U.S. Department of Agriculture, Center for Nutrition Policy and Promotion, "Expenditures on Children by Families," 2003. www.usda.gov/cnpp/using2.html

15. Baby Center, "College Savings Calculator," 2000.www.babycenter.com/calculator/1508.html

16. U.S. Department of Health and Human Services, *The Health Benefits of Smoking Cessation: A Report of the Surgeon General* (Washington, DC: Government Printing Office, 1990).

17. Ibid.

18. Centers for Disease Control and Prevention, "Smoking Cessation for Pregnant Women," July 2002. www.cdc.gov

19. National Center for Health Statistics, "Fertility, Family Planning, and Women's Health," 19.

20. National Down Syndrome Society, 1998. www.ndss.org

21. Eleena de Lisser, "Breast Feeding Boosts Adult I.Q., Research Suggests," *The Wall Street Journal,* May 2, 2002, D2.

22. M. Avery et al., "Factors Associated with Very Early Weaning among Primiparas Intending to Breastfeed," *Maternal and Child Health Journal* 2 (1998): 167–179.

23. Centers for Disease Control and Prevention, "U.S. Birth Rate Reaches Record Low," June 25, 2003. www.cdc.gov/nchs/releases/03news/lowbirth.htm

24. Centers for Disease Control and Prevention, "Pelvic Inflammatory Disease," 2002. www.cdc.gov.

25. Ibid.

26. M. Hansen, J. J. Kurinczuk, C. Bower, and S. Webb, "The Risks of Major Defects after Intracytoplasmic Sperm Injection and In Vitro Fertilization," *The New England Journal of Medicine* 346, no. 10 (2002): 725–730.

CHAPTER 7

1. U.S. Department of Health and Human Services, Substance Abuse and Mental Health Services Administration, "Substance Abuse: A National Health Challenge," October 4, 2001. www.samhsa.gov/oas/oas.html

2. Ibid.

3. H. F. Doweiko, *Concepts of Chemical Dependency* (Pacific Grove, CA: Brooks/Cole, 1993), 9.

4. C. Nakken, *The Addictive Personality* (Center City, MN: Hazelden, 1996), 24.

5. J. Shuster, "Insomnia: Understanding Its Pharmacological Treatment Options," *Pharmacy Times* 62 (1996): 67–76.

6. Food and Drug Administration, "Phenylpropanolamine (PPA) Information Page." www.fda.gov/cder/drug/ infopage/ppa/default.htm

7. U.S. Department of Health and Human Services, *2002 National Survey on Drug Use and Health.* (2003) www.samhsa.gov/oas/nhsda.htm

8. Ibid.

9. L. D. Johnston, P. M. O'Malley, and J. G. Bachman, *Monitoring the Future, National Survey Results on Drug Use 1975–2002*

Volume II: College Students and Adults Ages 19–40 (NIH Publication No. 03-5376) (Bethesda, MD: National Institute on Drug Abuse, 2003).

10. Ibid., 215.

11. M. Fishman and C. Johanson, "Cocaine," in *Pharmacological Aspects of Drug Dependence: Towards an Integrated Neurobehavior Approach (Handbook of Experimental Pharmacology),* ed. C. Schuster and M. Kuhar (Hamburg: Springer Verlag, 1996), 159–195.

12. Ibid.

13. National Institute on Drug Abuse, *Capsules* (1996).

14. H. C. Ashton, "Pharmacology and Effects of Cannabis: A Brief Review," *The British Journal of Psychiatry* 178 (2001): 101–106.

15. American Academy of Ophthalmology, Medical Library, "The Use of Marijuana in the Treatment of Glaucoma." www.medem.com/MedLB/article_detaillb.cfm?article_ID = ZZZXIEOMH4C&sub_cat-115

16. R. Mathias, "Marijuana Impairs Driving-Related Skills and Workplace Performance," *NIDA Notes* 11, no. 1 (January–February 1996): 6.

17. National Institute on Drug Abuse, "Heroin, 0-12," *Infofax* (1998): 1.

18. Johnston, O'Malley, and Bachman, *Monitoring the Future.*

19. National Institute on Drug Abuse, "NIDA Launches Initiative to Combat Club Drugs," *NIDA Notes* 14, no. 2 (2000).

20. National Institute on Drug Abuse, "Anabolic Steroid Abuse," *NIDA Research Report Series* (2000).

21. Office of National Drug Control Strategy, "National Drug Control Strategy: 2002," 2002. www.whitehousedrugpolicy.gov

22. Ibid.

23. National Institute on Drug Abuse, *Worker Drug Use and Workplace Policies and Programs: Results from the 1994 and 1997 National Household Survey on Drug Abuse* (Bethesda, MD: National Institute on Drug Abuse, 1999).

24. Ibid.

CHAPTER 8

1. L. D. Johnson, P. M. O'Malley, and J. G. Bachman, *The Monitoring the Future Study, 1975–1999,* Vol. 2 (Rockville, MD: National Institute of Drug Abuse, 2000), 71.

2. A. Cohen, "Battle of the Binge," *Time,* September 8, 1997.

3. H. Weschler et al., "Trends in College Binge Drinking during a Period of Increased Prevention Efforts: Findings from Four Harvard School of Public Health College Study Surveys: 1993–2001," *Journal of American College Health* 50, no. 5 (2002): 207.

4. L. D. Johnson, P. M. O'Malley, and J. G. Bachman, *The Monitoring the Future Study, 1975–2002,* Vol. 2 (Rockville, MD: National Institute of Drug Abuse, 2003).

5. Weschler et al., "Trends in College Binge Drinking."

6. Weschler et al., "College Binge Drinking in the 1990s: A Continuing Problem," *Journal of American College Health* 28 (2000): 202.

7. J. Knight et al., "Alcohol Abuse and Dependence among U.S. College Students," *Journal of Studies on Alcohol* 63, no. 3 (2002): 263–270.

8. T. Katsouyanni et al., "Ethanol and Breast Cancer: An Association That May Be Both Confounded and Causal," *International Journal of Cancer* 58, no. 3 (1994): 356–361.

9. C. Ikonomidou et al., "Ethanol-Induced Apoptotic Neurodegeneration and the Fetal Alcohol Syndrome," *Science* 287 (2000): 1056–1060.

10. National Highway Traffic Safety Administration, "Traffic Safety Facts 2002—Alcohol," 2003. www.nhtsa.dot.gov.

11. H. Wechsler et al., "Changes in Binge Drinking and Related Problems among American College Students between 1993 and 1997," *Journal of American College Health* 47, no. 2 (1998): 57–68.

12. Ibid.
13. National Highway Traffic Safety Administration, "Traffic Safety Facts 2002—Alcohol."
14. Ibid.
15. Ibid.
16. Ibid.
17. F. K. Goodwin and E. M. Gause, "Alcohol, Drug Abuse, and Mental Health Administration," *Prevention Pipeline* 3 (1990): 19.
18. Marc A. Shockit, "New Findings on Genetics of Alcoholism," *The Journal of American Medical Association* 281, no. 20 (1999): 1875–1976.
19. "Adult Children of Alcoholics," *Alcohol Issues and Solutions* 6, no. 2 (2000): 6.
20. B. F. Grant, "Estimates of U.S. Children Exposed to Alcohol Abuse and Dependence in the Family," *American Journal of Public Health* 90, no. 1 (2000).
21. U.S. Department of Health and Human Services, *Ninth Special Report to the U.S. Congress on Alcohol and Health* (1997): 261.
22. E. Gomberg, "Women and Alcohol: Issues for Prevention Research," *National Institute on Alcohol Abuse and Alcohol Research Monograph* 32 (1996): 185–214.
23. Ibid.
24. J. M. McGinnis and W. H. Foege, "Actual Causes of Death in the United States," *The Journal of the American Medical Association* 270 (1993): 2207–2212.
25. American Lung Association Epidemiology and Statistics Unit, "Trends in Tobacco Use," June 2003. www.lungusa.org/data/smoke/SMK1.pdf
26. Centers for Disease Control and Prevention, "Trends in Cigarette Smoking among High School Students—United States, 1991–2001," *Morbidity and Mortality Weekly* 51, no. 19 (2002): 409–412.
27. Centers for Disease Control and Prevention, *Annual Smoking-Attributable Mortality, Years of Potential Life Lost, and Economic Costs—United States* 51, no. 14.
28. N. Rigotti, J. Lee, and H. Wechsler, "U.S. College Students' Use of Tobacco Products," *The Journal of the American Medical Association* 284 (2000): 699–705.
29. S. A. Everett et al., "Smoking Initiation and Smoking Patterns among U. S. College Students," *Journal of American College Health* 48 (1999): 55.
30. American Cancer Society, "Harmful Effects of Tobacco," 2003, www.cancer.org.
31. American Lung Association, "Trends in Tobacco Use."
32. S. Hansen, "Bidis," University of Iowa's Student Health Service/Health Iowa. www.uiowa.edu/~shs
33. National Institutes of Health, *Smokeless Tobacco or Health,* Monograph 2 (May 1993): 3.
34. Oral Cancer Foundation, "Oral Cancer Facts," 2002. www.oralcancer.org.
35. American Cancer Society. "Cancer Facts and Figures 2003." 2003. www.cancer.org
36. American Cancer Society, "Harmful Effects of Tobacco."
37. "Study Links Smoking to Pancreatic Cancer," *Science News,* October 22, 1994, 261.
38. WHO Collaborative Study of Cardiovascular Disease and Steroid Hormone Contraception, "Acute Myocardial Infraction and Combined Oral Contraceptives: Results of an International Multicentre Case-Control Study," *The Lancet* (April 26, 1997): 1202–1209.
39. American Cancer Society, "Harmful Effects of Tobacco."
40. National Institute on Drug Abuse, "Nicotine Conference Highlights Research Accomplishments and Challenges," *NIDA Notes* (September/October 1995): 11–12.
41. American Lung Association, "Secondhand Smoke." www.lungusa.org

42. K. Steenland, "Passive Smoking and the Risk of Heart Disease," *The Journal of the American Medical Association* 267 (1992): 94–99.
43. P. Hilts, "Wide Peril Is Seen in Passive Smoking," *The New York Times,* May 9, 1990, A25.
44. American Lung Association, "Secondhand Smoke."
45. D. Mannino, "Children Exposed to ETS Miss More School," *Tobacco Control* (May 1996).
46. Tobacco Control Research Center, Tobacco Litigation Documents, "Multistate Settlement with Tobacco Industry." www.library.ucsf.edu/tobacco/litigation
47. "Nicotine Patches Seen to Help Smokers Quit," *The Boston Globe,* June 23, 1994, 3.
48. "Grounds for Breaking the Coffee Habit," *Tufts University Diet and Nutrition Newsletter* 7 (1990): 4.
49. "Fetal Loss Associated with Caffeine," *Fact and Comparisons Drug Newsletter* 13 (March 1994): 39.

CHAPTER 9
1. Oregon Dairy Council, Nutrition Education Services, "Quotable Nutrition: It's All About You," news release, 1998.
2. American Dietetic Association, "Nutrition and You Survey," 2002. www.eatright.org/pr/2002/052002a.html
3. J. Beary and R. Donatelle (doctoral dissertation, Oregon State University, 1994).
4. C. Georgiou et al., "Among Young Adults, College Students and Graduates Practiced More Healthful Habits and Made More Healthful Food Choices Than Did Non-Students," *Journal of the American Dietetic Association* 97 (1997): 754–762.
5. E. Whitney and S. Rolfes, *Understanding Nutrition, 8th ed.* (Belmont, CA: Wadsworth, 1999), 3–4.
6. National Center for Health Statistics, "Prevalence of Overweight and Obesity Among Adults: United States, 1999–2000," 2002. www.cdc.gov/nchs/products/pubs/pubd/hestats/obese/obse99.htm
7. Office of the Surgeon General, The Surgeon General's Call to Action to Prevent and Decrease Overweight and Obesity: The Health Consequences of Obesity," 2001. www.surgeongeneral.gov/topics/obesity
8. D. Ludwig, *Obesity: A New Dietary Treatment for a Major Public Health Threat,* Linus Pauling Institute International Conference on Diet and Optimum Health (Portland, OR: May, 2001).
9. American Dietetic Association, "American Dietetic Association Survey Shows Americans Can Use Some Help in Sizing Up Their Meals," 2002. www.eatright.org/pr/2002/052002b.html
10. "Proteins," *Harvard Women's Health Watch* 5 (1998): 4.
11. Ibid., 4.
12. J. W. White and M. Wolraich, "Effect of Sugar on Behavior or Cognition in Children: A Meta-Analysis," *The Journal of the American Medical Association* 274 (1995): 1617–1621.
13. "Is Sugar Really Addictive?" *Tufts University Health and Nutrition Letter: Special Report* 20, no. 8 (2002): 1–4.
14. "Do Potato Chips Cause Cancer? Don't Panic Yet, Say Experts," *Environmental Nutrition* 25, no. 6 (2002): 3.
15. Center for Science in the Public Interest, "New Tests Confirm Acrylamide in American Foods: Snack Chips, French Fries Show Highest Levels of Known Carcinogens," 2002. www.cspinet.org/new/200206251.html
16. World Cancer Research Fund/American Institute for Cancer Research, *Food, Nutrition, and the Prevention of Cancer: A Global Perspective* (Washington: World Cancer Research Fund/American Institute for Cancer Research, 1997); C. Fuchs et al., "Dietary Fiber and the Risk of Colorectal Cancer and Adenoma in Women," *The New England Journal of Medicine* 340 (1999): 169–176.
17. Fuchs et al., "Dietary Fiber," 170.
18. Ibid.

19. American Dietetic Association, "Position Statement: Diabetic Care," 22 suppl., no. 1 (1999): 542.

20. R. Mensink and M. Katan, "Effect of Dietary Trans-Fatty Acids on High-Density and Low-Density Lipoprotein and Cholesterol Levels in Healthy Subjects," *The New England Journal of Medicine* 323, no. 7 (1990): 439–445.

21. G. Ruoff, "Reducing Fat Intake with Fat Substitutes," *American Family Physician* 43 (1991): 1235–1242.

22. *Food, Nutrition and the Prevention of Cancer,* 532.

23. W. Willet and A. Ascherio, "Health Effects of Trans-Fatty Acids," *American Journal of Clinical Nutrition* 66 (1997): 1006S–1010S.

24. Whitney and Rolfes, *Understanding Nutrition,* 144.

25. American Heart Association, Nutrition Advisory Committee, "Trans-Fatty Acids," news release, May 13, 1994.

26. Willet and Ascherio, "Health Effects of Trans-Fatty Acids."

27. Whitney and Rolfes, *Understanding Nutrition,* 144.

28. E. Ward, R. D., "Balancing Essential Dietary Fats: When More Might Be Better," *Environmental Nutrition* 24, no. 12 (2002): 1–6.

29. Ibid.

30. J. Midgley et al., "Effects of Reduced Dietary Sodium on Blood Pressure: A Meta-Analysis of Randomized Controlled Trials," *The Journal of the American Medical Association* 275 (1996): 1590–1598.

31. "The CLA Paradox," *American Institute for Cancer Research Newsletter,* issue 78 (Winter 2003): 8–9.

32. "MUFAs and PUFAs," *Food and Fitness Advisor,* September 2002.

33. J. Midgley et al., "Effects of Reduced Dietary Sodium on Blood Pressure."

34. Whitney and Rolfes, *Understanding Nutrition,* 412.

35. A. C. Looker et al., "Prevalence of Iron Deficiency in the United States," *The Journal of the American Medical Association* 277 (1997): 973–976; "Recommendations to Prevent and Control Iron Deficiency in the United States," *Morbidity and Mortality Weekly Report* 47 (1998 supplement).

36. G. T. Sempos, A. C. Looker, and R. E. Gillum, "Iron and Heart Disease: The Epidemiological Data," *Nutrition Reviews* 54 (1996): 73–84.

37. Whitney and Rolfes, *Understanding Nutrition,* 412.

38. "Food as Medicine," *Harvard Women's Health Watch* 5 (1998): 4–5.

39. J. Blumber, *Changing Vitamin Requirements,* L. Kolonel, *Overview of Diet and Cancer Epidemiology,* M. Gould, *The Anticancer Effects of Plant Monoterpenes,* J. Potter, *Diet and Colorectal Cancer.* Papers presented at Linus Pauling Institute International Conference on Diet and Optimum Health (Portland, OR: May, 2001).

40. "Food as Medicine," 5.

41. M. Manore and J. Thomson, *Sport Nutrition for Health and Performance* (Champaign, IL: Human Kinetics Publishing, 2000), 278–283.

42. Ibid., 283.

43. E. Giovanucci et al., "Intake of Carotenoids and Retinol in Relation to Risk of Prostate Cancer," *Journal of the National Cancer Institute* 87 (1995): 1767.

44. "Kale, Collards, and Spinach Beat Carrots for Protecting Aging Eyes," *Environmental Nutrition* 24, no. 4 (2001).

45. Ibid.

46. J. Carper, R. D. "Eat Smart," *USA Weekend,* May 3–5, 2002, 6.

47. J. Smythies, *Every Person's Guide to Antioxidants* (Newark, NJ: Rutgers University Press, 1998).

48. Ibid.

49. B. Frei, *Closing Remarks Summary, 2001.* Paper presented at the Linus Pauling Institute International Conference on Diet and Optimum Health (Portland, OR: May, 2001).

50. Ibid.

51. R. Malinow, *Homocysteine, Folic Acid and CVD, 2001.* Linus Pauling Institute International Conference Diet and Optimum Health (Portland, OR: May, 2001).

52. Frei, *Closing Remarks Summary, 2001.*

53. Ibid.

54. R. Malinow, *Homocysteine, Folic Acid and CVD, 2001.*

55. N. T. Crane, V. S. Hubbard, and C .J. Lewis, "National Nutrition Objectives and Dietary Guidelines for Americans," *Nutrition Today* 33 (1998): 186–188.

56. Ibid.

57. L. K. Mahan and S. Escott-Stump, *Krause's Food, Nutrition, and Diet Therapy* (Philadelphia: Saunders, 2000): 343–345.

58. S. Loft, *Diet, Oxidative DNA Damage and Cancer, 2001.* L. Kolonel, *Overview of Diet and Cancer Epidemiology.* Papers presented at the Linus Pauling Institute International Conference on Diet and Optimum Health (Portland, OR: May, 2001).

59. K. M. Fairfield and R. H. Fletcher, "Vitamins for Chronic Disease Prevention in Adults: Scientific Review," *The Journal of the American Medical Association* 287, no. 23 (2001): 3116–3126.

60. D. Bender, "Daily Doses of Multivitamin Tablets," *British Medical Journal* 325 (2002): 173–174.

61. Centers for Disease Control and Prevention, Center for Infectious Diseases. "Food Borne Illnesses," 2002. www.cdc.gov

62. J. Stephenson, "Public Health Experts Take Aim at a Moving Target: Food-Borne Infections," *The Journal of the American Medical Association* 277 (1997): 97–102.

63. Ibid., 98.

64. Ibid.

65. Ibid., 99.

66. L. Hughes, "Don't Let Unexpected Visitors 'Spoil' Summer Meals," *Environmental Nutrition* 25, no. 6 (2002): 2.

67. P. Morris, Y. Motarjemi, and F. Kaferstein, "Emerging Food-Borne Diseases," *World Health* 50 (1997): 16–22.

68. "Special Report: Irradiation Plants Geared to 'Zap' Meat and Poultry—Is it Safe?" *Tufts University Health and Nutrition Letter* 18, no. 1 (2000): 4–7.

69. Ibid., 5.

70. National Institute of Allergy and Infectious Diseases, National Institute of Health, "Fact Sheet: Food Allergy and Intolerances," 2002. www.niaid.nih.gov/factsheets/food.htm

71. Ibid.

CHAPTER 10

1. National Center for Health Statistics, "Prevalence of Overweight and Obesity among Adults: United States, 1999–2000," 2002. www.cdc.gov/nchs/products/pubs/pubd/hestats/obese/obse99.htm; Weight-Control Information Network, "Statistics Related to Overweight and Obesity," July 2003. www.niddk.nih.gov/health/nutrit/pubs/statobes.htm

2. G. Cowley, "Generation XXL," *Newsweek,* July 3, 2000, 40–46; K. R. Fontaine et al., "Years of Life Lost due to Obesity," *The Journal of the American Medical Association* 289, no. 2 (2003): 187–193.

3. J. P. Boyle et al., "Projection of Diabetes Burden through 2050: Impact of Changing Demography and Disease Prevalence in the U.S.," *Diabetes Care* 24, no. 11 (2001): 1936–1940.

4. E. A. Finkelstein, I. C. Fiebelkorn, and G. Wang, "National Medical Spending Attributable to Overweight and Obesity: How Much, and Who's Paying?" *Health Affairs* (2003). www.healthaffairs.org/WebExclusives/Finkelstein_Web_Excl_051403.htm

5. National Center for Health Statistics, "Prevalence of Overweight and Obesity."

6. Centers for Disease Control and Prevention, "Defining Overweight and Obesity," 2002. www.cdc.gov/nccdphp/dnpa/obesity/defining.htm

7. Weight-Control Information Network, "Statistics Related to Overweight and Obesity."

8. Centers for Disease Control and Prevention, "Defining Overweight and Obesity."

9. Weight-Control Information Network, "Statistics Related to Overweight and Obesity."

10. Ibid.

11. Ibid.

12. Ibid.

13. D. Eberwine, "Globesity: The Crisis of Growing Proportions," *Perspectives in Health* 7, no. 3 (2003): 9.

14. Center for Nutrition Policy and Promotion, "Dietary Guidelines for Americans 2000, 5th Edition," 2000. www.usda.gov/cnpp/Pubs/DG2000

15. Centers for Disease Control and Prevention, "Defining Overweight and Obesity."

16. S. Cummings, E. S. Parham, and G. W. Strain, "Position Paper on Weight Management," *Journal of the American Dietetic Association* 102 (2002): 1145–1155.

17. J. G. Meisler and S. St. Jeor, "Summary and Recommendations from the American Health Foundation's Expert Panel on Healthy Weight," *The American Journal of Clinical Nutrition* 63 (1996): 474S–477S.

18. U.S. Department of Health and Human Services, "The Surgeon General's Call to Action to Prevent and Decrease Overweight and Obesity," 2001. www.surgeongeneral.gov/topics/obesity

19. Weight-Control Information Network, "Statistics Related to Overweight and Obesity."

20. U.S. Department of Health and Human Services, "The Surgeon General's Call to Action."

21. S. A. French, M. Story, and R. W. Jeffrey, "Environmental Influences on Eating and Physical Activity," *Annual Review Public Health* 22 (2001): 309–335.

22. Ibid., 312, 320.

23. M. W. Gillman et al., "Risk of Overweight among Adolescents Who Were Breastfed as Infants," *The Journal of the American Medical Association* 285 (2001): 2461–2467; M. L. Hediger et al., "Association between Infant Breastfeeding and Overweight in Young Children," *The Journal of the American Medical Association* 285 (2001): 2453–2460.

24. National Center for Health Statistics, "Prevalence of Overweight and Obesity."

25. C. J. Crespo et al., "Television Watching, Energy Intake, and Obesity in U.S. Children: Results from the Third National Health and Nutrition Examination Survey," *Archives of Pediatric and Adolescent Medicine* 155 (2001): 360–255; W. H. Dietz, "The Obesity Epidemic in Young Children: Reduce Television Viewing and Promote Playing," *British Medical Journal* 322 (2001): 313–324.

26. M. Dowda et al., "Environmental Influences, Physical Activity and Weight Status in 8–12 Year Olds," *Archives of Pediatrics and Adolescent Medicine* 155 (2001): 711–717.

27. Ibid., 715.

28. "Special Report: Weight Control," in *Women's HealthSource* (Mayo Clinic, 1997), 3.

29. A. Stunkard et al., "The Body Mass Index of Twins Who Have Been Raised Apart," *The New England Journal of Medicine* 322 (1990): 1477–1482.

30. C. Bouchard et al., "The Response to Long-Term Overfeeding in Identical Twins," *The New England Journal of Medicine* 322 (1990): 1483–1487.

31. Ibid.

32. Cummings, Parham, and Strain, "Position Paper on Weight Management," 73.

33. P. Jaret, "The Way to Lose Weight," *Health* (January–February 1995): 52–59.

34. A. Novitt-Morena, "Obesity: What's the Genetic Connection?" *Current Health* 24 (1998): 18–23.

35. "Genes and Appetite," *Harvard Women's Health Watch,* January 1996; L. Tartaglia et al., "Identification and Expression Cloning of a Leptin Receptor," *Cell* 83 (1995): 1263–1271.

36. "Special Report: Weight Control."

37. M. Turton et al., "A Role for Glucagon-Like Peptide 1 in the Central Regulation of Feeding," *Nature* 379 (1996): 69–72.

38. "Special Report: Weight Control," 4.

39. K. Brownell, *Comments on the Latest Study on Yo-Yo Diets by Steven Blair of the Institute for Aerobics Research* (paper presented in 1993, newer report presented Fall 1998 at Oregon State University by Steven Blair).

40. National Center for Health Statistics, "Prevalence of Sedentary Leisure-Time Behavior among Adults in the United States," December 2000. www.cdc.gov/nchs/products/pubs/pubd/hestats/3and4/sedentary.htm

41. Ibid.

42. Ibid.

43. "Special Report: Weight Control," 4.

44. N. Diehl, C. Johnson, and R. Rogers, "Social Physique Anxiety and Disordered Eating: What's the Connection?" *Addictive Behaviors* 23 (1998): 1–16.

45. "Special Report: Weight Control," 4.

46. G. K. Goodrick and J. P. Foreyt, "Why Treatments for Obesity Don't Last," *Journal of the American Dietetic Association* 91 (1991): 1243–1247.

47. C. F. Telch and W. S. Agras, "The Effects of Very Low-Calorie Diet on Binge Eating," *Behavior Therapy* 24 (1993): 177–193.

48. *USA TODAY Weekend,* July 14–16, 2000, 6.

49. Cummings, Parham, and Strain, "Position Paper on Weight Management," 75.

50. R. L. Atkinson, "Use of Drugs in Treatment of Obesity," *Annual Review of Nutrition* 17 (1997): 383–403.

51. Fen-Phen-Legal-Resources.com, "Advancing the Rights of Patients," 2002. www.fen-phen-legal-resources.com

52. Food and Drug Administration, "FDA Approves Orlistat for Obesity," 1999. www.fda.gov/bbs/topics/ANSWERS/ANS00951.html

53. U.S. Food and Drug Administration Center for Drug Evaluation and Research, "Phenylpropanolamine (PPA) Information Page," 2003. www.fda.gov/cder/drug/infopage/ppa/

54. E. Whitney and S. Rolfes, *Understanding Nutrition,* 9th ed. (Belmont, CA: Wadsworth, 2002), 279.

55. "Eating Disorders," *Harvard Mental Health Letter* 14 (1997): 4.

CHAPTER 11

1. U.S. Department of Health and Human Services, *The Surgeon General's Call to Action to Prevent and Decrease Overweight and Obesity* (Rockville, MD: U.S. Department of Health and Human Services, Public Health Service, Office of the Surgeon General, 2001); U.S. Department of Health and Human Services. "Physical Activity Fundamental to Preventing Disease." 2002. http://aspe.hhs.gov/health/reports/physicalactivity

2. U.S. Department of Health and Human Services. "Physical Activity Fundamental to Preventing Disease."

3. Ibid.

4. American Heart Association, *Heart and Stroke Statistical Update* (Dallas, TX: American Heart Association, 2003); U.S. Department of Health and Human Services. "Physical Activity Fundamental to Preventing Disease."

5. R. Gates, "Fitness Is Changing the World: For Women," *IDEA Today* (July–August 1992): 58.

6. U.S. Department of Health and Human Services, *Healthy People 2000: National Health Promotion and Disease Prevention Objectives* (DHHS [PHS] Publication No. 91-50213) (Washington, D.C.: Government Printing Office, 1991).

7. C. J. Caspersen, K. E. Powell, and G. M. Christianson, "Physical Activity, Exercise, and Physical Fitness: Definitions and Distinctions for Health-Related Research," *Public Health Report* 100 (1985): 126–131.

8. L. Bernstein et al., "Adolescent Exercise Reduces Risk of Breast Cancer in Younger Women," *Journal of the National Cancer Institute* (September 1994).

9. U.S. Department of Health and Human Services. "Physical Activity and Health: A Report of the Surgeon General," 2002. www.cdc.gov/nccdphp/sgr/mm.htm

10. Gates, "Fitness Is Changing the World."

11. W. McCardle, F. Katch, and V. Katch. *Exercise Physiology, 5th ed.* (Philadelphia: Lippincott, Williams, and Wilkins, 2001), 873.

12. C. B. Corbin and R. Lindsey, *Concepts in Physical Education with Laboratories, 8th ed.* (Dubuque, IA: Times Mirror, 1994).

13. U.S. Department of Health and Human Services, "Physical Activity and Health."

14. W. L. Haskell et al., "Cardiovascular Benefits and Assessment of Physical Activity and Physical Fitness in Adults," *Medicine and Science in Sports and Exercise* 24, no. 6, Supplement (1992): S201–S220.

15. K. Ishikawa-Takata, T. Ohta, and H. Tanaka, "How Much Exercise Is Required to Reduce Blood Pressure in Essential Hypertensives: A Dose-Response Study," *American Journal of Hypertension* 16, no. 8 (2003): 629–633.

16. C. Christmas, "Fitness for Reducing Osteoporosis," *The Physician and Sports Medicine* 28 (October 2000): 33–34.

17. C. M. Snow, J. M. Shaw, and C. C. Matkin, "Physical Activity and Risks for Osteoporosis," in *Osteoporosis,* eds. R. Marcus, D. Feldman, and J. Kelsy (San Diego: Academic Press, 1996), 511–528.

18. C. Snow and T. Hayes, *Bone Health Lecture* (Corvallis, OR: Modern Maladies Class, Oregon State University, 2001).

19. McCardle, Katch, and Katch, *Exercise Physiology,* 60–65.

20. *ACSM's Guidelines for Exercise Testing and Prescription, 6th ed.* (Philadelphia: Lippincott, Williams and Wilkins, 2000).

21. R. Ross, J. A. Freeman, and I. Janssen, "Exercise Alone Is an Effective Strategy for Reducing Obesity and Related Comorbidities," *Exercise and Sport Sciences Reviews* 28, no. 4 (2000): 165–170.

22. Ibid.

23. National Institutes of Health, "Consensus Development Conference Statement on Diet and Exercise in Non-Insulin-Dependent Diabetes Mellitus," *Diabetes Care* 10 (1987): 639–644.

24. S. P. Helmrich, D. R. Ragland, and R. S. Paffenbarger, Jr., "Prevention of Non-Insulin-Dependent Diabetes Mellitus with Physical Activity," *Medicine and Science in Sports and Exercise* 26 (1994): 824–830.

25. S. N. Blair et al., "Physical Fitness and All-Cause Mortality: A Prospective Study of Healthy Men and Women," *The Journal of the American Medical Association* 262 (1989): 2395–2401.

26. E. R. Eichner, "Infection, Immunity, and Exercise: What to Tell Patients?" *The Physician and Sportsmedicine* 21 (January 1993): 125–135.

27. W. A. Primos, Jr., "Sports and Exercise During Acute Illness: Recommending the Right Course for Patients," *The Physician and Sportsmedicine* 24 (January 1996): 44–53.

28. D. C. Nieman et al., "Infectious Episodes in Runners Before and After the Los Angeles Marathon," *Journal of Sports Medicine and Physical Fitness* 30 (1990): 316–328.

29. Eichner, "Infection, Immunity, and Exercise."

30. Ibid.

31. Gates, "Fitness Is Changing the World."

32. E. T. Howley and D. B. Franks, *Health Fitness Instructor's Handbook, 2nd ed.* (Champaign, IL: Human Kinetics Books, 1992).

33. U.S. Department of Health and Human Services, "Physical Activity and Health."

34. McCardle, Katch, and Katch. *Exercise Physiology,* 483.

35. Ibid.

36. B. Stamford, "Tracking Your Heart Rate for Fitness," *The Physician and Sportsmedicine* 21 (March 1993): 227–228.

37. U.S. Centers for Disease Control and Prevention and American College of Sports Medicine, "Summary Statement: Workshop on Physical Activity and Public Health," *Sports Medicine Bulletin* 28, no. 4 (1993): 7.

38. G. A. Klug and J. Lettunich, *Wellness: Exercise and Physical Fitness* (Guilford, CT: Dushkin Publishing Group, 1992).

39. P. D. Wood, "Physical Activity, Diet, and Health: Independent and Interactive Effects." *Medicine and Science in Sports and Exercise* 26 (1994): 838–843.

40. American College of Sports Medicine, "ACSM Position Stand on the Recommended Quantity and Quality of Exercise for Developing and Maintaining Cardiorespiratory and Muscular Fitness, and Flexibility in Adults." *Medicine and Science in Sports and Exercise* 30, no. 6 (1998): 975–991.

41. Ibid.

42. M. Cyphers, "Flexibility," in *Personal Trainer Manual, 2nd ed.* (San Diego: American Council on Exercise, 1996), 291–308.

43. P. A. Sienna, *One Rep Max: A Guide to Beginning Weight Training* (Indianapolis: Benchmark Press, 1989).

44. H. G. Knuttgen and W. J. Kraemer, "Terminology and Measurement in Exercise Performance," *Journal of Applied Sport Science Research* 1 (1987): 1–10.

45. M. S. Feigenbaum and M. L. Pollock, "Prescription of Resistance Training for Health and Disease," *Medicine and Science in Sports and Exercise* 31 (1999): 38–45.

46. M. L. Pollock and W. J. Evans, "Resistance Training for Health and Disease: Introduction," *Medicine and Science in Sports and Exercise* 31 (1999): 10–11.

47. American College of Sports Medicine, "ACSM Position Stand on the Recommended Quantity and Quality of Exercise."

48. C. L. Wells, *Women, Sport, and Performance: A Physiological Perspective, 2nd ed.* (Champaign, IL: Human Kinetics, 1991).

49. American College of Sports Medicine, "ACSM Position Stand on the Recommended Quantity and Quality of Exercise."

50. W. C. Whiting and R. F. Zernicke, *Biomechanics of Musculoskeletal Injury* (Champaign, IL: Human Kinetics, 1998).

51. D. M. Brody, "Running Injuries: Prevention and Management," *Clinical Symposia* 39 (1987).

52. J. C. Erie, "Eye Injuries: Prevention, Evaluation, and Treatment," *The Physician and Sportsmedicine* 19 (November 1991): 108–122.

53. R. C. Wasserman and R. V. Buccini, "Helmet Protection from Head Injuries among Recreational Bicyclists," *American Journal of Sports Medicine* 18 (1990): 96–97.

54. S. M. Simons, "Foot Injuries of the Recreational Athlete," *The Physician and Sportsmedicine* 27 (January 1999): 57–70.

55. J. Andrish and J. A. Work, "How I Manage Shin Splints," *The Physician and Sportsmedicine* 18 (December 1990): 113–114.

56. E. A. Arendt, "Common Musculoskeletal Injuries in Women," *The Physician and Sportsmedicine* 24 (July 1996): 39–48.

57. American Academy of Orthopaedic Surgeons, *Athletic Training and Sports Medicine, 3rd ed.* (Park Ridge, IL: American Academy of Orthopaedic Surgeons, 2000).

58. J. J. Mistovich, B. Q. Hafen, and K. J. Karren, *Prehospital Emergency Care, 6th ed.* (Upper Saddle River, NJ: Prentice-Hall, 2000).

59. American College of Sports Medicine, "Position Stand—Heat and Cold Illnesses During Distance Running," *Medicine and Science in Sports and Exercise* 28 (December 1996): i–x.

60. American College of Sports Medicine, "Position Stand—Exercise and Fluid Replacement," *Medicine and Science in Sports and Exercise* 28 (January 1996): i–vii.

61. P. R. Below et al., "Fluid and Carbohydrate Ingestion Independently Improve Performance During 1 Hr of Intense Exercise," *Medicine and Science in Sports and Exercise* 27 (1995): 200–210.

62. D. J. Casa et al., "National Athletic Trainers' Association Position Statement: Fluid Replacement for Athletes," *Journal of Athletic Training* 35, no. 2 (2000): 212–224.

63. J. S. Thornton, "Hypothermia Shouldn't Freeze Out Cold-Weather Athletes," *The Physician and Sportsmedicine* 18 (January 1990): 109–113.
64. American College of Sports Medicine, "Position Stand—Heat and Cold Illnesses During Distance Running."
65. N. Clark, "Muscle Cramps: Do They Cramp Your Style?' *Newsletter of the American College of Sports Medicine* (Summer 2001): 7.
66. Ibid.
67. Ibid.

CHAPTER 12

1. American Heart Association, *Heart Disease and Stroke Statistics—2003 Update* (Dallas, TX: American Heart Association, 2003).
2. Ibid., 4.
3. Ibid., 5.
4. Ibid., 5.
5. Ibid.
6. Ibid., 40.
7. Ibid.
8. R. Ross, "Atherosclerosis—an Inflammatory Disease," *The New England Journal of Medicine* 340 (1999): 115–126.
9. C. Napoli et al., "Fatty Streak Formation Occurs in Human Fetal Aortas and Is Greatly Enhanced by Maternal Hypercholesterolemia: Intimal Accumulation of Low-Density Lipoprotein and Its Oxidative Precede Monocyte Recruitment into Early Atherosclerotic Lesions," *Journal of Clinical Investigation* 100 (1997): 2680–2690.
10. J. L. Breslow, "Cardiovascular Disease Burden Increases, NIH Funding Decreases," *Nature Medicine* 3 (1997): 6000–6009.
11. Ross, "Atherosclerosis—an Inflammatory Disease," 115.
12. J. Danesh, R. Collins, and R. Peto, "Chronic Infections and Coronary Heart Disease: Is There a Link?" *The Lancet* 350 (1997): 430–436.
13. E. Braunwald, "Cardiovascular Medicine at the Turn of the Millennium: Triumphs, Concerns, and Opportunities," *The New England Journal of Medicine* 337 (1997): 1360–1369.
14. Ross, "Atherosclerosis—an Inflammatory Disease," 122.
15. A. Forman, "The Threat of Insulin Resistance to Your Heart," *Environmental Nutrition* 23, no. 8 (2000): 4–6.
16. American Heart Association, "Syndrome X or Metabolic Syndrome," 2002. www.americanheart.org/presenter.jhtml?identifier=534
17. American Heart Association, *Heart Disease and Stroke Statistics,* 11.
18. Ibid., 14.
19. Ibid., 23.
20. Ibid., 23.
21. Ibid., 23.
22. Ibid., 24.
23. Ibid., 44.
24. Ibid., 15.
25. Ibid., 26.
26. Ibid., 26.
27. Ibid., 26
28. Ibid., 28.
29. National Heart, Lung and Blood Institute, "Third Report of the National Cholesterol Education Program (NCEP) Expert Panel on Detection, Evaluation and Treatment of High Blood Cholesterol in Adults (Adult Treatment Panel III)," May, 2001. www.nhlbi.nih.gov/guidelines/cholesterol/index.htm
30. Ibid.
31. American Heart Association, *Heart Disease and Stroke Statistics.*
32. National Heart, Lung and Blood Institute, "Third Report of the National Cholesterol Education Program (NCEP)."

33. Ibid.
34. Ibid.
35. Center for Science in the Public Interest, *Nutrition Action Health Letter* 22 (1995): 4.
36. U.S. Department of Health and Human Services, *Surgeon General's Report on Physical Activity* (1996) www.cdc.gov/nccdphp/sgr/contents.htm; American Heart Association, *Heart Disease and Stroke Statistics,* 30.
37. American Heart Association, *2001 Heart and Stroke Statistical Update* (Dallas, TX: American Heart Association, 2001): 18.
38. Ibid. 18.
39. Ross, "Atherosclerosis—an Inflammatory Disease," 117.
40. R. Eliot, "Changing Behavior: A New Comprehensive and Quantitative Approach" (Keynote Address at the Annual Meeting of the American College of Cardiology on Stress and the Heart, Jackson Hole, Wyoming, July 3, 1987).
41. L. L. Yan et al., "Psychosocial Factors and Risk of Hypertension," *The Journal of the American Medical Association* 290, no. 16 (2003): 2138–2148.
42. American Heart Association, *Heart Disease and Stroke Statistics,* 4.
43. A. G. Boston et al., "Elevated Plasma Lipoprotein(a) and Coronary Heart Disease in Men Aged 55 Years and Younger: A Prospective Study," *The Journal of the American Medical Association* 276 (1996): 555–558.
44. Ibid., 555.
45. Ibid., 556.
46. National Heart, Lung and Blood Institute, "Heart Memo: The Cardiovascular Health of Women" (Bethesda, MD: NHLBI, 1995): 5.
47. Ibid., 5.
48. American Heart Association, *2001 Heart and Stroke Facts* (Dallas, TX: American Heart Association, 2001), 25.
49. J. E. Willard, R. A. Lange, and D. L. Hillis, "The Use of Aspirin in Ischemic Heart Disease," *The New England Journal of Medicine* 327 (1992): 175–179.
50. Agency for Health Care Policy and Research, "Cardiac Rehabilitation: Exercise, Training, Education, Counseling, and Behavioral Interventions" (Publication #96-0672, 1996).

CHAPTER 13

1. American Cancer Society, *Cancer Facts and Figures 2003* (Atlanta: American Cancer Society, 2003), 1–2.
2. Ibid., 1.
3. Ibid., 2.
4. Ibid., 29.
5. Ibid.
6. Ibid., 1.
7. Julian Peto, "Cancer Epidemiology in the Last Century and Next Decade," *Nature* 411 (2001): 390–395.
8. Ibid.
9. L. Remennick, "The Cancer Problem in the Context of Modernity, Sociology, Demography and Politics," *Current Sociology* 46 (1998): 144.
10. American Cancer Society, *Cancer Facts and Figures 2003,* 1.
11. Ibid., 1.
12. M. Osborne, P. Boyle, and M. Lipkin, "Cancer Prevention," *The Lancet* 349 (1997): 1–8 (special oncology supplement).
13. American Cancer Society, *Cancer Facts and Figures 2003,* 32.
14. Peto, "Cancer Epidemiology in the Last Century."
15. Ibid., 393.
16. Ibid.
17. American Cancer Society, *Cancer Facts and Figures 2003.*
18. Osborne, Boyle, and Lipkin, "Cancer Prevention."
19. IARC, *Hormonal Contraception and Post-Menopausal Hormonal Therapy* (IARC Monographs on the Evaluation of Carcinogenic Risks to Humans, 72) (Lyon: IARC, 1999).

20. Peto, "Cancer Epidemiology in the Last Century," 394.
21. American Cancer Society, *Cancer Facts and Figures 2003.*
22. Osborne, Boyle, and Lipkin, "Cancer Prevention."
23. Osborne, Boyle, and Lipkin, "Cancer Prevention"; Peto, "Cancer Epidemiology in the Last Century."
24. Peto, "Cancer Epidemiology in the Last Century."
25. American Cancer Society, *Cancer Facts and Figures 2003,* 13.
26. Ibid., 13–14.
27. Ibid., 32.
28. Ibid.
29. Ibid., 9.
30. Ibid.
31. Ibid.
32. Ibid.
33. Ibid., 10.
34. Ibid.
35. A. Bergstrom et al., "Overweight as an Avoidable Cause of Cancer in Europe," *International Journal of Cancer* 91, no. 3 (2001): 421–430.
36. American Cancer Society, *Cancer Facts and Figures 2003,* 11.
37. P. A. Janne and R. J. Mayer, "Chemoprevention of Colorectal Cancer," *The New England Journal of Medicine* 342 (2000): 1960–1968.
38. American Cancer Society, *Cancer Facts and Figures 2003,* 16.
39. Ibid., 16.
40. Ibid.
41. Ibid.
42. Ibid., 17.
43. Ibid.
44. American Academy of Dermatology, "Indoor Tanning, All the Dangers of the Outdoor Sun, Including Skin Cancer," 2002. www.aad.org/PressReleases/indoor.html
45. American Cancer Society, *Cancer Facts and Figures 2003,* 17.
46. Ibid.
47. Ibid., 15.
48. Ibid.
49. A. Harvey et al., "Dietary Fat Intake and Risk of Epithelial Ovarian Cancer," *Journal of the National Cancer Institute* 86 (1994): 21.
50. American Cancer Society, *Cancer Facts and Figures 2003,* 15.
51. Ibid., 19.
52. Ibid., 19.
53. Ibid.
54. Ibid., 20.
55. Ibid., 16.
56. Ibid.
57. Ibid., 12.
58. Ibid.

CHAPTER 14
1. K. Nelson, C. Williams, and N. Graham, *Infectious Disease Epidemiology: Theory and Practice* (Gaithersburg, MD: Aspen, 2001), 17–39.
2. Centers for Disease Control and Prevention, Division of Bacterial and Mycotic Diseases, "Group B Streptococcal Infections (GBS)," 2001. www.cdc.gov/ncidod/dbmd/diseaseinfo/groupbstrep_g.htm
3. Ibid.
4. U.S. Department of Health and Human Services, *Preventing Emerging Infectious Diseases: A Strategy for the 21st Century* (Atlanta: Centers for Disease Control and Prevention, 1998).
5. A. Evans and P. Brachman, *Bacterial Infections of Humans: Epidemiology and Control, 3rd ed.* (Atlanta: Plenum, 1998).
6. Centers for Disease Control and Prevention, *Reported Tuberculosis in the United States 2002* (Atlanta: U.S Department of Health and Human Services, 2003).
7. Ibid.

8. World Health Organization, "Tuberculosis Fact Sheet No. 104," 2002. www.who.int/mediacentre/factsheets/who104/en/
9. Ibid.
10. A. Evans and R. Kaslow, *Viral Infections in Humans: Epidemiology and Control, 4th ed.* (New York: Plenum, 1997), 6–11.
11. National Institutes of Health, National Institute of Allergy and Infectious Diseases, "The Common Cold," March 2001. www.niaid.nih.gov/factsheets/cold.htm
12. Ibid.
13. Ibid.
14. Centers for Disease Control and Prevention, "Flu Facts for Everyone," 2003. www.cdc.gov/NiP/Flu/public.htm#cold
15. National Digestive Diseases Information Clearinghouse, "Promote Prevention: Hepatitis—Education and Information for Patients and Professionals," 2000. www.niddk.nih.gov/health/digest/digest.htm
16. Ibid.
17. Ibid.
18. Ibid.
19. World Health Organization, *World Health Report 2002: Reducing Risks, Promoting Healthy Life,* 2003. www.who.int/whr/en
20. Nelson, Williams, and Graham, *Infectious Disease Epidemiology,* 17–39.
21. National Center for Infectious Disease, Centers for Disease Control and Prevention, "BSE and CJD Information and Resources," May 2003. www.cdc.gov/ncidod/diseases/cjd.cjd.htm
22. Ibid.
23. Nelson, Williams, and Graham, *Infectious Disease Epidemiology,* 315–318.
24. Ibid.
25. Centers for Disease Control and Prevention, Special Pathogens Branch. "Diseases–Ebola Hemorrhagic Fever," 2002. www.cdc.gov/ncidod/drvd/spb/mnpages/dispages/ebola.htm
26. Ibid.
27. R. Fenner, *The History of Smallpox and Its Spread around the World* (Geneva, Switzerland: World Health Organization, 1988).
28. Centers for Disease Control and Prevention, Division of Sexually Transmitted Diseases, *1999 Annual Report* (Atlanta: Centers for Disease Control and Prevention, 2000).
29. "Primary and Secondary Syphilis 2000–2001," *MMWR* 51, no. 43 (2002): 971–973.
30. K. Painter, "STI Rate Higher than Previously Believed," *USA Today,* December 3, 1998, D1.
31. Centers for Disease Control and Prevention, *Sexually Transmitted Disease Surveillance 2001 Supplement. Chlamydia Prevalence Monitoring Project* (Atlanta: U.S. Department of Health and Human Services, 2002).
32. J. Hill and E. Lockrow, "Pelvic Inflammatory Disease," eMedicine.com, Inc., 2002. www.emedicine.com/med/topic1774.htm
33. "PID: Guidelines for Prevention, Detection, and Management," *Clinical Courier* 10 (1992): 1–5.
34. National Institute of Allergy and Infectious Diseases, National Institutes of Health, "Gonorrhea Fact Sheet," May 2002. www.niaid.nih.gov/factsheets/stdgon.htm
35. Ibid.
36. Ibid.
37. National Institute of Allergy and Infectious Diseases, National Institutes of Health, "Genital Herpes Fact Sheet," September 2003. www.niaid.nih.gov/factsheets/stdherp.htm
38. Ibid.
39. Centers for Disease Control and Prevention, National Center for HIV, STD and TB Prevention, Division of HIV/AIDS Prevention, *HIV/AIDS Surveillance Report* 14 (October 27, 2003).
40. Ibid.
41. Ibid.
42. Centers for Disease Control and Prevention, *CDC Update: Critical Need to Pay Attention to HIV Prevention for Women* (July 24,

1998); G. Stine, *AIDS Update 2000* (Upper Saddle River, NJ: Prentice Hall, 2000), 349.

43. Stine, *Aids Update 2000,* 343–349; Society for the Advancement of Women's Health Research, "Some Ailments Found Guilty of Sex Bias," *The New York Times,* November 11, 1998, D12; B. M. Branson, "Home Sample Collection Tests for HIV Infection," *The Journal of the American Medical Association* 280 (1998): 1699–1701.

44. Centers for Disease Control and Prevention, National Center for HIV, STD and TB Prevention, Division of HIV/AIDS Prevention, *HIV/AIDS Surveillance Report.*

45. Centers for Disease Control and Prevention, "Revised Recommendations for HIV Screening of Pregnant Women," *MMWR* 50 (November 9, 2001), www.cdc.gov/mmwr/preview/mmwrhtml/rr5019a2.html

46. Centers for Disease Control and Prevention, "HIV and Its Transmission," Division of HIV/AIDS Prevention, September 2003. www.cdc.gov/hivpubs/facts/transmission.htm

47. Ibid.

48. Centers for Disease Control and Prevention, National Center for HIV, STD and TB Prevention, Division of HIV/AIDS Prevention, *HIV/AIDS Surveillance Report.*

49. R. Brownson, P. Remington, and J. Davis, eds., *Chronic Disease Epidemiology and Control* (Washington, D.C.: American Public Health Association, 1998), 379–382.

50. American Academy of Allergy, Asthma, and Immunology, February 2001. www.aaaai.org

51. Brownson, Remington, and Davis, *Chronic Disease Epidemiology,* 389.

52. American Lung Association, January 2001. www.lungusa.org

53. Brownson, Remington, and Davis, *Chronic Disease Epidemiology,* 516.

54. J. Adler and A. Rogers, "The New War against Migraines," *Newsweek,* January 11, 1999, 46–55.

55. Ibid., 48.

56. Ibid., 49.

57. Ibid., 52.

58. J. Koplan, "Diabetes Is a Growing Public Health Concern," Centers for Disease Control and Prevention, 2002. www.cdc.gov/diabetes/pubs/glance.htm

59. J. Adler and C. Kalb, "An American Epidemic: Diabetes," *Newsweek,* September 4, 2000, 40–48; Centers for Disease Control and Prevention, January 2001. www.cdc.gov

60. J. Koplan, "Diabetes Is a Growing Public Health Concern."

61. Brownson, Remington, and Davis, *Chronic Disease Epidemiology,* 424.

62. J. Koplan, "Diabetes Is a Growing Public Health Concern."

63. Adler and Kalb, "An American Epidemic: Diabetes," 42.

64. Arthritis Foundation, "Disease Center," 2002. www.arthritis.org/conditions/DiseaseCenter/oa.asp

65. Ibid.

66. Brownson, Remington, and Davis, *Chronic Disease Epidemiology,* 424.

67. "Prevalence of Low Back Pain in the United States: New Estimates," *The Back Letter* (Philadelphia: Lippincott, Williams, and Wilkins, 1998).

68. N. Hadler and T. Carey, "Low Back Pain: An Intermittent Predicament in Life," *Annals of the Rheumatic Diseases* 57 (1998): 1–3.

69. Nelson, Williams, and Graham, *Infectious Disease Epidemiology,* 348–349.

CHAPTER 15

1. J. Kavenaugh, *Adult Development and Aging* (Pacific Grove, CA: Brooks/Cole/ITP, 1996), 45.

2. Illinois Department on Aging. "Facts on Aging," June 1, 2002. www.state.il.us/aging/1news_pubs/onage53.htm

3. W. Madar, "Life Stories as Well as Theory Needed to Understand Aging," *Center for the Humanities Newsletter* (Consortium of Humanities Centers and Institutes, Oregon State University, spring 2000), 8.

4. Department of Health and Human Services, Administration on Aging, "A Profile of Older Americans: 2002," October 2003. www.aoa.gov//prof/statistics/profile/profiles2002.asp

5. Ibid.

6. U.S. Senate Special Committee on Aging, *Aging Committee: Hearing Finding Summary Report to Congress* (Washington, DC: U.S. Government Printing Office, 2002).

7. Department of Health and Human Services, Administration on Aging, "A Profile of Older Americans: 2002."

8. Ibid.

9. Ibid.

10. National Institutes of Health, Osteoporosis and Related Bone Diseases National Resource Center, "Osteoporosis Overview," December 2000. www.osteo.org/osteo.html

11. National Institutes of Health, Osteoporosis and Related Bone Diseases National Resource Center, "Fast Facts on Osteoporosis," February 2003. www.osteo.org/osteo.html

12. National Kidney and Urologic Diseases Information Clearinghouse, "Kidney and Urologic Disease Statistics," 2002. http://kidney.niddk.nih.gov/kudiseases/pubs/kustats/index.htm

13. Ibid.

14. National Council on Aging, "Half of Older Americans Report They Are Sexually Active, 4 in 10 Want More Sex, Says New Survey," news release, September 28, 1998. http://ncoa.org

15. National Institute of Mental Health, "Older Adults: Depression and Suicide Facts," May 2003. www.nimh.nih.gov/publicat/elderlydepsuicide.cfm

16. National Institute on Aging and National Institutes of Health, "2000 Progress Report on Alzheimer's Disease: Taking the Next Step," January 2002. www.alzheimers.org/pubs/prog00.htm

17. Ibid.

18. Alzheimer's Association, "Obesity after 70 Increases Risk for Alzheimer's Disease," July 14, 2003. www.alz.org/Media/newsreleases/current/071403obesity.htm

19. National Institute on Alcohol Abuse and Alcoholism, National Institute of Health, "Frequently Asked Questions," January 2002. www.niaaa.nih.gov/faq/faq.htm

20. Ibid.

21. *Oxford English Dictionary* (Oxford, UK: Oxford University Press, 1969), 72, 334, 735.

22. President's Commission for the Study of Ethical Problems in Medicine and Biomedical and Behavioral Research, *Deciding to Forgo Life-Sustaining Treatment* (New York: Concern for Dying, 1983), 9.

23. Ad Hoc Committee of the Harvard Medical School to Examine the Definition of Brain Death, "A Definition of Irreversible Coma," *The Journal of the American Medical Association* 205 (1968): 377.

24. L. R. Aiken, *Dying, Death, and Bereavement, 3rd ed.* (Boston: Allyn and Bacon, 1994), 4.

25. *Civilization* 6, no. 6 (2000): 30, 33–34.

26. E. Kübler-Ross, *On Death and Dying* (New York: Macmillan, 1969), 113.

27. R. J. Kastenbaum, *Death, Society, and Human Experience, 6th ed.* (Boston: Allyn and Bacon, 1998), 95.

28. Ibid., 336–337.

29. K. J. Doka, ed., *Disenfranchised Grief: Recognizing Hidden Sorrow* (Lexington, MA: Lexington Books, 1989).

30. "Last Rights: Why a 'Living Will' Is Not Enough," *Consumer Reports on Health* (September 1993): 5, 9.

31. J. G. Bachman et al., "Attitudes of Michigan Physicians and the Public toward Legalizing Physician-Assisted Suicide and Voluntary Euthanasia," *The New England Journal of Medicine* 334 (1996): 303.

32. M. A. Lee et al., "Legalizing Assisted Suicide: Views of Physicians in Oregon," *The New England Journal of Medicine* 334 (1996): 310–315.

CHAPTER 16

1. M. Renner, "Economic Features," *Vital Signs 1997: The Environmental Trends That Are Shaping Our Future* (New York: W. W. Norton & Co., 1997).

2. R. Caplan, *Our Earth, Ourselves* (New York: Bantam, 1990), 247.

3. United Nations, *Global Population Policy Database* (New York: UN Population Division, 1995); U.S. Census Bureau, "World POPClock Projection," July 17, 2003. http://www.census.gov/cgi-bin/ipc/popclockw

4. J. Abramovitz and S. Dunn, "Record Year for Weather-Related Disasters," in *Vital Signs Brief 98–5* (Washington, DC: Worldwatch Institute, 1998).

5. L. R. Brown, M. Renner, and C. Flavin, *Vital Signs 1998: The Environmental Trends That Are Shaping Our Future* (New York: W. W. Norton & Co., 1998).

6. Ibid.

7. L. Gordon, "Environmental Health and Protection: Century 21 Challenges," *Journal of Environmental Health* 57 (1995): 28–34.

8. U.S. Census Bureau, International Database, "Countries Ranked by Population: 2003," July 17, 2003. www.census.gov/cgi-bin/ipc/idbrank.pl

9. L. R. Brown, G. Gardner, and B. Halweil, *Beyond Malthus: Sixteen Dimensions of the Population Problem* (Washington, DC: Worldwatch Institute, 1998).

10. Environmental Literacy Council, "Population Dynamics," April 15, 2003. www.enviroliteracy.org/subcategory.php/30.html

11. J. Schwartz, "Health Effects of Particulate Air Pollution," *The Center for Environmental Health Newsletter* (University of Connecticut, College of Agriculture & Natural Resources) 7 (1998).

12. "Children's Blood-Lead Levels Declining, but Studies Show Exposure Causes Long-Term Risks," Children's Health Environmental Coalition, CHEC's Health*e*House, January 12, 2003. www.checnet.org/healthehouse/education/articles-detail.asp?Main_ID = 527

13. L. Brown, "A New Era Unfolds," in *State of the World, 1993*, ed. Lester Brown (New York: W. W. Norton Co., 1993), 107.

14. U.S. Environmental Protection Agency, "The Inside Story: A Guide to Indoor Air Quality" (EPA Document 402-K-93-007), 1995. http://epa.gov.iaq/pubs/insidest.html

15. Ibid.

16. U.S. Environmental Protection Agency, "Indoor Air–Radon," October 16, 2003. www.epa.gov/iaq/radon/radonqa1.html#What % 20are % 20the % 20Health % 20Effects % 20From % 20Exposure % 20to % 20Radon

17. U.S. Environmental Protection Agency, "The Inside Story."

18. B. Condor, "Alternative Watch: Clearing the Air in Classrooms," *Chicago Tribune,* August 20, 2000.

19. N. Carpenter, "'Sick' Buildings Can Be Root of Work-Related Maladies," *Boston Business Journal* 20 (2000): 36–37.

20. U.S. Environmental Protection Agency, *Questions and Answers on Ozone Depletion* (Washington, DC: Stratospheric Protection Division, 1998).

21. U.S. Environmental Protection Agency, "Global Warming–Climate," 2002. http://yosemite.epa.gov/oar/globalwarming.nsf/content/climate.html

22. Ibid.

23. Ibid.

24. J. Abramovitz, *Taking a Stand: Cultivating a New Relationship with the World's Forests* (Washington, DC: Worldwatch Institute, 1998).

25. Ibid.

26. M. Morgan. *Environmental Health* (Belmont, CA: Wadsworth, 2003), 73.

27. U. S. Environmental Protection Agency, *Water on Tap: A Consumer's Guide to the Nation's Drinking Water* (Washington, D.C.: Safe Drinking Water Information System, 1997).

28. Ibid.

29. Ibid.

30. Brown et al., op. cit.

31. Global Programme of Action for the Protection of the Marine Environment from Land-Based Activities, "Inputs of POPs in Coastal and Marine Environment," July 9, 2001. http://pops.gpa.unep.org/031marin.htm

32. Ibid.

33. A. Hoyer, "Organochlorine Exposure and Risk of Breast Cancer," *The Lancet* 352 (1998): 1816–1831.

34. Environment News Service, "Europe Secures Victory over Aircraft Noise," October 8, 2001. http://ens-news.com/ens/oct2001/2001-10-08-05.asp

35. Ibid.

36. B. L. Johnson and C. T. DeRosa, "The Toxicologic Hazard of Superfund Hazardous Waste Sites," *Environmental Health* 12 (1997): 242.

37. U.S. Environmental Protection Agency, "National Priorities List, Final National Priorities List (NPL) Sites," October 21, 2003. www.epa.gov/superfund/sites/query/queryhtm/nplfin1.htm

38. U.S. Environmental Protection Agency, *Meeting the Environmental Challenge: EPA's Review of Progress and New Directions in Environmental Protection* (EPA Publication No. 21K-2001, 1990), 4.

39. Environmental News Network. www.enn.com

40. The National Institute of Environmental Health Sciences, "EMF Questions & Answers June 2002," EMF*Rapid,* Electric and Magnetic Fields Research and Public Information Dissemination Program, "3 Results of EMF Research," October 1, 2002. www.niehs.nih.gov/emfrapid/booklet/results.htm#learned

CHAPTER 17

1. L. C. Baker and L. S. Baker, "Excess Cost of Emergency Department Visits for Nonurgent Care," *Health Affairs* (winter 1994): 162–180.

2. Hospital Health Network, "Emergency Care: The Number of Visits to U.S. Hospital Emergency Departments Has Declined," *Hospital Health Network* 70 (1996): 14.

3. R. M. Williams, "The Costs of Visits to Emergency Departments," *The New England Journal of Medicine* 334 (1996): 642–646.

4. J. Schmittdiel et al., "Choice of a Personal Physician and Patient Satisfaction in a Health Maintenance Organization," *The Journal of the American Medical Association* 278 (1997): 1596–1599.

5. C. Huggins, "Poll Shows Most Americans Trust Their Doctors," Medline Plus Health Information, 2002. www.nlm.nih.gov/medlineplus/news/fullstory_10844.html

6. G. Annas, *The Rights of Patients: The Basic ACLU Guide to Patient Rights,* 2nd ed. (Chicago: Southern Illinois University Press, 1989), 105.

7. "Use of Non-Physician Practitioners," *Pennsylvania Medicine* 101 (1998): 17–19.

8. C. Hafner-Eaton, "Patterns of Hospital and Physician Utilization among the Uninsured," *Journal of Health Care for the Poor and Underserved* 5 (1994): 297–315.

9. National Center for Chronic Disease Prevention and Health Promotion, "Chronic Disease Overview," 2003. www.cdc.gov/nccdphp/overview.htm

10. Ibid.

11. Centers for Medicare and Medicaid Services, "National Health Care Expenditures Projections: 2002–2012," 2003. http://cms.hhs.gov/statistics/nhe/projections-2002/highlights.asp; K. Levit et al., "Trends in U.S. Health Care Spending, 2001," *Health Affairs* 22, no. 1 (2003): 154–164.

12. L. Kohn, J. Corrigan, and M. Donaldson, eds., *To Err Is Human: Building a Safer Health System* (Washington, D.C.: The National Academies Press, 2000).

13. J. Rhoades and J. Cohen, "Statistical Brief #24: The Uninsured in America—1996–2002: Estimates for the Civilian Noninstitutionalized Population Under Age 65," Agency for Healthcare Research and Quality, September 2003. www.meps.ahrq.gov/papers/st24/stat24.htm

14. P. Lee and C. Estes, *The Nation's Health, 7th ed.* (Sudbury, MA: Jones and Bartlett, 2003).

15. *Medical Group Practice Digest: Managed Care Digest Series* 1998 (Kansas City: Hoechst Marion Roussel, Inc., 1998).

16. Ibid.

17. Ibid.

18. Ibid.

19. Ibid.

CHAPTER 18

1. E. Eisenberg et al., "Trends in Alternative Medicine Use in the United States, 1990–97: Results of a Follow-Up National Study," *The Journal of the American Medical Association* 280 (1998): 1569–1579.

2. L. C. Paramore, "Use of Alternative Therapies," *Journal of Pain and Symptom Management* 13 (1997): 83–89; Landmark Healthcare, *The Landmark Report on Public Perceptions of Alternative Care* (Sacramento, CA: Landmark Healthcare, 1998).

3. National Institute of Health, National Center for Complementary and Alternative Medicine (NCCAM), "Health Information." 2003. www.nccam.nih.gov/health

4. D. M. Eisenberg et al., "Unconventional Medicine in the United States," *The New England Journal of Medicine* 328 (1993): 246–252.

5. Eisenberg et al., "Unconventional Medicine," 247; Eisenberg et al., "Trends in Alternative Medicine," 1570.

6. NCCAM, "Health Information."

7. Ibid.

8. A. Weil, *Spontaneous Healing* (New York: Fawcett Columbine, 1995), 233.

9. NCCAM, "Health Information."

10. N. Rasmussen and J. Morgall, "The Use of Alternative Treatments in the Danish Adult Population," *Complementary Medicine Research* 4 (1990): 16–22; A. MacLennan, D. Wilson, and A. Taylor, "Prevalence and Cost of Alternative Medicine in Australia," *The Lancet* 347 (1996): 569–573; P. Fisher and A. Ward, "Complementary Medicine in Europe," *British Medical Journal* 309 (1994): 107–111; W. Miller, "Use of Alternative Health Care Practitioners by Canadians," *Canadian Journal of Public Health* 88 (1997): 154–158.

11. NCCAM, "Health Information."

12. M. Angell and J. P. Kassirer, "Alternative Medicine—The Risks of Untested and Unregulated Remedies," *The New England Journal of Medicine* 339 (1998): 839–841.

13. NCCAM, "Health Information."

14. Ibid.

15. Ibid.

16. Ibid.

17. Ibid.

18. J. Greenwald, "Herbal Healing," *Time,* November 23, 1998, 63–65.

19. NCCAM, "Health Information."

20. Weil, *Spontaneous Healing,* 233.

21. Food and Drug Administration, Center for Food Safety and Applied Nutrition, "Consumer Advisory: Kava-Containing Dietary Supplements May Be Associated with Severe Liver Injury," March 25, 2002. www.cfsan.fda.gov/~dms/addskava.html

22. Weil, *Spontaneous Healing,* 241.

23. J. Kleignene and P. Knipschild, "Ginkgo Biloba," *The Lancet* 340 (1992): 1136–1139.

24. M. Murray, "Ginkgo Biloba Extract and Ginkgo Phytosome," *Ask the Doctor, Vital Communication,* 1998.

25. P. L. LeBars et al., "A Placebo-Controlled, Double Blind, Randomized Trial of an Extract of Ginkgo Biloba for Dementia," *The Journal of the American Medical Association* 278 (1997): 1327–1332.

26. "The Pill that Helps You Think?" *Tufts University Health and Nutrition Letter* 15 (1997): 8–10.

27. H. Schultz, "St. John's Wort for Depression," *British Medical Journal* 7052 (1996): 313–319.

28. Schultz, "St. John's Wort," 314; R. J. Davidson, et al., "Effect of SJW in Major Depressive Disorder: A Randomized, Controlled Study," *The Journal of the American Medical Association* 287 (2002): 1807–1814.

29. K. D. Hansgen et al., "Multicenter Double Blind Study Examining the Anti-Depressant Effectiveness of the Hypericum Extract L1160," *Journal of Geriatric Psychiatry and Neurology* Supplement 1 (1994): S15–S18.

30. H. Schultz et al., "Effects of Hypericum Extract on the Sleep EEG in Older Volunteers," *Journal of Geriatric Psychiatry and Neurology* Supplement 1 (1994): S39–S43.

31. H. Martin, "St. John's Wort vs. Tricyclic Antidepressants," *American Journal of Naturopathic Medicine* 2 (1995): 42.

32. J. Blair, "Echinacea—New Wonder Drug?" *Archives of Family Medicine* (November 24, 1998): 1332–1339.

33. S. Momoyama, "Green Tea as Protection from Heart Attack," *American Journal of Cardiology* 909 (2002): 1150–1153.

34. U.S. Food and Drug Administration, "HHS Acts to Reduce Safety Concerns Associated with Dietary Supplements Containing Ephedra," February 28, 2003. www.fda.gov/bbs/topics/NEWS/ephedra/factsheet.html

35. "New Guides in Herbal Remedies," *Harvard Women's Health Watch* 41 (1999): 6–8.

36. P. A. DeSmet, "Health Risks of Herbal Remedies," *Drug Safety* 13 (1996): 81–93.

37. E. Ernst, "Harmless Herbs," *The American Journal of Medicine* 104 (1998): 170–178.

38. "New Guides in Herbal Remedies," 7.

39. Ernst, "Harmless Herbs," 172.

40. Ibid., 173.

41. Agency for Healthcare Research and Quality, *S-Adenosyl-L Methionine for Treatment of Depression, Osteoarthritis, and Liver Disease. Summary, Evidence Report/Technology Assessment: Number 64* (AHRQ Publication No. 02-E033) (August 2002). (AHRQ, Rockville, MD) www.ahrq.gov/clinic/epcsums/samesum.htm

42. Ibid.

43. Ibid.

44. S. Dixon, "Food for Thought: Prebiotic and Probiotics: What Are They and Why Should You Eat Them?" University of Michigan Comprehensive Cancer Center, January 15, 2003. www.cancer.med.umich.edu/news/pro09spr02.htm

45. C. Marwick, "Medical News and Perspectives: Alternatives Are Ahead of the OAM," *The Journal of the American Medical Association* 280 (1998): 1553–1554; D. Wilson, "Health Food Masquerade," *Corvallis Gazette Times,* August 11, 1999, C-4.

46. American Botanical Council, "The Complete German Commission E Monographs," January 2003. www.herbalgram.org/default.asp?c=comm_e_int

47. Ibid.

48. NCCAM, "NCCAM's Research Centers Program," 2003. www.nccam.nih.gov/training/centers/index.htm

49. "Health for Life: Inside the Science of Alternative Medicine," *Newsweek* (December 2, 2002): 45–70.

Credits

Chapter Opening Art

Chapter 1, **p. 1:** Paul Klee, *Color Shapes.* Reproduced with permission from the Artist Rights Society, NY, Superstock; Chapter 2, **p. 29:** Bob Commander, Stock Illustration Source, Inc.; Chapter 3, **p. 55:** *Racer,* Diana Ong, Superstock; Chapter 4, **p. 81:** Noma, Stock Illustration Source, Inc.; Chapter 5, **p. 105:** *Rainy Day Crowd,* Diana Ong, Superstock; Chapter 6, **p. 139:** Jose Ortega, Stock Illustration Source, Inc.; Chapter 7, **p. 171:** Russel Thurston/Getty Images; Chapter 8, **p. 199:** Stephanie Dalton Cowan/Getty Images; Chapter 9, **p. 231:** Images.com/CORBIS; Chapter 10, **p. 267:** Michael Shumate/ Getty Images; Chapter 11, **p. 295:** *The Runners,* Robert Delauney, Superstock; Chapter 12, **p. 315:** Gayle Ray/Superstock; Chapter 13, **p. 339:** Images.com/CORBIS; Chapter 14, **p. 361:** Bruno Budrovic, Stock Illustration Source, Inc.; Chapter 15, **p. 399:** Dave Cutler/Images.com, Inc.; Chapter 16, **p. 419:** John S. Dykes, Stock Illustration Source, Inc.; Chapter 17, **p. 439:** Timothy John, Stock Illustration Source, Inc.; Chapter 18, **p. 455:** Stephanie Dalton Cowan/Getty Images

Photo Credits

Chapter 1, **p. 3:** Digital Stock/CORBIS; **p. 12:** Scott Barbour/ ALLSPORT/Getty Images; **p. 22:** Tom Prettyman/PhotoEdit; Chapter 2, **p. 46:** Billy Barnes/Stock Boston; **p. 48:** Monte S. Buschbaum, M.D.; **p. 50:** Penny Tweedie/Stone; Chapter 3, **p. 68:** Ulrike Welsch/PhotoEdit; **p. 72:** Phil Cantor/IndexStock; **p. 77:** Robin Sachs/PhotoEdit; Chapter 4, **p. 88:** Rudi Von Briel/PhotoEdit; **p. 92:** Bill Aron/PhotoEdit; **p. 101:** AP/Wide World Photos; Chapter 5, **p. 109:** Jeff Greenberg/Stock Boston; **p. 111:** David Young-Wolff/PhotoEdit; **p. 116:** AP Photo/The Holland Sentinel, Dan Irving; **p. 120:** Ellen Senisi/The Image Works; **p. 130:** SAM MIRCOVICH/Reuters/Landov; Chapter 6, **p. 157:** Michael Newman/PhotoEdit; **p. 160a:** Claude Edelman/Photo Researchers; **p. 160b:** Petit Format-Nestle/Photo Researchers; **p. 160c:** Petit Format-Nestle/Photo Researchers; Chapter 7, **p. 186:** Michael Newman/PhotoEdit; **p. 193:** Courtesy of NIDA; **p. 195:** Luc Beziat/Getty Images; Chapter 8, **p. 202:** Andrew Lichtenstein/The Image Works; **p. 208:** Yva Momatiuk & John Eastcott/Stock Boston; **p. 216:** Courtesy of Romano & Associates Inc./Oral Health America; Chapter 9, **p. 243:** Reg Charity/ CORBIS; **p. 256:** Stone/Getty Images; Chapter 10, **p. 273:** Guang Niu/CORBIS; **p. 280:** Ariel Skelley/ CORBIS; **p. 291(left):** C Squared Studios/Getty Images; **p. 291(right):** James Noble/CORBIS; Chapter 11, **p. 304:** Image Source/SuperStock; **p. 308:** Mark Gamba/CORBIS; Chapter 12, **p. 318:** Mike Fiala/CORBIS; **p. 324:** Keith Brofsky/ Getty Images; **p. 331:** Thinkstock/Getty Images; Chapter 13, **p. 353 (left):** James Stevenson/SPL/Photo Researchers, Inc.; **p. 353 (middle and right):** Dr. P. Marazzi/SPL/Photo Researchers, Inc.; **p. 358:** Bill Greenblatt/ Newsamakers/ Liaison Agency; Chapter 14, **p. 364:** Rudi Von Briel/PhotoEdit; **p. 384:** A Ramy/Stock Boston; **p. 388:** John Miller/Stone; **p. 392:** Donna Day/Getty Images; Chapter 15, **p. 407 (left):** Fred Prouser/CORBIS; **p. 407 (middle):** AP/Wide World Photos; **p. 407 (right):** AP Photo/Eric Risberg; **p. 408:** Yva Momatiuk & John Eastcott/Stock Boston; Chapter 16, **p. 421:** AP/Wide World Photos; **p. 425:** Will and Demi McIntyre/Photo Researchers; **p. 431:** Seth Resnick/Stock Boston; Chapter 17, **p. 442:** Jim Sulley/Image Works; **p. 447:** Paul Conklin/PhotoEdit; **p. 448:** Superstock; Chapter 18, **p. 460:** Ron Sutherland/SPL/Photo Researchers; **p. 462:** Michael Newman/PhotoEdit; **p. 465:** Willie Hill, Jr./The Image Works.

Index

Page references followed by *t* indicate tables; *fig* illustrations; *p* photographs.

Behavior Change Contract

Complete the Assess Yourself questionnaire, and read the Skills for Behavior Change box describing the stages of change (page 17). After reviewing your results and considering the various factors that influence your decisions, choose a health behavior that you would like to change, starting this quarter or semester (see other side for a sample filled-in contract). Sign the contract at the bottom to affirm your commitment to making a healthy change, and ask a friend to witness it.

My behavior change will be:

_____

My long-term goal for this behavior change is:

_____

These are three obstacles to change (things that I am currently doing or situations that contribute to this behavior or make it harder to change):

1. _____

2. _____

3. _____

The strategies I will use to overcome these obstacles are:

1. _____

2. _____

3. _____

Resources I will use to help me change this behavior include:

a friend/partner/relative: _____

a school-based resource: _____

a community-based resource: _____

a book or reputable website: _____

In order to make my goal more attainable, I have devised these short-term goals:

short-term goal	target date	reward
short-term goal	target date	reward
short-term goal	target date	reward

When I make the long-term behavior change described above, my reward will be:

_____ target date: _____

I intend to make the behavior change described above. I will use the strategies and rewards to achieve the goals that will contribute to a healthy behavior change.

Signed: _____   Witness: _____

Sample Behavior Change Contract

Complete the Assess Yourself questionnaire, and read the Skills for Behavior Change box describing the stages of change (page 17). After reviewing your results and considering the various factors that influence your decisions, choose a health behavior that you would like to change, starting this quarter or semester. Sign the contract at the bottom to affirm your commitment to making a healthy change, and ask a friend to witness it.

My behavior change will be:

To snack less on junk food and more on healthy foods

My long-term goal for this behavior change is:

Eat junk food snacks no more than once a week

These are three obstacles to change (things that I am currently doing or situations that contribute to this behavior or make it harder to change):

1. The grocery store is closed by the time I come home from school

2. I get hungry between classes, and the vending machines only carry candy bars

3. It's easier to order pizza or other snacks than to make a snack at home

The strategies I will use to overcome these obstacles are:

1. I'll leave early for school once a week so I can stock up on healthy snacks in the morning

2. I'll bring a piece of fruit or other healthy snack to eat between classes

3. I'll learn some easy recipes for snacks to make at home

Resources I will use to help me change this behavior include:

a friend/partner/relative: my roommates: I'll ask them to buy healthier snacks instead of chips when they do the shopping

a school-based resource: the dining hall: I'll ask the manager to provide healthy foods we can take to eat between classes

a community-based resource: the library: I'll check out some cookbooks to find easy snack ideas

a book or reputable website: the USDA nutrient database at www.nal.usda.gov/fnic: I'll use this site to make sure the foods I select are healthy choices

In order to make my goal more attainable, I have devised these short-term goals:

Eat a healthy snack 3 times per week	September 15	new CD
short-term goal	target date	reward
Learn to make a healthy snack	October 15	concert ticket
short-term goal	target date	reward
Eat a healthy snack 5 times per week	November 15	new shoes
short-term goal	target date	reward

When I make the long-term behavior change described above, my reward will be:

Ski lift tickets for winter break   target date: December 15

I intend to make the behavior change described above. I will use the strategies and rewards to achieve the goals that will contribute to a healthy behavior change.

Signed: Elizabeth King   Witness: Susan Bauer

Lifelong Behavior Change Contract

Behavior change is a process that continues for a lifetime. The strategies that you begin to follow now can contribute to healthy benefits far into the future. Choose a change that will have long-term positive effects, then complete the contract and put your intentions into action (see other side for a sample filled-in contract). Sign the contract at the bottom to affirm your commitment to making a healthy change, and ask a friend to witness it.

My behavior change will be:

_____

My long-term goal for this behavior change is:

_____

These are three obstacles to change (things that I am currently doing or situations that contribute to this behavior or make it harder to change):

1. _____

2. _____

3. _____

The strategies I will use to overcome these obstacles are:

1. _____

2. _____

3. _____

Resources I will use to help me change this behavior include:

    a friend/partner/relative: _____

    a school-based resource: _____

    a community-based resource: _____

    a book or reputable website: _____

In order to make my goal more attainable, I have devised these short-term goals:

_____	_____	_____
short-term goal	target date	reward
_____	_____	_____
short-term goal	target date	reward
_____	_____	_____
short-term goal	target date	reward

When I make the long-term behavior change described above, my reward will be:

_____ target date: _____

I intend to make the behavior change described above. I will use the strategies and rewards to achieve the goals that will contribute to a healthy behavior change.

Signed: _____   Witness: _____

Sample Lifelong Behavior Change Contract

Behavior change is a process that continues for a lifetime. The strategies that you begin to follow now can contribute to healthy benefits far into the future. Choose a change that will have long-term positive effects, then complete the contract and put your intentions into action. Sign the contract at the bottom to affirm your commitment to making a healthy change, and ask a friend to witness it.

My behavior change will be:

To incorporate exercise into my daily life

My long-term goal for this behavior change is:

To maintain a healthy weight and feel fit

These are three obstacles to change (things that I am currently doing or situations that contribute to this behavior or make it harder to change):

1. I get bored doing the same exercise all of the time

2. I find myself watching TV I don't even enjoy and then not having time to exercise

3. I'm afraid I'll injure myself doing new activities

The strategies I will use to overcome these obstacles are:

1. I'll learn several activities so that I have variety in my exercise program

2. I'll give myself a set number of "TV hours" and use the extra time for exercise

3. I'll get a complete check-up by my physician before I start a new exercise program

Resources I will use to help me change this behavior include:

a friend/partner/relative: I'll ask friends to exercise with me so I stay motivated and don't get bored

a school-based resource: I'll find out what types of activities are offered by the PE department

a community-based resource: I'll join a local club that does the activity I enjoy most

a book or reputable website: I'll track my progress in the Fitness section of my Log Book and Wellness Journal

In order to make my goal more attainable, I have devised these short-term goals:

Walk to school 3 times a week	3 months from today	dinner out at my favorite restaurant
short-term goal	target date	reward
Learn a new activity to add to my exercise program	6 months from today	new outfit
short-term goal	target date	reward
Participate in the local 10k walk/run	1 year from today	weekend vacation
short-term goal	target date	reward

When I make the long-term behavior change described above, my reward will be:

vacation trip   target date: 2 years from now

I intend to make the behavior change described above. I will use the strategies and rewards to achieve the goals that will contribute to a healthy behavior change.

Signed: Barry Snow   Witness: Rob Santiago